RADIOLOGY TODAY

A Multinational Series

Proceedings of the Multinational Postgraduate Course,
held in Salzburg, June 24–27, 1982

Editors:

Professor Dr. Friedrich H. W. Heuck
Radiologisches Institut im Zentrum Radiologie
des Katharinenhospitals der Stadt Stuttgart
7000 Stuttgart 1, FRG

Professor Dr. Martin W. Donner
Department of Radiology and Radiological Science
The Johns Hopkins Medical Institutions
Baltimore, MA 21205, USA

ISBN-13: 978-3-642-68710-5 e-ISBN-13: 978-3-642-68708-2
DOI: 10.1007/978-3-642-68708-2

Library of Congress Cataloging in Publication Data. Main entry under title: Radiology today 2. (Radiology today ; a multinational series) "Proceedings of the Multinational Postgraduate Course, held in Salzburg, June 24–27, 1982"—T.p. verso. Bibliography: p. Includes index. 1. Diagnosis, Radioscopic–Congresses. I. Heuck, Friedrich. II. Donner, Martin W., 1920– . III. Title: Radiology today two. IV. Series: Radiology today. RC78.A2R22 1983 616.07'57 83-6570

2127/3130-543210

Proceedings of the Multinational Postgraduate Course,
held in Salzburg, June 24–27, 1982.

Editors

Professor Dr. Friedrich H. W. Heuck
Radiologisches Institut im Zentrum Radiologie
des Katharinenhospitals der Stadt Stuttgart
7000 Stuttgart 1, FRG

Professor Dr. Martin W. Donner
Department of Radiology and Radiological Science
The Johns Hopkins Medical Institutions
Baltimore, MA 21205, USA

ISBN-13: 978-3-642-68710-5 e-ISBN: 978-3-642-68708-2
DOI: 10.1007/978-3-642-68708-2

Library of Congress Cataloging in Publication Data. Main entry under title: Radiology today 2. (Radiology today: a multinational series) "Proceedings of the Multinational Postgraduate Course, held in Salzburg, June 24–27, 1982" – T.p. verso. Bibliography: p. Includes index. 1. Diagnosis, Radioscopic-Congresses. I. Heuck, Friedrich. II. Donner, Martin W., 1920–. III. Title: Radiology today two. IV. Series: Radiology today. RC78.A2R33 1983 616.07'57 83-6579

Softcover reprint of the hardcover 1st Edition 1983

2121/3140–543210

Preface

This book reflects the views of an international faculty and provides an authoritative appraisal of modern radiology. It represents the second volume in a planned series of competent overviews, and is modeled on the successful first volume, *Radiology Today*, which was enthusiastically received by an international readership. We were encouraged by the comments we received to continue blending the latest advances in radiology with comprehensive teaching material concerning modern radiological practice. The Radiology Today 1982 meeting again brought together outstanding radiologists from Europe and North America for the purpose of sharing their experiences and their viewpoints of the current position and opportunities of imaging in medicine.

Updating his/her knowledge of advances in medical imaging has become an integral part of continuing medical education for every radiologist. Because all imaging modalities are continuously being refined, new clinical applications develop and frequently replace more complex or more invasive procedures. Also, the relationship of imaging procedures to each other changes constantly, and with it the configuration of critical diagnostic pathways for investigation of clinical signs and symptoms. To recognize this trend is important, because it is expanding the role of the radiologist: our involvement in active guidance to the point of the patient's diagnostic workup has increased significantly where it has become strategic.

Progress in diagnostic radiology of the liver, the urinary tract, and the pelvis was demonstrated at the meeting, while special attention was drawn to renal trauma, renal transplant, and therapy planning. Swallowing disorders and functional analyses of the esophagus were also presented, and further advances in methods in cardiovascular and interventional radiology, as well as in diagnosis of the lympathic system and of mediastinal and lung diseases, were discussed. Diagnostic procedures in rare skeletal and soft tissue diseases were indicated. A selection of topics currently undergoing significant development were presented, including the new diagnostic methods of digital subtraction angiography and nuclear magnetic resonance.

The closing article of the book, a speech given during the opening ceremony of Radiology Today 1982 by Professor Sir Howard Middlemiss, Chairman of the International Comission on Radiological Education (ICRE), honours the memory of this well-respected radiologist, who died unexpectedly in April 1983. He was enthusiastic about our activities, and we shall remember his ideas on education in radiology as we carry on our work.

As we proceed with this series of timely updates in diagnostic radiology, we welcome suggestions and criticisms which might be included in future volumes.

Friedrich H. W. Heuck   Martin W. Donner

Contents

List of Contributors *

Ahn, H. S. 225[1]
Alerci, M. 212
Alessi Grassi, F. 212
Alken, P. 94
Atzinger, A. B. 71
Baert, A. L. 12, 40
Baretić-Kolar, E. 125
Bartelt, D. 340
Barth, K. H. 111
Bessler, W. 185, 266
Bockenheimer, S. 245
Bosniak, M. A. 49
Breit, A. 71
Burhenne, H. J. 40, 85
Campani, R. 212
Cox, P. H. 30
De Nile, D. 212
Di Giulio, G. 212
Donner, M. W. 6
Dorfman, H. D. 165, 266
Engels, P. H. C. 307
Feldberg, M. A. M. 76
Freedman, M. T. 171, 266, 339
Friedmann, G. 200, 311
Fromhold, H. 22
Fuchs, W. A. 133
Fudurić-Winter, I. 125
Fueger, G. F. 30, 40
Genant, H. K. 190
Gfirtner, H. 71
Grotemeyer, P. 315
Günther, P. 94
Gürtl, R. 125
Hacker, H. 339, 353
Heuck, F. H. W. 174, 311, 318
Hildell, J. 67
Hofmann, F. W. 311
Hübener, K. H. 298
Husberg, B. 67
Kaplan-Pavlovič, S. 125
Kaufman, S. L. 111
Kaufmann, H. J. 273
Klenkar, M. 125
Kormano, M. 324
Lipton, M. J. 298
Lissner, J. 145
Lombardi, M. 212
Ludwig, J. W. 307
Marchal, G. 12
Margulis, A. R. 3, 334
Marhoff, P. 283
Meyer-Ebrecht, D. 294
Middlemiss, J. H. 354
Neufang, K. F. R. 311
Nyman, J. 67
Obrez, I. 125
Overtoom, T. T. C. 307
Peters, P. E. 200, 311
Pfändner, K. 71
Pfeiler, M. 283
Pohlenz, O. 339, 340
Ponette, E. 12
Rau, W. S. 157
Reichardt, W. 40, 115
Reichelt, H. G. 30
Reiser, U. J. 318
Rosenbaum, A. E. 225
Rosenbloom, S. B. 255
Sanders, R. C. 58, 64, 91, 228
Sartor, K. 231
Schad, N. 315
Seemann, W.-R. 53
Seyler, G. 315
Šimunić, S. 125
Sommer, B. 145
Stoeter, P. 258

* The address of each first mentioned author is indicated below the according contribution heading

[1] Page, on which contribution begins

Gastrointestinal Radiology

Advances in Gastrointestinal Radiology

A. R. Margulis

Department of Radiology, University of California, San Francisco, CA 94143, USA

Gastrointestinal radiology has undergone dramatic changes in recent years. These changes result from the application of new medical knowledge and technology in radiological areas such as interventional radiology and from new equipment in fields such as ultrasound, X-ray, computer tomography (CT), digital radiography, and nuclear magnetic resonance (NMR) (Fig. 1).

Interventional gastrointestinal radiology has come of age in the past 3 years. The new procedures, which have changed radiologists from diagnostic consultants to therapeutic providers, include (1) dilation of narrow mesenteric vessels or strictures of the alimentary tube; (2) biopsy of organs or tissues guided by fluoroscopy, CT, or ultrasound; (3) occlusion of bleeding sites, arteriovenous communications, or arteries supplying neoplasms [2]; (4) drainage of cysts and abscesses; and (5) extraction of biliary stones [1]. These developments have resulted from the increasing radiologists in the delicate manipulation of instruments through catheters and needles and from the growing versatility of radiographic equipment, with particular reference to the introduction of digital equipment.

Digital radiography and digital fluoroscopy are proving to be beneficial to both patient and radiologist [4]. It is possible to store the last fluoroscopic image in a video memory. This significantly decreases radiation exposure levels. Since digital radiography allows better density discrimination, the relatively rapid and noninvasive intravenous injection of contrast material is already replacing many selective arteriographic procedures, reducing patient exposure, morbidity, and expense. Where selective studies are indispensable, digital arteriography with small injections (1–2 ml) gives superb detail.

Once the radiographic image is in digital form it is possible to process the image with many of the same computer techniques presently used in the space program to reduce noise and distortion in satellite pictures [7]. In the near future it will be possible to superimpose the image from one modality onto the image of another, e.g., ultrasound onto CT.

Images are increasingly stored on magnetic tape and viewed on video terminals, lessening the use

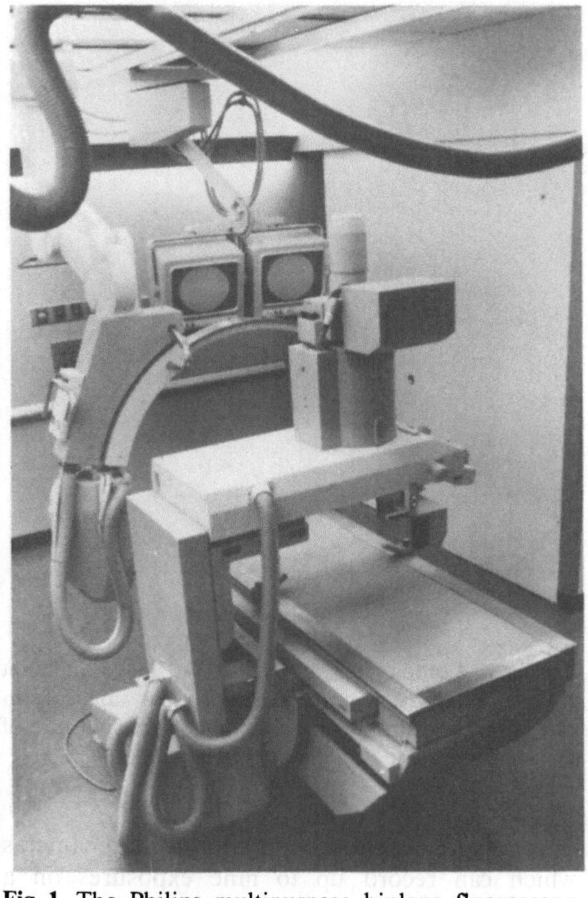

Fig. 1. The Philips multipurpose biplane fluoroscopy room with fluoroscopic tilt table. The room can be used for angiography, interventional procedures, myelography, arthrography, and digital subtraction fluoroscopy, as well as for all gastrointestinal studies. This is the busiest room at UCSF

Radiology Today 2. Ed. by F. H. W. Heuck and M. W. Donner

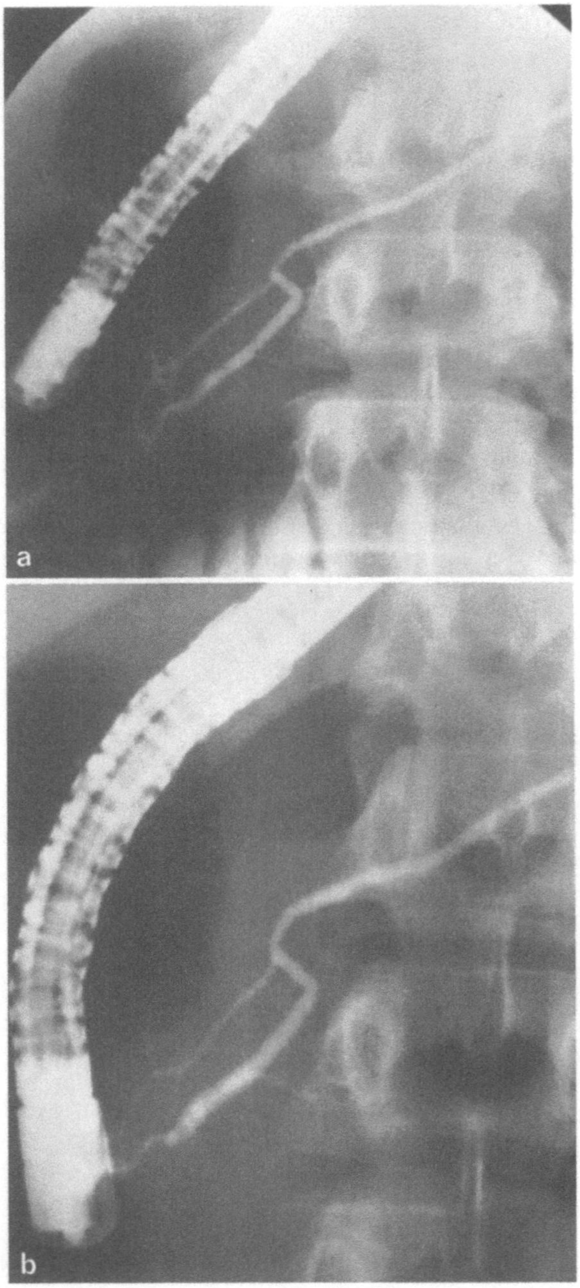

Fig. 2a, b. Comparison of multiformat image and spot film on a pancreatogram. **a** Multiformat image from one of six exposures on one film. **b** A single spot film of the same area. The film quality is very similar

of ever more expensive film. Multiformat cameras which can record up to nine exposures on a 14″×17″ film sheet are being developed and should be in general use within 1–2 years. These cameras will most likely replace conventional and 105-mm spot films. The multiformat cameras presently available produce images comparable in quality to conventional spot films and combine

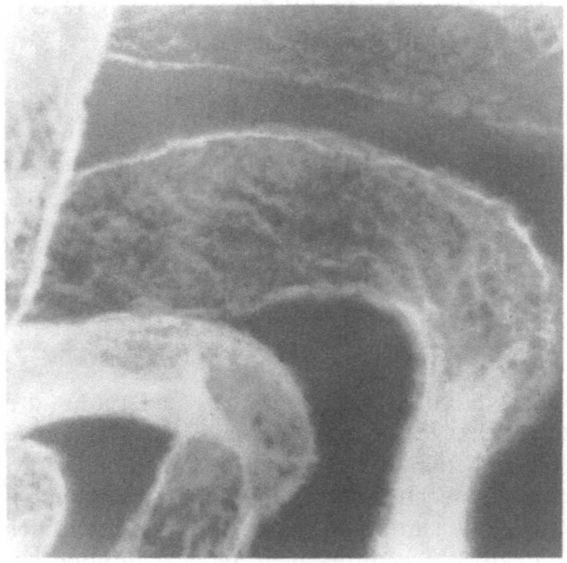

Fig. 3. Magnification film of the small bowel of a dog, showing villi in the jejunum. This type of magnification will open a new field: villography

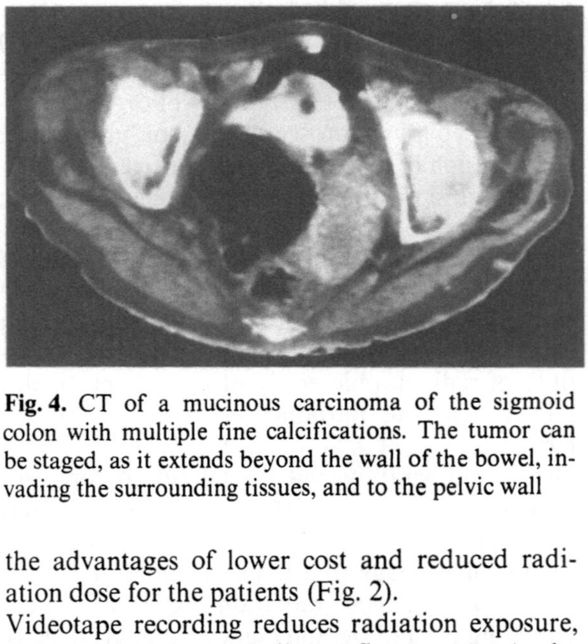

Fig. 4. CT of a mucinous carcinoma of the sigmoid colon with multiple fine calcifications. The tumor can be staged, as it extends beyond the wall of the bowel, invading the surrounding tissues, and to the pelvic wall

the advantages of lower cost and reduced radiation dose for the patients (Fig. 2).

Videotape recording reduces radiation exposure, as it replaces cine recording at fluoroscopy. As the quality of the recorded images improves, most fluoroscopy will be tape-recorded and the significant findings recorded permanently retrospectively from selected video frames. One-thousand-line videotape is already being used and 2000-line capability is available to the military.

Further improvements in the detail of images obtained from double-contrast examinations of the gastrointestinal tract will be achieved with new X-ray tubes having extra fine focal spots and targets capable of carrying the heat load. These finer

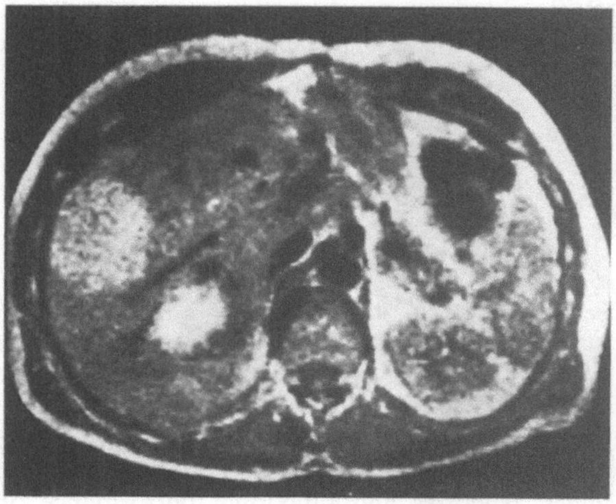

Fig. 5. Nuclear magnetic resonance image of a patient with multiple liver metastases from a carcinoma of the colon. The metastases are seen as white areas in the grey liver. The black streaks are hepatic blood vessels

detailed images of the gastrointestinal tract will improve pathologic correlation and open the field of studying the villi of the small bowel: villography (Fig. 3).

The role of CT in the examination of the liver, pancreas, and spleen has been well established for several years now. In the last few years, however, CT has also become an established procedure for the staging of carcinoma of the esophagus, stomach, and colon, particularly the rectum (Fig. 4) [5, 6]. It is also very valuable in the assessment of Crohn's disease, especially in the differentiation of abscesses from massive fibrolipomatous infiltration of the mesentery. Reformatting has also helped in the evaluation of perforations and in localization of abscesses.

Additional noninvasive pathologic correlation should be possible with NMR imaging [3], which maps the hydrogen protons in the body without X-rays and provides information about the molecular environment of the protons in the tissue. Further tissue characterization information can be obtained without the use of contrast media. The imaging modality permits direct imaging in any plane without reformatting. The liver, spleen, pancreas, and kidneys can be imaged with accuracy (Fig. 5). Metastatic nodes, mesentery, stomach wall, and large bowel are also seen. The relationship of NMR to CT will have to be worked out in the near future.

References

1. Burhenne HJ (1974) The technique of biliary duct stone extraction: experience with 126 cases. Radiology 113:567–572
2. Chuang VP, Wallace S (1981) Hepatic artery embolization in the treatment of hepatic neoplasms. Radiology 140:51–58
3. Crooks L, Arakawa M, Hoenninger J, Watts J, McRee R, Kaufman L, Davis PL, Margulis AR, DeGroot J (1982) Nuclear magnetic resonance whole-body imager operating at 3.5 KGauss. Radiology 143:169–174
4. Mistretta CA, Brummy AB, Strother CM (1981) Digital angiography: a perspective. Radiology 139:273–276
5. Moss AA, Schnyder P, Marks W, Margulis AR (1981) Gastric adenocarcinoma: a comparison of the accuracy and economics of staging by computed tomography and surgery. J Clin Gastroenterol 80:45–50
6. Moss AA, Schnyder P, Thoeni RF, Margulis AR (1981) A uniform, CT-based staging system for malignant neoplasms of the alimentary tube (Editorial). AJR 136:1251–1252
7. Selzer RH (1968) The use of computers to improve biomedical image quality. In: Proceedings of the Fall Joint Computer Conference, pp 817–834

Radiology in Swallowing Disorders

M. W. Donner

Department of Radiology and Radiological Science, The Johns Hopkins University School of Medicine and The Johns Hopkins Hospital, Baltimore, MD 21205, USA

Difficulties of swallowing occur in a wide variety of disorders and diseases, overlapping classical medical specialities such as gastroenterology, otolaryngology, neurology, rheumatology and orthopedic surgery. Whatever the disorder or disease, the radiologist's evaluation of a patient's swallowing process is strategic in determining which of usually several specialists should become involved in further investigations. Radiologists also participate increasingly in patient management decisions, including swallowing rehabilitation, surgical intervention, and application of feeding devices. The radiologist's role in the care of patients with swallowing disorders, therefore, is considerably greater than the traditional radiological reporting. This pattern compares with the increasing involvement of radiologists in the overall diagnostic process elsewhere in medicine and with their management of patients as exemplified by interventional radiology.

It is the purpose of this presentation to comment on anatomical and functional prerequisites of normal swallowing and to demonstrate, by example, typical radiographic observations of impaired swallowing affecting the pharynx and the esophagus.

Anatomy and Physiology

The task of safe transport of the bolus from mouth to distal esophagus is accomplished by a complex sequence of craniocaudal movements in a programmed order carried out by numerous muscles controlled by several cranial nerves [1, 2]. In the mouth and pharynx, other physiological processes, such as respiration and speech, share the same anatomical surroundings (Fig. 1). It is, therefore, essential that respiration and/or speech cease while swallowing occurs. In cases of abnormal swallowing, food and drink must not enter the larynx if the airways and lungs are to serve the vital functions of ventilation and exchange of respiratory gases.

Intact structures and functional performance of the tongue, palate, pharyngeal constrictors, larynx, and esophagus are all important for the successful completion of the normal swallowing sequence [5] and should therefore all be evaluated in every patient with swallowing difficulties. Included in this evaluation are:

1. Study of bolus configuration in the mouth with special attention to the effective apposition of tongue and palate
2. Displacement of the bolus into the pharyngeal cavity accomplished by movements of tongue and palate

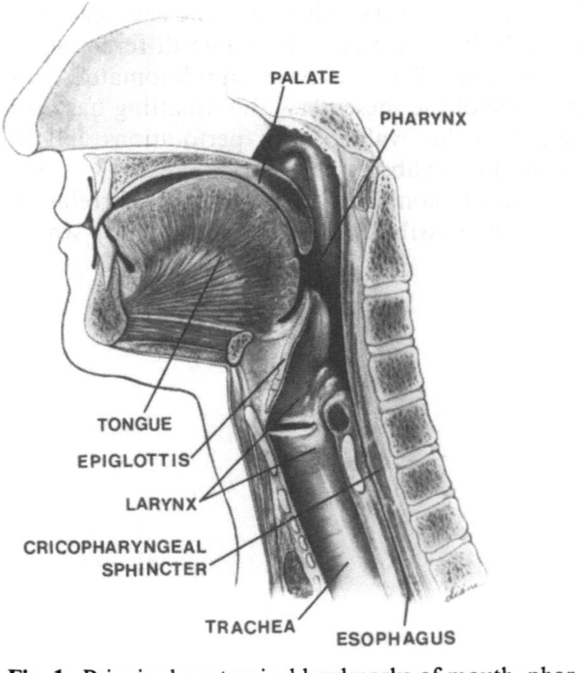

Fig. 1. Principal anatomical landmarks of mouth, pharynx and upper esophagus

Radiology Today 2. Ed. by F. H. W. Heuck and M. W. Donner

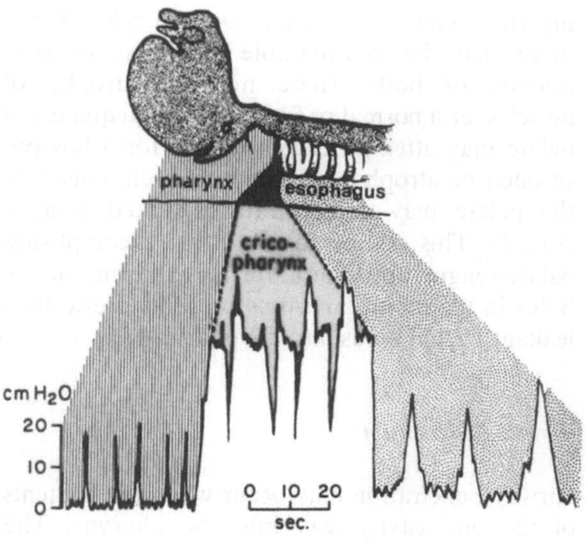

Fig. 2. Manometric recordings of the pharynx, cricopharyngeal sphincter, and esophagus during swallowing. Note the peaks of peristaltic contraction in the pharynx and esophagus, as well as relaxation of the increased sphincter tone prior to bolus arrival

3. Closure and upward movement of the larynx
4. Relaxation of the cricopharyngeal sphincter
5. Propulsion of the bolus through the pharynx into the esophagus

One of the single most important participants in pharyngeal swallowing is the cricopharyngeal sphincter. Located at the level of the sixth or seventh cervical vertebra, the sphincter normally relaxes to allow unobstructed passage of the bolus from the pharyngeal cavity into the esophagus. It protects the pharynx from regurgitation of esophageal or gastric contents and prevents aspiration of air into the esophagus during respiration (Fig. 2). The maintenance of an elevated sphincter pressure at rest is, therefore, vital in this dual function. During swallowing, the sphincter must relax early enough, i.e., in advance of a peristaltic contraction, to avoid spilling of the bolus into the airway.

Like the pistons of an automobile engine in operation, the soft tissue structures of the pharynx move up and down during swallowing, within a bony frame formed by the cervical spine and the base of the skull. Any interference with such motion may lead to swallowing difficulty. Adhesions, for example, may fix the prevertebral fascia to the adjacent cervical spine, rendering them incapable of participating in the normal descending posterior pharyngeal wave. Equally, severe deformities of the cervical spine proper may affect swallowing.

Important for the successful initiation of the swallowing reflex is the sensory innervation around the junction of mouth and pharynx. Sensory receptors are embedded in the mucosae of the tongue, soft palate, and posterior pharyngeal wall and connected by sensory nerves to the glossopharyngeal nerve in the upper portion of the pharynx and to the vagus nerve in the lower pharynx, larynx, and esophagus. Both of these nerves terminate in the nucleus tractus solitarii. Motor innervation of the swallowing function is accomplished by activation of motor nuclei, involving the fifth, seventh, ninth, tenth, and twelfth cranial nerves and the first, second, and third cervical nerves. These motor nuclei are also distributed in the brain stem. Both sensory and motor innervation are integrated in a swallowing center [10] which programs all muscles participating in deglutition, exciting them sequentially to accomplish transport of the bolus from the mouth to the entrance of the stomach [8].

Technique and Procedures of Radiographic Examination

Oropharyngeal swallowing studies are best carried out by employing video- or cineradiographic recordings in lateral and PA projections at rates of 24–40 frames per second. A preliminary radiograph of the neck in lateral projection serves to assess the position of the tongue and hyoid bone as well as the condition of the cervical spine and the distribution of air within the pharyngeal cavity. These scout films also serve as useful landmarks for further study. Individual frames from dynamic recordings show the step-by-step transport of each bolus from the mouth to the esophagus. These recordings require standardization, including positioning of the patient in straight lateral and PA projections. The oropharyngeal stage of swallowing is best examined with the patient upright, but if this is not possible the study can still be conducted with the patient recumbent. Contrast substances ranging in physical composition from watery liquids to solid food particles are given to the patient during the radiographic examination. The administration of these media should be matched to the patient's history of dysphagia. In our experience, a given patient's swallowing problem is usually limited to or prevalent for specific consistencies and does not range all the way from liquids to solid foods. Studies utilizing contrast materials of different consistencies also permit the selection of substances which the patient can safely swallow as part of his regular diet.

Frame-by-frame analysis of dynamic recordings displaying barium swallows enables the radiologist to make statements about the degree of oropharyngeal disability and, frequently, about the specific character of the disorder.

Radiographic Findings

The normal swallowing sequence of the oropharynx is shown and briefly discussed in Fig. 3.

Examples of impaired motor function involving the pharynx are presented according to area of involvement (soft palate, larynx, cricopharyngeal sphincter), according to specific functional abnormality (aspiration), or in terms of functional adaptation to motor impairment (compensation or decompensation).

Soft Palate Abnormalities

The principal muscles of the soft palate, the tensor and levator veli palatini, may not be functioning in proper equilibrium. On the other hand, there may be considerable weakness of contraction of both. There may be atrophy of muscles, or a normal or functionally adequate soft palate may attempt to compensate for a low-positioned or atrophic tongue; in this circumstance the palate may demonstrate a kinked contour (Fig. 4). This compensatory effort accomplishes palate-tongue apposition during gathering of the bolus in the mouth and thus prevents preswallow leakage of that bolus into the pharynx.

Airway Penetration

Airway penetration may occur when the contents of the oral cavity leak into the pharynx. The reason for such leakage may be a patient's loss of sensation along the back of the tongue or in the pharynx or motor impairment of these structures, which consequently are unable to come into apposition to effect closure of the oral cavity. Liquid retained in the pharyngeal cavity after completion of a swallow may be aspirated into the airway through spillage (Fig. 5). When solid particles leave the mouth uncontrolled or are re-

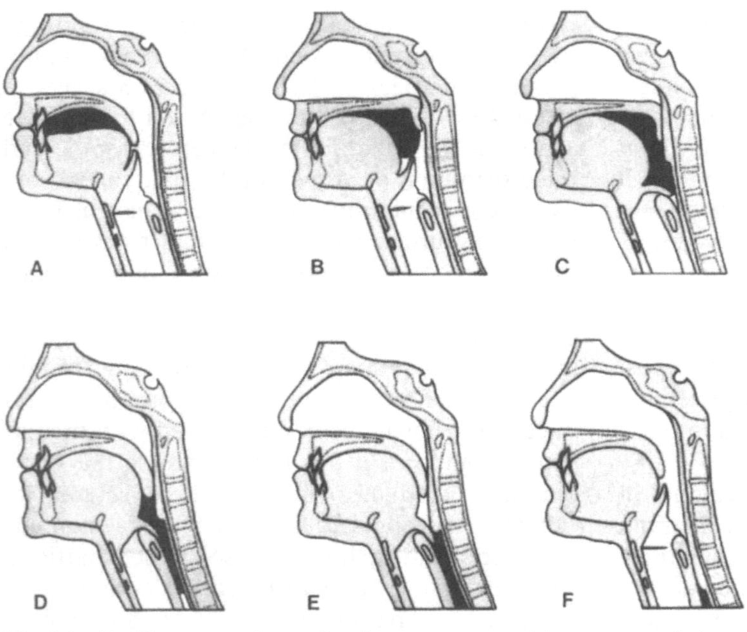

Fig. 3A–F. The normal swallowing sequence (cine barium swallow, 32 frames per second). **A** Bolus held in the mouth; note indentation of the tongue before swallow begins. **B** At this point swallowing becomes automatic; note movement of the palate upward and backward toward the posterior pharyngeal wall with its protruding muscle ridge (Passavant's cushion). **C** Note further progression of the bolus; the epiglottis has turned downward. **D** The epiglottis covers the larynx, which has risen above its resting position; a progressive wave is descending along the posterior pharyngeal wall. **E** The bolus has descended into the esophagus; the laryngeal muscles remain tightly constricted. **F** Upon completion of swallow, all structures return to their resting position

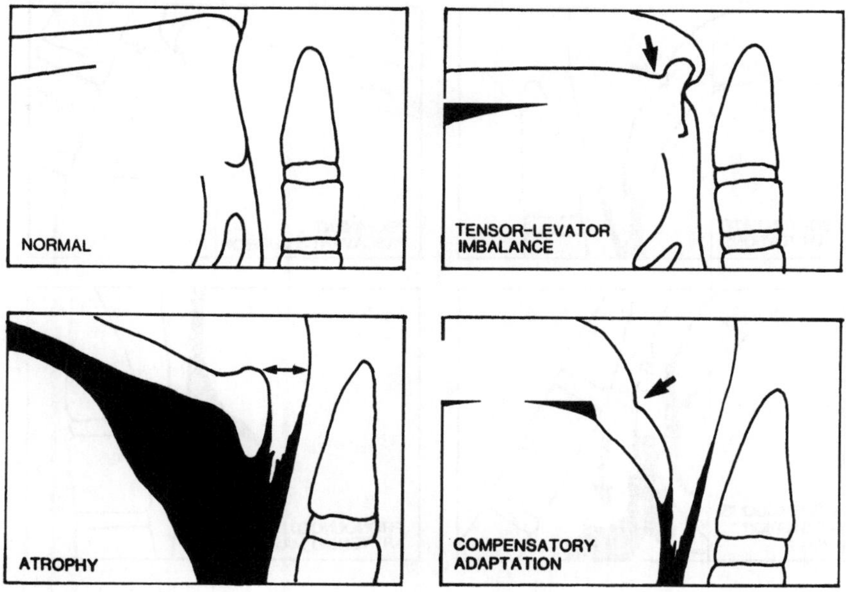

Fig. 4. Soft palate abnormalities

tained in the pharynx after swallowing, they may lodge in the aperture of the larynx, resulting in a life-threatening choking episode.

Compensation and Decompensation

For a considerable time during a patient's progressive disability, impairment of oropharyngeal swallowing may not be serious because compensatory measures partly or wholly correct the deficiency (Fig. 6). Examples are:

- Soft palate kinking towards the tongue
- A prominent Passavant's cushion coming into apposition with the palate to effect closure of the palatopharyngeal isthmus
- Increased extrusion of the constrictor wall, effecting constriction of the pharyngeal lumen in the event of impairment of the tongue
- Increased extrusion of the arytenoid mass into the space of the larynx

Decompensation of the pharyngeal swallow performance occurs when boluses are misdirected in-

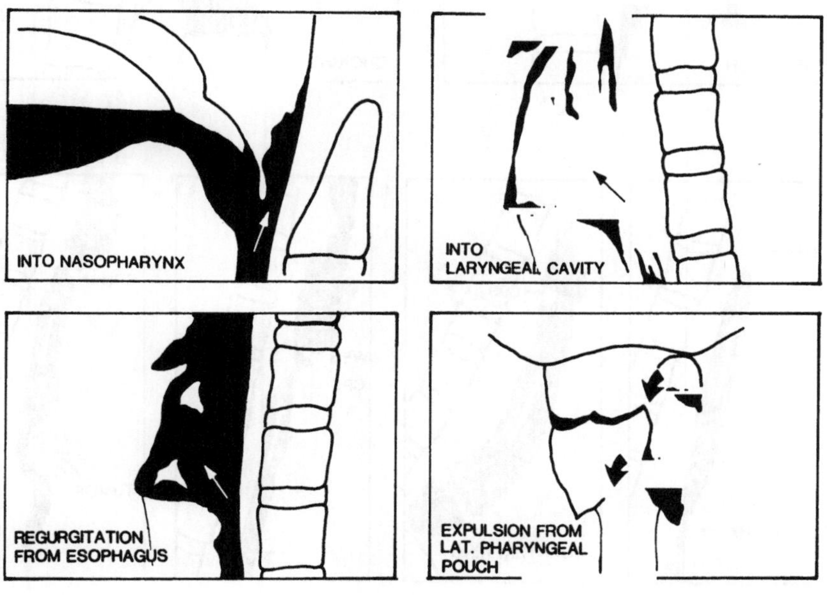

Fig. 5. Aspiration of retained bolus

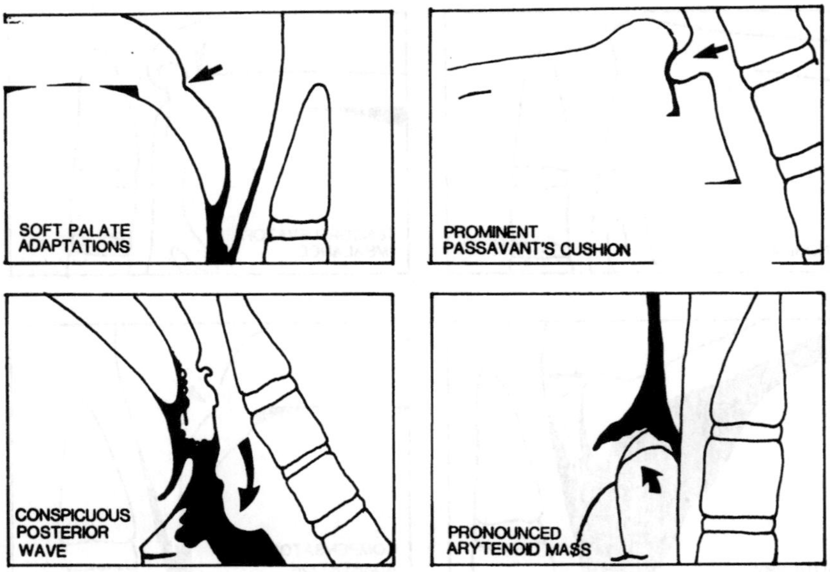

Fig. 6. Oropharyngeal compensation

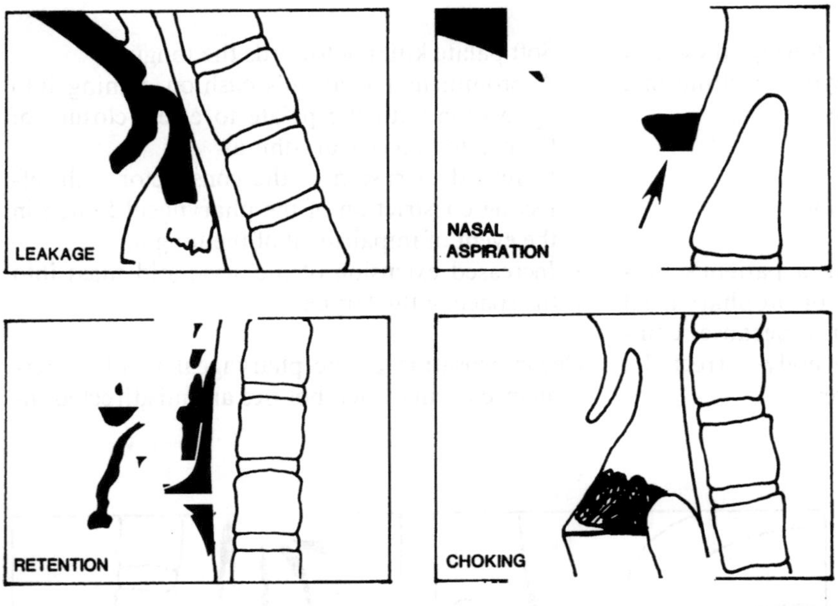

Fig. 7. Oropharyngeal decompensation

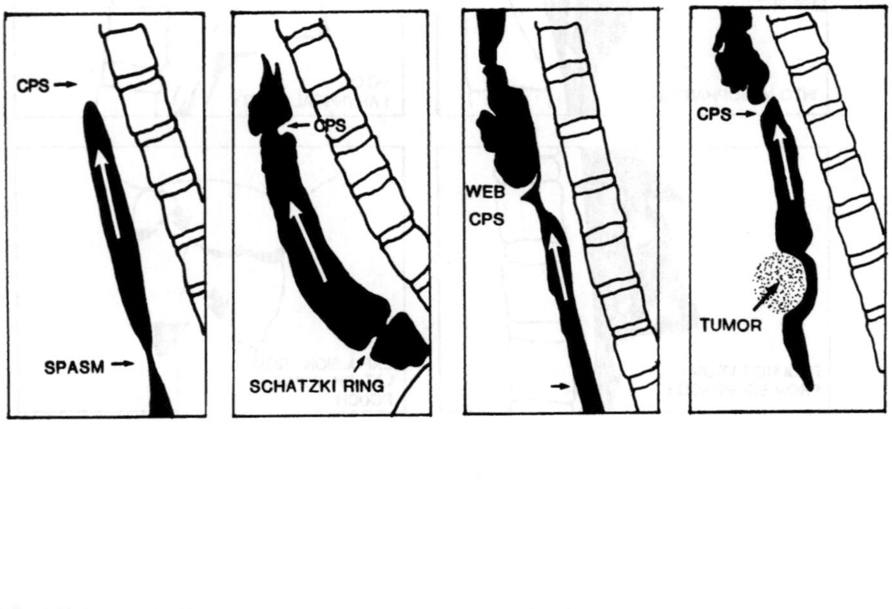

Fig. 8. Cricopharyngeal sphincter (*CPS*) response to esophageal disease

to the nasal cavity or the larynx and trachea before, during, or after swallowing. The patient is even more endangered if laryngeal penetration goes unnoticed, i.e., does not result in coughing. This latter circumstance may be caused by impairment of the larynx resulting from a stroke or peripheral neuropathy (Fig. 7).

Cricopharyngeal Sphincter Response to Esophageal Disease

In investigating patients with dysphagia, it is always important to examine all structures participating in deglutition – mouth, pharynx, and esophagus – regardless of where the patient localizes his symptoms. According to a study by Edwards [9], the patient is more often wrong than right in subjectively identifying the area of abnormality in the swallowing tract. For example, when segmental spasm of the esophagus occurs, bolus in the esophageal lumen is frequently displaced proximally toward the closed cricopharyngeal sphincter. Contact of the displaced bolus with the undersurface of the sphincter, results in a sensation frequently described by the patient as "lump in the throat" [3]. Unrecognized, this phenomenon may be referred to as "globus hystericus." It is seen in patients with gastroesophageal reflux, diffuse esophageal spasm, or organic obstruction of the more distal esophagus [4]. If such backup of liquids or food is allowed to exist over a period of time, the cricopharyngeal sphincter responds not merely with a reactive contraction to protect the pharyngeal mucosa from exposure to regurgitated material, but with a more sustained contraction consistent with a protrusion of sphincter tissue into the lumen of the hypopharynx. It needs to be determined whether this sort of visible sphincter defect in the barium column during fluoroscopic examination represents incomplete relaxation of the cricopharyngeal muscle or perhaps sphincter hypertrophy. In any case, radiological demonstration of a posterior filling defect at the sphincter level in the absence of other identifiable pharyngeal impairment or clinical history, e.g., bulbar poliomyelitis, usually implies an abnormality of the esophagus [6, 7].

Conclusion

From the foregoing, it is apparent that the radiologist's help is critical in determining the pattern and degree of swallowing impairment. More significantly, the radiologist is best able to suggest or identify the disease category producing the dysphagia, and can thus refer the patient to the appropriate consultants. His assistance is also required in patient management in terms of alternative modes of feeding, change of diet, optimal head and neck position, and perhaps surgical intervention. Follow-up recordings of the swallowing process usually determine whether the patient has adapted to the disability or is in the process of decompensation. Choking episodes and chronic aspiration may be reduced or prevented by careful radiological examination and advice to the patient based on the radiological information.

In recognizing the need for a multidisciplinary approach to patients with swallowing difficulties, a Swallowing Center has been established at The Johns Hopkins Medical Institutions with the participation of several clinical and basic science departments. In such a multidisciplinary group, the radiologist's role goes beyond traditional radiographic evaluation.

References

1. Bosma JF (1957) Deglutition, pharyngeal stage. Physiol Rev 37:275
2. Bosma JF, Donner MW (1980) Physiology of the pharynx. In: Paparella MM, Shumrick DA (eds) Otolaryngology, 2nd edn. Saunders, Philadelphia London Toronto
3. Cherry J, Siegel CI, Margulies SI, Donner MW (1970) Pharyngeal localization of symptoms of gastroesophageal reflux. Ann Otol 79:912
4. Delahunty JE, Margulies SI, Alonso UA, Knudson DH (1971) The relationship of reflux esophagitis to pharyngeal pouch (Zenker's diverticulum). Laryngoscope 81:570
5. Dodds WJ, Hogan WJ, Lyndon SB, Stewart ET, Stef JJ, Arndorfer RC (1975) Quantification of pharyngeal motor function in normal human subjects. J Appl Physiol 39:692
6. Donner MW (1976) Spezielle Röntgendiagnostik von Funktionsstörungen der Speiseröhre. In: Siewert R, Blum AL, Waldeck F (eds) Funktionsstörungen der Speiseröhre. Springer, Berlin Heidelberg New York
7. Donner WM (1980) Physiology of the esophagus. In: Paparella MM, Shumrick DA (eds) Otolaryngology, 2nd edn. Saunders, Philadelphia London Toronto
8. Doty RW, Bosma JF (1956) An electromyographic analysis of reflex deglutition. J Neurophysiol 19:44
9. Edwards DAW (1976) Discriminatory value of symptoms in the differential diagnosis of dysphagia. Clin Gastroenterol 5:49
10. Miller AJ (1982) Deglutition. Physiol Rev 62:129

Radiology of the Liver: Overview

A. L. Baert, G. Wilms, G. Marchal, E. Ponette, and R. Usewils

Department of Radiology, University Hospital St. Rafaël, Kapucijnenvoer 33, 3000 Leuven, Belgium

The advent of new imaging methods such as ultrasound and computed tomography (CT) has considerably changed the diagnostic radiologic approach to liver disease, reducing the role of nuclear medicine and the need for invasive diagnostic procedures.
Although CT and ultrasound are frequently complementary, each examination appears to have its specific indications. The different diagnostic possibilities for diffuse and focal liver lesions have to be considered.

Diffuse Parenchymatous Liver Disease

In diffuse parenchymatous liver disease, diffuse alterations in reflective pattern will be found on ultrasound and inhomogeneous density patterns will be found on CT. CT seems very accurate in hemochromatosis, where it shows a diffuse increase in attenuation values of the liver proportional to the iron content of the liver tissue [24].

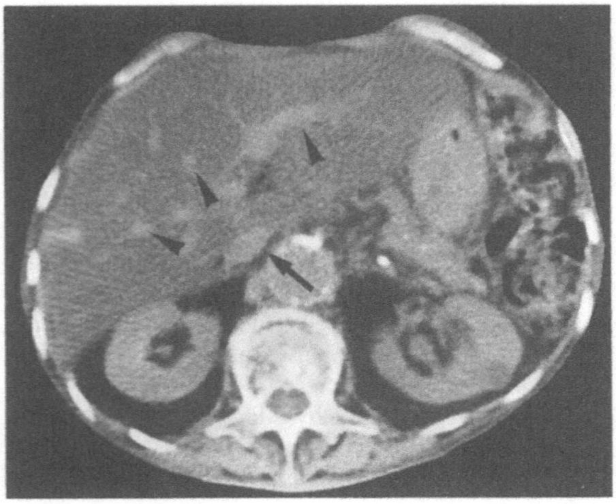

Fig. 1 Severe hepatic steatosis. A plain study shows a diffuse decrease in density of the liver parenchyma with negative attenuation values (−10 HU). The inferior vena cava (→) and the portal veins (►►) appear hyperdense in contrast with the liver

In hepatic steatosis a diffuse marked increased echogenicity will be observed on ultrasound. The degree of echogenicity of the liver can better be assessed by comparison with the adjacent right renal parenchyma (reversal of normal). This hyperechogenic liver pattern is not specific, however, and will also be seen in hepatic cirrhosis [19, 54−56] and in some types of glycogen storage disease. CT findings in fatty liver are quite characteristic: due to an overall decrease in attenuation coefficients of the liver parenchyma the vascular structures, especially the branches of the portal vein and the hepatic veins, will appear to be denser than the adjacent liver parenchyma and to stand out against it (Fig. 1). The density of the fatty liver will vary according to the degree of fatty replacement. Studies on tissue samples have proved that there is a linear relationship between hepatic triglyceride levels and the decrease in CT attenuation values. A fatty replacement of 10% will correspond to a decrease of 17 HU [48].
Fatty infiltrations can also be focally scattered within the liver [7, 40, 50] and can thereby mimic focal hepatic lesions on both ultrasound and CT. It has been noted that the CT values of the hepatic parenchyma rapidly revert toward normal following better nutrition, abstinence from alcohol, or elimination of exposure to hepatotoxic agents [3]. Repeat CT scans are therefore a useful clinical tool for assessing the evolution of hepatic steatosis (Fig. 2).
Glycogen in concentrations encountered in type I glycogen storage disease (von Gierke disease) has CT attenuation coefficients of 50−70 HU, but due to simultaneous infiltration with fat and glycogen a range of liver CT densities of 13−80 HU has been observed in patients with this disease [11].
In children, hyperechogenic livers can be related

Radiology Today 2. Ed. by F. H. W. Heuck and M. W. Donner

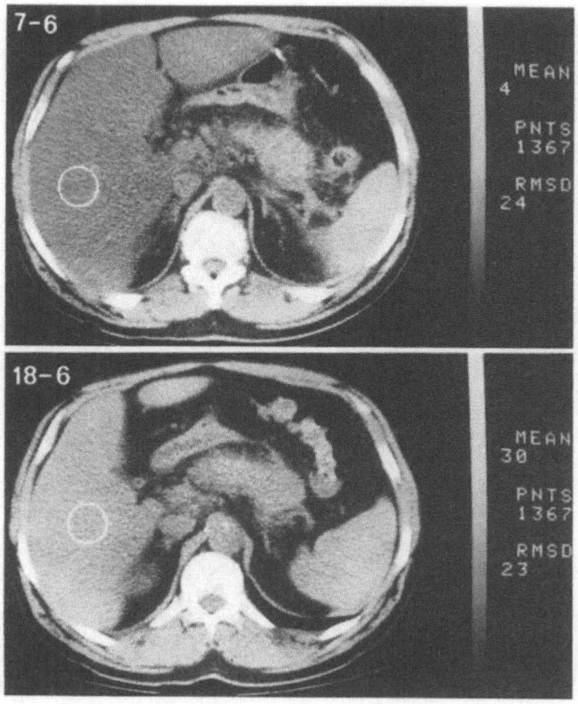

Fig. 2. Regression of liver steatosis after alcohol abstinence. *Above:* Homogeneous low density of the liver (4 HU) compared with normal density of pancreas and spleen. Enlargement of pancreatic tail due to acute alcoholic pancreatitis. *Below:* Control CT examination after 11 days. Increase of attenuation values of the liver to 30 HU, almost identical to pancreas and spleen

to metabolic disease, malnutrition, hyperalimentation, or chemotherapy [5, 23].

Other diffuse diseases of the liver, like cirrhosis or hepatitis, do not constitute indications for ultrasound or CT. Aspecific secondary findings that may be visualized with either method include macronodular outline, regional changes in hepatic morphology [22], and signs of portal hypertension such as portal dilatation, repermeabilized portal vein [14], portosystemic collateral vessels [9, 10], and ascites. In acute hepatitis ultrasound can demonstrate periportal edema [34].

Focal Hepatic Lesions

Benign

Hepatic cysts have a typical ultrasound and CT appearance, i.e., rounded well-defined lesions which are nonreflective on ultrasound and show the same density as water on CT. Solitary hepatic cysts are frequent incidental findings. Polycystic liver disease, in which multiple cysts are present, is shown dramatically by CT. In cases of multiple

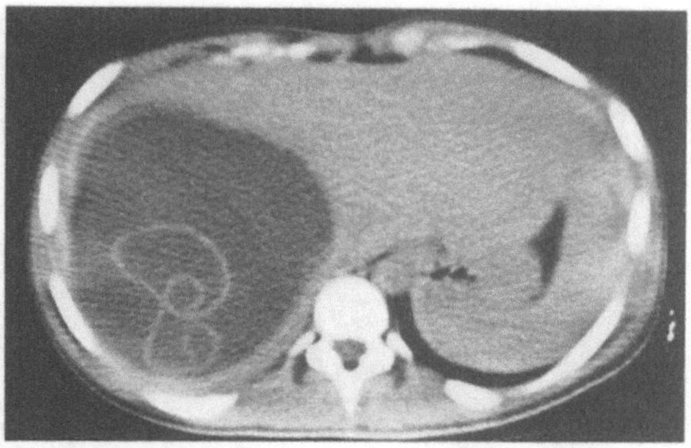

Fig. 3. Hepatic hydatid cyst. A contrast enhanced scan (1 min) shows a huge irregular oval hypodense area at the dorsal aspect of the right hepatic lobe. Presence of floating membranes in the center of the lesion

adjacent cysts the thinness of the cystic wall can be appreciated.

With ultrasound, differential diagnosis with bile ducts may occasionally present difficulties. On the other hand, ultrasound may be more accurate than CT in demonstrating wall thickness, mural nodules, septations, or fluid levels in pseudocystic necrotic metastasis [15] and in biliary cystadenomas, cystic hamartomas, hematomas, or abscesses [16].

Both methods show a high level of accuracy in hydatid liver disease [18, 46]. CT is more effective in alveolar hydatid lesions by showing the different types of calcification, whereas ultrasound provides a more accurate picture of the details of the internal structure of the cysts, such as intracystic septation, wall splitting, or daughter cysts, in cystic hydatid lesions (Fig. 3) [49].

Cavernous hemangiomas have an equally typical appearance on ultrasound and CT. Most are small single lesions, usually less than 5 cm in diameter, but multiple tumors occur in 10% of cases [27]. Cavernous hemangiomas occur in 0.4%–7.3% of the population and are the most common benign liver tumors, with a definite preponderance for females (70%–95%) [1]. Accurate diagnosis of the benign condition is of primary importance, both to differentiate it from liver metastasis in patients with a primary malignant tumor and to prevent massive or even portal bleeding after percutaneous biopsy [39].

On ultrasound, cavernous hemangiomas appear strongly hyperreflective. They have an homogeneous appearance if they are smaller than 2 cm in diameter, but the larger ones show a central hypoechogenic aspect. They are mostly located in the subcapsular area (Fig. 4).

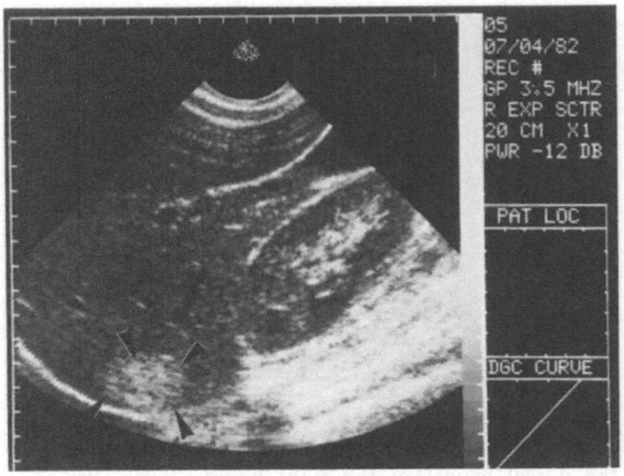

Fig. 4. Benign hemangioma of the right hepatic lobe. A longitudinal sonogram shows an oval strongly reflective lesion (►) of subcapsular location at the caudal aspect of the right hepatic lobe, near the diaphragm. The lesion is 3 cm in diameter

Cavernous hemangiomas appear on a nonenhanced CT scan as roughly spherical well-demarcated masses whose density is low but greater than that of hepatic cysts. Sequential CT imaging after intravenous bolus injection of contrast medium allows a specific diagnosis in most cases. Initially there is opacification of vascular structures in the periphery of the hypodense area but the central part of the lesion remains low in density. After 60–90 s there is gradual opacification ("filling in") of the center. On a delayed scan 3–4 min after injection the lesion is isodense or slightly hyperdense compared to the normal parenchyma (Fig. 5) [2, 30]. The sensitivity of both CT and ultrasound in displaying cavernous hemangiomas larger than 2 or 3 cm is very high, but due to the difficulty caused by respiration in imaging an identical slice constantly on sequential scanning, CT appears to be inferior to ultrasound for the detection of small hemangiomas.

Other benign solid tumoral lesions, such as adenomas or focal nodular hyperplasia, do not display any specific characteristics on ultrasound. They may be hyperechogenic or hypoechogenic.

On CT these lesions usually differ only slightly in density from normal liver and are similar in appearance to hepatoma. They can be missed due to their isodensity with the normal liver parenchyma, not only before intravenous contrast but also in the delayed phase after injection. Only during the early vascular phase after bolus injection will they be visible as hyperdense structures if they are well vascularized, as in the majority of cases [42, 47].

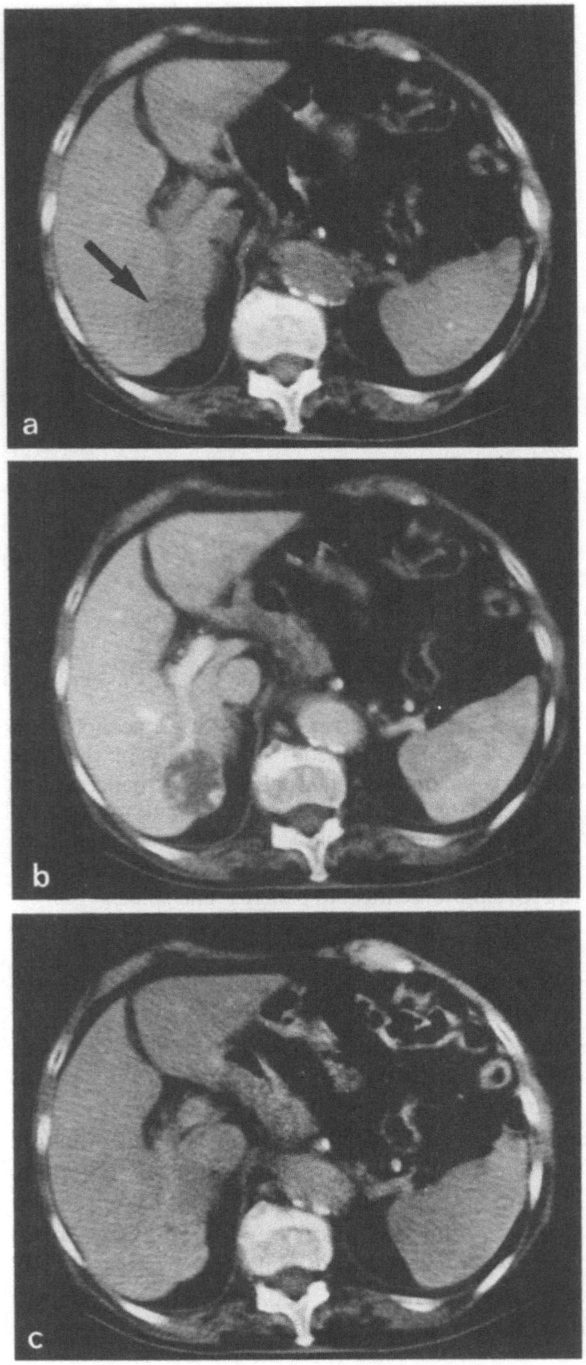

Fig. 5a–c. Hemangioma of the right lobe of the liver. **a** A plain scan shows an oval 2x3 cm diameter hypodense lesion ( ) at the dorsal aspect of the right hepatic lobe. Plain attenuation values of 30 HU compared with 60 HU of the normal hepatic parenchyma. **b** A contrast-enhanced scan in the early phase (25 s after bolus injection) gives visualization of multiple hyperdense spots at the periphery of the lesion, representing early filling venous lakes. **c** A contrast enhanced scan in the delayed phase (3 min) shows total filling of the center of the lesion with contrast, attenuation values reaching 120 HU

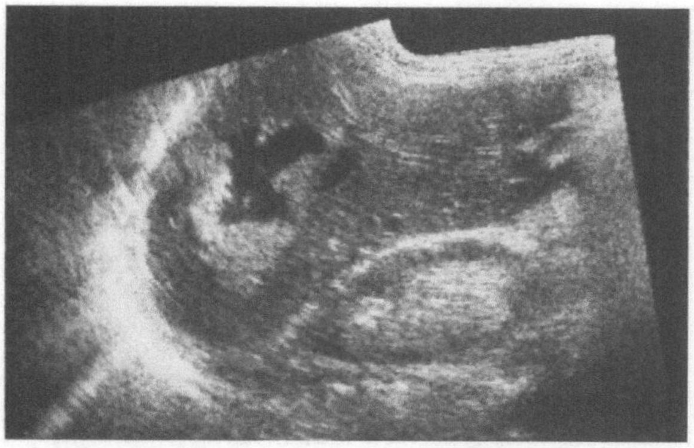

Fig. 6. Intrahepatic post-traumatic hematoma. A longitudinal sonogram shows an intrahepatic irregular area of decreased reflection. The surrounding hyperreflective area points to partial resolution of the hematoma

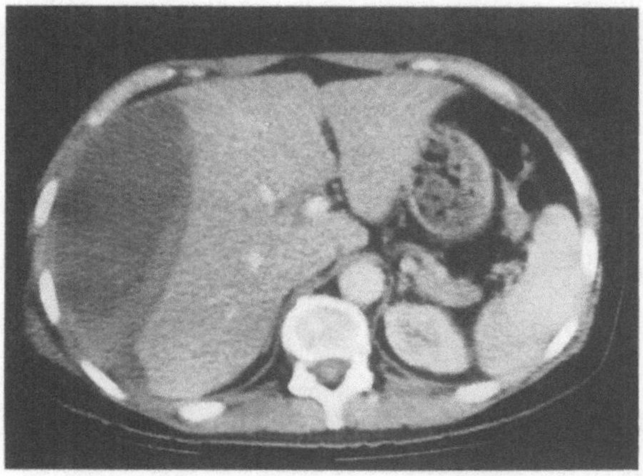

Fig. 7. Post-traumatic subcapsular hematoma of the liver. There is a huge, hypodense area at the lateral aspect of the right hepatic lobe, with typical biconvex shape. The center of the lesion is more hypodense due to a more advanced degree of hemolysis

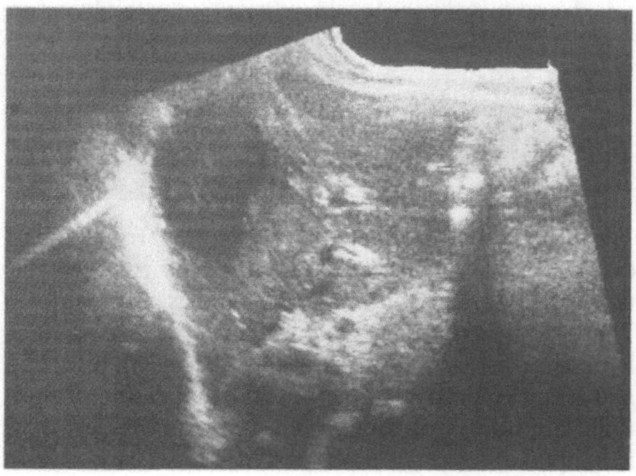

Fig. 8. Subcapsular hepatic abscess. A longitudinal sonogram shows a subcapsular irregular hyporeflective area containing multiple intraluminal hyperreflective spots. Total absence of posterior wall enhancement

Hepatic scintigraphy may contribute to the differential diagnosis between focal nodular hyperplasia and adenoma. As focal nodular hyperplasia is composed of normal hepatocytes, Kupffer cells, and bile ducts, a normal colloid uptake may be present. The use of a cholegraphic contrast agent to obtain selective enhancement of focal nodular hyperplasia by virtue of its functional activity has been proposed [25].

Hematomas vary, according to the age of the lesion, from strongly reflective to nonreflective on ultrasound (Fig. 6) and from hyper- to hypodense on CT. Fresh intrahepatic hematomas, however, can be missed by CT due to their isodense attenuation values with the normal liver parenchyma. The biconvex form of hematoma is typical for a subcapsular location (Fig. 7).

The diagnosis of pyogenic liver abscess continues to be a serious clinical problem, as the mortality is still between 20% and 50% [35, 36, 44]. The ultrasound appearance of pyogenic liver abscesses is nonspecific, varying from anechoic to highly echogenic and solid (Fig. 8) [32, 41].

On CT, hepatic abscesses present as mass lesions with a lower density than tumors and not as sharply circumscribed as benign cysts. They may be multilocular and hard to differentiate from necrotic malignant tumors. Due to their avascularity, they are visualized better after intravenous contrast enhancement. A thick enhancing rim may also be discernible and is quite specific, although it may also occur in some kinds of metastatic lesion. The presence of air within the abscess cavity is also highly suggestive, but spontaneous gas formation without inflammation can also be seen in necrotic malignant tumors and in liver infarction.

Malignant

For the detection of hepatic metastases, hepatic scintigraphy, ultrasound, and CT can be considered. It appears from studies published in 1978 and 1979 [6, 45, 52, 53] and reviewed by Freeny [17] that the sensitivities of hepatic scintigraphy and CT are 88% and 90% respectively and that both are more sensitive than ultrasound (79%). Since then important technical progress in ultrasound equipment has been made and the sensitivity of ultrasound may now be greater. However, the specificity of CT (91%) appears from these studies to be significantly greater than that of either ultrasound (74%) or hepatic scintigraphy. Although hepatic scintigraphy may still

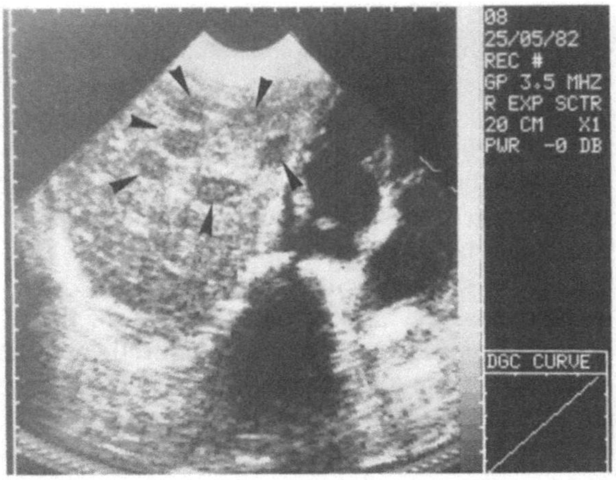

Fig. 9. Multiple hepatic metastases from breast carcinoma. A transverse sonogram shows multiple (►►) rounded nodular areas within the right hepatic lobe, with a peripheral sonolucent aspect and central isoreflection (bull's-eye lesion). The diffuse hyperreflective pattern of the hepatic parenchyma is due to moderate steatosis under the influence of chemotherapy

be preferred as the initial screening modality for liver metastases, there is now a tendency to apply ultrasound on a wider scale because of its availability and low cost (Fig. 9). CT will thus be most useful as the specific evaluation method when ultrasound gives an abnormal or equivocal result.

Most metastatic liver tumors are visible on a nonenhanced CT scan, because they are lower in density than normal parenchyma and greater in density, but usually less circumscribed and less uniform in density, than cysts. By virtue of its ability to detect minor density differences, calcified metastases originating mainly from primary breast or gastrointestinal tumors are more and more frequently demonstrated by CT [4]. They may have a punctate appearance or a more amorphous aspect, and will appear frequently during the course of chemotherapy. Calcification is a strong indicator of liver metastases, especially if not associated with an adjacent hypodense area.

After intravenous contrast administration, most metastatic lesions are equally well visualized (Fig. 10) [38]. In a minority of cases (about 5%–7%) they become more visible. Contrast enhancement should therefore be used only selectively in CT studies for metastatic liver disease. However, as some metastatic lesions may become isodense after contrast administration and therefore less visible, CT scanning must never be performed only after intravenous contrast, without previous plain scan series. In some rare instances, liver metastases which are isodense with the ad-

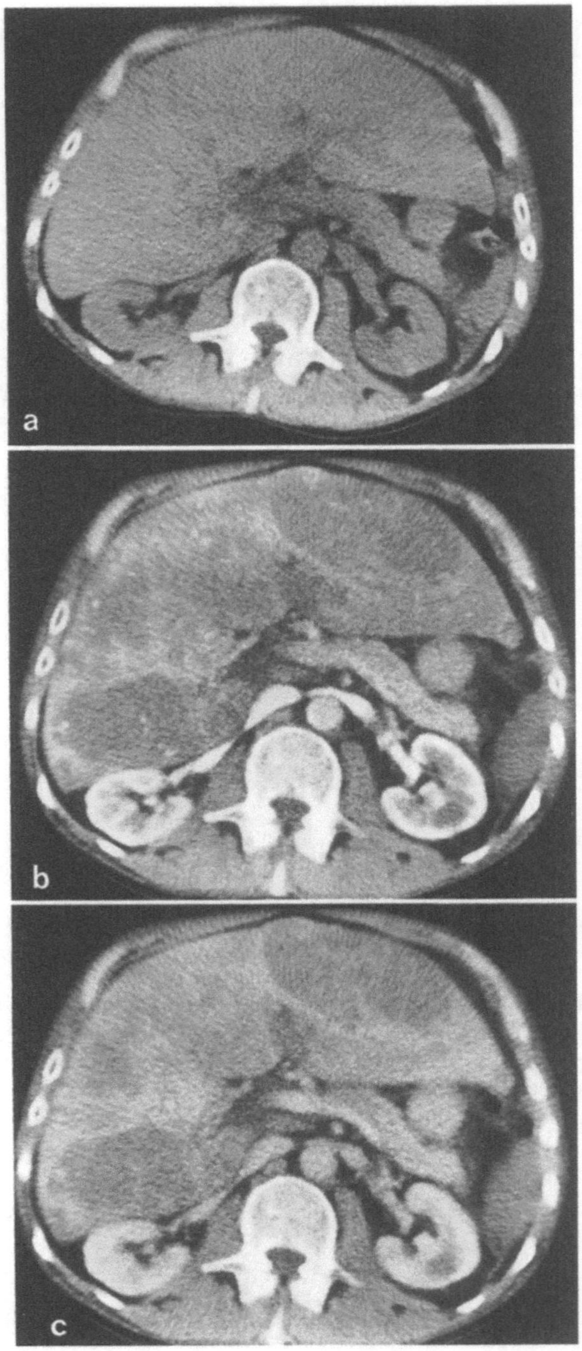

Fig. 10a–c. Diffuse hepatic metastases from breast carcinoma. **a** A plain scan shows diffusely enlarged volume of the liver with inhomogeneous parenchyma. There is suspicion of several large intraparenchymatous hypodense areas. **b, c** Contrast-enhanced scans after 25 s and 1 min respectively give better visualization of multiple large areas of diminished and pathological contrast uptake

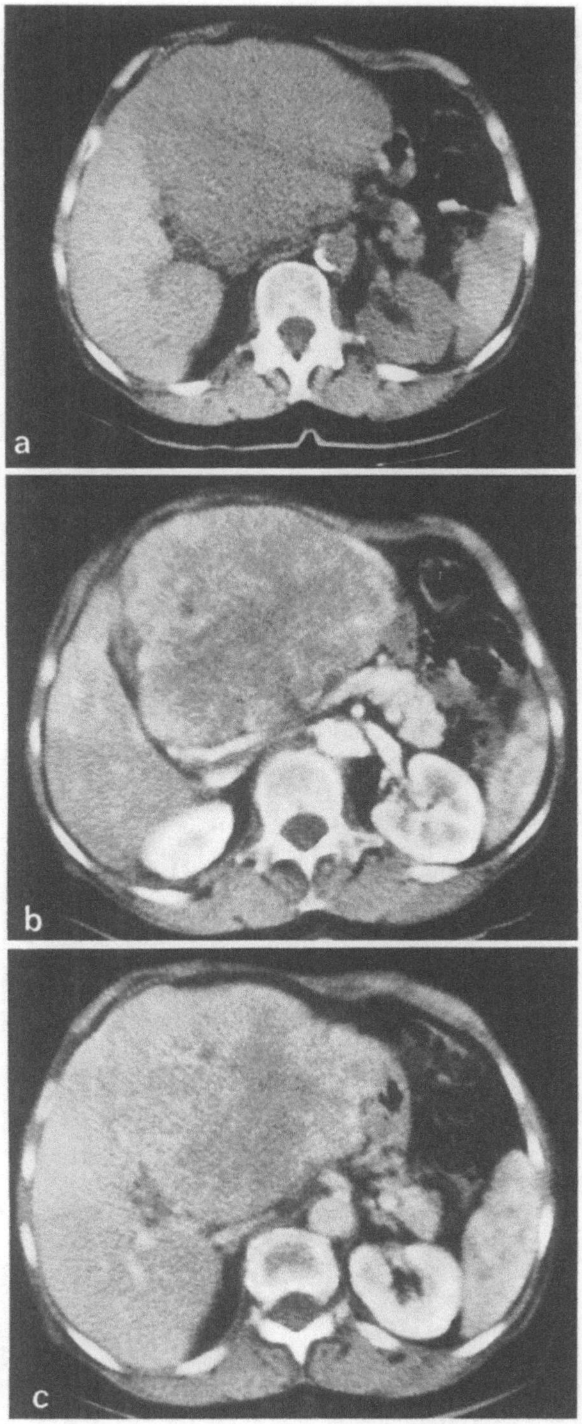

Fig. 11 a–c. Hepatocellular carcinoma. **a** A plain scan shows enormous enlargement of the left lobe of the liver with polylobular outline. The lesion appears hypodense towards the normal hepatic parenchyma of the right lobe with attenuation values of 35 HU. **b** A contrast-enhanced scan 25 s after bolus injection shows inhomogeneous contrast uptake in the lesion, characterised by an overall hypervascular pattern, alternating with areas of diminished contrast uptake. Note dorsal displacement and flattering of the main branch of the portal vein and lateral displacement of the pancreatic tail. **c** A contrast-enhanced scan 1 min after bolus injection shows the inhomogeneous "capillary phase" of the tumor, pointing to central necrosis

jacent liver parenchyma on a plain scan become transiently hyperdense for a very short period (about 30–60 s) due to their hypervascularity [37]. If they are small their detection is extremely difficult with the actual available scanning time and sequential scanning frequency. Ultrasound seems to be more accurate than CT in demonstrating very small and subcapsular metastatic lesions, mainly due to the artifacts related to normal motion [51]. Particularly difficult in this regard, due to contact motion at the liver-lung interface, is the evaluation of the dome of the right lobe of the liver. Respiratory motion, which is not always controllable, may cause considerable difficulties, as may artifacts due to air within the stomach or the colon and/or associated peristalsis.

Unfortunately, neither ultrasound nor CT appearance of liver metastases yet allows accurate prediction of the site or histologic type of primary tumor, although the presence of focal areas of increased density on CT or hyperechogenicity on ultrasound may suggest an origin in the gastrointestinal tract. Most primary hepatic malignant tumors have no typical ultrasound or CT appearance [13, 20, 26, 28, 29, 31, 33]. On CT they will present as either isodense or slightly hypodense mass lesions unless there is clear tumor necrosis. The patterns of enhancement observed after intravenous contrast administration do not allow a specific histopathologic diagnosis (Fig. 11).

Vascular Lesions

Both ultrasound and CT can demonstrate portal vein thrombosis, Budd-Chiari syndrome, or other vascular anomalies [43]. Nevertheless, ultrasound, by virtue of its echoscopic capacity, is superior in following the course of tortuous vessels and in the identification of respiratory influences. Moreover, it frequently allows determination of flow direction in portal hypertension and portacaval shunt.

Liver infarction presents mainly as a low-density area and can erroneously be interpreted as a mass lesion. In rare instances there may be noninflammatory gas formation due to tissue necrosis.

Angiography

Angiography maintains its place as a diagnostic procedure in the context of arterial hepatic lesions [5]. Small aneurysms of the hepatic artery and the typical arterial alterations in periarteritis nodosa require selective angiography (Fig. 12.).
In post-traumatic conditions, angiography will be the only way to detect a site of bleeding (Fig. 13).

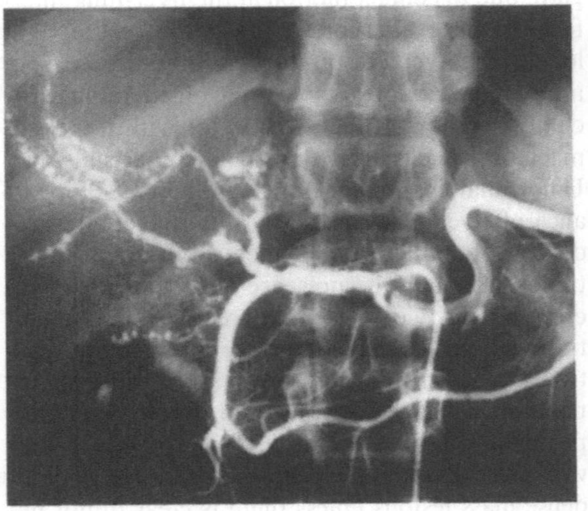

Fig. 12. Periarteritis nodosa. A selective hepatic angiogram shows diffuse narrowing of the intrahepatic branches of the hepatic artery with multiple short concentric stenoses, alternating with aneurysms

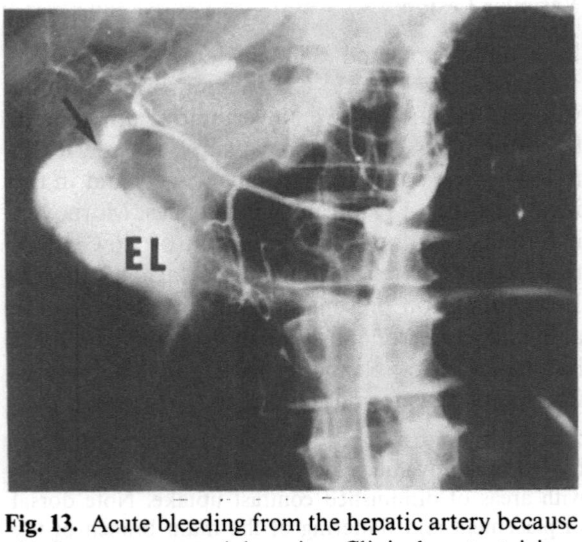

Fig. 13. Acute bleeding from the hepatic artery because of inflammatory arterial erosion. Clinical context: jejunal loop on bile ducts after cholecystectomy for acute cholecystitis. Selective angiogram of the coeliac trunk shows marked diffuse vascular collapse due to hypovolemia. The right descending branch of the right hepatic artery is interrupted (→). There is extensive contrast filling of the efferent loop (*EL*)

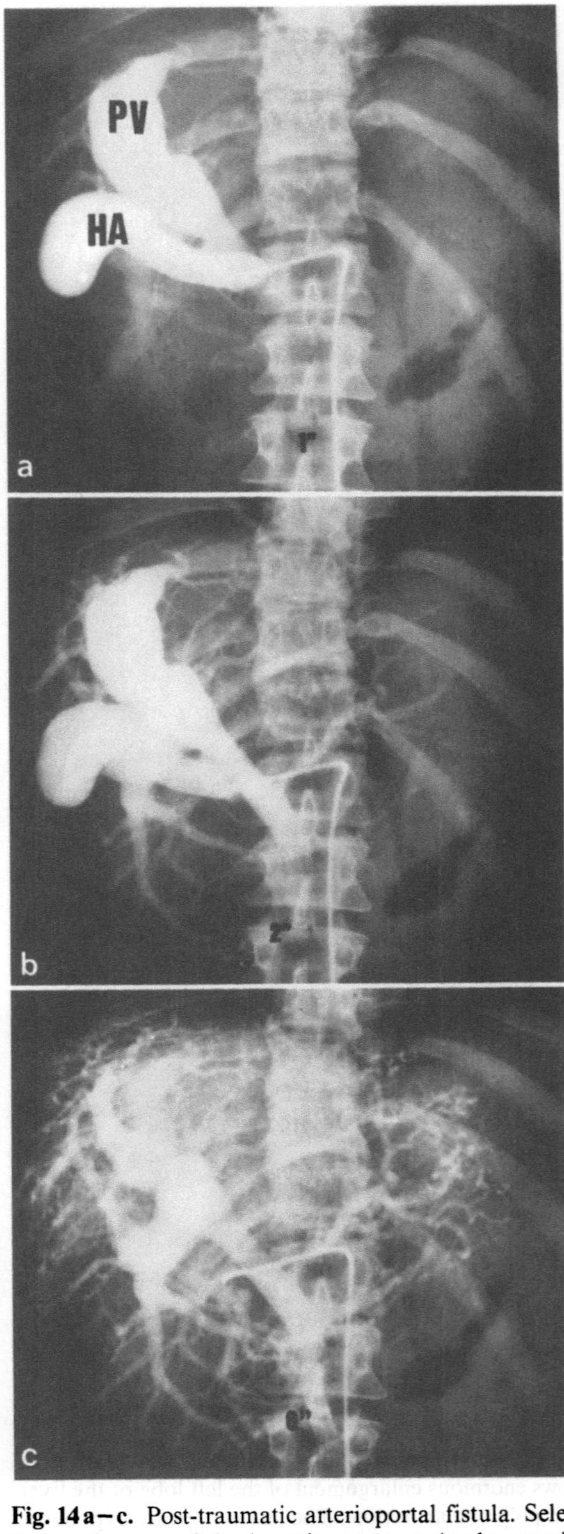

Fig. 14a–c. Post-traumatic arterioportal fistula. Selective angiogram of the hepatic artery. **a** At the arterial phase (1 s) there is a marked increase in caliber of the hepatic artery (*HA*) and immediate filling of a dilated portal vein (*PV*). **b** After 2 s there is further opacification of the portal system. **c** After 6 s there is opacification of the entire hepatic portal tree

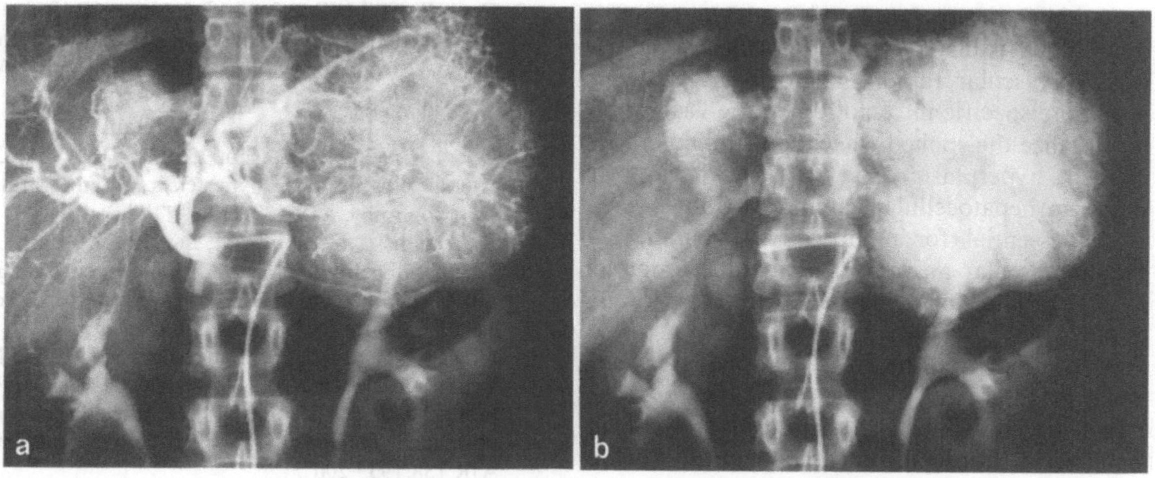

Fig. 15 a, b. Focal nodular hyperplasia of the liver: two localizations. Selective hepatic angiogram. **a** Arterial phase. Note the typical spoked wheel appearance of the vessels. The left lobe of the liver is considerably enlarged. **b** Capillary phase. The intense tumor stain in both lesions reflects their hypervascular character

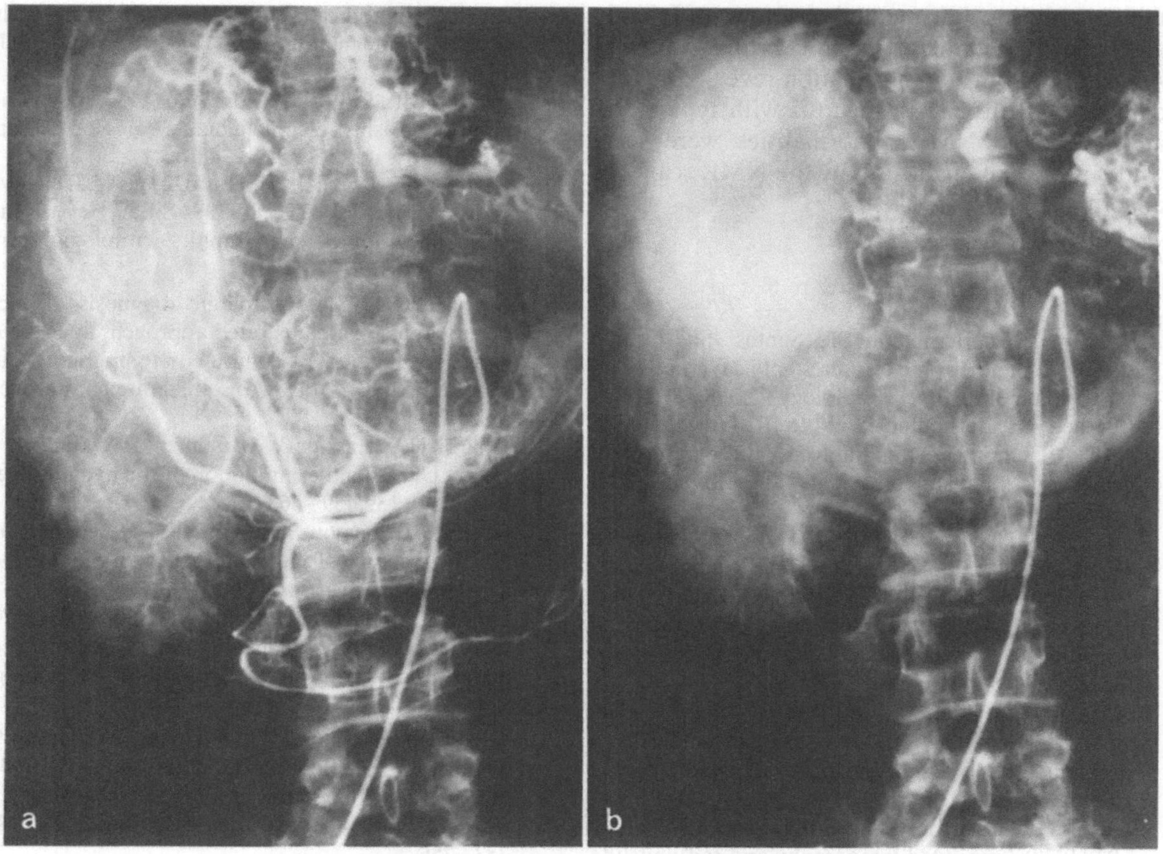

Fig. 16 a, b. Hepatocellular carcinoma. Selective hepatic angiogram. **a** Arterial phase. There is marked enlargement of the liver and important stretching of the intrahepatic branches of the hepatic artery with diffuse signs of neovascularization. **b** Capillary phase. These is intense tumor stain at the upper aspect of the lesion

To establish the presence and exact site of an arteriovenous fistula is shown in Fig. 14.
In hypervascular tumors, angiography may furnish more specific information on the vascularity, for instance the spoked wheel appearance in focal nodular hyperplasia (Fig. 15) or arterioportal shunts in hepatocellular carcinoma. Moreover, it is still essential for preoperative evaluation of hepatic vascular anatomy and for determination of resectability prior to selective hepatic lobectomy (Fig. 16).
Finally, more and more indications are being found for interventional therapeutic angiography, e.g., in the intra-arterial administration of chemotherapy, in transcatheter embolization of life-threatening bleeding from vascular lesions, and in palliative embolization of unresectable tumors [8].
Very recently, initial experience with nuclear magnetic resonance (NMR) imaging of the liver has been reported [12]. It appears that images obtained with this new method are now sufficiently anatomically detailed to permit serious comparison with CT, but the information revealed is fundamentally different: in steatosis with typical CT appearance no NMR abnormalities were seen, while in cases of cirrhosis only the NMR scan was abnormal.

References

1. Abrams RM, Bernbaum ER, Santos JS, Lipson J (1969) Angiographic features of cavernous hemangioma of the liver. Radiology 92:308–312
2. Barnett PH, Zerhouni EA, White RI, Siegelman SS (1980) Computed tomography in the diagnosis of cavernous hemangioma of the liver. AJR 134:439–447
3. Bashist B, Hecht HL, Harley WD (1982) Computed tomographic demonstration of rapid changes in fatty infiltration of the liver. Radiology 142:691–692
4. Bernardino ME (1979) Computed tomography of calcified liver metastases. J Comput Assist Tomogr 3:32–35
5. Bertrand PH, Baert AL, van Dooren W (1981) L'artériographie hépatique: un examen superflu à l'époque de la tomodensitométrie? Radiologie J CEPUR 1:23–31
6. Biello DR, Levitt RG, Siegel BA, Sagel SS, Stanley RJ (1978) Computed tomography and radionuclide imaging of the liver: a comparative evaluation. Radiology 127:159–163
7. Brauwer MK, Austin GE, Lewin KJ (1980) Focal fatty change of the liver, a hitherto poorly recognized entity. Gastroenterology 78:247–252
8. Chuang VP, Wallace S, Soo Chiu-Shiung, Charnsangavej C, Bowers T (1982) Therapeutic ivalon embolization of hepatic tumors. AJR 138:289–294
9. Dach JL, Hill MC, Pelaez JC, Le Page JR, Russell E (1981) Sonography of hypertensive portal venous system: correlation with arterial portography. AJR 137:511–517
10. Dökmeci AK, Kimura K, Matsutani S, Ohto M, Ono T, Tsuchiya Y, Saisho H, Okuda K (1981) Collateral veins in portal hypertension: demonstration by sonography. AJR 137:1173–1177
11. Doppman JL, Cornblath M, Dwyer AJ, Adams AJ, Girton ME, Sidbury J (1982) Computed tomography of the liver and kidneys in glycogen storage disease. J Comput Assist Tomogr 6:67–71
12. Doyle FH, Pennock JM, Banks LM, McDonnell MJ, Bydder GM, Steiner RE, Young IR, Clarke GJ, Pasmore T, Gilderdale DJ (1982) Nuclear magnetic resonance imaging of the liver: initial experience. AJR 138:193–200
13. Dunnick NR, Ihde DC, Doppman JL, Bates HR (1980) Computed tomography in primary hepatocellular carcinoma. J Comput Assist Tomogr 4:59–62
14. Fakhry J, Gosink BB, Leopold GR (1981) Recanalized umbilical vein due to portal vein occlusion: documentation by sonography. AJR 137:410–412
15. Federle MP, Filly RA, Moss AA (1981) Cystic hepatic neoplasms: complementary roles of CT and sonography. AJR 136:345–348
16. Forrest ME, Cho KJ, Shields JJ, Wicks JD, Silver TM, McCormick TL (1980) Biliary cystadenomas: sonographic–angiographic–pathologic correlations. AJR 135:723–727
17. Freeny PC (1981) Radiologic diagnosis of focal hepatic masses: an integrated approach. In: Moss A, Goldberg H (eds) Computed tomography, ultrasound and X-ray. An integrated approach. pp 253–264
18. Gharbi HA, Hassine W, Brauner MW, Dupuch K (1981) Ultrasound examination of the hydatid liver. Radiology 139:459–463
19. Gosink BB, Lemon SK, Scheible W, Leopold GR (1979) Accuracy of ultrasonography in diagnosis of hepatocellular disease. AJR 133:19–23
20. Green B, Bree RL, Goldstein HM, Stanley C (1977) Gray scale ultrasound evaluation of hepatic neoplasms: patterns and correlations. Radiology 124:203–208
21. Grossman H, Ram PC, Coleman RA, Gates G, Rosenberg ER, Bowie JD, Wilkinson RH (1981) Hepatic ultrasonography in type I glycogen storage disease (von Gierke disease). Radiology 141: 753–756
22. Harbin WP, Robert NJ, Ferruci JT Jr (1980) Diagnosis of cirrhosis based on regional changes in hepatic morphology. Radiology 135:273–283
23. Henschke CI I, Goldman H, Littlewood Teele R (1982) The hyperechogenic liver in children: cause and sonographic appearance. AJR 138:841–846
24. Houang MTW, Arozena X, Skalicka A, Huehns ER, Shaw DG (1979) Correlation between comput-

ed tomographic values and liver iron content in thalassaemia major with iron overload. Lancet 23:1322–1323
25. Hübener KH (1981) Computertomographie des Körperstammes. Thieme, Stuttgart
26. Inamoto K, Sugiki K, Yamasaki H, Nakao N, Miura T (1980) Computed tomography and angiography of hepatocellular carcinoma. J Comput Assist Tomogr 4:832–839
27. Ishak KG, Rabin L (1975) Benign tumours of the liver. Med Clin North Am 59:995–1013
28. Itai U, Nishikawa J, Tasaka A (1979) Computed tomography in the evaluation of hepatocellular carcinoma. Radiology 131:165–170
29. Itai Y, Araki T, Furui S, Tasaka A (1981) Differential diagnosis of hepatic masses on computed tomography, with particular reference to hepatocellular carcinoma. J Comput Assist Tomogr 5: 834–842
30. Johnson CM, Sheedy PF, Stanson AW, Stephens DH, Hattery RR, Adson MA (1981) Computed tomography and angiography of cavernous hemangiomas of the liver. Radiology 138:115–121
31. Kamin PD, Bernardino ME, Green B (1979) Ultrasound manifestations of hepatocellular carcinoma. Radiology 131:459–461
32. Kuligowska E, Connors SK, Shapiro JH (1982) Liver abscess: sonography in diagnosis and treatment. AJR 138:253–257
33. Kunstlinger F, Federle MP, Moss AA, Marks W (1980) Computed tomography of hepatocellular carcinoma. AJR 134:431–437
34. Kurtz AB, Rubin CS, Cooper HS, Nisenbaum HL, Cole-Beuglet C, Medoff J, Goldberg BB (1980) Ultrasound findings in hepatitis. Radiology 136: 717–723
35. Lee JF, Block GE (1972) The changing clinical pattern of hepatic abscesses. Arch Surg 104:465–470
36. Madayag MA, Lefleur RS, Braunstein P, Beranbaum E, Bosniak M (1975) Radiology of hepatic abscess. NY State J Med 75:1417–1423
37. Marchal G, Baert AL, Wilms G (1980) CT of noncystic liver lesions: bolus enhancement. AJR 135:57–65
38. Moss AA, Schrumpf J, Schnyder P, Korobkin M, Shimshak RR (1979) Computed tomography of focal hepatic lesions: a blind clinical evaluation of the effect of contrast enhancement. Radiology 131:427–430
39. Muehlbauer MA, Farber MG (1966) Hemangioma of the liver. Am J Gastroenterol 45:355–365
40. Mulhern CB, Arger PH, Coleman BG, Stein GN (1979) Nonuniform attenuation in computed tomography study of the cirrhotic liver. Radiology 132:399–402
41. Newlin N, Silver TM, Stuck KJ, Sandler MA (1981) Ultrasonic features of pyogenic liver abscesses. Radiology 139:155–159
42. Rogers JV, Mack LA, Freeny PC, Johnson ML, Sones PJ (1981) Hepatic focal nodular hyperplasia: angiography, CT, sonography and scintigraphy. AJR 137:983–990
43. Rossi P, Sposito M, Simonetti G, Sposato S, Cusumano G (1981) CT diagnosis of Budd-Chiari syndrome. J Comput Assist Tomogr 5:366–369
44. Rubin RH, Swartz MN, Malt R (1974) Hepatic abscess: changes in clinical, bacteriological and therapeutic aspects. Am J Med 57:601–610
45. Scherer U, Rothe R, Eisenburg J, Schildberg FW, Meister P, Lissner J (1978) Diagnostic accuracy of CT in circumscript liver disease. AJR 130:711–714
46. Scherer U, Weinzierl M, Sturm R, Schildberg FW, Zrenner M, Lissner J (1978) Computed tomography in hydatid disease of the liver: a report on 13 cases. J Comput Assist Tomogr 2:612–617
47. Schild H, Thelen M, Paquet KJ, Biersack HJ, Janson R, Bücheler E, Hansen HH, Grönniger J (1980) Fokal noduläre Hyperplasie. ROFD 133:355–364
48. Schmitt WGH, Hübener KH (1978) Dichtebestimmung normaler und pathologisch veränderter Lebergewebe als Basisuntersuchung zur computertomographischen Densitometrie von Fettlebern. ROFO 129:555–559
49. Schulze K, Hübener KH, Klott K, Jenss H, Bähr R (1980) Computertomographische und sonographische Diagnostik der Echinokokkose. ROFO 132:514–521
50. Scott WW, Sanders RC, Siegelman SS (1980) Irregular fatty infiltration of the liver. Diagnostic dilemmas. AJR 135:61–67
51. Sheedy P (1982) Liver CT: anatomy, mass lesions, technique. Syllabus Vth Course Computed Tomography Febr 1982, Tarpon Springs/Florida
52. Snow JH Jr, Goldstein HM, Wallace S (1979) Comparison of scintigraphy, sonography and computed tomography in the evaluation of hepatic neoplasms. AJR 132:915–918
53. Sullivan DC, Taylor KJW, Gottschalk A (1978) The use of ultrasound to enhance the diagnostic utility of the equivocal liver scintigraph. Radiology 128:727–732
54. Taylor KJW, Viscomi GN (1980) Hepatic ultrasonography. In: Moss AA, Goldberg HI (eds) Computed tomography, ultrasound and X-ray: an integrated approach. pp 169–176
55. Taylor KJW, Gorelick FS, Rosenfield AT, Riely CA (1981) Ultrasonography of alcoholic liver disease with histological correlation. Radiology 141:157–161
56. Yeh Hsu-Chong, Rabinowitz JG (1980) Ultrasonography and computed tomography of the liver. Radiol Clin North Am 18:321–338

Ultrasonographic Evaluation of Diffuse and Localized Liver Diseases

H. Frommhold

Universitätsklinik für Radiologie, Ordinariat für Strahlentherapie, Anichstrasse 35, 6020 Innsbruck, Austria

Diffuse Diseases

Diffuse diseases of the liver modify the entire organ in the same manner, hence changing its histologic and ultrasonographic characteristics. For visual evaluation by optimum gray-scale ultrasonograms the following criteria are taken into consideration:

1. Changes of size and contours of the liver
2. Changes involving the vessels
3. Most important, changes in the pattern of echoes within the organ, as well as the sound attenuation qualities

In advanced *fatty infiltration* of the liver the intrahepatic echo is diffuse or circumscribed, intensified, and rather coarse ("light liver"; Fig. 1).

Acute infective hepatitis, on the other hand, is found to be associated with a strikingly thin echographic appearance and low echosensitivity (Fig. 2).

Cirrhosis of the liver is characterized by a marked increase in the absorption of ultrasonic waves; this makes evaluation of the deeper segments of the organ more difficult (Fig. 3). Problems in differential diagnosis and in distinction of malignant processes in the liver arise with growing changes in the parenchymal pattern, particularly if regeneration products in the organ add to the already wide spectrum of echographic features.

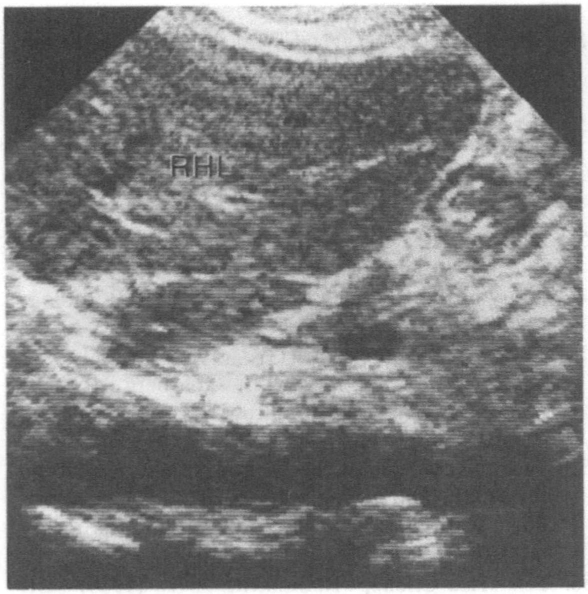

Fig. 1. Fatty liver: longitudinal section through the right hepatic lobe (*RHL*). Increased intrahepatic reflection with blurring of the lower edge of the liver and convex forward arching of the facies visceralis hepatis

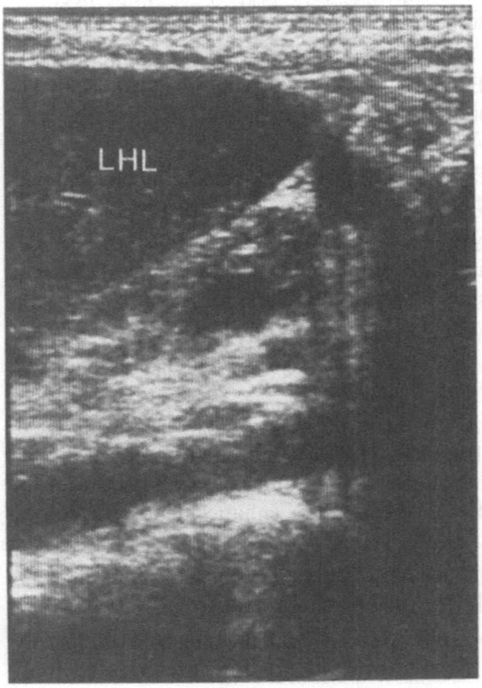

Fig. 2. Acute infectious hepatitis: longitudinal section through the left hepatic lobe (*LHL*). Sparse echogenicity of the LHL with blurring of the lower edge of the liver and bulging of the facies visceralis hepatis

Radiology Today 2. Ed. by F. H. W. Heuck and M. W. Donner

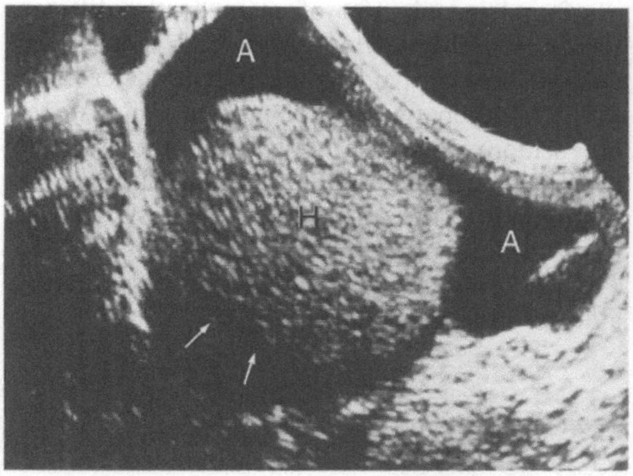

Fig. 3. Liver cirrhosis: longitudinal section through the right hepatic lobe. *H*, liver; *A*, ascites; →, incomplete imaging of the dorsal (deeper) parts of the shrunken and otherwise echodense right lobe

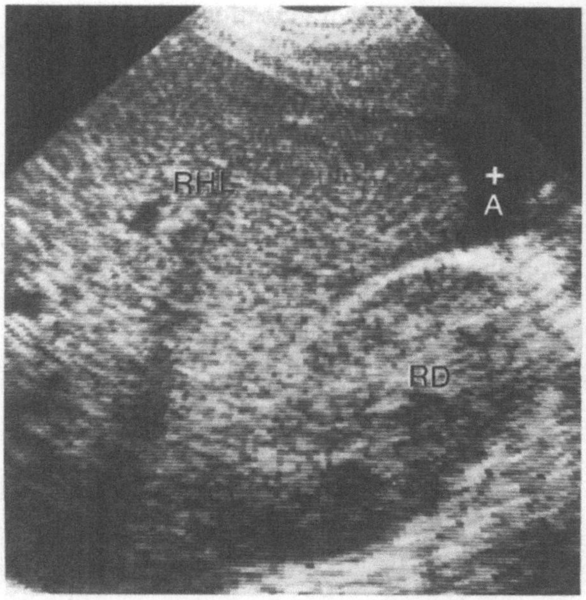

Fig. 4. Liver cirrhosis: longitudinal section through the right hepatic lobe (*RHL*). The RHL shows increased reflection and blurred lower edge of the liver. *RD*, right kidney; *A*, ascites

Ascites, which extends first into existing interspaces, i.e., between intestinal loops, into the perihepatic and paracolic areas, and into the true pelvis, is identifiable in the ultrasonographic scan in amounts as small as 100 ml (Fig. 4). Since there exist various possible pathways for ascites, differential diagnosis from other liquid or semiliquid structures may at times be rather difficult.

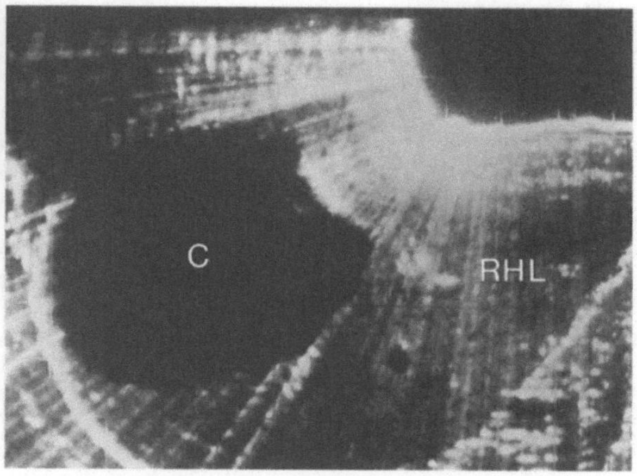

Fig. 5. Congenital liver cyst: longitudinal section through the right hepatic lobe (*RHL*). *C*, cyst

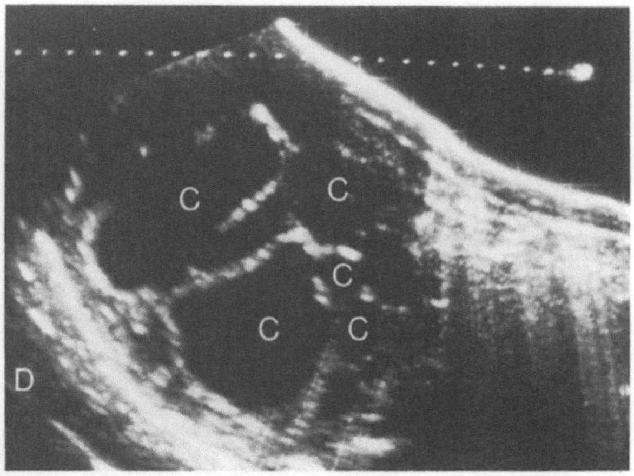

Fig. 6. Hepatic cystic echinococcus: longitudinal section through the right hepatic lobe. *C*, multilocular cyst formation caused by the parasite

Localized Diseases

Localized liver lesions of 1 cm or more in diameter can be demonstrated clearly by ultrasonography, with a diagnostic accuracy of more than 90%. For these reasons, ultrasonography is the investigative and diagnostic method of choice. Accuracy is greater in fluid-containing structures than in semisolid or solid formations.

Cystic

Congenital modifications of the liver are usually discovered only by chance, for they are not associated with any clinical symptoms. They mostly appear as unilocular cysts (Fig. 5); multiple cysts

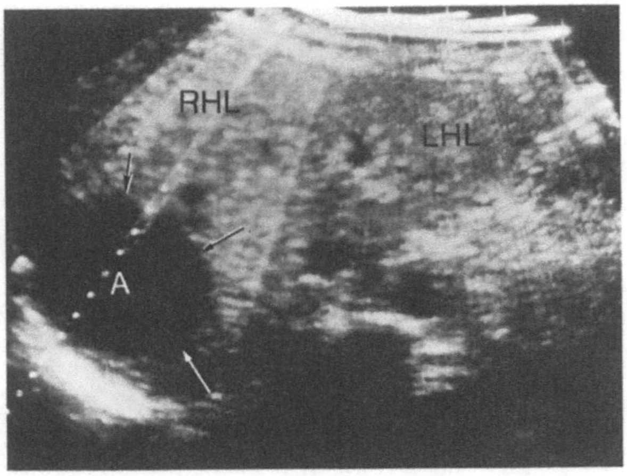

Fig. 7. Amebic abscess of the right hepatic lobe (*RHL*): transverse section through the liver. *LHL*, left hepatic lobe; *A*, abscess; →, poorly defined contours of the abscess

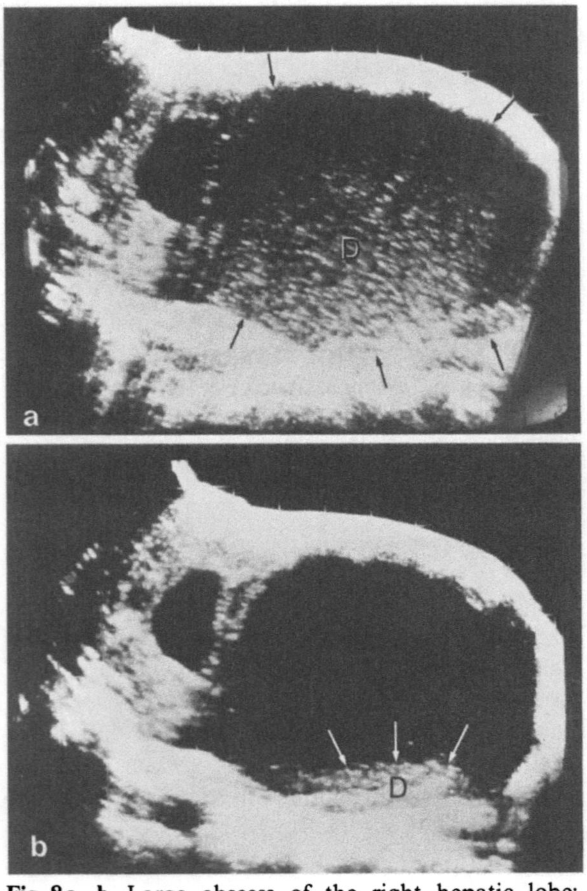

Fig. 8a, b. Large abscess of the right hepatic lobe: longitudinal section. **a** *D*, detritus in the abscess cavity; →, poorly defined border of the abscess. **b** with the patient at rest, the detritus (D) settles to the floor of the abscess cavity (→)

are found in only 10% of cases. In the differentiation of *post-traumatic cystic changes* special attention must be paid to the individual case history. Intrahepatic or subcapsular hematomas are seldom echo-free. They are not smoothly rounded, but have rather irregular outlines corresponding to the extension of the cystic process along the lines of rupture.

Parasitic cysts of the liver usually occur either alone or in conglomerates (Fig. 6).

Semiliquid

Abscesses of the liver, the majority of which can be classified as semiliquid, have blurred contours (Fig. 7) and are mostly intrahepatic, more rarely subhepatic or subphrenic. Sound-reflecting cell detritus may be found predominantly in the lower parts of the abscess, i.e., it may settle there during the ultrasonographic examination (Fig. 8).

Solid

The ultrasonographic diagnosis of solid intrahepatic space-occupying lesions is far more complicated than the evaluation of cystic changes, since the differences in density values between different tissue textures, and hence the differences in impedance qualities relevant to ultra-

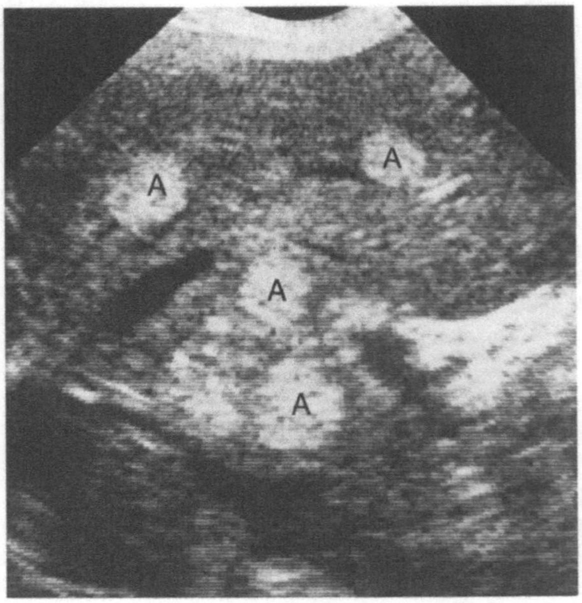

Fig. 9. Multiple hepatic adenoma: longitudinal section through the right hepatic lobe. *A*, multiple adenoma with well-defined border and echodense structure

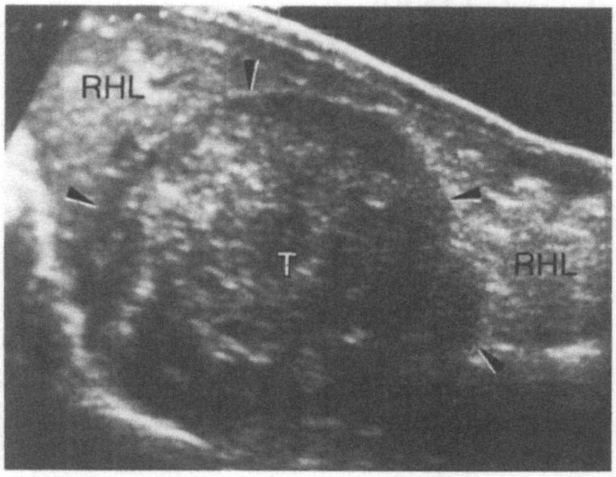

Fig. 10. Hepatoma of the right hepatic lobe (*RHL*): longitudinal section. T, tumor; ►, polycyclic, relatively well-defined border. The hepatoma exhibits irregular echo patterns

sonographic differential diagnosis, are smaller than those found between soft tissue structures and liquid components. Moreover, solid tumors of the liver do not show homogeneous echo patterns, but are rather characterized by great echomorphological variation.

Benign tumors of the liver are rare. The most frequent are hemangiomas and adenomas (Fig. 9). The most common *primary malignancy* of the liver is hepatocellular carcinoma, which may be multilocular or solitary (Fig. 10). In about 50% of cases, it is sonomorphologically identifiable by its increased echosensitivity and irregular contours. The echo patterns consist of both diminished and increased reflections. *Metastases* of the liver present a varied sonographic spectrum. After basic division into localized and diffuse tumor infiltration, further classification of localized tumors into various types can be made according to the degree of increased reflection.

At present, however, it is not possible even with the help of computer analysis based on evaluation of the amplitudinal pattern or on densitometric evaluation of the gray-scale patterns obtained in the two-dimensional echogram to differentiate malignant from benign tumors of the liver merely by ultrasonography. Puncture of the liver under ultrasonographic control to ensure correct localization for biopsy is then to be preferred.

Computer-Assisted Echographic Liver Tissue Characterization

G. van Kaick

Institut für Nuklearmedizin, Deutsches Krebsforschungszentrum, Im Neuenheimer Feld 280, 6900 Heidelberg 1, FRG

The original A-scan (video signal) is the result of a complex interaction between acoustic wave and tissue. It contains information which can be used to characterize different tissue states (Fig. 1). The first successful analyses of A-scans of patients with liver cirrhosis were performed in 1966 by Schentke and Renger [4] with the aid of graphic methods. In our institute we have developed a hardware system for computer-assisted analysis of A- and B-scans, working in cooperation with the Departments of Biophysics and Oncological Diagnostics [1–3, 5].

Material and Methods

The ultrasonic device is a compound scanner (Echoview VI, Picker) with a storage tube (Fig. 2). After analog-digital conversion the echo signals are conducted to the computer system. Each A-scan can be recorded with a maximum of 1024 words each consisting of 8 bits, i.e., 256 amplitude levels are available.

For the reproduction, processing, and analysis of the digitized B-scans an interactive color display system is used. From the magnetic tape the data are fed into a central VAX-11/780 computer, were the B-scans are built up in matrices consisting of 256 × 256 picture elements. These B-scans are displayed and analyzed by an interactive system, i.e., regions of interest can be selected in each B-scan for quantitative analysis (Fig. 3). The parts of the original digitized A-scans going through the individual region are stored on magnetic tape and can be analyzed by the central computer. Our computed echographic system has been applied in comparative studies involving patients with diffuse and focal liver and kidney diseases and control groups. In the liver study we examined healthy people and patients with cirrhosis, fatty infiltration, chronic hepatitis, primary tumors, metastases, and cystic lesion, each group consisting of 20–30 subjects. All diagnoses were confirmed by clinical examination, biopsy, or operation. During liver scanning the patients' respiration was suspended at full inhalation. Echograph-

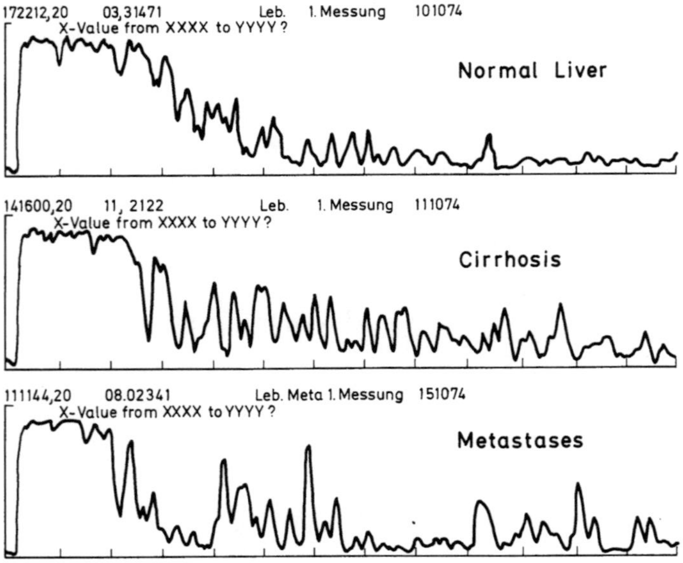

Fig. 1. A-scans of a normal liver, a cirrhotic liver, and a metastatic liver

Radiology Today 2. Ed. by F. H. W. Heuck and M. W. Donner

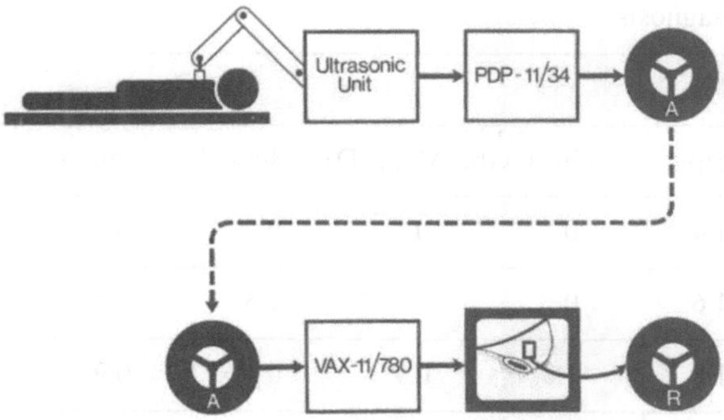

Fig. 2. The hardware system for computer-assisted echography

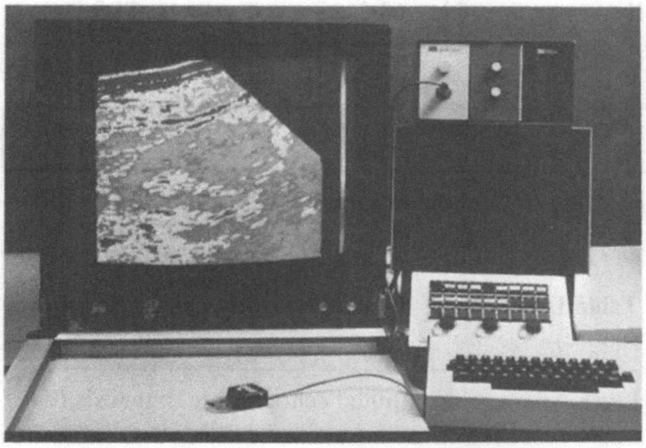

Fig. 3. The interactive system: RAMTEK 9000 color monitor, graphic tablet, function box

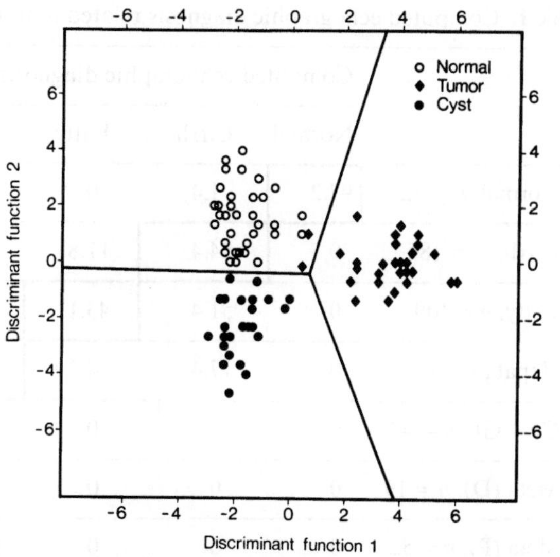

Fig. 4. Discriminant analysis of the kidney study using two discriminant functions

ic examination of the liver was performed by means of so-called sector scanning with the ultrasonic device at a constant setting. The standard time gain correction for the liver was an experimentally determined function.

Results

Altogether 150 parameters (e.g., peak distance, relative peak value and absolute peak value) were calculated and used for a quantitative description of the amplitude structures. From the different parameters the median and the 90% point can be calculated. Only a few of the parameters proved to be useful for separation of the different tissue states. For evaluation of the parameters we applied the concept of discriminant functions.

Figure 4 illustrates the mathematical procedure and demonstrates the results of discriminant analysis in the kidney study. The coordinates of the two-dimensional diagram are built up by two discriminant functions which are used for differentiation. These discriminant functions are linear combinations of the parameters that proved to be most powerful in differentiation.

The first discriminant function separates tumors from normal and cystic tissue, the second distinguishes cystic alterations from normal tissue. The two discriminant functions thus enable us to differentiate three different tissue states.

The same method was employed for the liver. Table 1 shows the computed echographic diagnosis in relation to the clinical diagnosis in normal tissue, cirrhotic liver, fatty liver, chronic hepatitis, cystic lesions, gallbladder, echodense and echopoor metastases, and primary tumors of the liver. We choose to display the results in table from because a graphic visualization of the discriminant function would require a seven-dimensional space referring to the liver diseases under consideration. It can be seen that 97.2% of the controls were correctly diagnosed. The differentiation between cirrhosis and fatty liver is rather limited, but 95% of these diffuse alterations were classed in one of the two categories. In hepatitis, however, the correct diagnosis was reached in only 58.7% of the cases! The diagnosis of liquid areas attained an accuracy level of 82.7%. Echodense metastases are classified correctly in 63.2% of cases and echopoor metastases in 79.2%. The accuracy in primary tumor diagnosis is 79.8%.

We wanted to simplify the data processing, thus making it possible to use the small PDP-11/34 computer, which is installed for data acquisition. Therefore we tested a hierarchical procedure for

Table 1. Computed echographic diagnosis related to true diagnosis

True diagnosis	Computed echographic diagnosis (%)							
	Normal	Cirrh.	Fatty	Hepat.	Cy. + Gb.	Meta (D)	Meta (P)	Tumor
Normal, $n = 72$	97.2	1.4	0	1.4	0	0	0	0
Cirrh., $n = 186$	0	84.4	11.8	1.6	0	0	1.6	0.5
Fatty, $n = 109$	0	51.4	43.1	1.8	1.8	0.9	0	0.9
Hepat., $n = 46$	0	17.4	4.3	58.7	0	2.2	15.2	2.2
Cy + Gb, $n = 43$	0	0	0	7.0	79.1	0	11.6	2.3
Meta (D), $n = 19$	0	0	0	21.1	0	63.2	0	15.8
Meta (P), $n = 52$	0	0	0	13.5	3.8	0	69.2	13.5
Tumor, $n = 40$	0	0	0	17.5	0	2.5	17.5	62.5

Cy + Gb, cysts + gallbladder; *Meta (D)*, echodense metastases; *Meta (P)*, echopoor metastases

Table 2. Results of the pilot study (hierarchical procedure)

Liver (True diagnosis)	Computed echographic diagnosis (%)		
	Normal	Fatty + ci	Tu + meta
Normal $n = 16$	88	12	0
Fatty + ci $n = 42$	5	93	2
Tu + meta $n = 21$	0	5	95

Table 3. Results of the clinical study (hierarchical procedure)

Liver (True diagnosis)	Computed echographic diagnosis (%)		
	Normal	Fatty + ci	Tu + meta
Normal $n = 30$	78	16	6
Fatty + ci $n = 53$	9	87	4
Tu + meta $n = 29$	0	30	70

the categories "normal," "fatty or cirrhotic liver," and "tumor or metastases." In the first step the diffuse and local tissue alterations are separated by means of 16 parameters, in the second normal and fatty or cirrhotic liver tissue are differentiated using six parameters. Table 2 summarizes the rates of correct classification: overall accuracy was 93%.

However, we must bear in mind that all these results are derived from a pilot study; we knew the histological results and tried afterwards to make a classification. It can be statistically predicted that the accuracy rate would be about 15% lower in a clinical study.

Table 3 shows the results of a clinical study in which the hierarchical procedure was used. We compared the results of computer tissue characterization with the histological findings, and saw that overall accuracy decreased 13% to 80%.

Concluding Remarks

This study suffered under two handicaps: a) the ultrasound examination was carried out with an old storage tube compound scanner, and b) the region of interest could often not be selected immediately after the examination. These disadvantages have now been eliminated by further improvement of the system, so we can expect better results. We hope that microprocessor development will allow us to append such an electronic system to commercial ultrasound devices such as real-time scanners, so that computed echographic tissue characterization will become a topic of general interest for medical diagnostics.

References

1. Geissler M, Johnson AF, Lorenz A, Zabel HJ, van Kaick G, Lorenz WJ (1978) Digitale Erfassung und Verarbeitung zweidimensionaler Ultraschallbilder. In: Kratochwil A, Reinold E (eds) Ultraschalldiagnostik. Thieme, Stuttgart, pp 204–206
2. Lorenz WJ, van Kaick G, Lorenz A, Stengel M, Malzacher P, Geissler M, Lorenz D, Weizel A (1980) B-Scan kontrollierte A-Scan-Computeranalyse bei Leber- und Nierenerkrankungen. In: Hinselmann M, Anliker M, Meudt R (eds) Ultraschalldiagnostik in der Medizin. Thieme, Stuttgart, pp 263–266
3. Lorenz WJ, Bihl H, van Kaick G, Lorenz A, Geissler M (1981) Methods of image analysis and enhancement. In: Hill CR, Kratochwil A (eds) Medical ultrasonic images: formation, display, and recording. Excerpta Medica, Amsterdam, pp 69–76
4. Schentke KU, Renger F (1966) Ultraschalluntersuchungen bei diffusen Leberkrankheiten. Dtsch Gesundheitswes 21:1013
5. Stengel M, Malzacher P, Lorenz A, Lorenz WJ, van Kaick G, Bihl A, Geissler M, Schlaps D (1981) Ergebnisse der Computer-Echographie (CE) bei der Diagnostik von Leber- und Nierenerkrankungen. In: Rettenmaier G, Loch EG, Hansmann M, Trier HG (eds) Ultraschalldiagnostik in der Medizin. Thieme, Stuttgart, pp 262–263

Cholescintigraphy

G. F. Fueger, H. G. Reichelt, and P. H. Cox

Abteilung für Nuklearmedizin, Universitätsklinik für Radiologie und Zentralröntgeninstitut, 8036 Graz, Austria

Introduction

Cholescintigraphy is a serial radionuclide imaging procedure able to visualize the transport of bile along the biliary tract and excretion of hepatobiliary tracers into the small bowel and their retrograde or anterograde intestinal propagation. Additional computer processing is required to assess certain functional aspects:

1. Dyskinetis of the common duct
2. The speed of hepatobiliary throughput
3. The degree of hepatic uptake
4. The relative contributions of the hepatic artery and the portal vein to total liver uptake (Fig. 4)

This potential has aroused keen interest during the past few years, and a large body of experience has been accumulated during a relatively short period of time. Three avenues of exploration have been used: (a) a variety of hepatobiliary tracers, (b) the scintigraphic findings in normal conditions and in various hepatobiliary diseases, and (c) the techniques of computer processing. This chapter deals mainly with the scintigraphic findings, discussing the present clinical role of cholescintigraphy. The variety of radionuclide tracers of the hepatobiliary eliminatory process, their biokinetics in various hepatobiliary diseases, and parametric imaging have been discussed in recent publications [4, 15]. The biologic behavior of various hepatobiliary agents relative to each other was discussed previously [1, 5, 6, 8, 9].

Technique

The overwhelming body of clinical experience has been accumulated with [^{99m}Tc]*N*-(2,6-diethylphenylcarbamoyl-methyl)-imino-diacetate, variously referred to as diethyl-ida, diethyl-hida, Hepato-bida, Solco-hida, diaida, de-ida, and ehida. The radioactivity of the ^{99m}Tc administered ranged between 2.5 and 7.5 mCi. There is no agreement in the literature on whether it is preferable to examine the patient in the fasting state or after a light breakfast or other meal. A light breakfast has the advantage of avoiding spasm of the sphincter of Oddi, which may suggest distal choledochal obstruction, but at the same time has the disadvantage of delaying or in rare cases even preventing visualization of the gallbladder. Serial imaging begins with the intravenous injection of the tracer, and can be carried out continuously to 45 min p.i. if there is an associated computer facility for parametric imaging. Intermittent imaging at 10- or 15-min intervals may suffice otherwise. Delayed images of the upper and lower abdomen are necessary at 2 h and 4 h, and at 24 h if no bowel activity is visible at 4 h (Fig. 3). In addition, an assay of the 4-h urinary excretion of ^{99m}Tc activity is carried out at our institution in all patients except children in whom urine collection may not be possible.

Computer-Assisted Evaluation

The following forms of computer processing have been described:

1. Classical region of interest (ROI) analysis for one, two, or more areas of the liver. Time activity curves are analyzed for half-times of upslope and downslope and for times to peak. A single region encompassing all of the liver yields an overall hepatic time-activity curve, a kind of hepatogram analogous to the renogram. It permits the diagnosis of prolonged transhepatic transit times. Peripheral ROIs excluding bile ducts or their major branches yield transparenchymal hepatic transit curves.
2. Parametric imaging. Rather than increasing the number of ROIs to four, eight, or more it is preferable to do parametric imaging using as parameters time to peak, downslope, and mean transit time [4].

Radiology Today 2. Ed. by F. H. W. Heuck and M. W. Donner

3. Common bile duct motor activity. Background-subtracted time-activity curves of the portal area, i.e., the common bile duct, reveal distinct dyskinetic motor patterns in some patients after cholecystectomy [12, 13, 14].
4. Relative contributions to total hepatic blood flow from hepatic artery and portal vein. The early influx of tracer occurs in two steps, the first flush of activity arriving via the hepatic artery, the second via the portal vein, delayed because of circulation through the stomach, gut, and spleen (Feine 1979, personal communication). Acquisition of 0.5 s frames is required for at least 1 min p.i.

Scintigraphic Findings

Normal Cholescintigraphy

The tracer is injected intravenously. The initially elevated intracardiac activity drops to a level below hepatic activity within 2 or 3 min p.i. and is undetectable after 10 min. Hepatic activity begins to increase within 1 min p.i. and continues increasing for several minutes. The initially diffuse hepatic activity changes to focal hyperactivity, located centrally as a consequence of tracer accumulation within bile ducts, within 10–15 min p.i. Most of the hepatic activity is cleared by 2 h p.i. The transfer of tracer into the duodenum begins between 10 and 20 min p.i. in nonfasting patients and is complete by about 2 h. Visualization of the gallbladder begins between 7 and 25 min p.i. in fasting patients and between 14 and 34 min in nonfasting subjects. Virtually all of the activity is present within gallbladder and bowel at 4 h p.i.

Cholecystitis

There is no tracer accumulation within the gallbladder in the vast majority of patients suffering from acute cholecystitis. The lack of accumulation may stem from the fact that the patient has eaten, but this occurs very rarely. The recently reported observation of tracer uptake into the inflamed gallbladder [7] indicates that there may be cases of cholecystitis without complete obstruction of the cystic duct from either stone or mucosal edema. Cholescintigraphy is particularly useful in the differentiation of cholecystitis from pancreatitis, in which case there is normal tracer uptake in the gallbladder. There may be delay in the clearance of the tracer from the hepatic parenchyma and bile ducts in acute cholecystitis, caused by associated cholangitis. A noteworthy variation was seen in one patient with surgically proven cystic duct obstruction whose gallbladder was visualized by [^{99m}Tc]diethyl-ida imaging via an accessory hepatic duct which entered the gallbladder directly [11]. Such "accessory" hepatic ducts are normal in certain animals, e.g., pigs.

Benign Biliary Obstruction

Some causes of biliary obstruction other than malignancy are calculi, strictures, and congenital anomalies. The findings on cholescintigraphy depend upon the degree and duration of the stenosis (or occlusion) and upon the absorbing capacity of the gallbladder epithelium.

Complete obstruction is recognized by the lack of intestinal activity at 24 h, poor hepatic tracer accumulation, and persistence of elevated blood levels of the [^{99m}Tc]chelate. The latter findings are complementary: the lower the hepatic extraction efficiency, the longer and higher the blood activity. It is presumably the duration of obstruction which determines the degree of hepatic uptake failure.

In incomplete obstruction there is definite transfer of tracer into the intestinal tract, but it begins later than normal (i.e., later than about 12 min p.i.) and takes longer to reach completion (more than 2 h).

The bile ducts usually appear dilated, and may show an hourglass-like narrowing or an interruption. A depot of radioactivity usually persists in the bile ducts proximal to the partial obstruction for about 2–4 h (Fig. 1).

Dilatation of the gallbladder with particularly high tracer uptake may indicate increased reabsorption of bile or water via the vesicular mucosa, a compensatory phenomenon in incomplete biliary obstruction. Serial imaging may reveal rapid clearance of the tracer from the hepatic parenchyma, but a delay in the emptying of the common duct. In other cases the transfer of tracer from the parenchymal periphery of the liver into the centrally located bile ducts may be prolonged, with only little appreciable change in hepatic activity during the first hour. These findings are interpreted as indicating full compensation of incomplete obstruction in the first situation (rapid parenchymal clearance), and incipient decompensation in the latter cases with delayed parenchymal clearance.

Causes of dilatation of the bile ducts are *cholecystectomy; incomplete obstruction* from fibrosis,

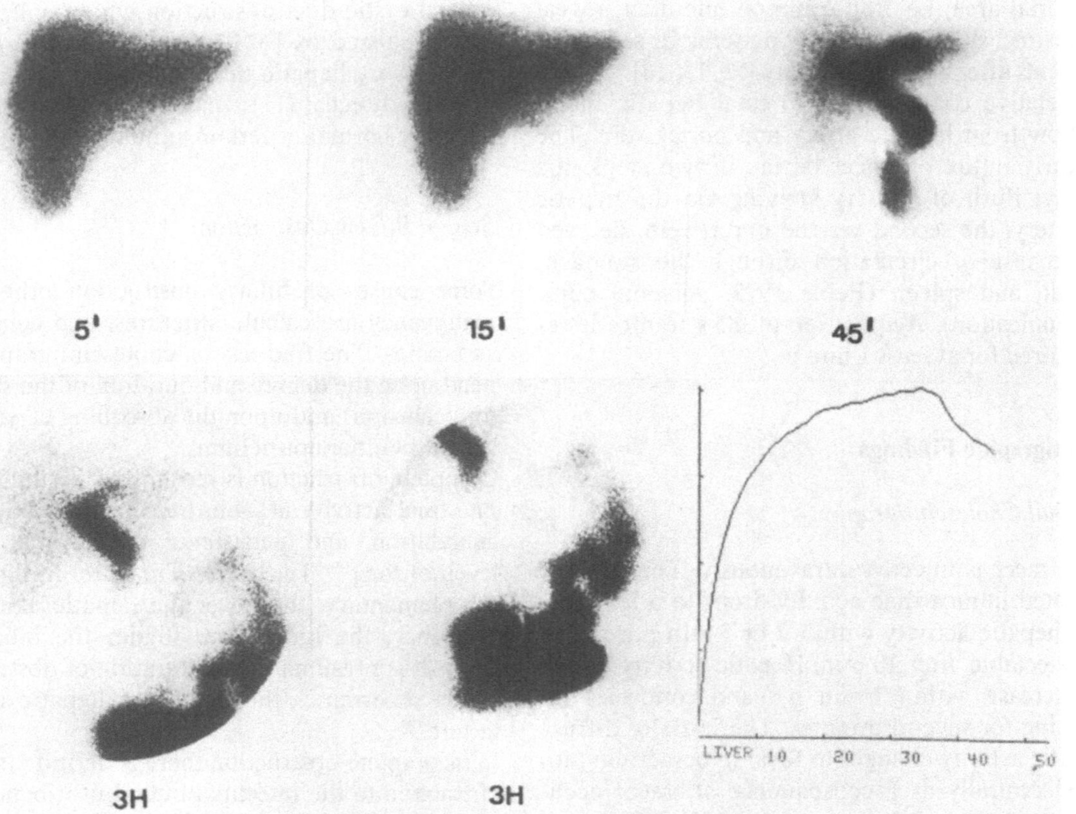

Fig. 1. Benign, fully compensated, incomplete obstruction in a 76-year-old male patient after cholecystectomy. Cholodochal calculi after choledochotomy; stenosis of common duct. Delay of transhepatic transport, ROI of total liver activity: T (max) 30 min; no tracer in duodenum by 15 min p.i., hyperactivity of bile ducts with dilatation and stenosis at 45 min; virtually complete clearance of hepatic parenchyma, but persistence of a depot of radioactivity in dilated common duct at 3 h. Full compensation of the obstruction: normal 4-h urinary excretion (10.3% of the administered activity), therefore no effect upon the extraction of tracer by hepatocytes

stone, tumor; *choledochal cyst* (the segmental dilatation of the common bile duct); *congenital hepatic diverticulum* (a cystic structure without smooth muscle fibers, lined with bile duct epithelium, communicating by a narrow stoma with the common duct); *congenital diaphragm* of the common bile duct; *segmental saccular dilatation* complicated by intrahepatic ductal calculi and recurrent cholangitis (also called Caroli's syndrome); *calculus in a cystic duct remnant* causing obstruction; (also called Mirizzi Syndrome); and chronic recurrent *cholangitis.*

Postcholecystectomy Syndrome

The postcholecystectomy syndrome is the postoperative persistence of the complaints for which cholecystectomy had been performed. Its intrinsic causes are *residual calculi* (in the common bile duct, in a long cystic duct stump, or in a gallbladder remnant); *malignancy* of the ampulla, the papilla, or the head of the pancreas; *stricture* of the common bile duct; and *dysfunction of the ampulla* of Vater with or without pancreatitis. Common to all of the intrinsic causes is a certain degree of dilatation of the common bile duct and various degrees of obstruction. Dilatation of the common bile duct does not occur as a normal consequence of cholecystectomy. Cholescintigraphy is particularly suitable for monitoring biliary drainage in ductal dilatation following cholecystectomy.

Cholangitis

There may be delayed clearance of the tracer from the biliary vessels associated with delayed visualization of the gallbladder. The bile ducts usually show no hyperactivity. Delayed parenchymal clearance may also occur.

Malignant Biliary Obstruction

In jaundiced patients with carcinoma of the head of the pancreas, cholescintigraphy may reveal persistence of high levels of activity in the intracardiac blood pool and in the general body background, a lack of uptake into the liver, and no intestinal activity at 24 h p.i. This "uptake failure" is the result of severe, secondary hepatocellular dysfunction as a consequence of complete obstruction of relatively long duration.

In other patients with carcinoma of the head of the pancreas in whom there is similarly no intestinal tracer accumulation by 24 h p.i., definite hepatic uptake may occur, but without transfer of tracer into bile duct or gallbladder. This again demonstrates complete obstruction with increased intraductal pressure, but some ability to accumulate the [^{99m}Tc]chelate into hepatocytes has been maintained. Only a minority of patients with carcinoma of the head of the pancreas display incomplete obstruction. The occasional patient will present a persisting extrahepatic depot, the result of a segment of intestine without adequate motor propagation of the tracer, or other signs of incomplete biliary obstruction.

Very similar findings are observed in cholangicarcinoma, carcinoma of the papilla of Vater, and space-occupying lesions of the porta hepatis.

Segmental Biliary Obstruction

The obstruction of one intrahepatic bile duct or one of its (major) branches is called segmental biliary obstruction and is usually the consequence of focal intrahepatic space-occupying disease. If the obstruction is complete it manifests itself as a photon- deficient area [18] within the liver. In its early form it is recognizable as an intrahepatic focus of delayed clearance. It should not be confused with the normal visual dominance of the left intrahepatic bile duct, which shows up more prominently than its right counterpart in 80% of all cases [2].

Biliodigestive Anastomoses

The purpose of anastomosing a bile-draining stoma of the biliary tract to a segment of the upper intestinal tract is to facilitate unobstructed and well-contained bile flow. Dehiscence of a suture, primary obstruction, or significant stenosis from mucosal edema can be visualized reliably by cholescintigraphy in a physiologic way during the immediate postoperative period without undue mechanical strain, like that from ERCP, or pharmacologic burden, including induced hypotension such as that resulting from administration of intravenous biliary X-ray contrast media. Possible late sequelae of biliodigestive anastomoses include stenosis from cicatricial shrinkage, obstruction due to the Roux-en-Y blind loop syndrome or the "strangulation phenomenon," and recurring cholangitis, all of which can be diagnosed advantageously by cholescintigraphy, as shown by one of us [10]. Diagnostic uncertainty may be introduced by secondary hepatocellular dysfunction associated with chronic decompensated obstruction from stenosis or with destructive cholangitis.

Orthotopic Liver Transplants

The establishment and maintenance of unhindered bile flow in orthotopic transplantation of the liver is imperative to acceptance of the transplant by the body. Immunosuppression may lead to cholestasis by increasing viscosity of the bile or to cholangitis by lowering resistance against infections; there may be obstruction to bile flow from surgical complications of biliobiliary or biliodigestive anastomoses.

Traumatic Changes

Early detection of rupture of a bile duct can reduce the incidence of mortality. Since every trauma to the liver may be accompanied by rupture of the bile duct or one of its (major) branches, noninvasive cholescintigraphy should be used for screening. Typical findings are localized depots of [^{99m}Tc]diethyl-ida which do not clear rapidly from the liver. In case of extravasation in the region of the porta hepatis, cholescintigraphy shows a juxtahepatic irregular depot of tracer. The demonstration of normal bile flow should obviate the need for more invasive studies such as ERCP.

Postoperative cholescintigraphy is valuable in demonstrating bile production and well-contained bile flow without obstruction or extravasation.

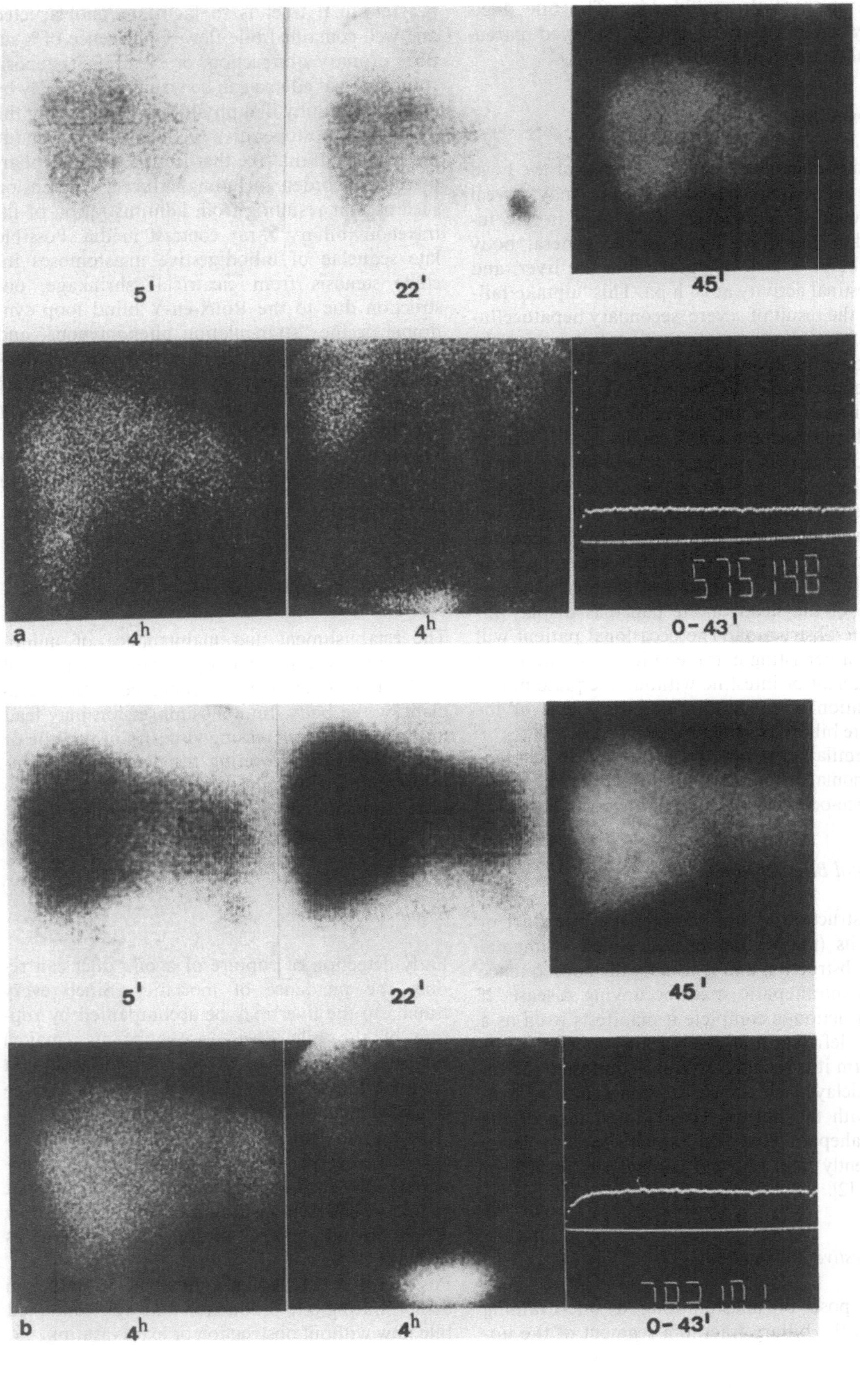
5'
22'
45'
a
4h
4h
0-43'
575,148
5'
22'
45'
b
4h
4h
0-43'

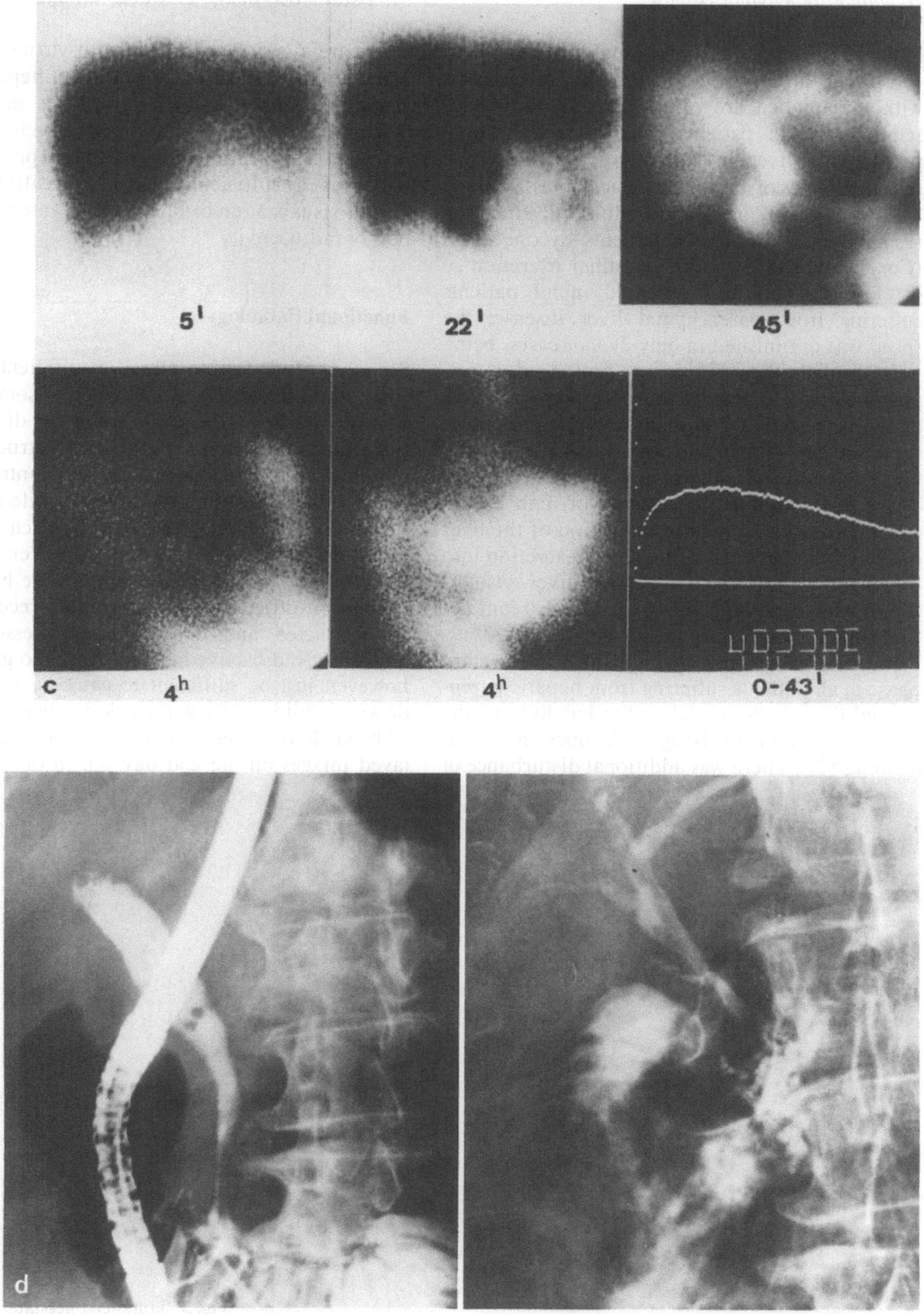

Fig. 2a–d. Follow-up of return of hepatobiliary function after depression from obstruction due to calculi. **a–c** Cholescintigraphy and parenchymal transit time from peripheral ROI at 8. Nov 1979 (**a**), 4. Jan 1980 (**b**), and 13. Feb 1980 (**c**). The respective 4-h urine excretions were 53%, 21% and 8.5%. **d** Endoscopic retrograde cholangiography: 12. Nov 1979 (*left*) threadlike stenosis of common bile duct; 24. Jan 1980 (*right*) T-tube insertion after cholecystectomy

Hepatic Parenchymal Disease

Patients with hepatic parenchymal disease such as chronic hepatitis, toxic hepatopathy, or cirrhosis without jaundice are rarely referred for cholescintigraphy. In patients with jaundice due to parenchymal liver disease, cholescintigraphy will reveal patency of the biliary tract unless there is a high degree of hepatocellular dysfunction (Fig. 3). In a study of 38 patients by one of us (Cox, unpublished work), intestinal excretion of [^{99m}Tc]diethyl-ida was observed in all patients suffering from parenchymal liver disease; the speed was diminished in only 29% of cases, being normal in all others. There was prolonged detectable intracardiac activity (beyond 10 min) in 33% of the patients with normally rapid excretion of the tracer into the small bowel and intrahepatic bile ducts were visualized in 63% of this group. There was pathologic persistence of high bloodstream activity and poor visualization of the liver in 82% of the patients with delayed excretion into the intestine and relatively good liver visualization with persistence of slight bloodstream activity in the other 18% of the group.
Parametric images revealed a disturbed excretory phase in all patients suffering from hepatic parenchymal disease, restricted to the left lobe of the liver in 18% and involving both lobes in the remaining 82%. There was additional disturbance of the parametric image of tracer uptake in 45% of patients.
There are a very few patients with virtually complete hepatic uptake failure in acute hepatitis or acute dystrophy. Cholescintigraphy is unable to distinguish the causes of jaundice in such patients if there is no elimination of the hepatobiliary tracer at a sufficiently high concentration to permit visualization of bile ducts or intestinal depots of radioactivity.

Functional Pathology

Secretion of ^{99m}Tc into bile at a sufficiently high concentration and the maintenance of some measure of bile flow is a prerequisite for diagnostically adequate cholescintigraphy. Obstruction to bile flow with consequent increase in intraductal pressure decreases the production of bile and the secretion of [^{99m}Tc]diethyl-ida. In such a situation, despite maintained hepatic tracer uptake, the degree of radioactive labeling of the bile may become insufficient for scintigraphic recognition of obstructed and dilated biliary vessels; the amount of radioactive label passing into gut may, however, just be sufficient to cause a detectable depot of radioactivity in the colon between 18 and 30 h p.i. It is therefore mandatory to obtain delayed images on the 2nd day p.i. in order to es-

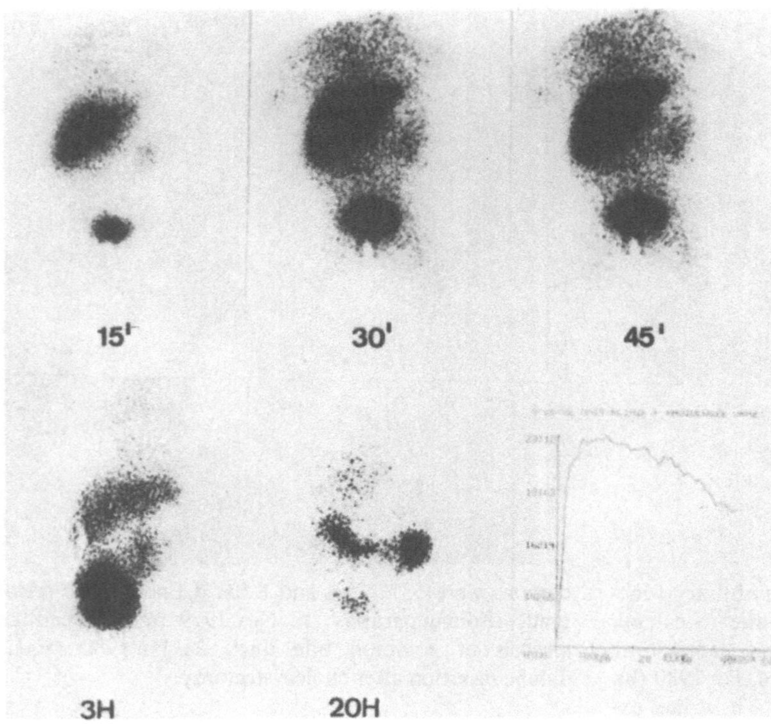

Fig. 3. Jaundiced neonate. Cholescintigraphy reveals ^{99m}Tc in colon at 20 h p.i. and increased urinary excretion: intrahepatic cholostasis with hepatocellular dysfunction and no obstruction

tablish the cause of the (obvious) functional impairment: a lack of intestinal tracer depots indicates obstruction (Fig. 3).

An even more pronounced decrease in the concentration of ^{99m}Tc in bile may arise as a consequence of hepatic uptake failure or of too low a dose being administered. In such cases cholescintigraphy may not reveal any depots of tracer within the intestinal or biliary tract, and a differentiation between obstruction and hepatocellular dysfunction is not possible.

The degree of failure to transport [^{99m}Tc]diethyl-(or dimethyl- or diisopropyl-)-ida from the blood across the hepatocytes into biliary canaliculi may be so pronounced that scintigraphically the radioactivity of the liver may remain equal to that of the intracardiac blood pool, indicating that it is only the great intrahepatic blood content which allows recognition of this organ on cholescintigraphy. This finding points to uptake failure of the liver. Computer- based techniques may demonstrate minimal degrees of hepatic uptake.

A lack of recognizable biliary and/or intestinal radioactivity indicates obstruction. It may be associated with various degrees of hepatic tracer uptake, which ranges between relatively well maintained and almost totally lacking. This impaired secretion of [^{99m}Tc]diethyl-(or dimethyl- or diisopropyl-)-ida may be caused by primary hepatocellular dysfunction or by obstruction leading to secondary depression of hepatobiliary elimination. Differentiation between these two causes will not be possible in such cases by imaging alone. Computer-based analysis of tracer transport will permit accurate diagnosis in a majority of patients [4, 16]. If there is hepatocellular dysfunction (primary or secondary), the tracer extraction efficiency of the liver is diminished, and as a parallel phenomenon the 4-h urinary excretion of [^{99m}Tc]diethyl-ida is increased. Although the renal extraction efficiency remains the same, urinary output of the tracer increases because of the longer persistence of higher blood levels, the consequence of lowered hepatic extraction efficiency.

The 4 h urinary elimination of [^{99m}Tc]diethyl-ida is a very sensitive parameter for monitoring the degree of hepatocellular dysfunction, which may well improve upon surgical intervention enabling unobstructed bile flow (Fig. 2). In a collective of more than 300 cases, the 4 h urinary excretion of [^{99m}Tc]diethyl-ida was found to remain below ca. 11% of the administered radioactivity in normal patients and to increase to as much as 70% in severe hepatic failure. Follow-up cholescintigraphy in patients recovering from jaundice (medical or surgical) revealed not only improvement in the labelling of bile, but also a decrease in the amount of ^{99m}Tc found in the 4-h urine (Fig. 2).

The level of bilirubin is less of an indicator of the likelihood of successful cholescintigraphy than is the duration of jaundice. Sucessful visualization of patent bile ducts has been reported with bilirubin levels as high as 12 mg%, but much lower bilirubin levels were associated with non-diagnostic cholescintigraphy performed later than 2 weeks after the onset of jaundice. This is particularly true in jaundice of obstructive origin.

Obstruction may be followed by an increase in biliary intraductal pressure. Biliary secretion is maintained up to a pressure of about 35 mmH_2O, but perhaps only at a reduced volume of secretion. The hepatobiliary eliminatory function decompensates as intraductal pressure increases. This is a gradual process: the extreme form consists of failure of the hepatocyte to accumulate the tracer, and an intermediate stage of failure to elaborate the tracer into bile while hepatic uptake is maintained at a diminished rate. The diminution is recognizable by the increase in urinary excretion. Compensatory mechanisms in partial biliary obstruction are increased reabsorption of bile by the gallbladder, dilatation of the gallbladder and bile ducts, and hypocholia, the diminution of bile secretion.

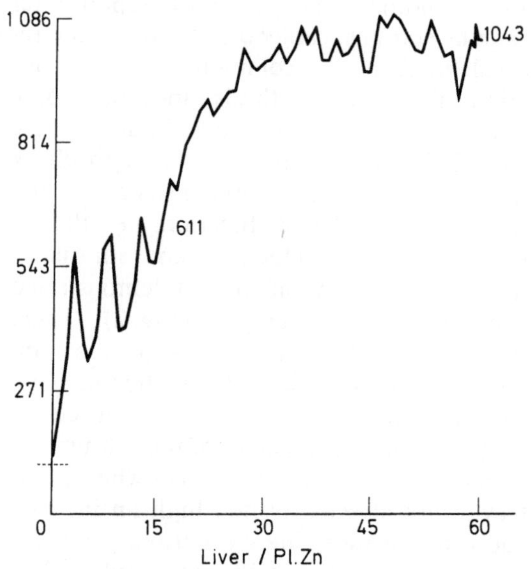

Fig. 4. Relative contribution to total liver blood flow by hepatic artery and portal vein: Activity-time curve during first minute after injection (120 frames): Initial upslope (to 611) represents tracer uptake via hepatic artery, second upslope that via portal vein, diminished in cirrhosis

Diminished hepatic tracer uptake with prolonged transhepatic transit time and increased urinary tracer output is also observed in cardiac failure. Relative diminution of the fraction of tracer delivered via the hepatic artery occurs in cirrhosis, and may be studied during the initial uptake phase (Fig. 4).

Discussion

The advent of ^{99m}Tc-labeled hepatobiliary tracers has enabled noninvasive radionuclide imaging of the flow of bile if there is adequate elaboration of the labeled chelate by the hepatocytes (Fig. 1). The biliary excretion of the hida analog [^{99m}Tc]diethyl-ida was found to be the least depressed among a large number of analogs by obstruction or hepatocellular dysfunction [9]. Cholescintigraphy with [^{99m}Tc]diethyl-ida appears most useful clinically in acute cholecystitis, after surgery involving the biliary tract, in postcholecystectomy dilatation of the common bile duct, and, last but not least, in monitoring the return of liver function after depression of any origin. In the differentiation between acute cholecystitis and pancreatitis, a lack of tracer accumulation in the gallbladder establishes to a very high degree of probability that one is dealing with cholecystitis. Surgical procedures involving the biliary tract include biliodigestive anastomosis (including transplantation), repair after traumatic lacerations, choledochotomy for the removal calculi from the common bile duct, implantation of an endoprosthesis, and endoscopic papillotomy or similar procedures. In all of these instances cholescintigraphy serves well to check the integrity of the biliary draining structures and monitor the return of liver function, i.e., the resumption of bile production and drainage. Changes in bile elaboration are best demonstrated on follow-up cholescintigraphy (Fig. 2). There may be narrowing of the anastomosis of the common bile duct at some later time after surgery. Other studies can visualize a stenosis, but cholescintigraphy with measurement of the 4-h urinary excretion will at the same time reveal whether the hepatocytes are affected by too high an increase in intraductal pressure. There is normally low urinary excretion (which can be measured easily), and normal hepatic uptake (which can be assessed only with difficulty) in compensated partial obstruction, and there is a pathologic increase in the 4-h urinary excretion of [^{99m}Tc]diethyl-ida in decompensating partial biliary obstruction. Dilatation of the common bile duct is not a "normal" sequela to cholecystectomy [17]. Cholescintigraphy reveals the speed of drainage, and assisted by computer analysis, also demonstrates dyskinesis during emptying; the 4-h elimination indicates whether there is associated hepatocellular dysfunction with depression of tracer extraction by the liver. Parenchymal diseases of the liver are amenable to diagnostic evaluation by cholescintigraphy, particularly if supported by computer-assisted parametric imaging.

In cholestasis of whatever etiology, including biliary atresia, differentiation between intrahepatic and posthepatic origin may be aided by cholescintigraphy unless the pathologic alteration overwhelmingly depresses the tracer elimination, a phenomenon well known to radiologists accustomed to dealing with X-ray contrast media (Fig. 3).

Relating cholescintigraphy to sonography and diagnostic X-ray procedures, including computer-assisted tomography, it becomes evident that all of the latter procedures are descriptive of anatomy, a characteristic much desired prior to surgery, whereas cholescintigraphy is the only imaging procedure describing a physiologic mechanism. This is a disadvantage only in complete depression of hepatobiliary secretion; more often than not it is an advantage yielding functional information. When ultrasound or some other technique yields the diagnosis of "dilatation of the common duct" or "calculi", it is only inferred that these are the cause of the patient's complaints. Based on the results of a study of 3000 patients by Reichelt (to be published), cholescintigraphy is the procedure of choice for demonstrating the pathogenetic effect of ductal dilatation or calculi, except, of course, in acute biliary colic with or without jaundice. Combined cholescintigraphy and sonography has been most useful in:

- Right upper quadrant complaints of obscure nature
- Suspected cholecystitis
- Differentiation between obstructive and parenchymal jaundice
- All kinds of complaints after cholecystectomy

Last but not least, cholescintigraphy is noninvasive, innocuous, applicable during the immediate postoperative period, unburdened by hypersensitivity reactions, usable in elevated bilirubin levels of up to about 12 mg% (occasionally even higher), and has a radiation dose which is low even in children and infants.

References

1. Bähre M, Biersack JH, Hofmann S, Winkler C (1979) Cholescintigraphy in experimentally-induced obstructive and parenchymatous jaundice. In: Cox PH (ed) Progress in radiopharmacology, vol 1. Elsevier, Amsterdam
2. Biersack HJ (ed) (1978) Hepatobiliary scintigraphy by means of IDA derivatives. Proceedings of the symposium of the Rheinisch-Westfälische Gesellschaft für Nuklearmedizin. Giebeler, Darmstadt
3. Cox PH (ed) (1979) Progress in radiopharmacology, vol 1. Elsevier, Amsterdam
4. Cox PH (ed) (1981) Cholescintigraphy. Developments in nuclear medicine, vol 1. Nijhoff, The Hague
5. Dietrich G, Fueger GF (1979) Diethyl-, trimethyl- and P- butyl- derivatives of 99m-Tc-hepatoiminodiacetic acid in 5 volunteers and 5 patients with hepatobiliary disease. In: Cox PH (ed) Progress in radiopharmacology, vol 1. Elsevier, Amsterdam
6. Dudczak R, Angelberger P, Kletter K, Frischauf H, Pamperl H (1979) Comparison of IDA derivatives in patients with liver cirrhosis. In: Cox PH (ed) Progress in radiopharmacology, vol 1. Elsevier, Amsterdam
7. Echevarria RA, Gleason JL (1980) False-negative gallbladder scintigram in acute cholecystitis. J Nucl Med 21:841–843
8. Erjavec M, Pahor S, Simcic V, Bano Poreko D, Cernej I, Praprotnik A, Snajder J (1979) Computer-assisted clearance calculations of diethyl-IDA in dogs with induced liver damage. In: Cox PH (ed) Progress in radiopharmacology, vol 1. Elsevier, Amsterdam
9. Popescu HI, Chia HL, Rohr HP (1979) Bilary elimination of various *N*- (acetanilido) -iminodiacetic acid (IDA) derivatives in rabbits with induced liver cell damage. In: Cox PH (ed) Progress in radiopharmacology, vol 1. Elsevier, Amsterdam
10. Reichelt HG (to be published) Combined use of cholescintigraphy and sonography in the evaluation of 3000 patients with right upper quadrant complaints
11. Reimer DE, Donald JW (1981) Technetium-99m-HIDA visualization of an obstructed gallbladder via an accessory hepatic duct. Am J Radiol 137:610–611
12. Schindler G (1981) Radiologische Gallenwegsdiagnostik nach Cholezystektomie. Fortschr Geb Röntgenstr Nuklearmed Ergänzungsband 135:181–187
13. Schindler G, Küper K (1982) Radiologische Gallenwegsdiagnostik nach Cholezystektomie, II. Mitteilung: Klinische Untersuchungen, Fortschr Geb Röntgenstr Nuklearmed Ergänzungsband 136: 64–73
14. Schindler G, Küper K, Müller-Schauenburg W (1982) Radiologische Gallenwegsdiagnostik nach Cholezystektomie, III. Mitteilung: Die nuklearmedizinische Weitenbestimmung des Hauptgallengangs. Fortschr Geb Röntgenstr Nuklearmed Ergänzungsband 136:254–260
15. Taavitsainen M (1980) Cholescintigraphy with 99m-Tc-Diethyl-IDA. Dissertation, University of Helsinki, Helsinki
16. Tjen HSLM (1979) Cholescintigraphy. The clinical application of 99m-Technetium-diethyl-IDA to the investigation of the liver and biliary tract. Dissertation of the University of Utrecht, Utrecht
17. Wise RE (1962) Intravenous cholangiography. Thomas, Springfield
18. Zeman RK, Gold JA, Gluck L, Caride VJ, Burrel M, Hoffer PB (1981) Tc-99m hida scintigraphy in segmental biliary obstruction. J Nucl Med 22:456–458

Diagnosis and Management of Obstructive Biliary Disease

H. J. Burhenne, A. Baert, G. F. Fueger, and W. Reichardt

Department of Radiology, University of British Columbia and Vancouver General Hospital, 855 West 12th Avenue Vancouver, British Columbia V5Z 1M9, Canada

Burhenne: This panel is concerned with the different radiologic modalities for the diagnosis of obstructive disease of the biliary tract. We shall also cover some of the aspects of radiologic interventional management of the same disease entity.

In order to get the discussion started, I shall propose that patients with suspected or undiagnosed obstructive biliary disease be best examined initially by real-time ultrasonography, followed by percutaneous transhepatic cholangiography (PTC) if indicated.

I shall first ask Professor Fueger to discuss the contribution of nuclear medicine studies in the diagnosis of obstructive biliary disease.

Fueger: Physicians in nuclear medicine are reasonably confident that cholescintigraphy can indirectly visualize the patency of bile ducts in a high percentage of cases with jaundice and hepatic parenchymal impairment. Although the tracer may be secreted at too low a concentration to see the common duct or the upper small bowel, the storage effect of the colon causes local concentration of the tracer between 18 and 30 h. The 24-h images together with suitable parametric images enable cholescintigraphy to differentiate intrahepatic from posthepatic causes of jaundice. Despite this, the present consensus appears to favor ultrasound and contrast cholangiography, either retrograde or transhepatic or both, to diagnose biliary obstruction.

Follow-up after therapy, particularly if there is protracted jaundice and a complicated postoperative course, requires the monitoring of liver function, as well as of bile production and drainage. It is in this setting that cholescintigraphy plays a most useful role: the bile ducts may still be dilated, and a repeat contrast cholangiography may be undesirable, but cholescintigraphy is noninvasive and true to function.

Causes of biliary obstruction other than malignancy are calculi, strictures, congenital anomalies, etc. The findings on cholescintigraphy depend upon the degree and duration of the stenosis (or occlusion) causing the obstruction, and upon the absorbing capacity of the gallbladder epithelium.

Complete obstruction is recognized by the lack of intestinal activity at 24 h, poor hepatic tracer accumulation, and persistence of elevated blood levels of the 99m-Tc-chelate. The latter findings are complementary to each other: the worse the hepatic extraction efficiency, the longer and the higher the blood activity. It is presumably the duration of obstruction which determines the degree of hepatic uptake failure.

In incomplete obstruction, there is definite transfer of tracer into the intestinal tract, but it begins later than normal (later than about 12 min. p.i.) and takes longer to be completed (more than 2 h).

In jaundiced patients with carcinoma of the pancreatic head, cholescintigraphy may reveal persistence of high levels of activity in the intracardiac blood pool, the general body background, a lack of uptake into the liver, and no intestinal activity at 24 h. This "uptake failure" is the result of severe, secondary hepatocellular dysfunction as a consequence of complete obstruction, and its relatively long duration.

The obstruction of one intrahepatic bile duct or one of its (major) branches is called segmental biliary obstruction. It is usually the consequence of focal intrahepatic space-occupying disease. If the obstruction is complete, it manifests itself as a photon-deficient area [22] within the liver. In its early form, it is recognizable as an intrahepatic focus of delayed clearance. It should not be confused with the normal visual preponderance of the left intrahepatic bile duct which shows up more prominently than its right counterpart in 80% of all cases [2].

Radiology Today 2. Ed. by F. H. W. Heuck and M. W. Donner

Relating cholescintigraphy to sonography and diagnostic X-ray procedures including computer-assisted tomography [4, 19], it becomes evident that all of the latter procedures are descriptive of anatomy, a characteristic much desired prior to surgery, whereas cholescintigraphy is the only imaging procedure describing a physiological mechanism. This is a disadvantage only in complete depression of hepatobiliary secretion; more often than not, it is an advantage yielding functional information. Whenever ultrasound or some other technique yields the diagnosis of "dilatation of the common duct" or "calculi," it is only inferred that these signs are the cause of the patient's complaints. Based on a study of 3 000 patients by Reichelt [15], cholescintigraphy is the procedure of choice to demonstrate the pathogenetic effect of ductal dilatation or calculi, expecting, of course, the acute biliary colic with or without jaundice. The combined use of cholescintigraphy and ultrasound has been most useful.

Cholescintigraphy's role in biliary obstruction therefore appears to be the monitoring of hepatobiliary function after therapy, particularly during the postoperative period. It is also quite useful during late postoperative follow-up, particularly after cholecystectomy, endoprosthesis insertion, or bilidigestive anastomoses.

Burhenne: In our experience, ultrasonography rather than scintigraphy is the preferred noninvasive procedure for the initial radiologic diagnosis of cholestasis. We agree with Weissman [21] that scintigraphy serves best as a complementary procedure, particularly if functional information is desired. Scintigraphy is often most informative in patients following surgery with anastomosis of the biliary and alimentary tract. Shuman and his colleagues [17] have pointed out that the accuracy of sonography in obstructive biliary disease is higher than that of scintigraphy. The modality of real-time ultrasonography provides the radiologist with a sensitive method for detecting bile duct dilatation in cases with obstruction. It often also reveals the level of obstruction. Ultrasonography is therefore the initial procedure of choice in patients with suspected biliary obstruction.

Is there a comment from the panel before we move to the next step of direct cholangiography by either the transhepatic or endoscopic approach.

Barth: Diagnostic ultrasonography is the most frequently used screening procedure to differentiate between obstructive and nonobstructive jaundice. If dilated ducts are found, obstruction is assumed [3]. Early obstruction may not be detectable by ultrasound since ductal dilatation lags behind [7]. In some instances, even long-standing obstruction does not go along with dilated bile ducts, in particular in sclerosing cholangitis and scirrhous cholangiocarcinomas [20]. If ultrasound does not demonstrate dilated bile ducts, a radionuclide biliary excretion study might be helpful in establishing obstruction.

After these preliminary tests, PTC appears to be the method of choice due to its relative simplicity, its high rate of success when compared to endoscopic retrograde cholangiopancreatography (ERCP), its proven safety and its ability to adequately visualize intrahepatic ducts and in particular, a high obstruction [6]. With the thin-needle study, intraperitoneal hemorrhage is not a problem, however seeding of contaminated bile into the blood stream during the procedure still remains an obstacle [9]. Since an obstructive biliary system is frequently infected even in the absence of clinical symptoms, PTC should always be performed under coverage with antibiotics effective against the common biliary organisms such as *E. coli,* enterococci, and *Klebsiella* [8]. Adequate blood levels can be a achieved after intravenous injection starting one hour before the study. Coverage should be continued for 24 h.

Burhenne: We use transhepatic cholangiography for the next and more specific step in the investigation of obstructive biliary disease. It is more readily available as a radiologic modality and it requires less operator experience and dexterity than ERCP. But there are preferred indications for both techniques. I will now ask Professor Baert to give us his experience on comparative morphologic information provided by PTC and ERCP.

Baert: The indications and diagnostic yield for PTC and ERCP depend on the area of interest, namely bile ducts and pancreatic ducts.

If the lesion or obstruction is located in the bile ducts, PTC provides generally better visualization for identification of the point of obstruction and for visualization of the bile duct segment proximally to the lesion. The segment of the bile duct distal to the lesion is generally better visualized by ERCP. ERCP and PTC are therefore complementary procedures in cases of total occlusion. In cases of partial obstruction of the bile ducts, PTC appears to be superior to ERCP (Fig. 1). More-

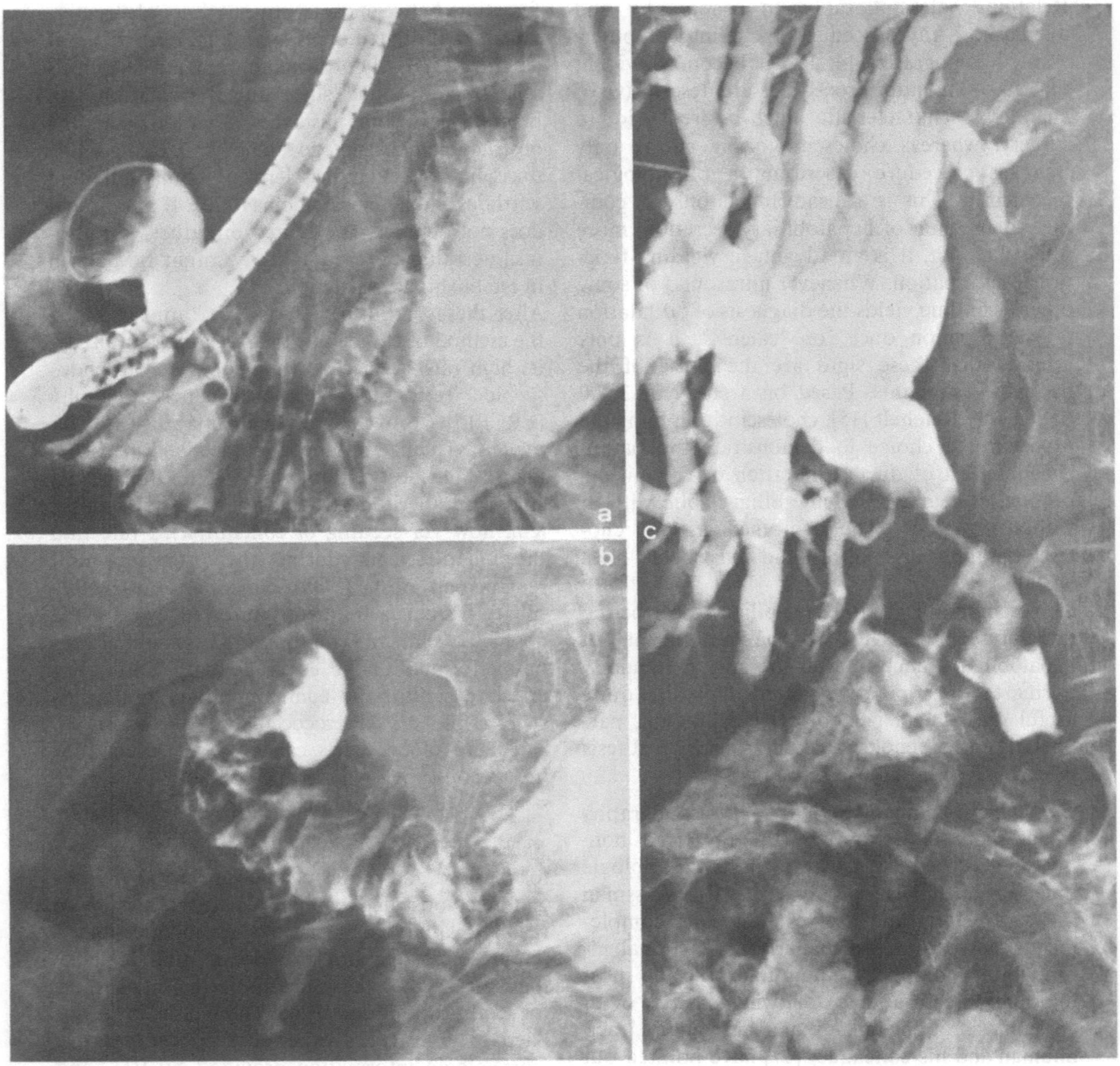

Fig. 1 a–c. Adenocarcinoma of the gallbladder extending to the common bile duct. **a, b** ERCP visualizes an irregularly bordered occlusion in the distal portion of the common bile duct but no opacification of the portion proximal to the lesion is obtained. **c** PTC visualizes the total extent of the lacunar narrowed segment and the degree of dilatation of the bile ducts proximal to the lesion. Moreover, the segment distal to the lesion is visualized as well as with ERCP

over, ERCP may erroneously suggest an image of stenosis of the distal portion of the common bile duct proximal to the papilla of Vater. Our experience with ERCP and PTC obtained in 25 patients is presented in Table 1.

Morphologic information about the pancreatic ducts can be provided by ERCP only.

Burhenne: The experience in our institution in Vancouver corresponds to the material just presented from Leuven. Our success rate of PTC is higher than that of ERCP and more diagnostic information is obtained in common duct lesions above the papilla, particularly if evaluation of the entire biliary tract is required in cases with

Table 1. Comparison of ERCP and PTC

Common bile duct visualized with both techniques $n = 11$				Common bile duct only by PTC but visualization by ERCP of Wirsung $n = 14$
Lesion of bile ducts $n = 10$			Normal bile ducts $n = 1$	• Contribution of ERCP to diagnosis $n = 8$
	ERCP	PTC	• Common bile duct	• Normal Wirsung $n = 6$
– lesion	+ 2	9	ERCP : 1	
	± 8	1	PTC : 1	
	– 0	0		
– proximal	+ 0	10	• Above bifurcation	
	+ 2	0	ERCP : 0	
	– 8	0	PTC : 1	
– distal	+10	6		
	± 0	0		
	– 0	4		

subsequent catheter placement for internal drainage.
Dr. Reichardt, would you like to comment on what has so far been discussed. We would then like you to go on and make some comments on external and internal drainage of bile duct obstructions.

Reichardt: The diagnostic separation of hepatocellular and obstructive jaundice based on laboratory examination is not definitive in about 40% of patients [12]. Ultrasound and computed tomography (CT), however, will demonstrate bile duct dilatation in over 90% of cases. We proceed first with ultrasonographic evaluation. PTC gives diagnostic results in these patients in over 94% [11, 13], whereas ERCP gives a lower yield of 76% [16]. PTC also offers the better modality for subsequent drainage catheter application.
If ultrasound or CT demonstrate obstruction due to tumor, we proceed to PTC; if common duct stones are evident on the initial study, we proceed to either PTC or ERCP, but ERCP is our preferred technique for direct cholangiography if ultrasonography or CT suggests an ampullary tumor [12].
If a tumor is demonstrated, we then proceed to fine-needle aspiration for histologic verification. In our opinion, needle biopsy is best performed during ultrasonography or after PTC.
If PTC examination demonstrates a low obstruction of the common bile duct, the most common cause is a carcinoma of the head of the pancreas. Typical tapering of the common duct with a "rat-tail" image is usually present. Decompression of the bile ducts should then be established for palliation of pruritus, for improvement of the nutritional state of the patient, for recovery of the liver, and for internal drainage of bile.
If the point of malignant stricture cannot be passed with the drainage catheter on the first session, the bile is drained externally. Two or three days later, a repeat attempt is undertaken to pass the obstruction for internal drainage. This is usually possible at that time. The drainage catheter is then fixed on the skin and closed to permit only internal drainage.
Catheter drainage is also indicated as a preoperative procedure for patients with high-grade bile duct obstruction due to common duct stones. Two recent publications stressed the use of preoperative drainage in patients with obstructive biliary disease [5, 14]. Denning et al. compared the number of complications in patients with and without preoperative drainage and found a 28% versus 56% incidence. Also, the number of patients with a fatal outcome was twice as high without preoperative drainage.
Internal drainage for malignant obstruction of the bile ducts can also be palliated with the use of an endoprosthesis. More evaluation of prosthesis placement is required, as the complication rate is higher than with transhepatic percutaneous catheter placement. The operative mortality for malignant tumors with high-grade obstruction is significant, and radiologic interventional catheter drainage is therefore done in our institution routinely if a high-grade icterus is present.
CT, arteriography, and even portography should be performed if the pancreatic tumor is con-

sidered resectable. This may aid in the selection of the small group of patients in whom radical surgery can be performed. Patients with non-resectable tumors all require permanent internal catheter drainage or placement of an endoprosthesis.

Burhenne: In addition to low common bile duct obstruction just discussed, the interventional radiologist is often confronted with obstruction high in the biliary ducts. Dr. Barth will carry on with points about percutaneous biliary drainage in the latter situation.

Barth: Diagnostic PTC is no longer considered a procedure on its own and is often logically followed by percutaneous transhepatic biliary drainage (PBD). Not only does placement of a drainage catheter relieve the obstruction and drain infected bile, but it also has been shown to reduce perioperative mortality dramatically [10]. Obstruction by unresectable tumor, in particular advanced carcinoma of the pancreas and metastatic tumors, can be definitely palliated in most instances by PBD.

Biliary obstruction proximal to the common hepatic duct (high obstruction) introduces the problem of noncontiguous bile ducts. Scirrhous cholangiocarcinoma, so-called Klatskin's tumors, typically produce this kind of ductal obstruction [10]. The tumor has a tendency to grow along the major ducts at intrahepatic bifurcations. The most frequent cause of high biliary obstruction is probably metastatic lymph nodes in the porta hepatis, rarely carcinoma of the gallbladder or the common bile duct. Patients with Klatskin's tumors may have a prolonged survival time once adequate biliary drainage can be reestablished due to the slow growth of the tumor. Surgical anastomosis in such cases is notoriously difficult, if not impossible. In this situation, percutaneous catheter drainage has a major advantage.

Drainage catheters may serve as a conduit for interstitial radiation therapy, e.g., with Iridium wires. Drainage in patients with sclerosing cholangitis is difficult. Frequently, right and left hepatic drainage catheters are required and brought into the duodenum for internal drainage (Fig. 2). Sometimes passage of one catheter through the obstruction is not possible so that one catheter may be draining externally and the other catheter internally. Both catheters can be connected externally to establish drainage of bile into the duodenum. We have been able to maintain such patients on long-term drainage up to two years. Ultimately, tumor growing along the intrahepatic ducts will prevent effective drainage. Late sequelae may be infection and sepsis, as well as liver abscess due to total or partial obstruction of intrahepatic ducts [1].

Catheter checks for adequacy of drainage in monthly intervals and routine catheter exchanges every three months are recommended. 10 French catheters are generally sufficient to maintain long-term drainage. These catheters can usually be introduced after the first 8 to 10 days of drainage through a smaller (8 French) catheter. For long-term catheter maintenance, the softest available catheter material is preferable, such as polyvinyl over polyurethane.

In general, a drainage problem is suspected if the patient develops pain, fever and, of course, rising bilirubin. Catheter exchange is the first measure to be taken and antibiotics might be started as

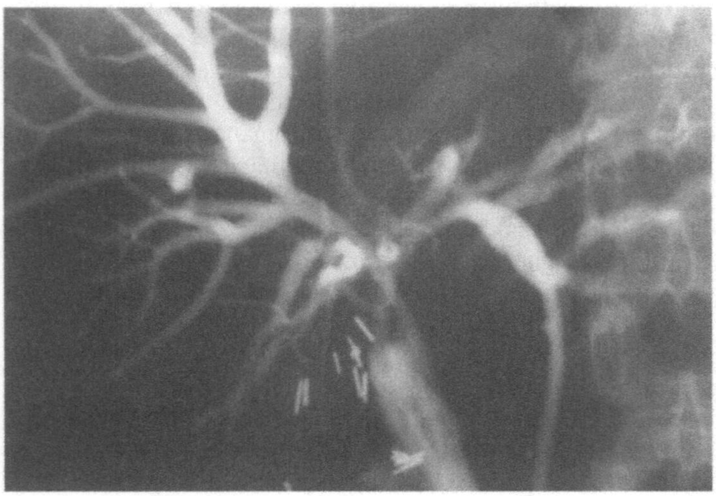

Fig. 2. 57-year-old women with cholangiocarcinoma of the porta hepatis (Klatskin's tumor) after failed surgical drainage. Two percutaneous catheters are draining the right and left ductal system internally

well. Once adequate drainage is reestablished, infection can usually be controlled. Presence of enteric organisms in the catheter is common and does not necessarily mean infection. Infection will only become a problem if obstruction to flow occurs, even by sludge accumulation in side holes.
Extended survival of patients with high biliary obstruction, particularly due to Klatskin's tumor and sclerosing cholangitis, will compensate the effort of the interventional radiologist to follow these patients carefully and maintain their vital biliary drainage.

Burhenne: I would like to close by thanking the panelists for their participation. We have had time only to discuss some of the features of diagnosis and interventional treatment of biliary obstruction, but it became apparent that radiologists from five different countries on this panel agree that patients with undiagnosed jaundice require ultrasonography as early as possible as a screening procedure to identify biliary obstructive disease. If indicated, ultrasonography is then followed by PTC as the modality of choice for direct cholangiography in the majority of patients. It is also satisfying to see that PBD has received international recognition as the treatment of choice in the majority of malignant biliary duct obstructions.

References

1. Barth KH, Au WF, Kaufman SL et al. (1981) Paper presented at the 67th scientific assembly and annual meeting, Radiological Society of North America, Chicago, 15–20 Nov 1981
2. Biersack HJ (1978) Hepatobiliary scintigraphy by means of IDA derivatives. Proceedings of the Symposium of the Rheinisch-Westfälische Gesellschaft für Nuklearmedizin. Giebeler, Darmstadt
3. Cooperberg PL, Li D, Wong P, Cohen MM, Burhenne HJ (1981) Accuracy of hepatic duct size in the evaluation of extrahepatic biliary obstruction. Radiology 135:141–144
4. Cox PH (ed) (1981) Developments in nuclear medicine, vol 1, Cholescintigraphy. Nijhoff, The Hague
5. Denning DA, Ellison EC, Carey LC (1981) Preoperative percutaneous transhepatic biliary decompression lowers operative morbidity in patients with obstructive jaunice. Am J Surg 141: 61–65
6. Elias E, Hamlyn AN, Jain S, Long RG, Summerfield JA, Dick R, Sherlock S (1976) Liver physiology and disease. Gastroenterology 71:439–443
7. Fried AM, Bell RM, Bivins BA (1981) Biliary obstruction in a canine model: sequential study of the sonographic threshold. Invest Radiol 4:317–319
8. Fritsch WP, Strohmeyer G (1980) Cholangitis. Zur Fortbildung aktueller Medizin 24:1841–1846
9. Harbin WP, Mueller PR, Ferrucci JT (1980) Transhepatic cholangiography: complications and use patterns of the fine-needle technique. Radiology 135:15–22
10. Klatskin G (1965) Adenocarcinoma of the hepatic duct at its bifurcation within the porta hepatis. Am J Med 38:241–256
11. Okuda K, Tanikawa K, Emura T, Kuratomi S, Jinmouchi S, Urabe K, Sumikoski T, Kanda Y, Fukuyama Y, Musha H, Mozi H, Shimokawa Y, Yakushiji F, Matsuura Y (1974) Nonsurgical percutaneous transhepatic cholangiography-diagnostic significance in medical problems of the liver. Am J Dig Dis 19:21
12. Owman T, Reichardt W (1979) Perkutane transhepatische Diagnostik und Therapie beim Stauungsikterus. Radiologe 19:376–384
13. Pereiras R, White P, Dusal M, Loven G, Hutsun D, Liberman B, Schiff ER (1976) Percutaneous transhepatic cholangiography utilising the Chiba University needle. Radiology 121:219
14. Pitt HA, Cameron JL, Postier RG, Gadacz TR (1981) Factors affecting mortality in biliary tract surgery. Am J Surg 141:66
15. Reichelt HG (to be published) Combined use of cholescintigraphy and sonography in the evaluation of 3000 patients with right upper quadrant complaints.
16. Seifert E (1977) Endoscopic retrograde cholangiopancreatography. Am J Gastroenterol 68:542
17. Shuman WP, Mack LA, Rudd TG, Rogers JV, Gibbs P (1982) Evaluation of acute right upper quadrant pain: Sonography and 99m-Tc-PIPIDA cholescintigraphy. AJR 139:61–64
18. Takada T, Hanyu F, Kobayashi S, Yashiko U (1976) Percutaneous transhepatic cholangial drainage: Drainage approach under fluoroscopic control. J Surg Onc 8:83–87
19. Then HSLM (1979) Cholescintigraphy. The clinical application of 99m-Technetium-diethyl-IDA to the investigation of the liver and biliary tract. Dissertation, University of Utrecht
20. Thomas JL, Zornoza J (1980) Obstructive jaundice in the absence of sonographic biliary dilatation. Gastrointest Radiol 5:357–360
21. Weissman HS (1982) In: Berk RN, Ferrucci JT, Leopold GR (eds) Radiology of the gallbladder and bile ducts, diagnosis and intervention. Saunders, Philadelphia, pp 261–314
22. Zeman RK, Gold JA, Gluck L, Caride VJ, Burrel M, Hoffer PB (1981) Tc-99m Hida scintigraphy in segmental biliary obstruction. J Nucl Med 22:456–458

Urogenital Radiology

Comparison of Imaging Modalities in the Kidney: Overview

M. A. Bosniak

New York University Medical Center, 560 First Avenue, New York, NY 10016, USA

Further developments in imaging of the kidneys (and the entire urinary tract) have occurred in the past few years. New techniques have been introduced and greater experience in the use of existing modalities has been accumulated. With the escalating costs of medical practise, it becomes increasingly important to use these newly developed radiologic tools to the best possible advantage. The goal is obviously to achieve diagnostic accuracy in the safest, least invasive, and most economical way possible. The radiologic approach taken to achieve this goal will depend on a number of factors, including the particular problem to be solved and the relative accuracy and invasiveness of the radiologic techniques available.

The current modalities for imaging the kidney (and urinary tract) are as follows:

1. *Totally noninvasive*
   Sonography
   Nuclear magnetic resonance (NMR)
2. *Relatively noninvasive*
   Intravenous urogram (with tomography)
   CT with or without intravenous contrast
   Nuclear renal scintigraphy
   Digital intravenous angiography (DIVA)
3. *Invasive*
   Venography – Arteriography
   Pyelography (anterograde, retrograde)
   Needle aspiration

A comparison of these techniques is not possible in this overview. Instead we will limit discussion to the impact of sonography and CT on renal imaging, particularly as these techniques relate to each other and to the use of angiography, especially in the evaluation of renal neoplasms.

Intravenous Urogramm

Even with the expanded use of sonography and CT, it should be emphasized that the intravenous urogram still remains the standard screening procedure in evaluation of the urinary tract. This is because urography images the entire urinary tract and its surroundings in a relatively safe, noninvasive, and economical manner. While the number of urograms performed in most medical centers has decreased as other imaging techniques have appeared, and while the indications for the technique have narrowed somewhat, the information obtained continues to make it an essential examination in many instances. It hardly needs to be stated that the caliber of urography should not be allowed to deteriorate as we get more involved in sonography and CT. Tomography as part of urography is essential, and as in any radiographic procedure, high-quality images should be obtained with proper preparation, adequate contrast media, and excellent radiographic technique.

In a patient with hematuria, the excretory urogram remains the initial examination, with other techniques then used as necessary to determine the cause of the disorder if it is not evident from the urogram. On the other hand, an excretory urogram would not be indicated (as it once was) to evaluate a patient with systemic symptoms such as anemia, weight loss, or fever of unknown origin (FUO). In such a case CT would be far more revealing, since not only the urinary tract would be imaged, but also the rest of the abdomen. At the same time, the CT examination might be definitive. For example, if a renal tumor is discovered as the cause of a patient's systemic symptoms, CT not only detects the disease process but also diagnoses and stages it.

Sonography

It is becoming more and more obvious that at present the ideal technique for imaging the kidney is in many instances sonography [10]. This is because it is totally noninvasive, relatively inex-

Radiology Today 2. Ed. by F. H. W. Heuck and M. W. Donner

pensive, and accurate and definitive in many conditions. As with any radiologic technique, one must know when it should be used, when it is definitive, and what its limitations are. Sonography has proven to be exceedingly valuable in assessment of the kidney in the following applications:

1. When radiation is to be avoided (e.g., pregnant women, children, young adults)
2. When intravenous contrast media is to be avoided (e.g., allergy, renal failure, diabetes)
3. As the initial study in the evaluation of patients with renal failure of uncertain etiology
4. As the initial study in evaluating a renal mass found on urography (unless the lesion is clearly not a simple cyst, in which case CT should be performed directly)
5. To study the urographically nonfunctioning (nonvisualized) kidney
6. To evaluate a renal pelvic filling defect seen on urography (determine stone by shadowing)
7. To help distinguish edema (lobar nephronia) and necrosis (abscess)
8. To help localize the kidney for puncture (e.g., needle aspiration, biopsy, anterograde pyelography, nephrostomy)
9. In combination with CT:
   a) Particularly when intravenous contrast cannot be used in the CT examination
   b) To increase specificity of diagnosis of lymphoma
   c) To detect small angiomyolipomas that can be proven by CT

Sonography is in many of the above instances specific and definitive, often requiring no further studies. For example, if a renal mass found on urography is found to have all the sonographic criteria for a simple cyst(s) and the patient is asymptomatic, no further study is performed for evaluation. This constitutes well over 80% of renal mass lesions seen. If the patient is symptomatic (pain, hematuria, metastatic disease, etc.), then further evaluation by CT is performed for confirmation. In no instance in our own experience has a lesion that was classically a cyst on sonography proved to be a renal tumor, although this has been described elsewhere. Renal artery aneurysms, infected cysts, and hydrocalices could be mistaken for renal cysts by sonography [9]. Of course, any lesion that is *not absolutely classically* a cyst by sonography will be studied by CT.

Computed Tomography

As more third- and fourth-generation scanners become available, the diagnostic capability and reliability of CT is becoming more widely appreciated. This is because exquisite anatomic delineation of the kidney and the perinephric spaces is achieved. Tissue density discrimination is available ranging from calcium through blood and fat to gas. CT can also evaluate blood flow sensitively (by contrast enhancement).

The technique is relatively noninvasive with a high degree of accuracy. It is definitive in a wide range of disorders and diseases and therefore obviates more invasive studies in many cases. The range of diagnostic uses of CT in imaging of the kidney continues to expand, and includes mass lesions, inflammatory disease, perirenal processes, trauma, some vascular diseases, and the evaluation of hydronephrosis and its etiology [1, 4, 7].

The Decreased Need for Angiography

The use of angiography for diagnosis of renal disease in general continues to decrease as dynamic CT scanning and more third- and fourth-generation scanners become available. The need for angiography in the diagnosis of renal mass lesions has been particularly affected [3, 5, 12, 13]. Prior to CT, almost all patients with renal mass lesions underwent angiographic evaluation for diagnosis and staging, but now angiography is indicated in probably less than half of these patients. In a retrospective study performed at the New York University Medical Center of over 100 consecutive patients with neoplasms of the kidney presenting as renal masses, in which CT and angiography were both performed, angiography was felt unnecessary in 60% of the cases [3]. CT proved to be extremely accurate in renal mass diagnosis and the staging of renal neoplasms, making angiography unnecessary in the majority of cases. Angiography was indicated if:

1. The CT examination was not clearly diagnostic or definitive.
2. There was any reason to suggest that the renal mass was a lesion other than renal cell carcinoma, e.g., a metastatic neoplasm, invasion by an adjacent neoplasm such as adrenal carcinoma or lymphoma, or extension into the renal parenchyma by a renal pelvic neoplasm.

3. Surgery was to be performed and:
   a) The cava or renal vein was definitely or possibly involved by tumor on the basis of CT.
   b) Partial nephrectomy was to be performed.
   c) The tumor was very large and bulky, in which case the vascular anatomy of the kidney had to be outlined.
4. Tumor embolization was to be performed for therapy.

Angiography was not felt necessary for diagnosis or staging if:

1. The tumor was localized to the kidney and there was no evidence of extension of the tumor into the renal vein or vena cava.
2. The patient was found to have metastatic disease and surgery was not to be performed. If tissue diagnosis is needed, percutaneous needle aspiration biopsy can be obtained.

Combination of CT and Sonography

The previous discussions have outlined how the combination of CT and sonography has been very effective in the evaluation of renal mass lesions. There are three other specific areas where the combination of these techniques has been particularly helpful.

CT Without Intravenous Contrast

Occasionally CT examination of the abdomen is performed without intravenous contrast. The vascularity of a renal mass seen in such an examination cannot be ascertained. In these instances, sonographic evaluation of the mass can add greatly to the accuracy of diagnosis, which is particularly helpful when CT criteria for diagnosis of the lesion are not clear. The additional information obtained from sonography can make the diagnosis definitive in a noninvasive way.

Detection and Diagnosis of Angiomyolipomas

The opportunity to detect and diagnose small angiomyolipomas of the kidney has been afforded through the specific imaging pattern of these fat-containing tumors [2, 11]. These lesions have been detected by sonography because of their intense echogenicity and then specifically diagnosed by CT by means of their fat content. Figure 1a, b demonstrates a small angiomyolipoma of the kidney which was detected by sonography when the patient was being scanned for gallbladder disease. CT was then performed and established the fat content and the exact nature of the tumor.

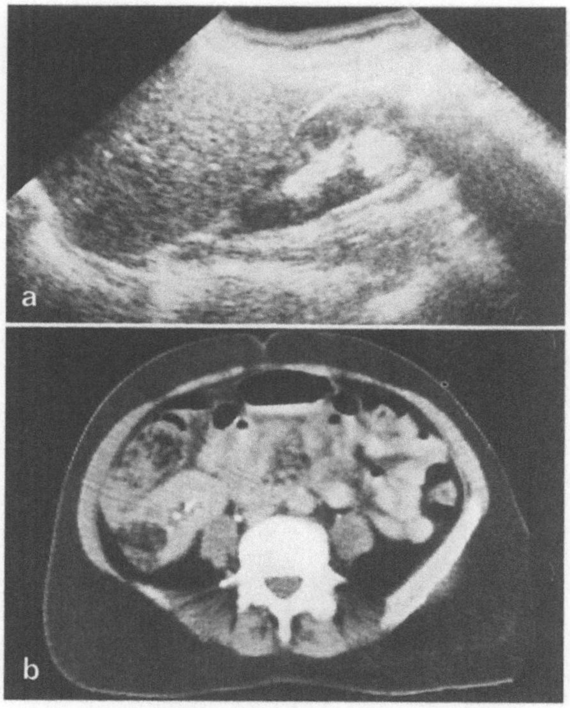

Fig. 1a, b. Angiomyolipoma of right kidney. A 40-year-old female with symptoms of gallbladder disease had a mass in the right kidney. **a** On sonogram of the right kidney, a highly echogenic mass is seen in the lower pole. **b** On intravenous-contrast-enhanced CT of the right kidney a mass with an attenuation value of −80 HU is seen at the lower pole. At surgery a 3-cm diameter angiomyolipoma was removed by tumorectomy

Lymphoma of the Kidney

Because of the characteristic CT and sonographic findings in lymphoma involving the kidneys, histologic diagnosis of this disease can be made with a relatively high degree of accuracy [6, 8]. Figure 2a, b depicts such a case. The patient underwent CT examination for FUO, and the scan demonstrated some retroperitoneal and renal masses. The diagnosis of lymphoma was suspected because of the distribution of the disease, and sonography demonstrated a homogeneously sonolucent mass which confirmed this impression. Aspiration needle biopsy was performed for definitive diagnosis.

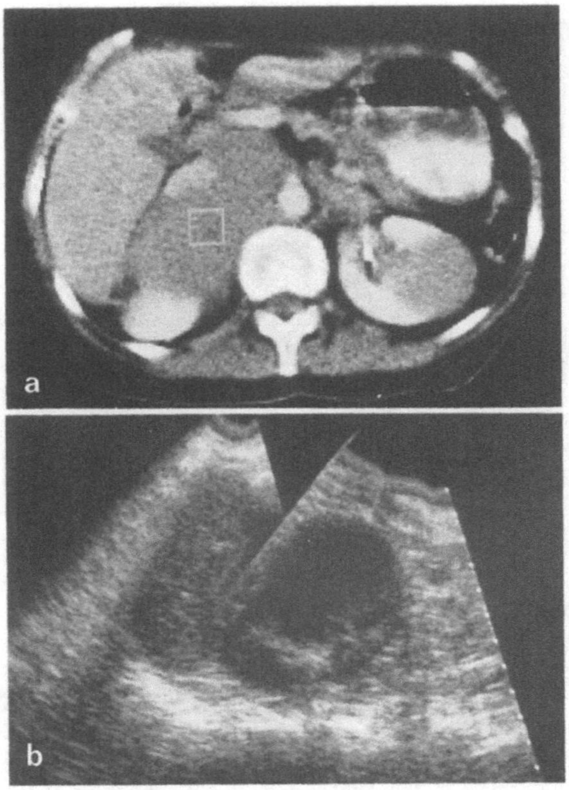

Fig. 2 a, b. Lymphoma. A 46-year-old female had an FUO. **a** An intravenous- and oral-contrast-enhanced CT scan of upper abdomen reveals a large mass of diminished attenuation (50 HU) displacing the IVC anteriorly and occupying the space between the upper pole of the right kidney, the aorta, and the IVC. Also noted is an area of diminished attenuation in the left kidney. **b** A sonogram of the left kidney shows a large homogeneous sonolucent mass in the left kidney. The combination of the CT and sonographic findings is highly suggestive of retroperitoneal and renal lymphoma. Percutaneous aspiration biopsy proved this diagnosis

Conclusion

Achieving an accurate diagnosis in the safest and most economical way possible is the goal. Newer less invasive techniques must replace older, expensive, more invasive ones. This presentation has discussed some of the changes in radiologic diagnosis of the kidney which have occurred in the past few years in this regard.

References

1. Baert AL, Wilms G, Usewils R, Marchal G (1982) Dynamic CT of the urogenital tract. Urol Radiol 2–3:69–84
2. Bosniak MA (1981) Angiomyolipoma of the kidney. A preoperative diagnosis is possible in virtually every case. Urol Radiol 3:135–142
3. Bosniak MA, Megibow AJ, Ambos MA, Mitnick JS, Lefleur RS, Rothberg M, Rosen RJ (in preparation) Analysis of seventy-one neoplasms of the renal parenchyma studied by CT and angiography. Proceedings of the 67th Scientific Program RSNA Nov. 15–20, Chicago
4. Bosniak MA, Megibow AJ, Ambos MA, Mitnick JS, Lefleur RS, Gordon R (1982) Computed tomography of ureteral obstruction. AJR 138:1107–1113
5. Cronan JJ, Zeman RK, Rosenfield AT (1982) Comparison of computerized tomography, ultrasound and angiography in staging renal cell carcinoma. J Urol 127:712–715
6. Falappa P, Trodella L, Maresca G (1980) Lymphomatous involvement of the kidney: computed tomography and ultrasound demonstration. Diagn Imaging 49:266–268
7. Goldman SM, Siegelman SS (1982) Computerized tomography in the scheme of things (eds). J Urol 127:724–727
8. Jafri SZH, Bree RL, Amendola MA, Glazer GM, Schwab RE, Francis IR, Borlaza G (1982) CT of renal and perirenal non-Hodgkins lymphoma. AJR 138:1101–1105
9. Pollack HM, Banner MP, Arger PH, Peters J, Mullhern CB Jr (1982) The accuracy of grey-scale renal ultrasonography in differentiating cystic neoplasms from benign cysts. Radiology 143:741–745
10. Rosenfield AT (1982) Ultrasound evaluation of renal parenchymal disease and hydronephrosis. Urol Radiol 2–3:125–135
11. Totty WG, McClennan BL, Melson GL, Patel R (1981) Relative value of computed tomography and ultrasonography in the assessment of renal angiomyolipoma. J Comput Assist Tomogr 5:173–178
12. Wadsworth DE, McClennan BL, Stanley RJ (1982) CT of the renal mass. Urol Radiol 2–3:85–94
13. Weyman P, McClennan BL, Stanley RJ, Levitt RG, Sagel SS (1980) Comparison of computed tomography and angiography: The evaluation of renal cell carcinoma. Radiology 137:417–424

Renal Trauma: Diagnosis and Management of Renal Injuries

W. Wenz, W.-R. Seemann, and U. Wetterauer

Institut für Röntgendiagnostik, Universitäts-Klinik, Hugstetterstrasse 55, 7800 Freiburg, FRG

The kidneys are among the most frequently injured abdominal organs in patients submitted to blunt trauma. Recognition of the renal lesion is far easier than the choice of correct treatment. Nevertheless, diagnosis – especially with modern imaging methods – and treatment are inseparably connected.
Our experience at the University of Freiburg and the reports published in the literature form the background for a review of modern trends in diagnosis and treatment of renal trauma.

Clinical Signs and Symptoms

The same three leading symptoms have consistently been noted in acute renal trauma over the past decades:

1. Hematuria is the most common clinical feature.
2. Flank pain or tenderness to palpation may indicate injury to the abdominal wall or the lower ribs.
3. Palpation of a mass may indicate a significant extravasation of blood or urine into the retroperitoneal space.

Classification

Clinical diagnosis of renal trauma should not only identify the organ lesion but also enable staging of the injury. It is very interesting that many past classifications of renal injury basically used radiologic signs (Table 1). We shall see if modern imaging also allows certain systematization.
Figure 1 shows a possible three-grade classification of renal injury and represents a simplification of classification proposals regarding clinical signs and pathomorphology.

In our own series of 89 patients during the past 4 years, traffic accidents were by far the most frequent cause of renal trauma (Table 2).

Table 1. Past classifications of renal ruptures

1943: Adams [1]
1. Contusion with or without subcapsular hematoma
2. Fracture, incomplete or complete
3. Tears in the renal vessels or ureter

1949: McKay et al. [19]
1. Intact pyelogram: no exploration!
2. Rupture of the renal collecting system: exploration within 72 h!
3. Unresponsive shock: operation as immediate lifesaving measure

Table 2. Etiology in 89 cases of renal trauma

	n	Mean age (years)
Traffic	45	19
Sport	19	22
Occupational	12	41
Other	13	23
Total	89	24

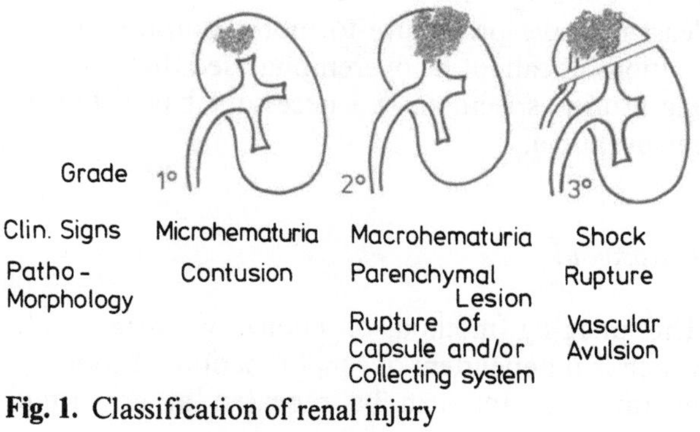

Fig. 1. Classification of renal injury

Radiology Today 2. Ed. by F. H. W. Heuck and M. W. Donner

Table 3. Pathomorphology in 89 cases of renal trauma

	n
Contusion	53
Laceration	24
Pedicular injury	5
Renal pelvic rupture	4
Renal dislocation (extrarenal hemorrhage)	3

Table 4. Concomitant lesions in 89 cases of renal trauma

	n	Contusion	Laceration	Pedicular injury
Splenic laceration	12	1	8	3
Hepatic laceration	1	0	1	0
Bone fractures	52	25	19	8

Contusion and laceration were very common but severe pedicular injury with partial avulsion of the renal artery was also observed in no less than five cases (Table 3).

It is tacitly assumed that in most cases blunt abdominal trauma results in a number of concomitant organ lesions (Table 4).

Splenic laceration occurred in 12 cases, all together with left renal trauma. The frequent bone fractures must not be overlooked!

Diagnostic Approach

The prognosis of patients with renal trauma is dependent on their clinical status immediately following the traumatic episode. Most patients are able to undergo the full range of studies, from the least invasive procedure to more complex examinations. It cannot be overemphazised that obtaining a urine specimen is a necessary basic step in renal trauma.

Ultrasound

The imaging method of choice is ultrasound, which is independent of renal function, absolutely noninvasive, and can be repeated at any time (Table 5).

Three major mass-imaging patterns may be demonstrated in the renal area: cystic, complex, or solid.

Intracapsular hematomas present as cystic lesions, developing the complex pattern when clotting occurs. When they are associated with renal parenchymal injuries such as contusion, there is disruption of the renal capsule with extra echoes within the renal parenchyma [16].

Fluid within the retroperitoneal cavity can easily be detected, as can urinomas secondary to hydronephrosis or post-traumatic cysts. Ultrasound-guided puncture and drainage is now routine, as in our one case of post-traumatic pyonephrosis.

Ultrasound control at regular intervals is of great significance in deciding whether surgical intervention is necessary.

Plain-Film and Excretory Urography

Plain-film studies together with excretory urography will continue to be the basic examination in renal trauma for demonstrating injuries of the associated supporting structures, i.e., fractures of the ribs and the transverse processes of the lumbar vertebrae. In addition, scoliosis of the spine to the side of injury with an associated loss of the ipsilateral psoas margin is suggestive of significant abdominal trauma. Further findings are: ipsilateral renal enlargement, loss of renal outline, deviation of the renal axis, and displacement of the kidney. Excretory urography is an excellent and simple means of evaluating both kidneys separately.

High-quality pyelographic examinations will give satisfactory visualization of the kidneys, ureters, and bladder. Nonvisualization of one or both kidneys does not necessarily indicate severe renal injury; there may be prior renal disease, unilateral absence of a kidney, or acute renal shutdown secondary to post-traumatic reflex vasospasm. In our own series decreased function was the most frequent finding (Table 6).

Table 5. Ultrasound findings in renal trauma

Injury	n
Subcapsular hematoma	27
Perirenal hematoma	8
Hydronephrosis	5
Laceration	2
Other	3
No pathology	7

Table 6. Urographic findings in renal trauma

Finding	*n*
Decreased function	15
No delineation of psoas	14
Extravasation	13
Renal hypertrophy	11
Silent kidney	9
Hydronephrosis	6
Scoliosis	6
Renal dislocation	3
Blood clots	2
Traumatic cyst	1
Tumor	1
No pathology	23

Extravasation of contrast medium, whether intraparenchymal, perirenal, or pararenal, is one of the most reliable sign of significant injury. Obstruction or defects in the renal collecting system may be indicative of blood clots or extrarenal hematoma producing a disruptive stricture.

Angiography

Angiography remains the most accurate diagnostic tool in traumatized renal parenchyma. It can establish the presence, extent and significance of renal trauma. The indications for angiography are:

1. Nonvisualization of the kidney
2. Clinical evidence of severe renal trauma
3. Need for evaluation of vascular supply
4. Prior to surgery
5. Late complications (infarction!)

Angiography can demonstrate injury to the renal pedicle better than other techniques. Complete obliteration of the renal vascular supply may lead to shock and of course loss of the kidney. Partial avulsion may result in extravasation of blood or the development of a pseudoaneurysm or arteriovenous fistula. Trauma to the vessels within the renal parenchyma can lead to extensive cortical necrosis, since the renal vessels are end-arteries. Renal artery thrombosis is demonstrated by abrupt cutoff of the affected vessels and/or the presence of intraluminal defects. Fractures and lacerations of the kidney are angiographically demonstrated by separation and stretching of the vascular branches, sequestration of renal fragments, and contrast medium extravasation.
Our angiographic findings are presented in Table 7. Note the frequency of laceration, subcapsular hematoma, and concomitant – especially splenic – lesions.
Interventional angiography also allows treatment of severe post-traumatic hemorrhage by renal artery occlusion, first described by Richman et al. [21], and dilatation of post-traumatic renal artery stenosis.

Computed Tomography

Computed tomography (CT) is a noninvasive method which allows exact anatomical localization of focal contusion, subcapsular and perirenal hematoma and renal rupture.
CT findings in renal trauma are listed in Table 8. Very important additional signs are enlargement of the psoas and quadratus lumborum muscles and irregular dissection of the perirenal, retroperitoneal fat tissue. Sometimes the kidneys can be displaced anteriorly together with loops of intestine.

Table 7. Angiographic findings in renal trauma

	n
Kidneys	
Parenchymal laceration	19
Subcapsular hematoma	13
Pedicular injury	5
Renal pelvic rupture	4
Traumatic cyst	1
Traumatic aneurysm	1
Traumatic infarction	1
No pathology	6
Concomitant lesions	
Laceration of spleen	8
Subcapsular splenic hematoma	1
Subcapsular hepatic hematoma	1

Table 8. CT findings in renal trauma [11]

Injury	Findings
Subcapsular hematoma	Hyperdense, lentiform areas
Perirenal hematoma	Marked perirenal fascia, renal dislocation
Fragmentation	No contrast enhancement of parenchymal fragments
Rupture of collecting system	Contrast enhancement around the collecting system

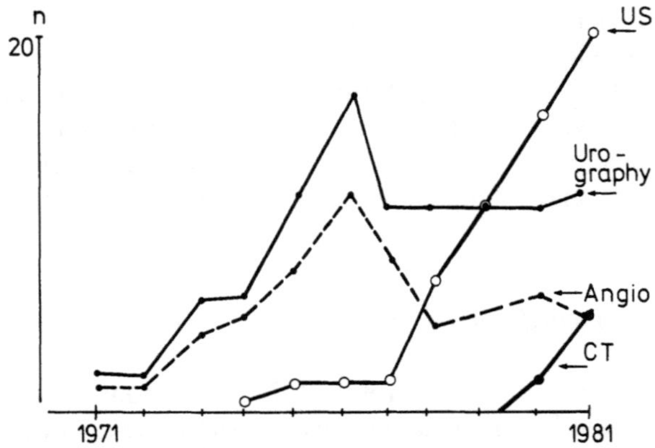

Fig. 2. Imaging in renal trauma 1971–1981 (University of Freiburg)

Contrast-enhanced scans allow differentiation of the opacified, mostly enlarged renal silhouette from the nonenhanced hematoma. Perirenal hematoma can also have various other causes, such as anticoagulants (the most important), tumors, and aneurysms.

Figure 2 shows the frequency of the most important imaging techniques in renal trauma during the past 10 years in Freiburg. The number of IVPs and angiograms has decreased in favor of ultrasound and CT, but they will retain their significance in special indications.

Angiography is the most sensitive and specific method, with a diagnostic accuracy of 88%. It is followed by ultrasound with 83%, CT with 80%, and urography with 67%.

Treatment

Though modern imaging allows optimal demonstration of renal injury, there is no agreement on whether renal laceration with or without lesion of the collecting system should be treated surgically.

Among our 89 patients, 52 were treated without surgical intervention. The number of operations

Table 9. Treatment of 89 cases of renal trauma

Injury	*n*	Nephrectomy	Organ-preserving surgery	Conservative treatment
Contusion	53	0	1	52
Laceration	24	9	11	4
Renal pelvic rupture	4	0	3	1
Pedicular injury	5	5	0	0

was divided almost equally between organ-preserving interventions and total nephrectomy.

According to Carlton [4], 90% of late complications are caused by conservative treatment. The urologists in our institution are also rather conservative, as shown by the following list of the types of treatment employed in descending order of frequency:

1. Intensive care
2. Hemostasis by transcatheter embolization
3. Organ-preserving surgery
4. Nephrectomy

Post-Therapeutic Complications

The high complication rate (Table 10) has encouraged many urologists to intervene more aggressively with a preference for transabdominal over translumbar access to allow better inspection of the peritoneal cavity.

Table 10. Complications in 89 cases of renal trauma

	n
Persisting microhematuria	2
Traumatic cyst: persistent hypertension	2
Hydronephrosis: decreased function	2
Epididymitis	1
Urinary tract infection	1

Our own experience has led us to propose the following therapeutic schedule according to our imaging findings:

1. Focal contusion or circumscribed subcapsular hematoma (ultrasound, CT): conservative treatment.
2. Intrarenal rupture of the renal collecting system and/or mild extracapsular extravasation (ultrasound, CT, I.V.P.): conservative treatment under ultrasound control.
3. Laceration, fragmentation, avulsion, or severe extracapsular hemorrhage (ultrasound, CT, IVP, angiography): operation.

Last but not least there is a long list of possible pathologic changes after treatment of renal injury: sclerosing perinephritis, hydronephrosis, cyst formation, infarction, loss of renal function, hypertension. Two of our eight patients with persistent complications had hypertension of post-traumatic origin. Both patients had roentgenologically verified laceration of the renal parenchyma, but had refused surgical intervention. Treatment of late complications consisted of:

1. Dilatation of renal vascular stenosis
2. Catheter drainage of post-traumatic hydronephrosis, cyst, or abscess
3. Surgery (infarction)

Summary

Diagnosis of renal trauma by modern imaging techniques has changed fundamentally within the past decade. Nowadays the method of choice is ultrasound, documenting the morphology of the kidneys and its neighboring structures, including collections of blood. Ultrasound-guided puncture and drainage of post-traumatic cysts and hydronephrosis, with possible removal of obstructions or dilatation of post-traumatic ureteral stenosis under fluoroscopic control, are further applications of this diagnostic tool. Renal function and details of the collecting system are best visualized by excretory urography. If available, CT gives excellent topographic information on extra- and intrarenal structures; whereas angiography still remains the method of choice when vascular avulsion, aneurysm, or arteriovenous fistula is suspected. Angiography is mandatory when post- traumatic hemorrhage or vascular stenosis are considered for catheter treatment. The decision between conservative or surgical treatment rests nowadays on the results of our logical diagnostic work-up.

References

1. Adams P (1943) Traumatic rupture of the kidney. Am J Surg 61:316
2. Baert AL, Wackenheim A, Jeanmart L (1980) Abdominal computer tomography. Springer, Berlin Heidelberg New York
3. Braedel HV, Rzehak L, Schindler E, Polsky MS, Döhring W (1980) Computertomographische Untersuchungen bei Nierenverletzungen. ROFO 132:49
4. Carlton CE (1978) Injuries of the kidney and ureter. In: Campell MF, Harrison JH (eds) Urology, vol 1, 4th edn. Saunders, Philadelphia, pp
5. Cockett ATK, Frank IN, Davis RS, Linke CA (1975) Recent advances in the diagnosis and management of blunt renal trauma. J Urol 113:750
6. Delany HM, Jason RS (1981) Abdominal trauma: surgical and radiologic diagnosis. Springer, Berlin Heidelberg New York
7. Elkin M, Meng CH, Paredes RG (1966) Correlation of intravenous urography and renal angiography in the kidney injury. Radiology 86:496
8. Federle MP, Goldberg HI, Kaiser JA, Moss AA, Jeffrey RB, Mall JC (1981) Evaluation of abdominal trauma by computed tomography. Radiology 138:637
9. Finkedick A-R, Müller RP (1982) Bedeutung der Computertomographie bei Nierenverletzungen. Röntgenblätter 35:218
10. Freth C, Haertel M (1981) Computertomographie nach Nierentrauma. ROFO 135:635
11. Friedmann G, Mödder H (1982) Computertomographie bei Bauchtraumen. Radiologe 22:112
12. Goldberg BB (1977) Abdominal gray scale ultrasonography. Wiley & Sons, New York
13. Guerriero WG, Carlton CE Jr, Scot R Jr, Beall AC Jr (1971) Renal pedicle injuries. J Trauma 11:53
14. Hauenstein KH, Wimmer, B, Billmann P, Nöldge G, Zavisic D (1982) Die Rolle der Sonographie beim stumpfen Bauchtrauma. Radiologe 22:106
15. Kaufman JJ, Brosman SA (1972) Blunt injuries of the genito-urinary tract. Surg Clin North Am 52:7747
16. Kay CJ, Rosenfield AT, Armm M (1980) Grayscale ultrasonography in the evaluation of renal trauma. Radiology 134:461
17. Lang EK (1975) Arteriography in the assessment of renal trauma. J Trauma 15:553
18. Lucey DT, Smith MJV, Coontz WW (1971) A plea for the conservative treatment of renal injuries. J Trauma 11:306
19. McKay HW, Baird HH, Lynch KJ Jr (1949) Management of injured kidney. JAMA 141:557
20. Olsson O (1973) Röntgendiagnostik des Urogenitalsystems. Springer, Berlin Heidelberg New York (Handbuch der medizinischen Radiologie, vol 13/ 1)
21. Richman S, Green W, Kroll R, Casarella W (1977) Superselective transcatheter embolisation of traumatic renal hemorrhage. AJR 128:843
22. Richter MW, Lytton B, Myerson D, Gruja V (1973) Radiology of genito-urinary trauma. Radiol Clin North Am 11:593
23. Schindler E, Pressler M, Braedel HV (1981) Kombinierte nichtinvasive Diagnostik beim Nierentrauma. Urologe [Ausg A] 20:85
24. Schmoller H, Kunit G (1979) Ultraschallbefunde beim stumpfen Bauchtrauma. ROFO 131:36
25. Sultzeyer W (1981) Traumatologie des Urogenitaltraktes. Springer, Berlin Heidelberg New York
26. Wenz W (1974) Abdominal angiography. Springer, Berlin Heidelberg New York
27. Wenz W, Reinbold WD (1982) Diagnostische und therapeutische Ergebnisse der Angiographie beim stumpfen Bauchtrauma. Radiologe 22:117

Renal Transplant Problems as Assessed by Ultrasound and Nuclear Medicine

R. C. Sanders

Department of Radiology and Radiological Science, The Johns Hopkins Medical Institutions, 601 N. Broadway, Baltimore, MD 21205, USA

Complication rates for renal transplants have been diminishing over the past few years as better tissue typing has become possible and surgical techniques have improved. Nevertheless, there are serious urological complications in the postoperative period and diagnosis of these complications is often confusing [2, 18]. The correct use of the various radiological imaging modalities at our disposal constitutes a challenge.

Worsening Renal Failure

Rejection

Rejection remains the commonest cause of renal failure in a patient with a renal transplant, but a number of other conditions such as acute tubular necrosis, hydronephrosis, and vascular accidents, may have an identical clinical appearance. Specific patterns for rejection have been developed with arteriography and renal biopsy, but both of these techniques carry a significant morbidity and are only used if more benign techniques have failed to yield a diagnosis and a trial of therapy has been ineffective. It has recently been shown that there are specific sonographic findings in rejection (Fig. 1) [5, 9, 11, 13, 14, 17]. In a patient who undergoes acute rejection, the kidney increased in size in a globular fashion with particular increase in the size of the cortex. The renal pyramids become enlarged and more obvious than usual, although the corticomedullary junction is poorly defined and the sinus echoes are diminished in size because there is replacement of the sinus fat by inflammatory tissue [13]. (Fat is considered responsible for the sinus echoes in the normal individual.) These findings are quite distinct from those seen in acute tubular necrosis [10]. Similar findings to those seen in rejection are, however, seen in acute suppurative pyelonephritis and acute interstitial nephritis. The progress of acute rejection can be followed by periodic sonograms.

Nuclear medicine findings are also helpful in the diagnosis of acute rejection. In rejection there is poor perfusion and function (Fig. 2a–c). Confusion between rejection and hydronephrosis in renal vein thrombosis is possible, especially if hydronephrosis is severe. Hyperacute rejection and infarction can look very similar [6, 23, 25, 27].

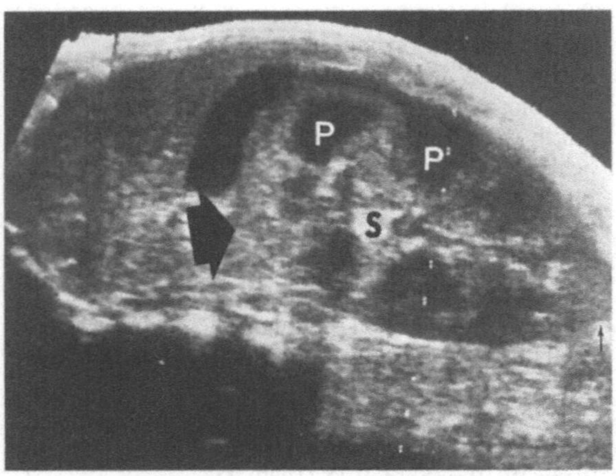

Fig. 1. Diagram showing the sonographic appearances of rejection. Note the great renal length (*arrows*), prominent pyramids (*P*), and the relatively insignificant sinus echoes (*S*)

Acute Tubular Necrosis

Acute tubular necrosis may have a similar or even identical clinical presentation to acute rejection, but has a very different sonographic appearance. The kidney remains virtually unchanged morphologically although the gross size increases. The pyramids do not enlarge and the sinus echoes remain normal. The isotopic appearances also differ from those seen in rejection since perfusion is adequate but excretion is poor.

Radiology Today 2. Ed. by F. H. W. Heuck and M. W. Donner

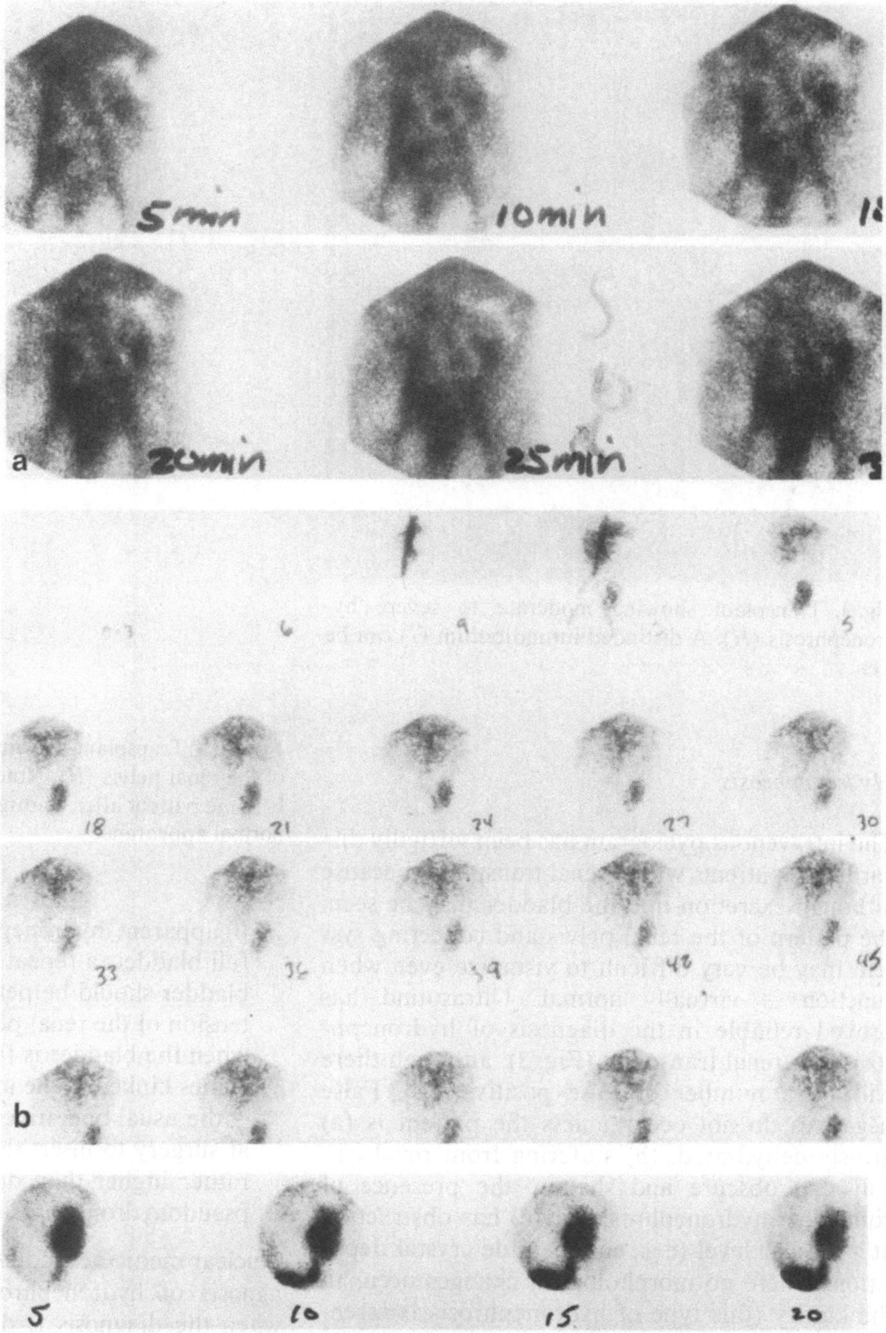

Fig. 2. a Nuclear medicine scan showing poor perfusion on a technetium DTPA scan in rejection. **b** Technetium DTPA scan showing poor function in rejection. **c** Normal technetium DTPA scan in transplant

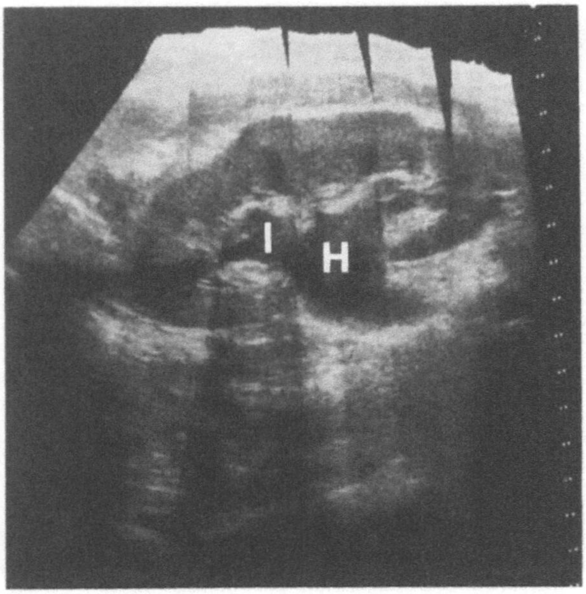

Fig. 3. Transplant showing moderate to severe hydronephrosis (*H*). A distinded infundibulum (*I*) can be seen

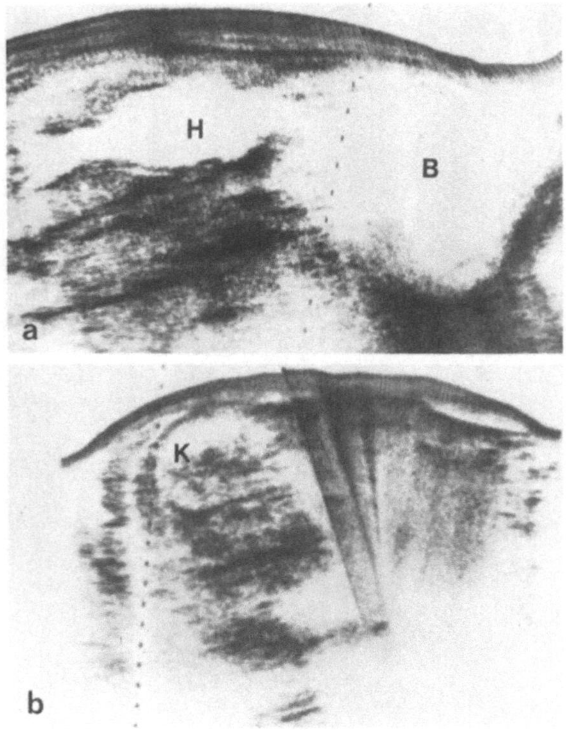

Fig. 4. a Transplant showing apparent gross dilatation of the renal pelvis (*H*). Note the very large bladder (*B*). **b** Same patient after voiding. The kidney (*K*) now has a normal appearance

Hydronephrosis

The intravenous pyelogram has been virtually discarded in patients with a renal transplant, because although excretion into the bladder may be seen, the pattern of the renal pelvis and collecting system may be very difficult to visualize even when function is virtually normal. Ultrasound has proved reliable in the diagnosis of hydronephrosis in a renal transplant (Fig. 3), although there will be a number of false positives [1]. False negatives do not occur unless the patient is (a) grossly dehydrated, (b) suffering from renal calculi that obscure and shadow the presence of coincident hydronephrosis, or (c) has obstruction at a tubular level (e.g., sulfonamide crystal deposition) where no morphological changes occur in the kidney (this type of hydronephrosis is essentially undiagnosable by any imaging technique). False positives are not uncommon but can be excluded if the following precautions are taken:

1. A baseline study should be performed shortly after the transplant procedure so that any morphological changes in the fashion in which the pelvis is connected to the kidney (e.g., a large extrarenal pelvis) due to operative techniques may be detected. This baseline study should be available for comparison whenever subsequent sonograms are performed in which the question of hydronephrosis arises.
2. If apparent hydronephrosis is present with a full bladder, a repeat study after emptying the bladder should be performed (Fig. 4a, b). Distension of the renal pelvis and ureter can occur when the bladder is full because the ureter becomes kinked at the ureterovesical anastomosis – the usual operative site. It is often necessary at surgery to insert the ureter into the bladder rather higher than desirable, resulting in this pseudohydronephrosis.

Nuclear medicine studies can be helpful in the diagnosis of hydronephrosis but there are times when the diagnosis is difficult to make because the findings are nonspecific. If function is poor it can be hard to distinguish between acute rejection, hydronephrosis, and severe acute pyelonephritis. False positives can occur with nuclear medicine studies, as with ultrasound, if there is an extrarenal pelvis. To diagnose the exact site of the obstruction, it may be necessary to perform an anterograde pyelogram. This technique has been used extensively in renal transplant patients and has proved to be essentially without hazard. It is probably preferable to retrograde pyelography since it is less traumatic to the ureter at the site of the ureterovesical anastomosis, where the stricture usually occurs [7, 15, 24].

Vascular Accidents

Infarcts. Noninvasive diagnosis of vascular accidents in transplant kidneys can be difficult if the lesion is only partial. Complete infarction of a kidney is relatively simple to diagnose, because although there will be no function whatsoever on a nuclear medicine study and no perfusion, the sonogram will have a normal appearance, at least in the first few days. Eventually shrinkage will occur, but this process only takes place over several weeks. A focal infarct gives rise to local swelling of the kidney with a sonolucent area on a sonogram. Later an echogenic area may develop which shows no perfusion on the isotope study. Confusion between focal infarction and acute pyelonephritis can occur sonographically [4, 21] and to a lesser extent on the nuclear medicine study. Gallium studies may be helpful in showing that the worrisome area is actually an area of infection [8, 19]. Computed tomography (CT) may show gas bubbles in infected areas.

Renal Vein Thrombosis. Renal vein thrombosis is perhaps the most difficult of the vascular problems to diagnose noninvasively. Sonographic appearances are somewhat confusing, with an overall enlargement of the kidney and either an increase or a diminution in the number of sinus echoes [12, 22], the former being the more common pattern. Nuclear medicine studies are no more specific; there is diminished perfusion and excretion confusable with hydronephrosis. CT can be helpful, as one may sometimes be able to demonstrate thrombosis within the vein. One may, nevertheless, be forced as a last resort to submit the patient to venography when renal vein thrombosis is a possibility.

Fever

The second major problem in which imaging techniques are valuable is fever of unknown origin. Because transplant patients are immunosuppressed, possibly life-threatening abscesses can develop in a subtle fashion without much in the way of local tenderness [16].

Many patients with renal transplants have hemorrhages in the region of the kidney, and abscesses often develop at these sites [26]. Sonographic detection of the hemorrhages is relatively simple, though not without the occasional inaccuracy, since they vary considerably in acoustic appearance (Fig. 5a). In some instances the hemorrhage can be densely echogenic, changing its character rapidly and becoming less echogenic over a period of hours (Fig. 5b). In the echogenic phase it can be mistaken for surrounding gut. In such patients CT can be very helpful in showing the typical increased density of hemorrhage [20].

Abscesses usually develop at the site of hemorrhage formation around the transplant kidney, but can also occur where the native kidney nephrectomy was performed or even in a subphrenic location. Percutaneous aspiration of such collections under ultrasonic control is a simple technique without complications that yields information as to whether the collection is infected

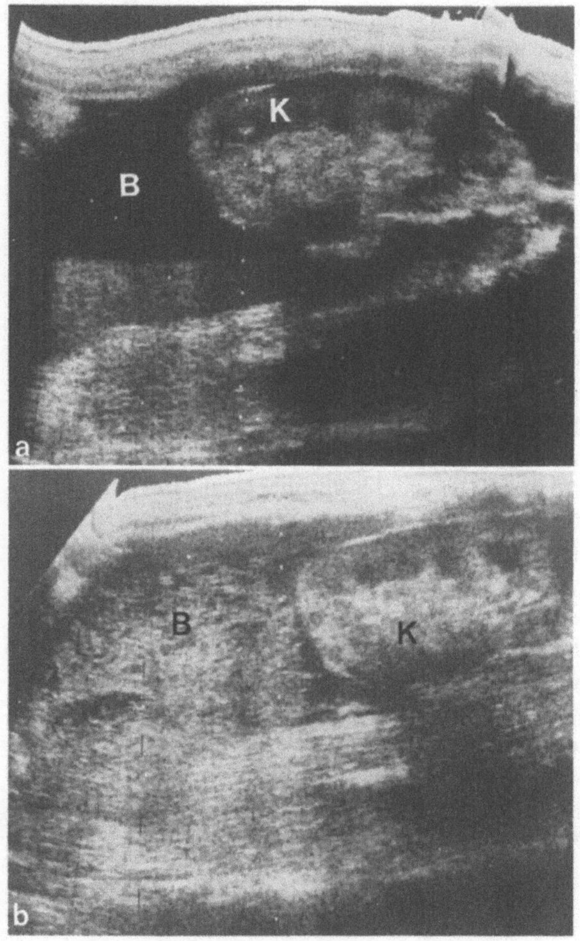

Fig. 5. a Sonogram on a patient with a renal transplant inserted 24 h previously. The kidney (*K*) is surrounded by blood (*B*). **b** The same patient was reexamined a few hours later. The hematoma (*H*) has developed a number of internal echoes

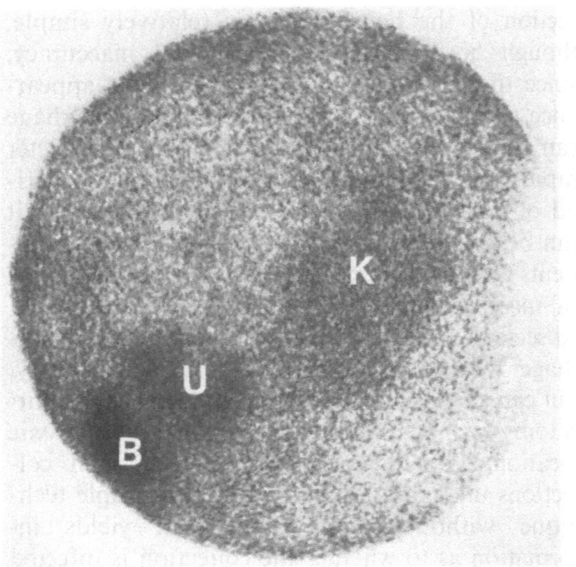

Fig. 6. Urinoma (*U*) demonstrated on a technetium DTPA nuclear medicine study. The kidney (*K*) and bladder (*B*) have an area of uptake between them due to the urinoma

or is merely a hemorrhage. If it is infected percutaneous catheter insertion for drainage under ultrasonic or CT guidance is now standard practice in many laboratories.

Other types of collections are much rarer than they used to be thanks to improved surgical techniques. Urinomas still occur and can be diagnosed definitively with the aid of nuclear medicine scans (Fig. 6) [3, 28]. Isotope accumulation within the collection will occur on delayed views. Such urinomas are frequently associated with hydronephrosis, as are lymphoceles. The sonographic appearance and the fluid obtained are identical in lymphocele and urinoma. The problem with lymphoceles lies in ascertaining whether the collection is responsible for or secondary to the hydronephrosis.

Surgical removal is becoming relatively rare; lymphoceles usually regress spontaneously and often recur following surgery or aspiration.

References

1. Balchunas WR, Hill MC, Isikoff MB et al. (1982) The clinical significance of dilatation of the collecting system in the transplanted kidney. J Clin Ultrasound 10:221–225
2. Becker JA, Kutcher R (1978) Urologic complications of renal transplantation. Semin Roentgenol 13:341–351
3. Burt RW, Reddy RK (1979) Evaluation of nuclear imaging for detecting posttransplant fluid collection. JR 133:91–95
4. Edell S, Bonavita JA (1979) The sonographic appearance of acute pyelonephritis. Radiology 132:683–685
5. Frick MP, Feinberg SB, Sibley R, Idstrom ME (1981) Ultrasound in acute renal transplant rejection. Radiology 138:657–660
6. Frodin L, Grefberg N, Hemmingsson A, Johansson A, Jung B, Lindgren PG, Wicklund H (1981) Computed tomography, ultrasonography and gamma camera scintigraphy after renal transplantation. Scand J Urol Nephrol 15:299–302
7. Goldstein I, Cho SI, Olsson CA (1981) Nephrostomy drainage for renal transplant complications. J Urol 126:159–163
8. Hampel N, Class RN, Persky L (1980) Value of gallium scintigraphy in the diagnosis of localized renal and perirenal inflammation. J Urol 124:311–314
9. Hillman BJ, Birnholz JC, Busch GJ (1979) Correlation of echographic and histologic findings in suspected renal allograft rejection. Radiology 132:673–676
10. Hricak H, Toledo-Pereyra LH, Eyler WR, Madrazo BL, Zammit M (1979) The role of ultrasound in the diagnosis of kidney allograft rejection. Radiology 132:667–672
11. Hricak H, Cruz C, Eyler WR, Madrazo BL, Romanski R, Sandler MA (1981) Acute post-transplantation renal failure: differential diagnosis by ultrasound. Radiology 139:441–449
12. Hricak H, Sandler MA, Madrazo BL, Eyler WR, Guat SS (1981) Sonographic manifestations of acute renal vein thrombosis: An experimental study. Invest Radiol 16:30–35
13. Hricak H, Romanski RN, Eyler WR (1982) The renal sinus during allograft rejection: sonographic and histopathologic findings. Radiology 142:693–699
14. Hricak H, Cruz C, Eyler WR, Madrazo BL, Sandler MA (1982) Post-transplant renal failure: Differential diagnosis by ultrasound – experimental and clinical observations. Med Ultrasound 6:1–9
15. Lieberman RP, Crummy AB, Glass NR, Belzer FO (1981) Fine needle antegrade pyelography in the renal transplant. J Urol 126:155–158
16. Lorber MI, Campbell DA, Konnak JW, et al. (1981) Etiology and management of early and late peritransplant infections. J Urol 127:870–872
17. Maklad NF, Wright CH, Rosenthal SJ (1979) Gray scale ultrasonic appearances of renal transplant rejection. Radiology 131:711–717
18. Malek GH, Uehling DT, Daouk AA, et al. (1973) Urologic complications of renal transplantation. J Urol 109:173–176
19. Mendez G, Morillo G, Alonso M, Isikoff MB (1980) Gallium-67 radionuclide imaging in acute pyelonephritis. AJR 134:17–22

20. Nghiem DD, Goldman MH, Mendez-Picon G, Rao KG, Woodlief RM, Fields WR, Lee HM (1981) Noninvasive assessment of the transplanted kidney: ultrasound vs. computerized tomography. Am Surg 47:492–494
21. Rosenfield AT, Glickman MG, Taylor KJ, Crade M, Hodson J (1979) Acute focal bacterial nephritis (acute lobar nephronia). Radiology 132:553–561
22. Rosenfield AT, Zeman RK, Cronan JJ, Taylor KJ (1980) Ultrasound in experimental and clinical renal vein thrombosis. Radiology 137:735–741
23. Rosenthall L, Mangel R, Lisbona R, Lacourciere Y (1974) Diagnostic applications of radiopertechnetate and radiohippurate imaging in post-renal transplant complications. Radiology 111:347–358
24. Schiff M, Rosenfield AT, McGuire EJ (1979) The use of percutaneous antegrade renal perfusion in kidney transplant recipients. J Urol 122:246–248
25. Shanahan WS, Klingensmith WC III, Weil R III (1981) 99m Tc-DTPA renal studies for acute tubular necrosis: specificity of dissociation between perfusion and clearance. AJR 136:249–253
26. Silver TM, Campbell D, Wicks JD, Lorber MI, Surace P, Turcotte J (1981) Peritransplant fluid collections. Radiology 138:145–151
27. Singh A, Cohen WN (1980) Renal allograft rejection: sonography and scintigraphy. AJR 135:73–77
28. Spigos DG, Tan W, Pavel DG, Mozes M, Jonasson O, Capek V (1977) Diagnosis of urine extravasation after renal transplantation. AJR 129:409–413

Sonography of Hydronephrosis

R. C. Sanders

Department of Radiology and Radiological Science, The Johns Hopkins Medical Institutions, 601 N. Broadway, Baltimore, MD 21205, USA

In the last few years there has been a transformation in the way in which renal failure is radiologically investigated. The prime goal remains the differentiation of hydronephrosis from a small or large kidney affected by a medical cause of renal failure. Obstructive causes of renal failure are treatable by either percutaneous or surgical drainage techniques and are associated with progressive destruction of glomeruli and nephrons if left untreated. Possible renal obstruction represents a radiological emergency. Sonography has proved to be reliable in the diagnosis of hydronephrosis [3, 6, 7, 11, 12], relegating the retrograde pyelogram to a limited role, i.e., showing the precise level of the obstruction and the nature of the obstructing lesion once the diagnosis of hydronephrosis has been established by other imaging modalities.

The sonographic features of hydronephrosis are as follows: As a rule, multiple peripherally located cystic lesions of approximately the same size connect with one large central cystic lesion representing the pelvis (Fig. 1). In some instances the predominant feature may be a distended pelvis with only limited evidence of remaining calices because the obstruction is so severe. In other cases the predominant pattern is one of caliceal distension and the pelvis is relatively small (Fig. 2). If the kidney has previously been affected by chronic pyelonephritis, the pattern of the distended calices and pelvis may be distorred, but the diagnosis can still be made with real-time sonography since it will be possible to trace the distended calices to the enlarged pelvis (Fig. 3). Another confusing situation is a double collecting system. A second obstructed collecting system may resemble a large cyst, although as a rule a rim of renal parenchyma can be seen surrounding the dilated pelvis. The echogenic outline of the displaced sinus fat is helpful, but a centrally placed cyst can give the same appearance.

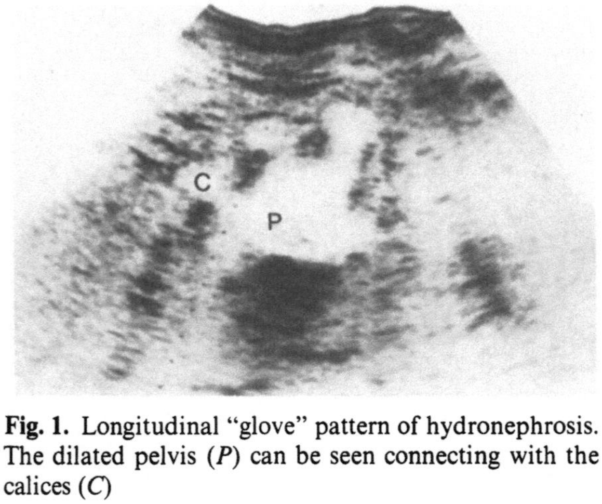

Fig. 1. Longitudinal "glove" pattern of hydronephrosis. The dilated pelvis (*P*) can be seen connecting with the calices (*C*)

In the neonate, distinction between a grossly hydronephrotic kidney and a multicystic kidney is important. As a rule, the pelvis of the hydronephrotic kidney, unlike the multicystic kidney, is centrally placed and renal parenchyma can be seen. On occasion, the two conditions may be indistinguishable.

Accuracy rates in the detection of hydronephrosis using sonography have proved to be satisfactory. The number of false negatives is exceedingly low (less than 1%); a false negative can be suspected if renal calculi are seen or the patient is grossly dehydrated. Renal calculi can obscure dilated calices by acoustic shadowing (Fig. 4), or may themselves be mistaken for a renal pelvis if the acoustic shadowing is overlooked in the presence of gross hydronephrosis. False positives, however, are reasonably common (approximately 15%) [3], occurring when a cystic structure is seen at the center of the kidney. In most instances an extrarenal pelvis is present (Fig. 5), but in other cases there are centrally located peripelvic cysts. Occasionally a renal artery aneurysm can mimic a renal pelvis [1]. In some individuals, particularly those with a renal transplant or in small children, overdistension of the bladder can cause secondary

Radiology Today 2. Ed. by F. H. W. Heuck and M. W. Donner

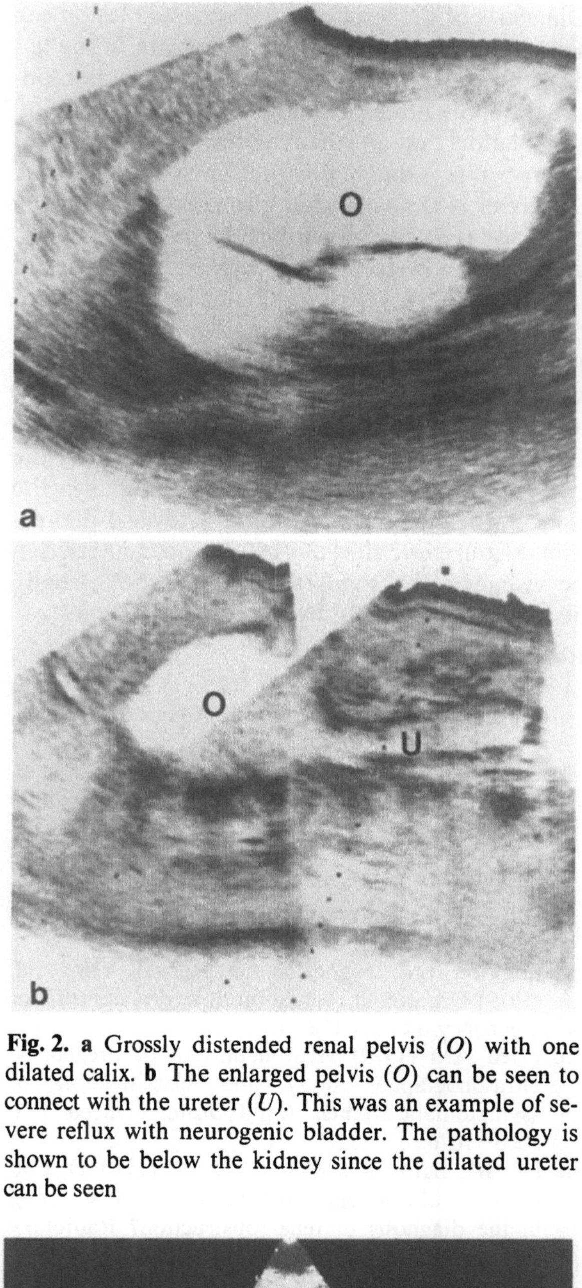

Fig. 2. a Grossly distended renal pelvis (*O*) with one dilated calix. **b** The enlarged pelvis (*O*) can be seen to connect with the ureter (*U*). This was an example of severe reflux with neurogenic bladder. The pathology is shown to be below the kidney since the dilated ureter can be seen

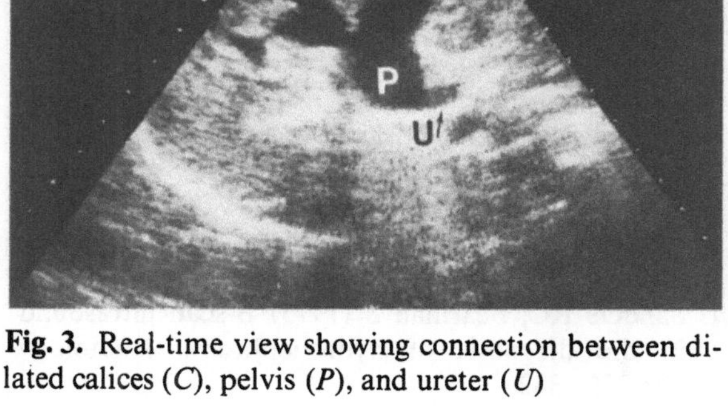

Fig. 3. Real-time view showing connection between dilated calices (*C*), pelvis (*P*), and ureter (*U*)

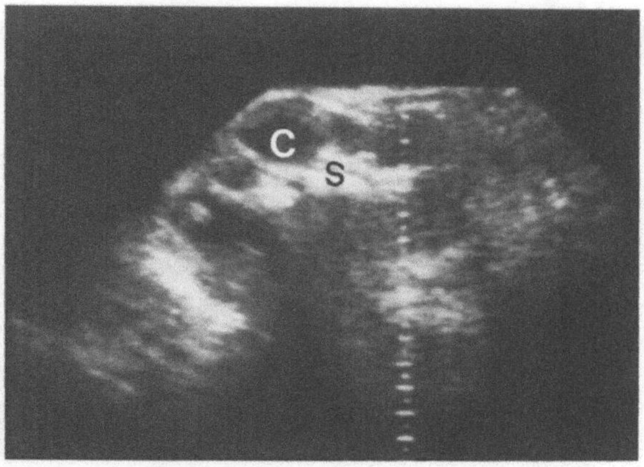

Fig. 4. Mild hydronephrosis was present in this case but the dilated calices (*C*) are hard to see due to an obscuring renal calculus (*S*). Note shadow behind staghorn calculus

renal pelvic distension, a transient reversible hydronephrosis [9]. During a normal pregnancy, the right renal pelvis can become relatively distended, particularly around the 28th week, as a normal variant. The left renal pelvis is not frequently involved [4, 5]; one cannot be certain that a distended pelvis is not a consequence of reflux rather than obstruction (Fig. 2). In the neonate, renal pyramids have been mistaken for hydronephrosis because they stand out more prominently at that time than they do later. This is thought to be due to parenchymal echogenicity induced by an alteration in the ratio of glomeruli to nephrons in the cortex.

Sonography is also useful in assessing the size of the kidney. It is more accurate than the IVP because the degree of tilt of the kidney does not cause confusion on a purely AP view. It is, however, important that the longest axis of the kidney should be sought using real-time sonography.

A crude assessment of parenchymal width can be made. If it is diminished from the norm of approximately 2.5 cm in an adult, there has been destruction of glomeruli and nephrons. Alternately, a useless kidney can be diagnosed by the lack of a surrounding rim of renal parenchyma. Assessment of function is not possible by sonography, but sonography may be as accurate as a nuclear medicine study in showing whether or not the kidney is salvageable, by displaying the quantity of remaining renal parenchyma; nuclear medicine studies are hard to assess in the presence of hydronephrosis.

Real-time sonography has an additional advantage in the patient in whom renal failure is being investigated in that, it can be used on a por-

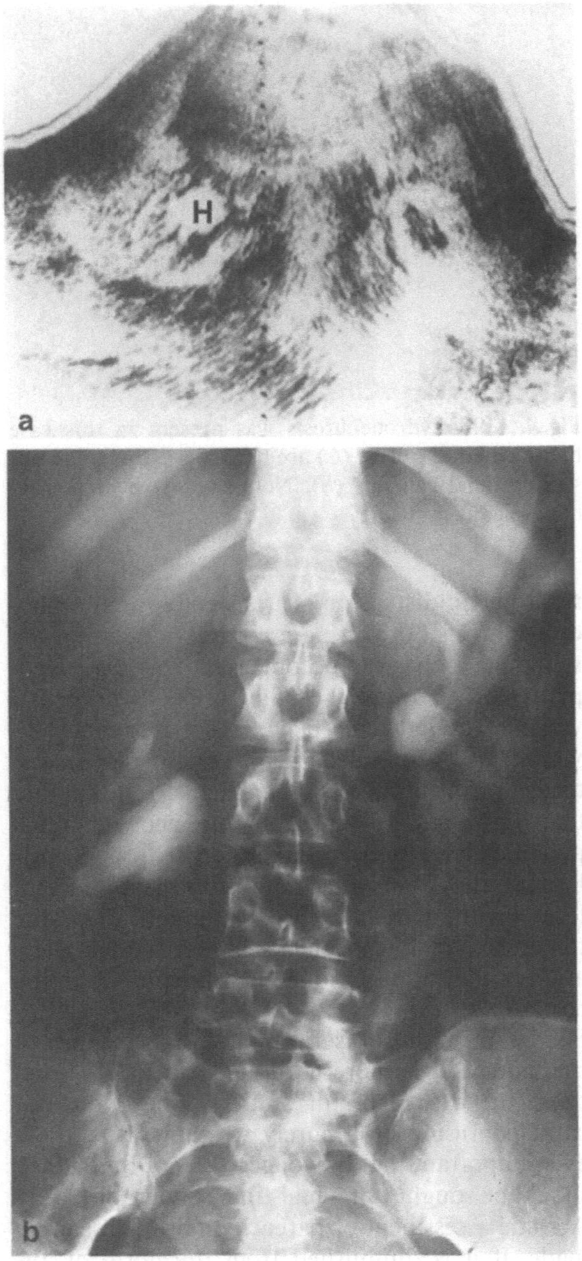

Fig. 5. a Apparent dilated renal pelvis (*H*) suggesting hydronephrosis. **b** IVP showing extrarenal pelvis with normal calices

table basis in the intensive care unit. If the kidney is small, then it is possible in some instances to show evidence of focal scarring, indicating that the patient has chronic pyelonephritis or multiple renal emboli. If the kidney is normal-sized or large, findings are less specific. An increase in cortical echogenicity is found with medical renal failure of many different causes. Focal masses causing renal failure may be seen with lymphoma or tuberosclerosis.

Diagnosis of the level of the obstructed lesion can sometimes be made from the sonogram. If the hydronephrosis is due to uretero-pelvic junction obstruction, the ureter will not be seen either behind the bladder or in the region of the kidney, whereas if it is due to obstruction at a lower level, the ureter is almost always glimpsed at one or the other site (Fig. 2). Sometimes the cause of the obstruction can be recognized, especially in cases of ureterocele [2, 8, 10] or a calculus in the region of the bladder. If the obstructing lesion is localized in the posterior urethra and is due to urethral valves, it may be visualized sonographically by angling the transducer toward the patient's feet. Prostatic enlargement is easily recognized by the presence of a prominent mass bulging into the floor of the bladder or posteriorly toward the rectum. Midureteric sites of obstruction cannot often be visualized by sonography, since they usually lie in an area obscured by gas.

References

1. Amis ES, Cronan JJ, Pfister RC et al. (1982) Ultrasonic inaccuracies in diagnosing renal obstruction. Urology 19:101–105
2. Brenner RJ, DeMartini WJ, Gooding GA et al. (1978) Ultrasonographic demonstration of a simple ureterocele and dilated ureter in an adult. J C U 6:377–456
3. Ellenbogen PH, Scheible FW, Talner LB et al. (1978) Sensitivity of gray scale ultrasound in detecting urinary tract obstruction. AJR 130:731–733
4. Erickson LM, Nicholson SF, Lewall DB et al. (1979) Ultrasound evaluation of hydronephrosis of pregnancy. J C U 7:128–132
5. Fried AM (1979) Hydronephrosis of pregnancy: ultrasonographic study and classification of asymptomatic women. Am J Obstet Gynecol 135: 1066–1070
6. Lee JK, Baron RL, Melson GL et al. (1981) Can real-time ultrasonography replace static B-scanning in the diagnosis of renal obstruction? Radiology 139:161–165
7. Malave SR, Neiman HL, Spies SM et al. (1980) Diagnosis of hydronephrosis: comparison of radionuclide scanning and sonography. AJR 135:1179–1185
8. Mascatello VJ, Smith EH, Carrera GF et al. (1977) Ultrasonic evaluation of the obstructed duplex kidney. Am J Roentgenol 129:113–120
9. Morin ME, Baker DA (1979) The influence of hydration and bladder distension on the sonographic diagnosis of hydronephrosis. J C U 7:192–194
10. Rose JS, McCarthy J, Yeh HC (1979) Ultrasound diagnosis of extopic ureterocele. Pediatr Radiol 8:17–20
11. Sanders RC, Bearman S (1973) B-scan ultrasound in the diagnosis of hydronephrosis. Radiology 108:375–382

Control of Renal Transplant Function by Diagnostic Imaging

H. Treugut, U. Nyman, J. Hildell, and B. Husberg

Katharinenhospital, Zentrum für Radiologie, Radiologisches Institut, Kriegsbergstrasse 60, 7000 Stuttgart, FRG

The kidney allograft is subject to a range of complications that can threaten its function. In addition to the surgical and urological complications, particularly rejection, ischemic damage and acute renal failure (ARF) are worthy of mention. Recognizing the type of functional disorder is of vital importance to the survival of transplant and patient; the methods of imaging available up to now, however, do not always provide the necessary diagnostic certainty. This study investigates the diagnostic possibilities of a new radiological diagnostic method, dynamic CT, based on about 300 examinations performed on more than 100 patients of the General Hospital in Malmö, Sweden (University of Lund), starting in the fall of 1979.

Dynamic CT is a simple extension of the conventional CT examination. Fast repeating scans are made at the same scan level after an intravenous bolus injection of contrast medium. The density changes (enhancement) of individual body structures can be determined with the aid of a special computer program, the course being recorded in the form of a curve. A series of parameters that cannot be provided by a conventional CT examination are obtained in this way. On the one hand, they include morphological and functional details of renal and perirenal structures, on the other, features of the enhancement curves.

It was found right at the beginning of the study that the renal cortex plays a key role in diagnosis. This is because the cortex is the central renal structure, where perfusion is at a maximum and where urine is produced. It can therefore be assumed that alterations in other parts of the kidney result from cortical changes. Especially with the present diagnostic problem of distinguishing between rejection and ARF, there further exists the peculiarity that during rejection a significant selective underperfusion of the cortex occurs, in addition to other modifications of the intrarenal blood distribution [2, 5]. All these physiological phenomena, some previously known and some observed during the study, led to a concentrated recording of cortical parameters, which were then correlated with the clinical status of the transplant (Figs. 1, 2).

The clinical transplant status available at the time of the respective examination as reference standard for the results of dynamic CT resulted from the synopsis of all individual data, giving consideration to clinical symptoms, laboratory values, other radiological investigative methods, occasionally histological findings, and the retrospective assessment of the course *ex juvantibus*.

The parameters used for evaluation in the area of renal morphology and function included size of the kidney, width, structure, and demarcation of the cortex, uniformity of cortex enhancement, intensity and time of appearance of contrast-enhanced urine in the collecting system, and so-called papillary stasis. The parameters taken from the density curves were the maximum slope of the cortex enhancement curve and the period of density difference between cortex and medulla, i.e., the corticomedullary density gradient (Fig. 3) [3, 7].

No problems were encountered in recording and interpreting the morphological parameters, since they directly reflected the gross anatomical alterations. They had a different diagnostic value, which follows from the discriminance analysis described below. Assessing the phenomena of the enhancement curves period to be more difficult, because their course depends on several functionally related factors. Thus the enhancement is not only determined by the perfusion of blood with contrast medium throughout the measured volume, but also results from eliminated contrast medium diffused into the renal interstitium and into the excretory structures [6]. Further, enhancement is a function of the plasma concentration of contrast medium, which can be determined from the form of contrast medium bolus resulting after the injections [1].

Radiology Today 2. Ed. by F. H. W. Heuck and M. W. Donner

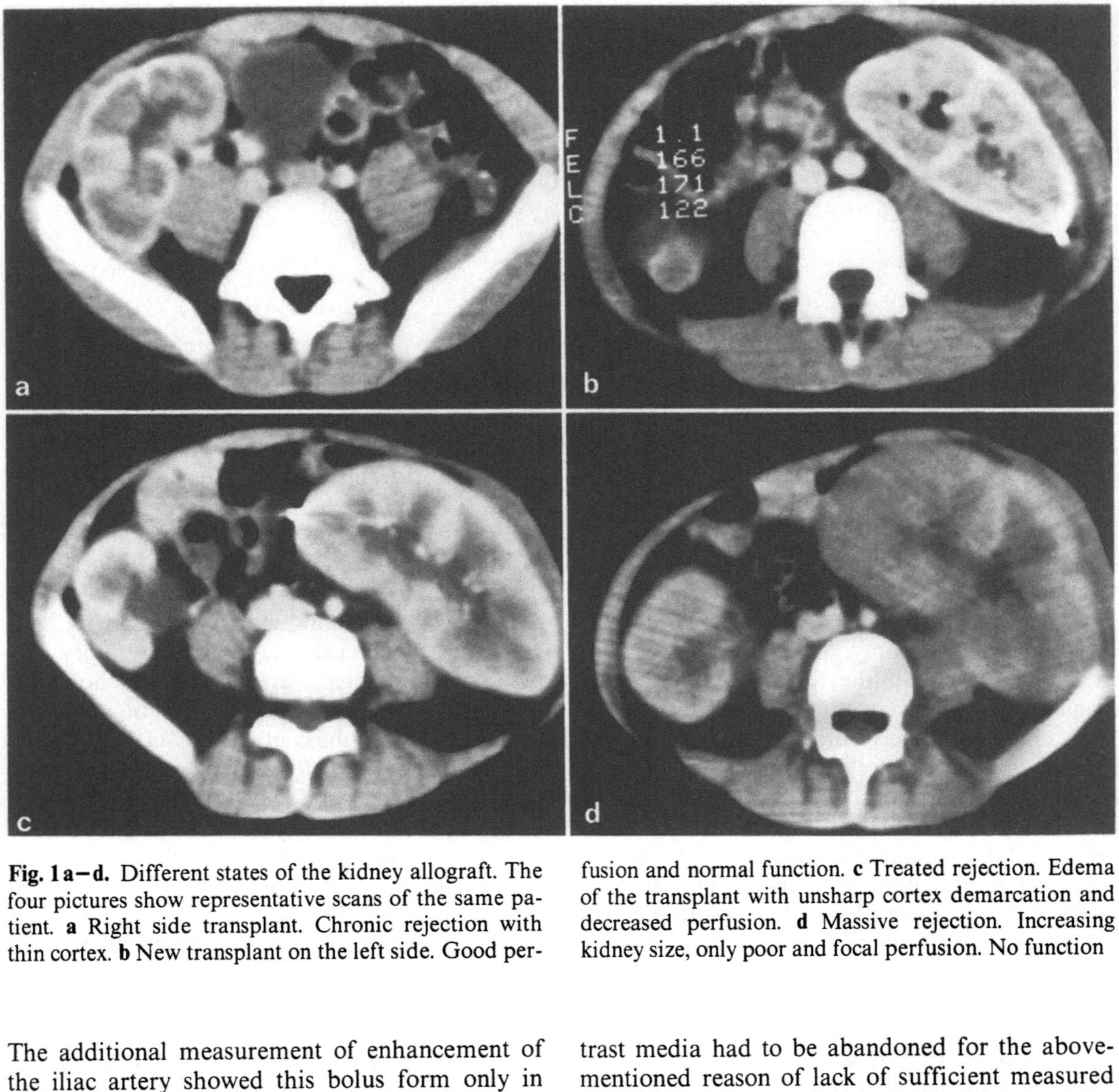

Fig. 1 a–d. Different states of the kidney allograft. The four pictures show representative scans of the same patient. **a** Right side transplant. Chronic rejection with thin cortex. **b** New transplant on the left side. Good perfusion and normal function. **c** Treated rejection. Edema of the transplant with unsharp cortex demarcation and decreased perfusion. **d** Massive rejection. Increasing kidney size, only poor and focal perfusion. No function

The additional measurement of enhancement of the iliac artery showed this bolus form only in very gross characteristics, due to the long measuring intervals (15 s). As expected, there was a clear relationship between the cortical blood flow and the behavior of the enhancement curve. In the group with rejection there was initially a gentler curve slope, which was most pronounced for irreversible rejection with cortical blood flow almost cut off. However, the exact mathematical correlation of enhancement curve and bolus form presented problems caused by the relatively long measuring intervals, which provided only one or at most two measured values for defining the initial artery enhancement course. Early attempts to form a ratio from the graphically determined angles of rise for the cortex and artery curves were not satisfactory [7]. Also, attempts to obtain a blood flow value, possibly disease specific, by calculating the cortical distribution volume for contrast media had to be abandoned for the above-mentioned reason of lack of sufficient measured values [4]. This lack of values caused a "phase displacement" of the enhancement differences of cortex and artery used to calculate the distribution volume; thus the precondition of their relationship, synchronism, no longer existed. On the other hand, this appears to be a very promising starting point for an elegant future solution to the problem of quantification in dynamic CT, since the determination of the distribution volume of a body tissue or of the increase in this distribution volume will be possible when more measuring points are provided by improved CT technology with a higher scan rate.

The value for the maximum density increase of the cortex enhancement curve and, almost more so, the period of the corticomedullary density gradient, showed a marked relationship to the type of functional disturbance. Thus in all groups

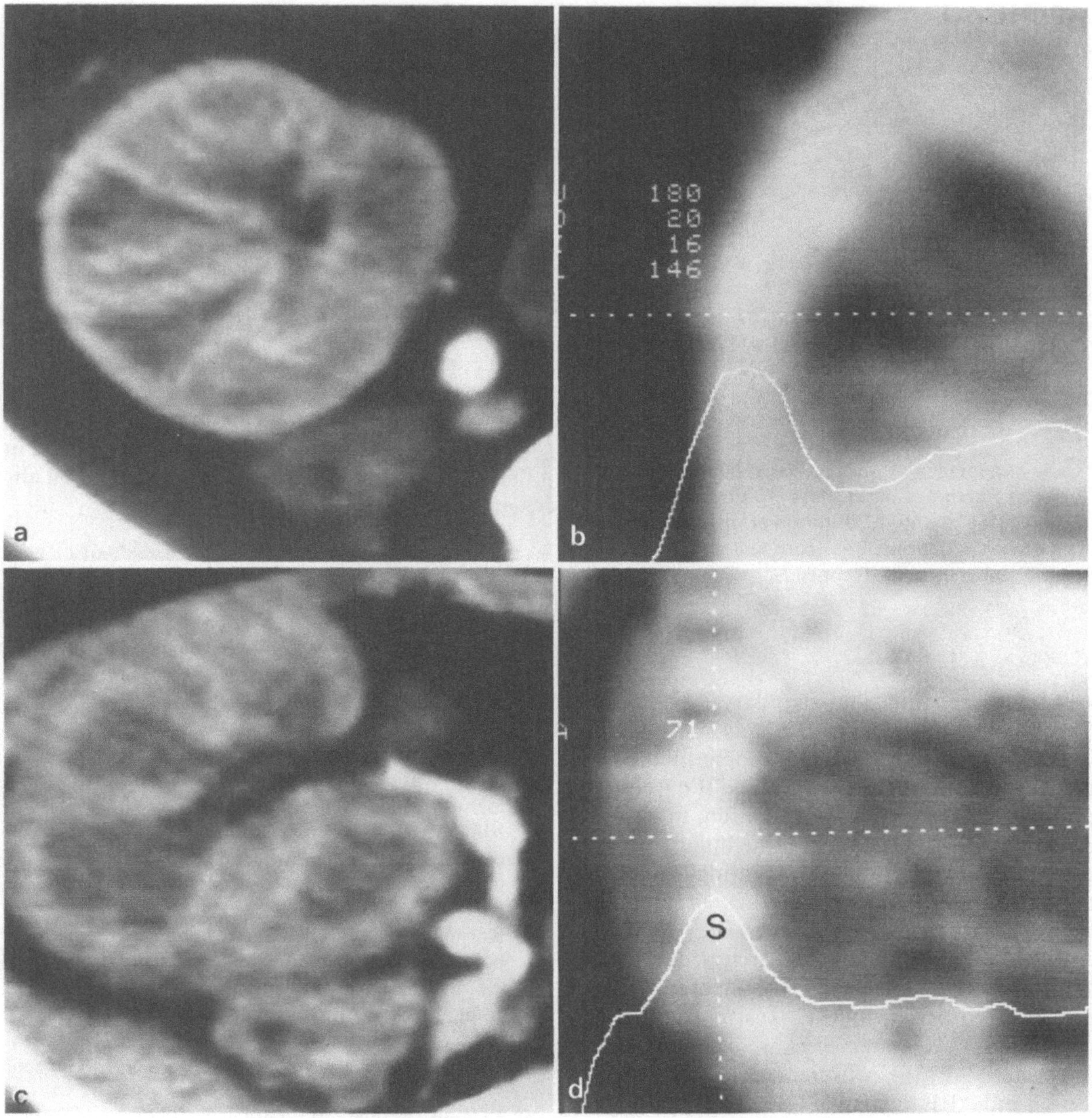

Fig. 2 a–d. Cortical flow diversion after rejection period. Normal function of the allograft. The profile shows a plateau-like density of the cortex. **b** After rejection period (same patient). There is marked variation of the perfusion to the corticomedullary border *S*

of rejection, a gentler slope of the cortex enhancement curve existed than in the groups with ARF. Likewise, a longer period of the corticomedullary density gradient was observed in the rejection groups as opposed to the more shortened period in the ARF groups. The diagnostic significance of the parameters, alone and combined, was determined by discriminance analyses ("direct" and "Mahalanobis" methods), which were based on the change of the parameters as a consequence of transitions from one clinical group to another. Because of the relative infrequency and thus low case rate of these transitional situations, only three could be subjected to discriminance analysis: the changes from normal function to acute rejection, from acute to subsiding rejection, and from ARF to subsiding ARF.

This resulted in the following weighting of the parameters using the direct method: intensity of excretion, intensity of papillary stasis, initial rise of the cortex enhancement curve, period of corticomedullary density gradient, size of renal cross-

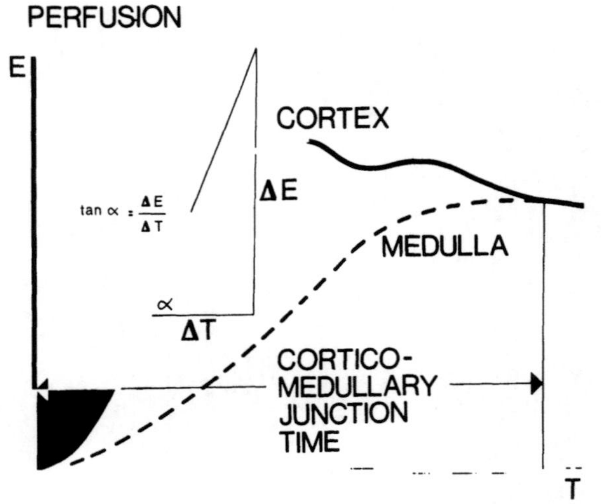

Fig. 3. Parameters of the cortex enhancement curve. The most important parameters are the initial slope of the curve (tan α) and the duration of different enhancement of cortex and medulla (corticomedullary junction time). *E*, enhancement; *T*, time

sectional area, time that papillary stasis occurs. The classification result, or diagnostic certainty, was 81.25%. Using the Mahalanobis method the diagnostic certainty was 68.75% and the weighting of parameters was: time of excretion, intensity of excretion, period of corticomedullary density gradient. The order of both weightings refers only to the discrimination possibilities in the transitional situations examined here. The specific accuracy of the cortical flow parameters, such as initial slope of the cortex enhancement curve and period of corticomedullary density gradient, indicates that these parameters are of much greater importance in the differentation between rejection and ARF. Dynamic CT of kidney allograft is thus similar to most other imaging modalities in that it, too, provides individual parameters of different specificity. Since the group-specific parameters overlap because of their deviation, diagnosis is possible only after a summarized evaluation of them. The diagnostic certainty increases in the presence of a comparable baseline examination. Thus in addition to the determination of transplant status, the course can be checked; however, prognostic statements, e.g., those related to transplant survival in the case of a rejection, are not possible.

The noninvasive and simple technique does not present any danger to the patient if consideration is given to the usual contraindications for use of contrast medium. The physical and chemical stress of radiation and contrast medium is insignificant or tolerable. The diagnostic certainty appears to be superior to that of other imaging methods, with the exception of sonography, and improvement can be expected upon further development of CT technology. The study is a model in that it is an initial experiment in functional diagnosis by means of dynamic CT.

References

1. Dean P, Kormano M (1977) Intravenous bolus of ^{125}J labeled meglumine diatrizoate. Early extravascular distribution. Acta Radiol [Diagn] (Stockh) 18:293–304
2. Hollenberg N, Retik A, Rosen S et al. (1968) The role of vasoconstriction in the ischemia of renal allograft rejection. Transplantation 6:59–69
3. Ishikawa J, Onorchi Z, Saito Y et al. (1981) Renal cortex visualisation and analysis of dynamic CT curves of the kidney. J Comput Assist Tomogr 5:695–701
4. Kormano M (1981) Kinetics of contrast media after bolus injection and infusion. In: Contrast media in CT. International workshop Berlin 14.–17. 1. 81. Excerpta Medica, Amsterdam, pp 38–46
5. Retik A, Hollenberg N, Rosen S (1967) Cortical ischemia in renal allograft rejection. Surg Gynecol Obstet 124:989–998
6. Treugut H, Nyman U, Hildell J (1980) Sequenz-CT: Frühe Dichteveränderungen der gesunden Niere nach Kontrastmittelapplikation. Radiologe 20:558–562
7. Treugut H, Nyman U, Hildell J, Molde A (1981) Funktionskontrolle des Nierentransplantats durch Sequenz-CT. Erste Ergebnisse. ROFO 135:133–142

Therapy Planning with Computed Tomography in Pelvic Tumors: Overview

A. B. Atzinger, H. Gfirtner, K. Pfändner, and A. Breit

Radiologische Abteilung, Städtisches Krankenhaus, Bischof-Pilgrim-Strasse 1, 8390 Passau, FRG

The treatment of many tumors in the pelvic region is well established. We will briefly discuss some of the most frequent, concentrating on some points of importance.

Prostate Carcinoma

Over the past 15 years, researchers such as Bagshaw [3], Ray and Bagshaw [21], and Van der Werf-Messing [31, 32] have developed radiation treatment into an effective form of therapy and shown that it is equivalent to surgery at stage B and to hormonal treatment at stage C. If staging lymphadenectomy has preceded radiation therapy and no lymph node metastases have been found, the prostate and the periprostatic tissues are treated with the rotational technique only up to 70 Gy in the 80% isodose.

If no lymphadenectomy has been carried out in a patient clinically classified as stage B or C, the *entire* pelvis is treated up to 50 Gy in the 80% isodose homogeneously with parallel opposed portals using ^{60}Co or a 10-MV X-ray beam, and after a 2- to 3-week interval (split course) an additional dose is administered by the rotational technique, with the dose at the prostate itself being increased by 20 Gy in the 80% isodose.

If no lymphadenectomy has been done we think that because of the unknown adenopathy the *whole* pelvis should be irradiated up to a dose of 50 Gy. McGowan [15] found in cases with more advanced disease, i.e., in patients with involvement of more than one lobe or extraprostatic extension, that extended field radiation improved the disease-free 5-year survival rate to 63% compared with 35% in cases treated with localized radiation. This is due to the fact that if the prostatic capsule has been penetrated, the incidence of pelvic adenopathy rises markedly. For example, according to Pistenma et al. [20], in a series of 93 patients who underwent lymph node resection, the incidence of lymphadenopathy in those with extracapsular extension was 59%.

The target volume for the boost dose according to involvement of the seminal vesicles causes a great problem in cases in clinical stages B and C. Carcinoma of the prostate frequently extends into the seminal vesicles, which cannot be visualized radiographically; their lateral extension, in particular, is completely undetectable. On computed tomography (CT) scan, however, their full extension is well demonstrated. Pilepich et al. [19] recently reported that the impact of CT data on treatment plan modification was most dramatic in stage C patients with seminal vesicle involvement. Fifty- three percent of these patients would not have had the entire tumor volume adequately irradiated if only conventional treatment planning procedures had been performed.

Bladder Carcinoma

Surgery or radiotherapy alone gives a 5-year survival rate of 15%–30% [26]. Therefore once the diagnosis of a high-grade or muscle-invading tumor has been established and no evidence of metastatic disease is found, aggressive therapy should be planned.

Following Whitmore et al. and others [16, 30, 34], we usually perform integrated irradiation followed by radical cystectomy 5 or 6 weeks later. Sometimes urinary diversion is carried out before the preoperative irradiation [7], which consists of 40–45 Gy delivered over a 6-week period [23], using ^{60}Co radiation or 10-MV X-ray beams in a three-field technique. The fields encompass the bifurcation of the common iliac vessels. Patients with cancers unsuitable for cystectomy are considered for radiation therapy alone. In these cases an additional boost dose of about 20–25 Gy in the 80% isodose is given by the rotational technique with reduced fields to the bladder itself.

Radiology Today 2. Ed. by F. H. W. Heuck and M. W. Donner

A major difficulty in radiation treatment is exact and reproducable positioning, especially with reduced fields. As Hendrickson [11] has said, the precision required of radiation treatment is probably the most critical of all oncologic disciplines. To miss the tumor once or twice during a treatment course or to have the tumor moved out of the treatment beam during an individual treatment could well produce a 10% or even greater reduction in dose below that believed to have been delivered.

If one side of a patient is elevated by some degrees during treatment, the bladder may be well included within the high isodose but the dose to the lymph nodes of the elevated side may be insufficient. This is even more important if the tumor is small and located deep in the body, as is the case with small local recurrences or lymph node metastases. If a patient with a small tumor deep within the body is twisted by 10°, more than 50% of the tumor volume moves out of the high isodose [22].

In order to make sure that the tumor remains at the same location during treatment planning with CT and the subsequent treatment course, and to *guarantee* that positioning of the patient can be exactly reproduced daily, we have installed laser strip devices *identically* in the CT room and the treatment room (Figs. 1, 2).

These three laser strips – a vertical line and left and right horizontal lines – define exactly the patient's positioning in three dimensions. The defined positioning is daily reproduced on the treatment couch if the laser strips of the treatment room fit the skin markings drawn in the CT room [1].

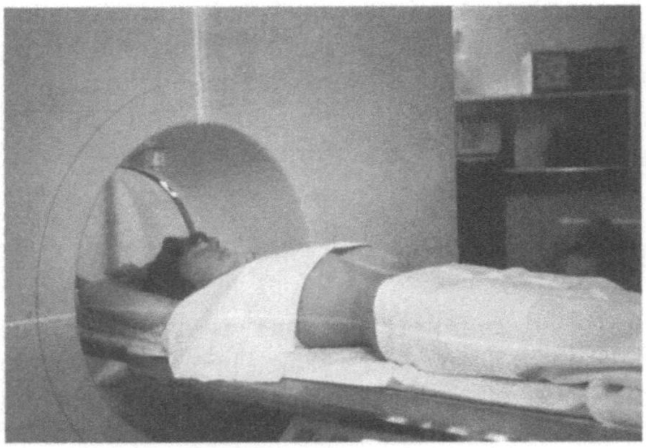

Fig. 1. Laserstrips in the CT-room

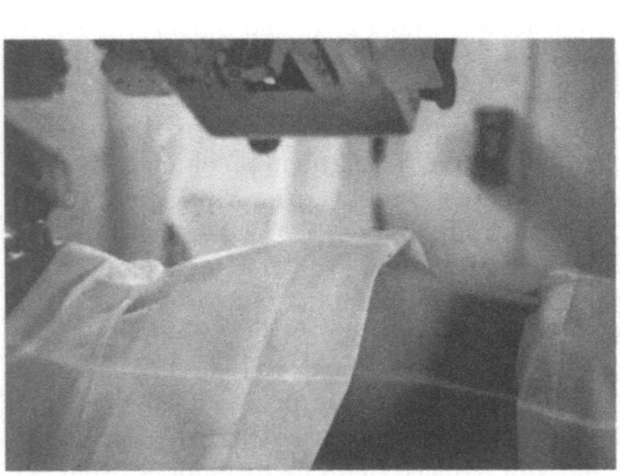

Fig. 2. Laserfacility in the treatment room

Rectal Carcinoma

Mortality rates for carcinoma of the colon and the rectum have remained unremittingly high for almost 30 years and total survival is under 30% [27]. Preoperative radiation has been standard in our department since randomized studies carried out in Great Britain, the USA, and Mainz, Federal Republic of Germany, showed its advantages [4, 13, 24].

We administer a dose of 30 Gy within 3 weeks through ventral and dorsal fields to cover the tumor and the collecting lymph trunks. Surgery is carried out 1 week later. In cases in stages A and B1, no further course of radiation therapy is planned after surgery. In cases in stages B2 and C, radiation treatment is administered 4 weeks after surgery, with the tumor dose increased to 55 Gy.

If the patient is for any reason inoperable, radiation therapy is carried out alone using the three-field technique, administering 45 Gy with the fields extending cranially up to the fourth lumbar vertebra.

As soon as a dose of 45 Gy is reached, the fields are limited to the original tumor and surrounding tissue and the tumor dose increased to 65 Gy at the 80% isodose.

There are a few patients with small rectal tumors that can be treated definitively with local contact irradiation. In these cases, we apply Iridium-AL once a week with a single contact dose of 8 Gy and repeat the treatment 6–10 times up to a total contact dose of 50–80 Gy (Fig. 3) [18]. At this point I would like to mention another problem; that of control of therapy planning during a course of treatment and the necessary modifications. A patient with inoperable carcinoma of the rectum underwent a 4-week course of radiation therapy. At a dose of 45 Gy at the 80% isodose, the patient had lost 16 kg in weight; shrinkage of the sagittal cross section by 3 cm was seen

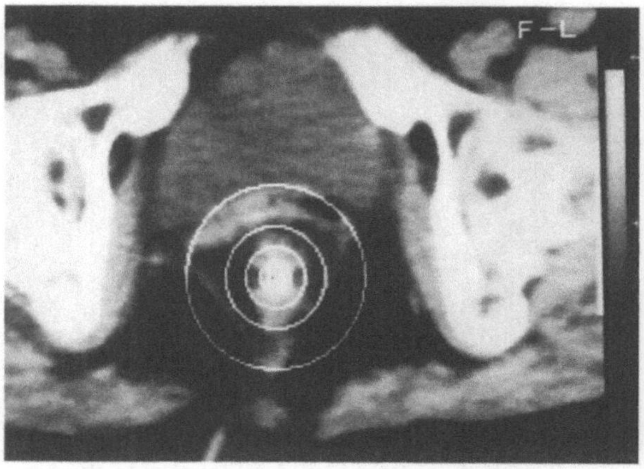

Fig. 3. Iridium afterloading applicator in the rectum with isodose overlay

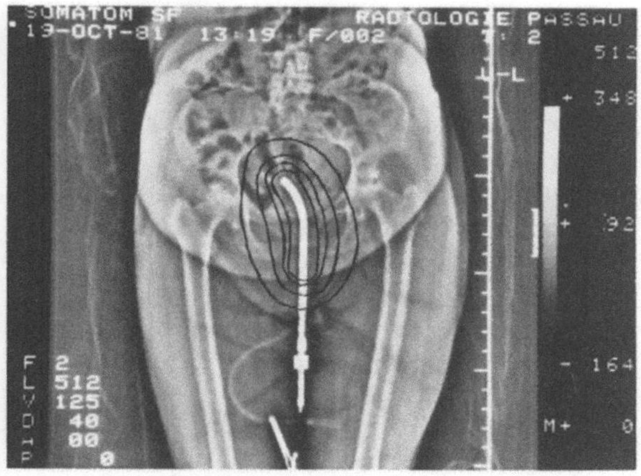

Fig. 5. Frontal scoutview of the pelvis with Iridium afterloading applicator in the uterus. Slight displacement of the uterus and applicator to the right

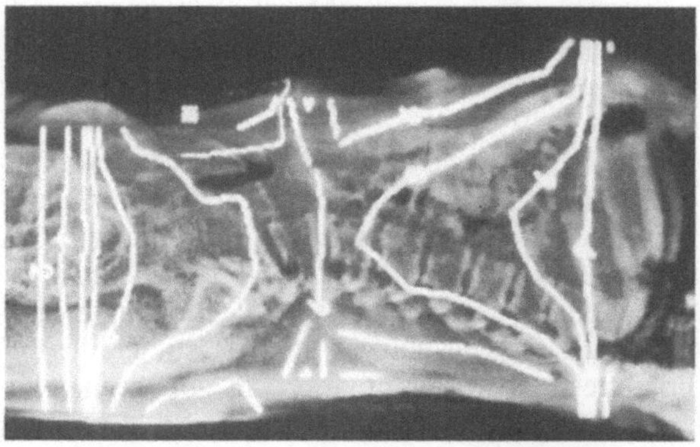

Fig. 4. Lateral scout view showing the dose distribution at the connection of adjacent field borders

on the control CT scan. Further application of the primary treatment plan would have led to deviation of dose distribution due to the changed body circumference. In order to include the target volume unchanged into the 80% isodose it was necessary to change the treatment plan. The new treatment plan resulted in reduced irradiation time using the ventral tangential fields. Penetratio n sites of the central beam related to the pelvic bones lie at identical points, but in relation to the body circumference, and compared to the initial situation, more ventral. CT furnishes, without doubt, the most exact basis for follow-ups and modifications as treatment progresses.

Field connections have to be considered a further problem in irradiation of the pelvic region [10, 12, 17, 33]. To solve this problem we use digital radiography, the so-called topograms or scout views [2]. Let me explain this with an example: We are currently treating a patient with teratoma of the testicle and a large tumor mass in the pelvis of testicular origin. The whole pelvis was irradiated with 40 Gy, administering an additional boost dose of 10 Gy to the tumor. The para-aortal field then had to be connected, so the field borders were marked on the patient's skin with opaque material and lateral scout views taken. With the help of the planning computer the fields are projected on the scout view and the dose distribution is calculated and graphically printed, thus enabling us to plan very well and avoid hot or cold spots. We are able to vary the adjacent field borders according to whether fields from one side or opposed fields are used and dependent upon the patient's body thickness, the field lengths, and the focus-skin distance (Fig. 4).

Gynecologic Tumors

It is common knowledge that in gynecologic tumors intracavitary therapy is used in combination with external beam radiation. Current dosimetric procedures for intracavitary therapy use input from orthogonal radiographs. In this approach, however, the ability to fully define anatomic structures is severely limited by blurring inadequate resolution, and film mangnification. To circumvent these limitations, we have been investigating, treatment planning on transverse and axial as well as coronal and sagittal reconstructed CT images for intracavitary therapy. Recently, Sewchand et al. [25], and Woon Sang et al. [35] reported on a similar approach. The disadvantages of this method are that the procedure is time consuming and that one needs about 25–30 CT scans for reconstruction. Therefore, for dose distri-

bution evaluation we now use some transverse CT scans and AP and lateral scout views. With this method one can easily see displacement of the applicator to any side and the lead block can be localized exactly. On displacement of the applicator, under- or overdosage to the pelvic wall can be seen and boost irradiation be carried out (Fig. 5). The dose-rate gradient across the bladder and rectum is shown in Fig. 5.
The advantages of this method of dosimetry planning lie in the following features:

1. Minimal image destruction and blurring compared to radiographic imaging
2. Direct one-to-one data transfer from imaging to treatment planning
3. Better three-dimensional evaluation of dosage to various reference points: cervix, parametrium, pelvic wall, bladder, rectum, and lymph-node-bearing regions
4. Direct dose adjustment to cover the tumor volume adequately and avoid excessive dose to adjacent organs

Recurrences

In treating the bladder, identical positioning is of tremendous importance, as we have already shown. We favor positioning with the laser strips discussed. This problem is even greater in cases with small local recurrences and lymph node metastases due to the fact that with limited dosage the dose must be administered effectively and precisely. With small tumors and small fields, parts of the tumor move out of the high isodoses even on slight displacement. These local recurrences and lymph node metastases are best recognized on CT, which therefore represents the best basis for therapy planning.

Nuclear Magnetic Resonance

Nuclear magnetic resonance (NMR) is a method which has not yet found its way into clinical routine. Radio-oncologists, however, have great hopes for its future development. In NMR images, the densities of protons are reproduced, whereas in CT images the differences in absorption density are reflected. In the field of radiologic diagnosis, the efficacy of NMR has already been established [5, 6, 14, 28]. Now, there is a chance that with the help of the additional biochemical information given by NMR, detection of recurrences in the pelvis, which are often quite

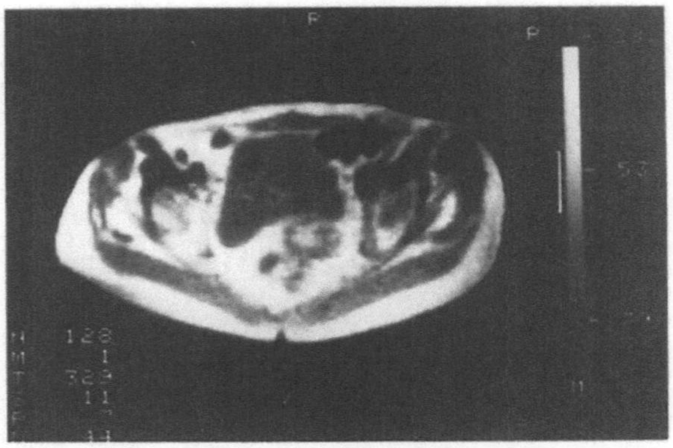

Fig. 6. Transaxial NMR-image at the level of the cervix uteri. The thickened cervix and infiltration to the parametrium is visualized

difficult to diagnose will be made easier. CT mostly shows space-occupying lesions in cases of tumor recurrence, but often differentiation between scarring and recurrence cannot be made [29].
Since early 1982 we have carried out comparative NMR and CT studies in 12 patients with primary and secondary gynecologic tumors. The tumors were recognized equally on CT and NMR studies, but a apparent advantage of NMR imaging is that tumor tissue is visualized at different grades of brightness at different intervals between two measurements, whereas the brightness of normal tissue does not change to this extent. This obviously represents specific visualization of tumor tissue.
Figure 6 shows a transaxial NMR image at the level of the cervix uteri. At a long interval the thickened cervix and infiltration to the parametrium (stage IIb) is visualized and appears light. Dorsally on the left the thickened bladder wall can be seen.
In therapy planning it is interesting that the NMR technique – unlike CT – is not restricted to transverse cross sections: any plane may be chosen [8, 9, 36]. Truly three-dimensional therapy planning seems to be imminent. In conclusion, our experience has shown very reliable demonstration and exact delineation of gynecologic tumors and recurrences on NMR studies. The advantages of NMR for radiation therapy and therapy planning may not yet be fully realized.

References

1. Atzinger A, Breit A (1982) Vier Jahre Erfahrung in der Strahlentherapie auf der Grundlage von CT-Schnitten. Strahlentherapie 158:97–102

2. Atzinger A, Pfändner K, Rohde U (1981) Der Wert des Topogramms für die Patientenlagerung bei der Bestrahlungsplanung. Röntgenpraxis 134:487–498
3. Bagshaw MA (1980) External radiation therapy of carcinoma of the prostate. Cancer [Suppl] 1912–1921
4. Brückner R, Kempf P (1978) Vorbestrahlung beim Rektumkarzinom. Dtsch Arztebl 41:2327–2332
5. Damadian R (1971) Tumor detection by nuclear magnetic resonance. Science 171:1151–1153
6. Doyle FH, Pennock JM, Banks LM, McDonnell MJ, Bydder GM, Steiner RE, Young IR, Clarke GJ, Pasmore T, Gilderdale DJ (1982) Nuclear magnetic resonance imaging of the liver: initial experience. AJR 138:193–200
7. Ellingwood KE, Drylie DM, de Ture FA, Million RR (1979) Postdiversion precystectomy irradiation for cancer of the bladder. Cancer 43:1032–1036
8. Gudden F (1981) Bildgebende Systeme heute und morgen. Electromedica 2:64–67
9. Gunby P (1982) The new wave in medicine: nuclear magnetic resonance. JAMA 247:151–159
10. Hackl A, Krispel F (1980) Untersuchungen über die Problematik der Dosisverteilung im Feldgrenzbereich. Strahlentherapie 156:115
11. Hendrickson FR (1982) Precision in radiation oncology. Int J Radiat Oncol Biol Phys 8:311–312
12. Kaplan HS (1972) Hodgkin's disease. Harvard University Press, Cambridge/Mass
13. Kligerman MM (1977) Radiotherapy and rectal cancer. Cancer 39:896
14. Koutcher JA, Goldsmith M, Damadian R (1978) NMR in Cancer. X.A. malignancy index to discriminate normal and cancerous tissue. Cancer 41:174–182
15. McGowan DG (1981) The value of extended field radiation therapy in carcinoma of the prostate. Int J Radiat Oncol Biol Phys 7:1333–1339
16. Miller LS (1977) Bladder cancer: superiority of preoperative irradiation and cystectomy in clinical stages B2 and C. Cancer 39:973–980
17. Page V, Gardner A, Karzmark CJ (1970) Physical and dosimetric aspects of the radiotherapy of malignant lymphomas. II. The inverted-y technique. Radiology 96:619
18. Papillon J, Montarbon JF (1975) La curie-thérapie interstitielle à l'iridium 192, appliqué aux petits cancers du rectum. J Radiol Electrol 56:439
19. Pilepich MV, Prasad SC, Perez CA (1982) Computed tomography in definitive radiotherapy of prostatic carcinoma, part 2: definition of target volume. Int J Radiat Oncol Biol Phys 8:235–240
20. Pistenma DA, Bagshaw MA, Freiha FS (1979) In: Johnson DE, Samuels ML (eds) Cancer of the genitourinary tract. Raven, New York, pp 229–247
21. Ray GR, Bagshaw MA (1975) The role of radiation therapy in the definitive treatment of adenocarcinoma of the prostate. Annu Rev Med 26:567–588
22. Rödel K (1972) Vermeidung von Fehlern bei der Bestrahlungsplanung. Rontgenpraxis 3:55–65
23. Scherer E (1976) Therapeutische Probleme bei der Radiotherapie der Harnblasentumoren. Strahlentherapie 151:387–398
24. Scherer E, Sack H (1979) Probleme der Strahlenbehandlung des Rektumkarzinoms. Strahlentherapie 155:300–306
25. Sewchand W, Prempree T, Patanaphan V, Whitley NO, Heidtman B, Scott RM (1982) Value of multiplanar CT images in interactive dosimetry planning of intracavitary therapy. Int J Radiat Oncol Biol Phys 8:295–301
26. Skinner DG (1980) Current perspectives in the management of high-grade invasive bladder cancer. Cancer [Suppl] 45:1866–1873
27. Smith AN (1980) Vorbestrahlung operabler Rektumkarzinome. Radiotherapie-Forum, Teil 1. Coloproctology 5:327–328
28. Smith FW, Reid A, Hutchison JMS, Mallard JR, Path FRC (1982) Nuclear magnetic resonance imaging of the pancreas. Radiology 142:677–680
29. Steinbrich W, et al. (1982) Wert der Computertomographie für die Diagnostik der Uterustumoren und ihrer Rezidive. Radiologe 22:154–161
30. Van der Werf-Messing BHP (1975) Carcinoma of the bladder T3-NxMo treated by preoperative irradiation followed by cystectomy. Cancer [Suppl] 36:718–722
31. Van der Werf-Messing BHP (1978) Prostatic cancer treated at the Rotterdam Radiotherapy Institute. Strahlentherapie 154:537–541
32. Van der Werf-Messing BHP, Sourek-Zikova V, Blonk DI (1976) Localized advanced carcinoma of the prostate: radiation therapy versus hormonal therapy. Int J Radiat Oncol Biol Phys 1:1043
33. Voss AC, Baier N (1980) Zur Strahlentherapie der Lymphogranulomatose. Strahlentherapie 156:105
34. Whitmore WF Jr, Batata MA, Hilaris BS, Reddy GN, Unal A, Ghoneim MA, Grabstald H, Chu F (1977) A comparative study of 2 preoperative radiation regimes with cystectomy for bladder cancer. Cancer 40:1077–1086
35. Woon Sang Y, Sagerman RH, Chung TC, King GA, Dala PS, Bassano DA, Ames TE (1982) Anatomical relationships in intracavitary irradiation demonstrated by computed tomography. Radiology 143:537–541
36. Zeitler E, Schittenhelm R (1981) Die Kernspintomographie (KST) und ihre klinischen Anwendungsmöglichkeiten. Electromedica 3:134–143

Direct Coronal and Direct Sagittal Whole Body Computed Tomography

P. F. G. M. van Waes, F. W. Zonneveld, and M. A. M. Feldberg

Academisch Ziekenhuis Utrecht, Universiteitsafdeling voor Röntgendiagnostik, Catharijnesingel 101, 3500 GV Utrecht, The Netherlands

The importance of the application of computed tomography (CT) in planes other than the axial transverse plane by means of multiplanar reformatting (MPR), first tested for the brain and orbits [4, 10, 11, 14, 16], has also been well documented for the study of the torso [1–3, 5, 7, 12, 15, 18]. Direct multiplanar views of the body have recently been suggested [8, 19], but limitations imposed by construction of the gantry, the table, and the size of the scanned area have prevented application on a routine basis. However, there are at least three reasons why direct coronal CT of the body is in many cases a unique alternative to MPR: improved image quality, improved definition of coronal anatomy, and shorter examination time.

There are several reasons why direct coronal CT yields better images than MPR. Partial volume averaging tends to degrade the quality of the MPR scans [6], and the possibility of patient motion at any moment during a series of axial transverse scans is always present, with resulting discrepancies in the multiplanar reconstruction. Direct coronal CT gives a better definition of the coronal anatomy because patient positioning requires stretching of the lordotic parts of the vertebral column; this results in scanning planes that are truly parallel to the spine. Finally, with direct coronal CT shorter examination times can be achieved, especially in cases of lesions with large dimensions, such as some abdominal masses. Here the full extent of the lesion can be covered with a few axial transverse and a few coronal scans, whereas if only the axial transverse modality is used, a large number of scans will be needed. Direct sagittal views are indicated, just as in classical radiology where lateral views or tomograms are helpful. This technique has proved to be feasible, especially in complicated cases involving lesions in the region of the pelvis, lower abdomen, or retroperitoneal space.

Materials and Methods

In order to cover most areas of the torso, three different patient positions have been developed: position A, pelvis including retroperitoneal space and lower abdomen (Fig. 1a); position B, upper abdomen and lower chest (Fig. 2); and position C, upper chest including neck and posterior fossa (Fig. 3). Position D is now available to obtain direct sagittal views, including perirenal space, pelvis, lower abdomen, and retroperitoneal space (Fig. 4).

For the pelvis (position A), a special seat has been developed. This device, which can be attached to the patient table for slice incrementation, incorporates a saddle, footrests, and handgrips. A cushioned, extendable sternum rest defines the degree of bending (Fig. 1b). After the patient seat has been slid into the gantry, a lateral scanogram is made, and the accurate site and angle for direct coronal slices can be selected with the help of a light pen. In order to examine the upper abdomen and lower chest (position B), the patient is seated directly on the gantry cover in the cone-shaped opening, reclining backward. Positioning is done by hand and the light visor in the scan plane is used for orientation (Fig. 2). For analysis of the upper chest, neck, and posterior fossa (position C), the patient is seated on the rear side of the gantry, allowing for more space to stretch the legs (Fig. 3). For direct sagittal views, including the contents of the bony pelvis, lower abdomen, and retroperitoneal space (position D), the patient is seated directly, legs spread, within the gantry with the reinforced rear side. A true sagittal view of the upper parts of the abdomen is not feasible, since the patient has to twist his body in order to mount the gantry in a horseback manner, resulting in a more oblique sagittal view (Fig. 4).

Radiology Today 2. Ed. by F. H. W. Heuck and M. W. Donner

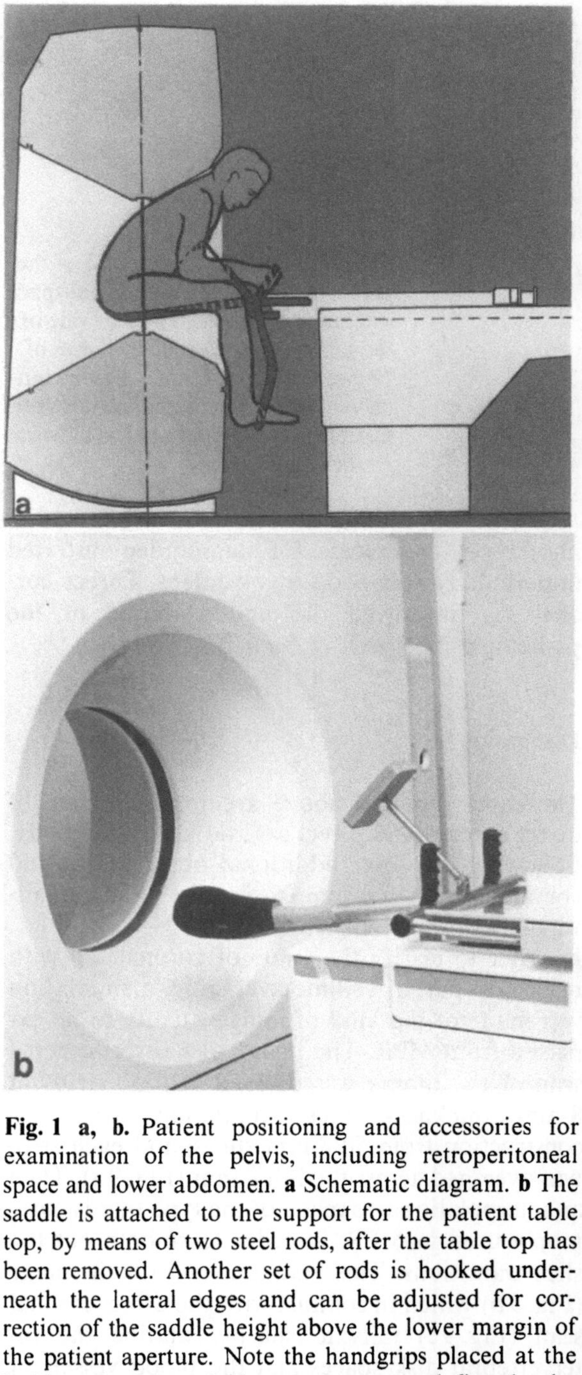

Fig. 1 a, b. Patient positioning and accessories for examination of the pelvis, including retroperitoneal space and lower abdomen. **a** Schematic diagram. **b** The saddle is attached to the support for the patient table top, by means of two steel rods, after the table top has been removed. Another set of rods is hooked underneath the lateral edges and can be adjusted for correction of the saddle height above the lower margin of the patient aperture. Note the handgrips placed at the inside and an extendable sternum rest to define the degree of body flexion. Accurate selection of the coronal plane can also be achieved by a slight gantry tilt

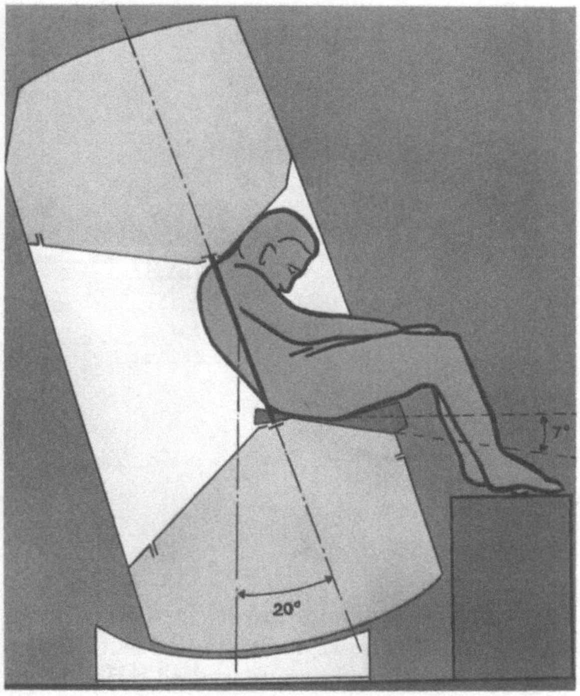

Fig. 2. Position for coronal CT of the upper abdomen and lower chest. This is the least comfortable position. The chin is pushed against the sternum. Only in relatively small or flexible patients can the anterior parts of the chest be analyzed. Backward tilt of the gantry and a silastic or rubber sheet prevents the patient slipping out

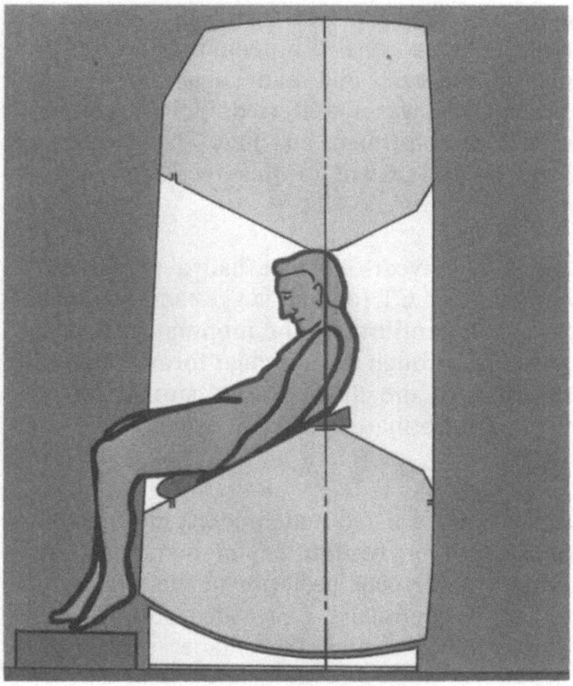

Fig. 3. Position for coronal CT of the upper chest, neck, and posterior fossa. The patient is seated on the rear side of the gantry. A silastic sheet prevents slipping

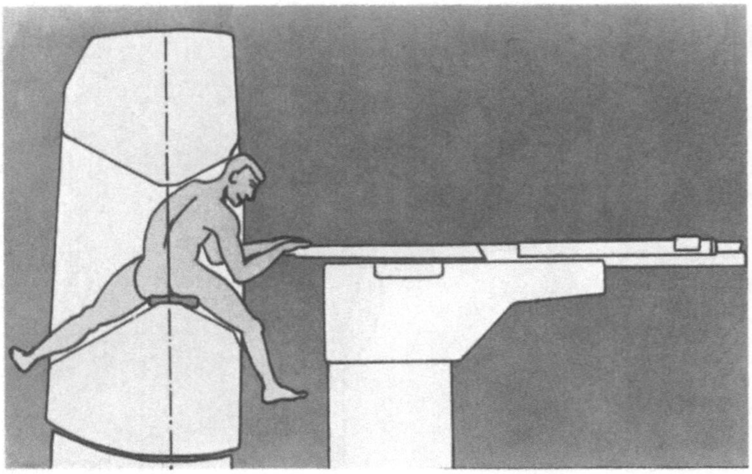

Fig. 4. Position for sagittal CT of the pelvis, including retroperitoneal space and lower abdomen. The rear side of the gantry is reinforced (thickness of 10 mm instead of 4 mm). A true sagittal view of the upper abdomen is not feasible, since the patient has to twist his/her shoulders

Case Reports

The following examples are selected from more than 1500 patients we have studied with direct coronal body CT and a more limited series of patients we have studied by means of direct sagittal CT.

Case 1. A 37-year-old male was admitted with evidence of rectal blood loss. Barium enema revealed an almost totally stenosed rectum. A pronounced mucosal fold prevented proper endoscopic inspection of the tumor. Transverse CT could not exclude involvement of the bladder dome. Direct coronal CT demonstrated the pronounced mucosal fold and suggested that the bladder dome was not affected. Only direct sagittal CT demonstrated an intact fatty interface along the full extent of this rectosigmoid carcinoma (Fig. 5).

Case 2. A 42-year-old male had a palpable abdominal mass. CT findings suggested a malignant schwannoma infiltrating the iliopsoas muscle and protruding through the muscular foramen into the soft tissue of the thigh. Three coronal sections were as informative as 23 transverse scans (Fig. 6).

Case 3. A 61-year-old male underwent pneumonectomy and was readmitted for hemoptysis. CT showed a recurrence posterior to the left pulmonary artery. Coronal CT provided additional information concerning the shape and extent. (Fig. 7).

Case 4. A 62-year-old male had endoscopic evidence of a large supraglottic carcinoma obliterating the piriform recess. CT staging demonstrated important lymph node involvement. Direct coronal CT improved the understanding of the pathologic changes (Fig. 8).

Discussion

The cases reported above are representative of direct coronal and direct sagittal CT of the body. Following are some additional observations and comments that will emphasize the inherent advantages of this technique.

In order to clarify the value of coronal CT with respect to partial volume averaging, a simulation was made of the kind of image quality to be expected from MPR. The image of a direct coronal scan of the thorax was divided into 50 strips of 8-mm thickness, thus simulating MPR reconstruction from 50 8-mm slices, and each strip was averaged across the full 8 mm (Fig. 9a). Then an interpolation was made of the type that is commonly used in MPR, in order to smooth out the slice transitions. This results in a smooth image (Fig. 9b) which in contrast with the direct coronal scan (Fig. 9c) fails to sharply outline the intervertebral disk spaces and the blood vessels of the lungs. This simulation does not demonstrate the problem of patient motion, another argument in favor of direct coronal CT. In order to illustrate the anatomy of a coronal cross section of a recumbent patient, i.e., the anatomical display to be expected from MPR, Fig. 10b shows an anatomical cut along the line indicated in Fig. 10a. When the patient bends slightly forward, as in the case with our positioning technique, the lordotic parts of the cervical and lumbar spine are stretched, as shown in Fig. 11a.

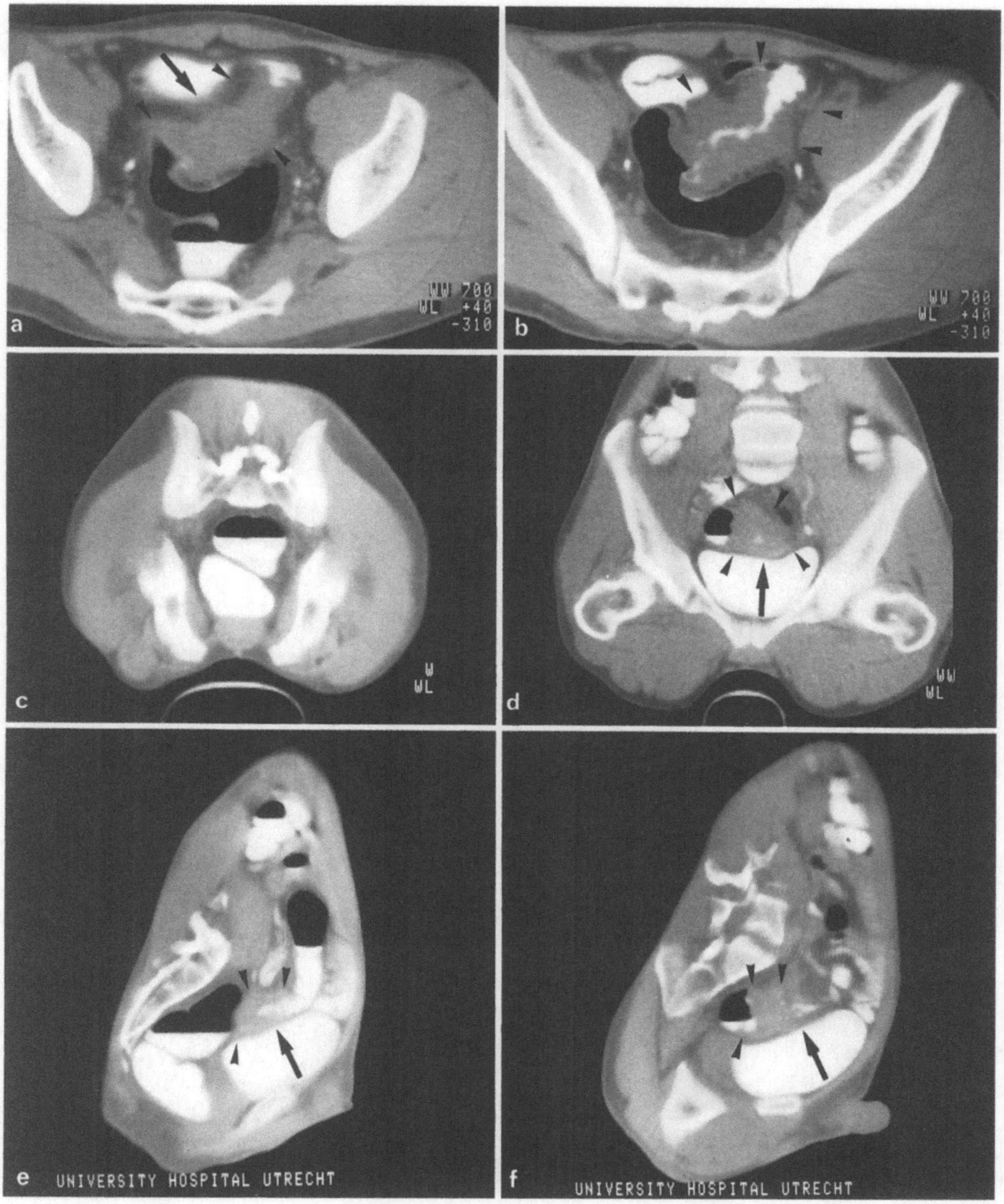

Fig. 5a–f. Staging of carcinoma involving the rectosigmoid junction (Case 1). Positions A and D. **a** Due to the partial volume effect, infiltration of the bladder dome (*arrow*) by the tumor (*arrowheads*) cannot be excluded. **b** The lumen of the rectosigmoid junction is almost totally stenosed due to intrinsic growth of the tumor (*arrowheads*). **c** Direct coronal CT reveals the normal outlines of pelvic diaphragm, external anal sphincter, and rectum. Note large mucosal fold. **d** Direct coronal CT demonstrates that the bladder dome (*arrow*) has not been infiltrated by the carcinoma (*arrowheads*). **f** Direct sagittal CT demonstrates the carcinoma (*arrowheads*) in its full length and the interface with the bladder dome (*arrow*). No obvious infiltration

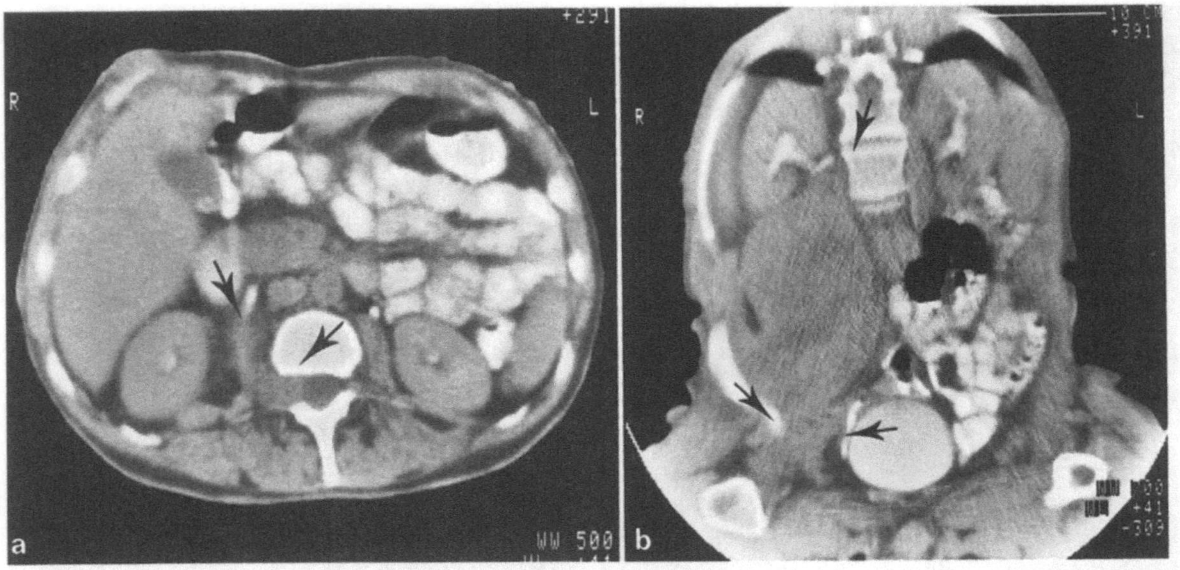
+291
R
L
a
WW 500
+391
R
L
b

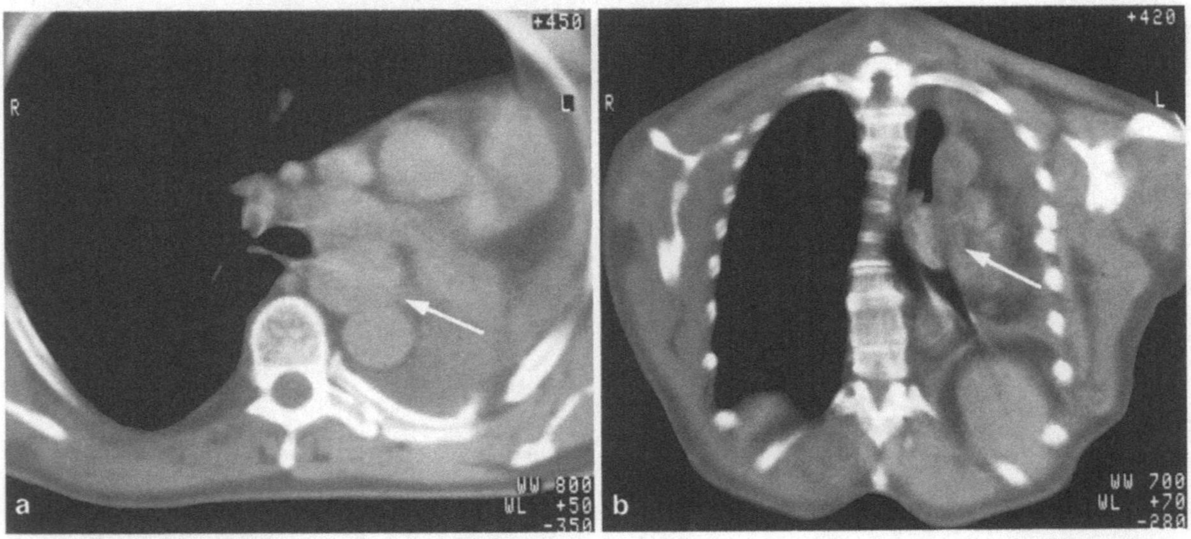
+450
R
a
WW 800
WL +50
-350
+420
R
L
b
WW 700
WL +70
-280

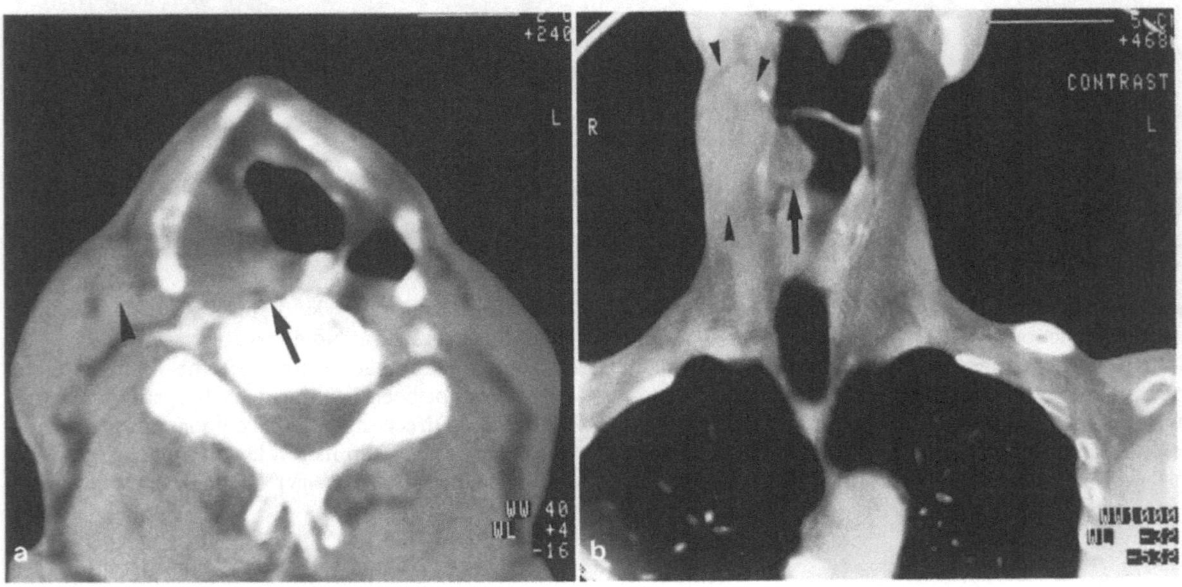
+240
L
a
WW 40
WL +4
-16
CONTRAST
R
L
b

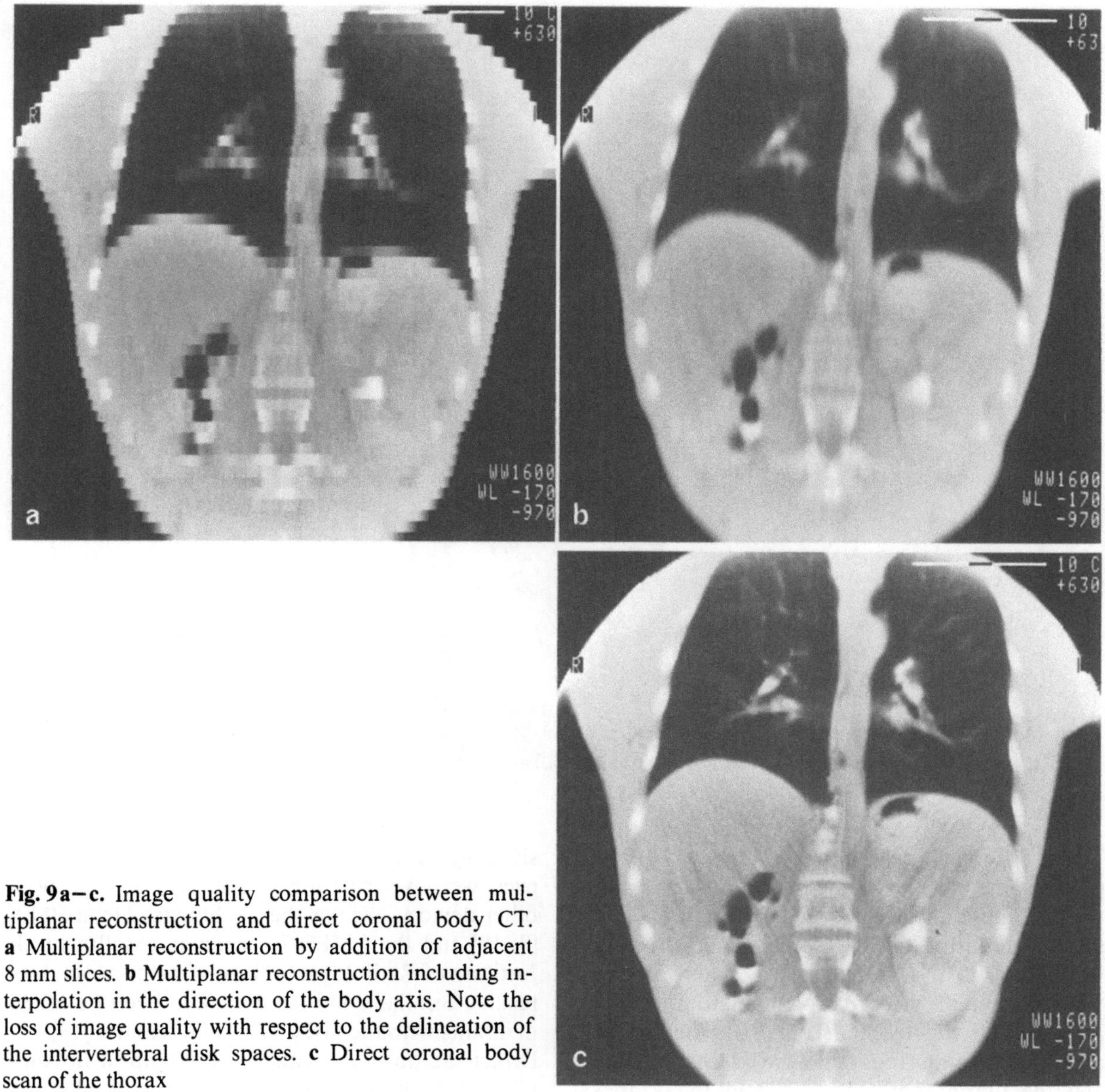

Fig. 9a–c. Image quality comparison between multiplanar reconstruction and direct coronal body CT. **a** Multiplanar reconstruction by addition of adjacent 8 mm slices. **b** Multiplanar reconstruction including interpolation in the direction of the body axis. Note the loss of image quality with respect to the delineation of the intervertebral disk spaces. **c** Direct coronal body scan of the thorax

Fig. 6a, b *(Above).* Malignant schwannoma originating from the nerve root at the level of the second and third lumbar vertebrae (Case 2). Position A. **a** Note the widened foramen and the biliary stone. **b** One single direct coronal CT reveals the origin of the tumor and its infiltration of the iliopsoas muscle and protrusion into the thigh (*arrows*)

Fig. 7a, b *(Middle).* Recurrent carcinoma of the left bronchus (Case 3). Position B. **a** The recurrence (*arrow*) is located behind the left pulmonary artery. **b** Coronal CT demonstrates the extent within the aortic window

Fig. 8a, b *(Below).* Supraglottic carcinoma with lymph node involvement (Case 4). Position C. **a** The piriform recess is totally obscured by the tumor (*arrow*). Note the swollen lymph node (*arrowhead*). **b** Coronal CT shows the true extent (*arrow*) and the nodal involvement (*arrowheads*) of this malignancy

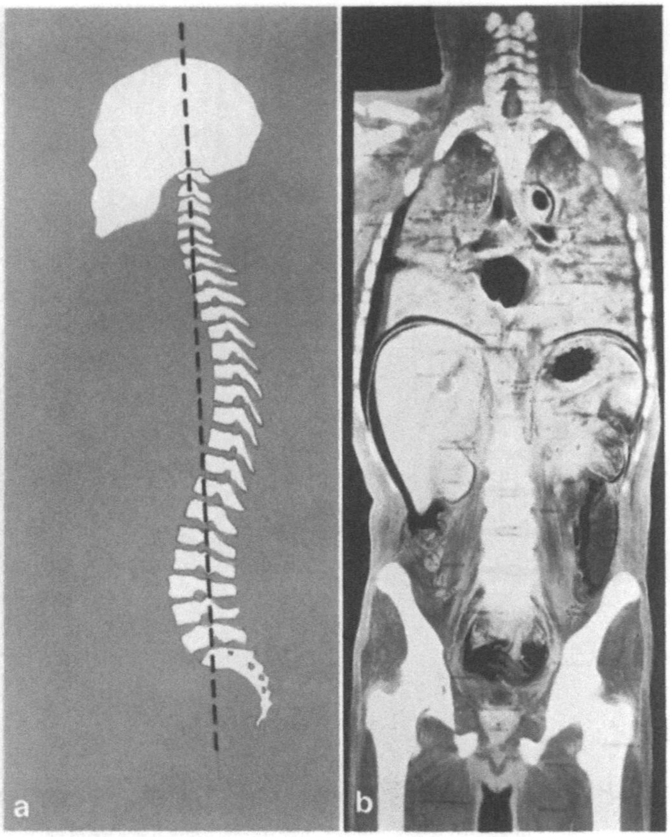

Fig. 10 a, b. The problem of imaging an S-shaped spine in one coronal plane. **a** Schematic diagram of a coronal plane traversing the S-shaped spine in the recumbent body. **b** Radiography of an anatomical coronal section of a frozen corpse (courtesy of P. E. Billimoria, M.D., and colleagues, Loma Linda University, California). Due to the kypholordotic curvature of the spine, a coronal section (**b**) and coronal reformatting (**a**) will result in images of a plane obliquely traversing spine, musculature, and viscera

Three different lines demonstrate how segments of the spine can be scanned in the exact coronal plane. Figure 11 b shows a combination of two scans demonstrating the spinal canal from the level of T6 to the first coccygeal body. Detailed visualization of direct coronal anatomy can be achieved for the trachea (Fig. 8 b), the thoracic and lumbar spine (Fig. 11 b), the descending aorta and the diaphragm (Fig. 9 c), and the kidneys, ureters, and psoas muscle (Fig. 6 b).

Patient throughput plays an important role in the cost effectiveness of a CT department. Direct coronal CT of the body markedly improves patient throughput by decreasing examination time. This is particularly true in cases with lesions of large dimensions in which a great number of axial transverse scans would be needed and also in patients in whom coronal scans are a must (e.g., certain lesions of the vertebral column). Here the MPR coronal images would be excessively time consuming.

The technique of direct coronal body CT was developed on the Philips Tomoscan 300 and 310, which have a large, deep conic aperture and a modified, reinforced rear side (thickness 10 mm). These features proved to be ideal for patient positioning in direct coronal CT of the torso. However, we have tried direct coronal body CT with other devices, such as the Technicare Delta 50 FS [8, 18] and the EMI 7070 scanners (Mallinckrodt Institute of Radiology, St. Louis) with satisfactory results. Similar good studies have been obtained in infants with the GE CT/T 8800 scanner [13].

Direct sagittal views can be very helpful in complicated cases, when midline or parasagittal structures are involved. In staging of carcinoma of the rectum, bladder, or reproductive system, defining the degree of local infiltration can be difficult due to partial volume effects and/or minimal interfaces (Fig. 5).

The oblique sagittal view has proved to facilitate the analysis of diseases affecting the dorsal or ventral side of the kidneys.

Positioning can be difficult in disabled or arthrotic patients. In order to obtain a true direct sagittal view, it is mandatory that the patients can rotate their lumbar spine and pelvis in a true lateral way into the gantry and can bend the thoracic spine and chest obliquely outward. The comfort in this positioning technique could be increased by constructing CT scanners with a shallower gantry cone and/or wider aperture.

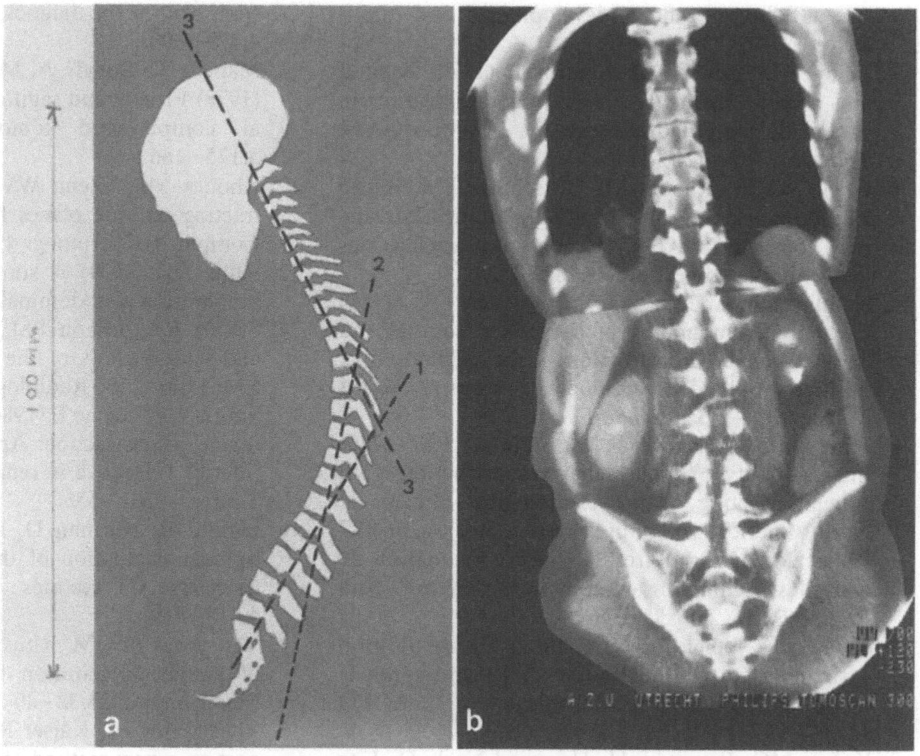

Fig. 11 a, b. Imaging the spine in the coronal plane by means of proper body flexion. **a** The three positioning possibilities for direct coronal imaging of *1* pelvis including retroperitoneal space and lower abdomen, *2* upper abdomen and lower chest, and *3* upper chest including neck and posterior fossa. **b** This combination of two direct coronal CT scans of a sitting patient 6 feet 3 inches (1.90 m) tall shows the spinal canal from the level of T6 to the upper coccy

Summary

Three patient position techniques have been developed for direct coronal CT covering the complete torso: position A, to study the pelvis including the retroperitoneal space and lower abdomen; position B, to study the upper abdomen and lower chest; and position C, to study the upper chest including the neck and posterior fossa. In comparison with MPR, direct coronal CT has three basic advantages: (a) image quality is improved as a result of a lack of partial volume averaging and patient motion disturbance; (b) the direct coronal planes can be truly parallel to the spinal axis, due to stretching of the lordotic segments of the spine; and (c) examination time is reduced, since a large number of overlapping slices and time-consuming MPR are not required. Direct coronal CT of the body has been carried out in more than 1500 cases and was often uniquely informative. Direct sagittal CT is extremely helpful in the region of the pelvis and lower abdomen and is obtained by position D, seating the patient sideways directly against the reinforced side of the gantry with the legs on each side. In our institution, the use of MPR CT is now restricted to small lesions and disabled patients.

Acknowledgments. We gratefully acknowledge the valuable suggestions of Carlo Panhuyzen, engineer, and Anneke Hamersma, head CT technician, on increasing patient comfort during positioning; the realization of the direct coronal body scans on the EMI 7070 scanner by R. J. Stanley, M.D. and B. L. McLennan, M.D. of the Mallinckrodt Institute, St. Louis; and the considerations concerning the direct sagittal body CT scans by Dr. R. Blümm of the University of Bochum.

References

1. Anderson RE, Koehler PR (1979) An accessory patient table for multidirectional CT scanning. Radiology 130:802–803
2. Federle MP, Moss AA, Boyd DP, Royal ST (1979) Coronal and sagittal reconstructions using a 4.8 sec-

ond CT body scanner: developments and applications. AJR 133:625–632

3. Foley WD, Lawson TL, Quiroz F (1979) Sagittal and coronal image reconstruction: application in pancreatic computed tomography. J Comput Assist Tomogr 4:717–721
4. Glenn WV Jr, Rhodes ML, Altschuler EM, Wiltse LL, Kostanek C, Kuo YM (1979) Multiplanar display computerized body tomography applications in the lumbar spine. Spine 4:282–323
5. Hamlin DJ, Cockett ATK, Burgener FA (1981) Computed tomography of the pelvis: sagittal and coronal image reconstruction in the evaluation of infiltrative bladder carcinoma. J Comput Assist Tomogr 5:27–33
6. Johnson GA, Korobkin M, Breiman RS (1980) Image quality in multiplanar reconstruction. 66th Annual Meeting of the Radiological Society of North America, "Work in Progress" Session, pp 497
7. Kaiser MC, Veiga Pires JA (1980) Evaluation de nouvelles techniques en tomodensitométrie. Ann Radiol (Paris) 23/7:559–563
8. Kaiser MC, Veiga Pires JA (1981) Sitting position variation of direct longitudinoaxial (semi coronal) mode in CT-scanning (technical note). ROFO 134:97–99
9. Kaiser MC, Petterson H, Harwood-Nash D, Fitz CR, Armstrong E (to be published) Direct coronal CT mode of spine in infants. Am J Neuroradiol
10. Lancourt JE, Glenn WV Jr, Wiltse LL (1979) Multiplanar computerized tomography in the normal spine and in the diagnosis of spinal stenosis. Spine 4:379–390
11. Manelfe C, Bonafé A, Morel C, Sancier A, Treil J (1978) Frontal and sagittal reconstructions in cranial computerised tomography. J Neuroradiol 5:175–186
12. Rhodes ML, Glenn WV, Azzawi YM (1980) Extracting oblique planes from serial CT sections. J Comput Assist Tomogr 4:649–657
13. Ruijs JHJ (1979) A simple procedure for patient preparation in abdominal CT. AJR 133:551
14. Schulz RA, Joseph PM, Hilal SK (1977) Frontal and lateral views of the brain reconstructed from EMI axial slices. Radiology 125:701–710
15. Smith WP, Levine E (1980) Sagittal and coronal CT image reconstruction: Application in assessing the inferior vena cava in renal cancer. J Comput Assist Tomogr 4:531–535
16. Unsöld R, Norman D, Berninger W (1980) Multiplanar evaluation of the optic canal from axial transverse CT sections. J Comput Assist Tomogr 4:418–419
17. Van Waes PFGM, Ruijs JHJ (1979) Some aspects of patient preparation for abdominal CT scans. Medicamundi 24:38–40
18. Veiga Pires JA, Kaiser MC (1980) Preliminary report on a new method of whole body CT scanning. Computerized Tomography 3:221–224
19. Veiga Pires JA, Kaiser MC (1980) Preliminary report on a new mode of CT scanning of the thorax. Comput Tomogr 4:139–143

Percutaneous Extraction of Gallstones and Other Interventional Techniques Using the T-Tube Tract

H. J. Burhenne

Department of Radiology, University of British Columbia and Vancouver General Hospital, 855 West 12th Avenue Vancouver, British Columbia V5Z, 1M9, Canada

General Considerations

Access to the biliary tract for interventional procedures follows one of three routes: retrograde via gastrointestinal endoscopy, anterograde through the liver, or through the postoperative drainage tract. The latter or subhepatic approach is less time consuming and less technically demanding than the transhepatic or endoscopic procedures (Fig. 1).

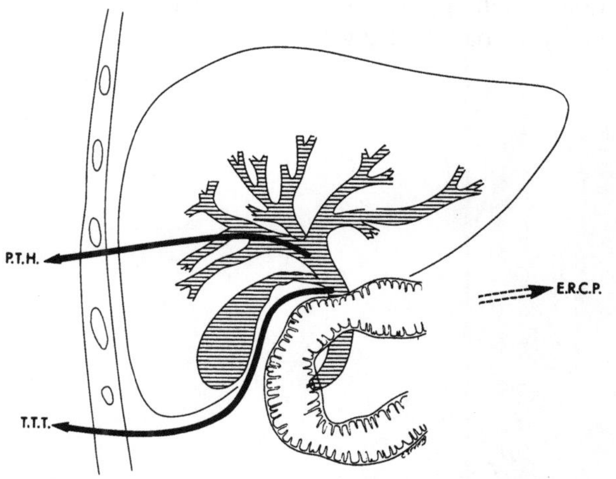

Fig. 1. Access routes to the biliary tract for interventional techniques. *P.T.H.*, percutaneous transhepatic route; *T.T.T.*, postoperative through the T-tube tract; *E.R.C.P.*, endoscopic retrograde approach

In 1972 the availability of a steerable catheter [1] made postoperative instrumentation of the biliary tract practical as a radiologic procedure. It is applicable to patients with indwelling tubes after surgery on the biliary tract and has significant diagnostic and therapeutic advantages. The complication rate is markedly low when compared to that of reoperation, the alternative [5]. The postoperative sinus tract is used for access to the biliary tract for the following procedures:

1. Nonoperative extraction of retained stones from extrahepatic or intrahepatic bile ducts [14]
2. Extraction of gallbladder stones through cholecystostomy tracts [2]
3. Transcholecystic removal of common bile duct stones [13]
4. Stricture dilatation [3, 4]
5. Internal biliary drainage [6]
6. Biopsy [2]
7. Reinsertion of drainage tubes [10]

Postoperative subhepatic interventional procedures through the surgical drainage tract are usually done without anesthesia and in the ambulatory patient. It requires about 4–5 weeks for the drainage tract to mature with a good fibrous reaction surrounding the surgical tube. The tract is easily negotiated with a steerable catheter at that time. Earlier postoperative procedures usually require initial placement of a guide wire through the drainage tube.

There exists the possibility of excessive radiation to the radiologist's fingers during prolonged interventional procedures [8]. Proper precautions include:

1. Fingers outside the primary beam
2. Collimation to the smallest possible field, preferably 3×5 cm
3. Under-table X-ray tube
4. Lead apron with window draped over the patient
5. Moving of instruments between fluoroscopies as much as possible

Nonoperative Extraction of Retained Stones from Extrahepatic or Intrahepatic Ducts

Stone retention in the bile ducts after bile duct surgery continues to be a problem, even with the routine use of choledochoscopy and operative

Radiology Today 2. Ed. by F. H. W. Heuck and M. W. Donner

cholangiography. Until recently, reexploration was required for removal of retained bile duct stones, but this second operation, which carries a higher mortality and morbidity than the initial procedure, can now be avoided through the use of interventional radiologic techniques. The technique of radiologic intervention for retained stone removal has been well described [6, 11, 16].

We have recommended that surgeons use routinely at least a 14F T tube after common duct exploration [2], thus permitting insertion of the 13F steerable catheter for interventional instrumentation. If 10F T tubes or smaller are indwelling, we first dilate the sinus tract [7].

Retained stones or fragments measuring 3–4 mm may pass spontaneously through the distal common duct into the duodenum. This is facilitated if the T tube is clamped or the intraductal fluid pressure raised. Saline infusions are satisfactory for this purpose. Small stones may also be expelled into the duodenum with the use of the catheter [12].

After insertion of the steerable catheter through the sinus tract, its tip is manipulated to the stone and the retrieval basket is opened distally to it. The open basket should ideally touch the walls of the duct, in order to engage stones readily on withdrawal. Baskets are available in three different sizes. After stone engagement by the basket, the entire assembly is slowly but continuously withdrawn through the sinus tract. We no longer try to close the basket over the stone after engagement, as this often results in fragmentation and prolongs the extraction procedure (Fig. 2).

However, stones of more than 10 mm usually require fragmentation. The stone is first engaged and extracted as far as the junction of bile duct and sinus tract. Strong traction on the basket is then needed for fragmentation. The wires of the basket are sufficiently sharp to accomplish this.

Impacted stones at the distal end of the common duct require a variety of maneuvers for successful extraction [6]. If basket engagement of distally impacted stones is difficult, another maneuver to mobilize and engage distal common duct stones employs the Fogarty balloon catheter. The balloon is inflated with contrast for fluoroscopic visualization just distally to the stone. Gentle traction is then applied to move the stone more proximally for basket engagement.

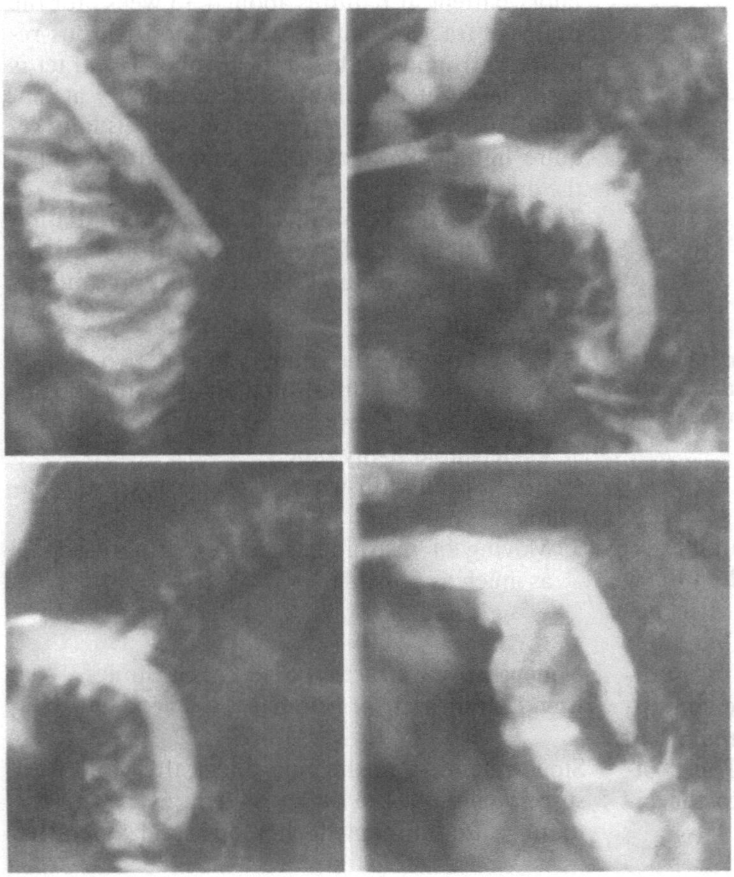

Fig. 2. Removal of 3-mm retained common duct stone through the T-tube tract. *Top left:* the steerable catheter is advanced beyond the stone. *Top right:* the stone is engaged in the basket. *Bottom left:* the stone is extracted through the sinus tract. *Bottom right:* normal common duct after stone removal

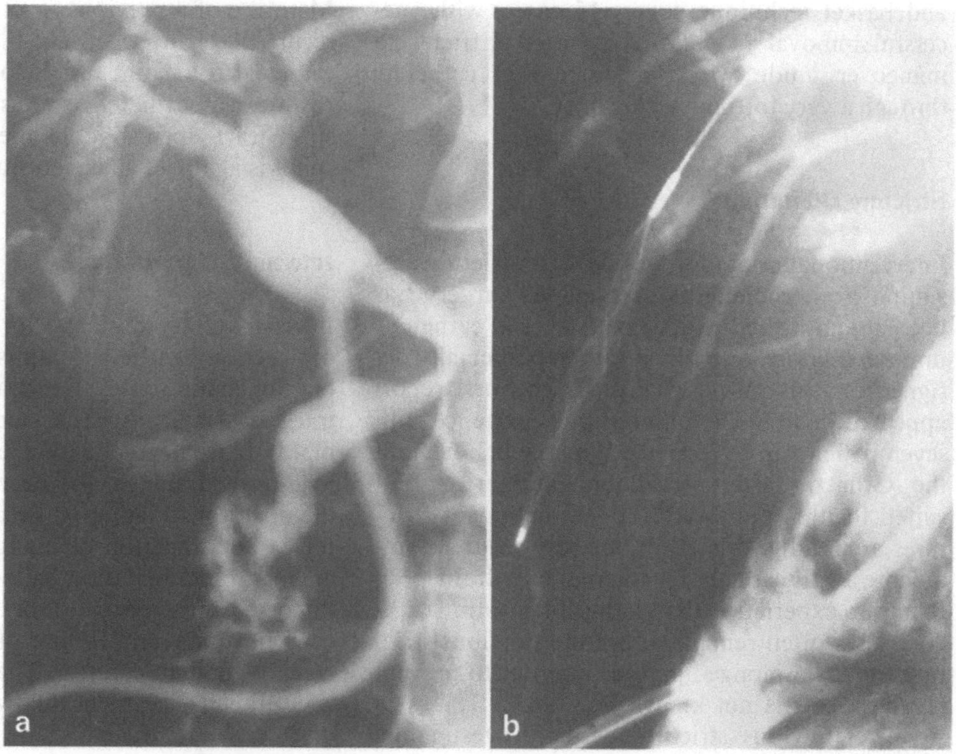

Fig. 3. a Multiple retained stones in dorsocaudal branch of left hepatic duct. **b** Basket in place after completion of stone extraction

The maneuver with the Fogarty balloon catheter may also be required for extraction of impacted intrahepatic stones. If stones are seen in hepatic radicles on postoperative cholangiography, however, a wait-and-see attitude will usually permit a more distal movement of the stone. It is easier to extract the stones from an extrahepatic position. Multiple interventional sessions may be required in patients with complicated or multiple retained stones (Fig. 3).

Our experience now comprises attempted stone extractions in 1125 patients, with a success rate of 96%. This implies that all stones have been removed successfully as demonstrated on careful cholangiography. Failure to remove retained stones usually involves patients with multiple impacted intrahepatic stones, where stone mobilization from small hepatic radicles is impossible.

Our morbidity amounted to 5%, with post-extraction fever, sepsis, pancreatitis, vasovagal reaction, and subhepatic bile collection. No perforation of the bile ducts occurred, but perforation of the sinus tract was present in seven patients. All patients were placed on antibiotics and all signs and symptoms disappeared after 48 h of treatment. We now place patients on antibiotic therapy before instrumentation if there is a history of previous pancreatitis or if instrumentation of impacted intrahepatic stones is to be attempted [5].

Nonoperative stone removal as a interventional radiologic procedure through the postoperative sinus tract carries a significantly higher success rate and lower complication rate than other methods, such as endoscopic procedures or stone dissolution techniques.

Extraction of Gallbladder Stones Through Cholecystostomy Tract

If stones remain in the gallbladder after cholecystostomy, access with a steerable catheter is gained postoperatively through the drainage tract. Stones may be removed with the basket technique or with forceps. The cholecystostomy tract may require enlargement with the use of angiographic dilatation balloons.

Access through postoperative cholecystostomy tracts may also be utilized to remove retained common duct stones. Instruments are manipulated through the cystic duct into the common duct [13]. Our experience of transcholecystic removal of common duct stones with the steerable catheter and basket technique covers 15 cases, with successful removal in eight. It is often difficult to maneuver guide wires and steerable catheters through a very tortuous cystic duct.

Stricture Dilatation

Interventional dilatation of bile duct strictures resulting from cholangitis or previous surgery has been accomplished with coaxial arterial catheters, ureteral dilators, or balloon catheters specially designed for this purpose (Fig. 4). The first report appeared in 1974 [2], followed by experience with seven patients in 1975 [3, 4]. We now believe that the Grüntzig arterial balloon catheter is best suited for this purpose [7]. Even malignant strictures are readily dilated in one session to accommodate a 14F catheter for internal bile drainage.

It is our experience that indwelling splint catheters must often remain within the previous stricture site for prolonged periods in order to prevent recurrence. It is not known how long it takes to stabilize previous strictures. Other investigators have had good results from a single dilatation procedure [16].

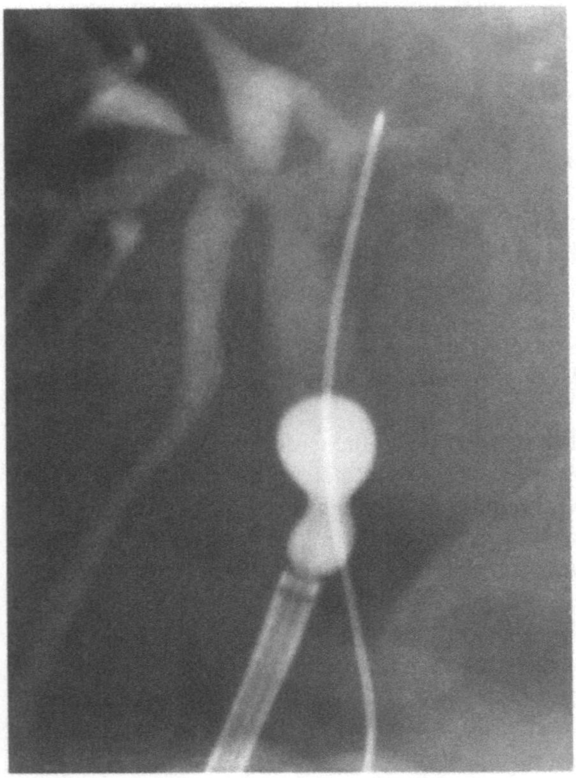

Fig. 4. Balloon catheter inflated with contrast during dilatation of hepatojejunostomy stricture

Maturing of a previous stricture site and possible recurrence can be checked by withdrawing the catheter to a point just below the previous narrowing. The catheter remains in place to keep the sinus tract open. Should the stricture recur, the splint is again advanced through it.

Internal Biliary Drainage

Internal biliary drainage for relief of malignant obstruction can be accomplished by transhepatic or subhepatic routes, but drainage through sinus tracts is technically easier and has the advantages of (a) placement of larger catheters with better long-term drainage, (b) decrease in exposure of the operator to radiation because of easier access, (c) easier dilatation of malignant strictures with angiographic dilatation balloons [7], (d) less likelihood of inadvertent tube removal, (e) fewer complications, and (f) use of softer rubber catheters for patient comfort. The technique of drainage catheter placement follows the same sequence of steerable catheter, guide wire, balloon dilatation, and catheter insertion with side holes above and end holes below the malignant stricture (Fig. 5).

Biopsy

Biopsy specimens of lesions in the biliary tract can be obtained by the subhepatic approach, using the postoperative sinus tract [3, 4]. The biopsy forceps employed with a bronchial or duodenal fiberscope had been successfully used for this purpose [15].

After cholangiographic identification of the filling defect in the bile duct, the steerable catheter is moved so that its tip is directly on the lesion. The endoscopic biopsy forceps is then moved through the steerable catheter and the biopsy specimen is obtained under fluoroscopic control. The technique is applicable for biliary masses in hepatic and extrahepatic ducts, including carcinoma of the pancreas involving the distal common duct. Our experience of biopsy through the subhepatic approach now comprises 18 patients. No bleeding or perforation has resulted.

Reinsertion of Drainage Tubes

Indwelling tubes may require reinsertion because of dislodgement or inadvertent extraction or re-

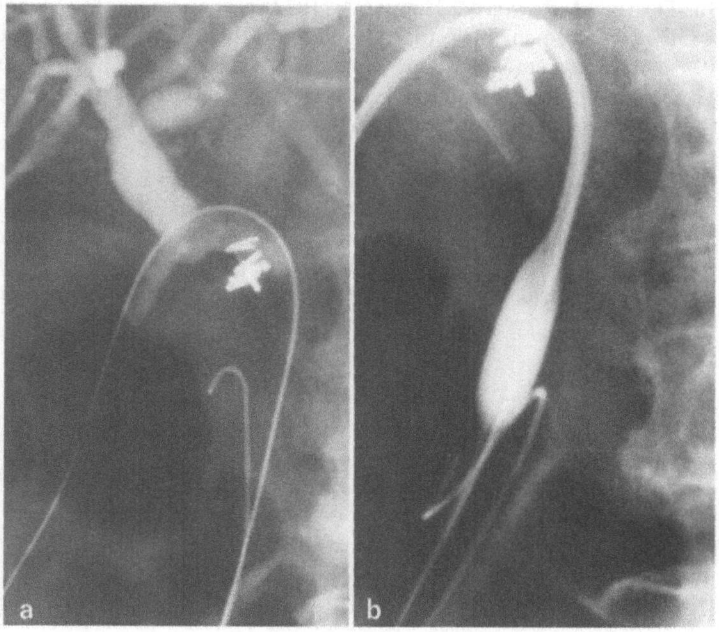

Fig. 5. a A guide wire has been placed through the malignant common duct stricture due to carcinoma of the pancreas using a postoperative T-tube tract for access. **b** The malignant stricture is dilated with an angiographic balloon catheter prior to placement of an internal drainage catheter through the sinus tract into the duodenum

placement because of obstruction by encrustation of bile sediment. This can be accomplished with the Seldinger technique [10], with the use of the steerable catheter, over a guide wire [9], or over a stiffer Teflon dilator [17].

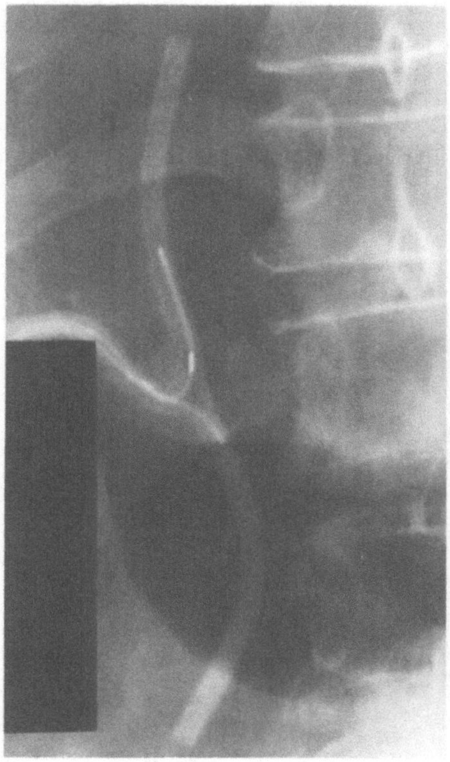

Fig. 6. T-tube exchange over two guide wires

We find insertion of T tubes easier with the use of two guide wires. Separate guide wires are placed through the T tube tract into the proximal and distal bile duct. The two shorter arms of the T tube are then inserted one over each guide wire and both guide wires are fed through the long arm of the T tube (Fig. 6).

References

1. Burhenne HJ (1972) Extraktion von Residualsteinen der Gallenwege ohne Reoperation. ROFO 117:425–428
2. Burhenne HJ (1974) Nonoperative roentgenologic instrumentation technics of the postoperative biliary tract. Am J Surg 128:111–117
3. Burhenne HJ (1975) Dilatation of biliary tract strictures. Radiol Clin 44:153–159
4. Burhenne HJ (1975) Bile duct biopsy with the stone extraction basket. Radiol Clin 44:178–181
5. Burhenne HJ (1976) Complications of nonoperative extraction of retained common duct stones. Am J Surg 131:260–262
6. Burhenne HJ (1980) Percutaneous extraction of retained biliary tract stones: 661 patients. AJR 134:888–898
7. Burhenne HJ, Morris DC (1980) Biliary stricture dilatation: use of the Grüntzig balloon catheter. J Can Assoc Radiol 31:196–197
8. Cruikshank JG, Fraser GM, Law J (1980) Finger doses received by radiologists during Chiba needle percutaneous cholangiography. Br J Radiol 53:584–585
9. Crummy AB, Turnipseed WD (1977) Percutaneous replacement of a biliary T tube. AJR 128:869–870

10. Dorsey TJ, Rowen M, Hepps SA (1972) Nonoperative replacement of T tube in common duct after inadvertent removal. Surgery 71:97–98
11. Ferrucci JT, Wittenberg J (1981) Interventional radiology of the abdomen. Williams & Wilkins, Baltimore
12. Lamis PA (1969) Retained common duct stones: a new nonoperative technique for treatment. Surgery 66:291–289
13. Mazzariello RM (1974) Transcholecystic extraction of residual calculi in common bile duct. Surgery 75:338–347
14. Mondet AF (1962) Tecnica de la extracction incruenta de los calculos en la litiasis residual del coledoco. Bol Soc Cir B Aires 46:278–290
15. Palayew MH, Stein L (1978) Postoperative biopsy of the common bile duct via the T tube tract. AJR 130:287–289
16. Ring EJ, McLean GK (1981) Interventional radiology. Little Brown, Boston
17. Sniderman KW, Baxi RK, Rumburg KN, Sos TA (1979) A modified technique for percutaneous insertion of a biliary T tube. Radiology 131:539–540

Mass Biopsy Using Ultrasound

R. C. Sanders

Department of Radiology and Radiological Science, The Johns Hopkins Medical Institutions, 601 N. Broadway, Baltimore, MD 21205, USA

Mass biopsy has reached a point where no accessible mass or organ in the body has not been subjected to percutaneous puncture using a small-bore needle [1, 2, 12]. Since morbidity is minimal, mass biopsy under ultrasound control is indicated under the following circumstances:

1. To confirm the diagnosis in a mass too extensive to resect, e.g., a carcinoma of the pancreas surrounding the superior mesenteric vein.
2. When in a patient with a previous neoplasm it is uncertain whether a new mass represents a metastatic lesion or a fresh primary.
3. When proof that a mass is a metastatic lesion is required prior to the commencement of a chemotherapy protocol.
4. When it is uncertain whether a mass represents a neoplasm, an abscess, or a hematoma; therapy for the latter two possibilities would be conservative rather than surgical and the ultrasonic and computed tomographic (CT) appearances can be identical.

The performance of the procedure varies depending on the site of the lesion. If the lesion is close to the skin with no intervening bowel or liver, a large-bore needle can be used and a cutting approach is employed. We commonly use a Truecut needle (16 gauge) which takes a large-core tissue specimen, as long as we are confident that no intervening bowel is present and, on the basis of an arteriogram or CT scan, that the lesion is hypovascular. If the lesion is vascular or there is intervening bowel or blood vessels in the region of the lesion, we use a 22-gauge needle. Such needles have been extensively investigated and there have been virtually no significant side effects with this small size [6]. There does not appear to be any significant difference between different needle tips in obtaining adequate specimens [11]. When a cutting needle is used, the needle is inserted into the mass and the mass is sliced to obtain a core of tissue. When a 22-gauge needle is used, aspiration techniques are employed. The needle is placed within the mass and, using negative pressure induced by a Camaco plunger, tissue is pulled into the needle. As the material is being aspirated, the needle is moved in and out and rotated within the suspect area. In a second approach the needle is moved slowly in a curved fashion while being inserted into the tissue.

When the needle is inserted into the tissue under ultrasonic control, several techniques can be employed to visualize its path. If it is inserted from an anterior approach, it can be seen with the transducer viewing from a lateral approach (or vice versa), providing it is inserted into sonographically homogeneous tissue such as liver or kidney at right angles to the transducer. This sort of approach is only available in the upper abdomen.

Various transducers are now available which allow one to see the needle as it is being inserted through the transducer or at an oblique axis alongside the transducer. The use of the B-scan transducer with a hole at the center has been more or less abandoned because the needle cannot be seen ultrasonically during insertion.

However, this technique has the advantage that one can plot the axis and depth of insertion in advance and maintain the correct oblique axis by putting the needle through the center of the transducer. Problems with the technique exist in that the inserted needle is held rigidly in place by the transducer and the needle target, so that laceration of tissues will occur if the patient moves. If the B-scan transducer is of the keyhole variety, the needle can be removed from the transducer while it is in the tissues, but because the keyhole allows some obliquity of the needle, insertion is less accurate. The system is cumbersome and difficult to use.

An alternative piece of equipment, which we use widely in the kidney and other organs which show respiratory motion, is the A-mode transducer with

Radiology Today 2. Ed. by F. H. W. Heuck and M. W. Donner

a central hole. This transducer is connected to the ultrasound system by a cable and can therefore move freely with the target organ. A-mode allows visualization of the needle tip within a fluid-filled structure such as a cyst or abscess, but unfortunately, the needle tip cannot be seen within solid masses. Needles smaller than 20 gauge are not visible at all with a 3.5-MHz transducer, but 18-gauge needle tips can be seen with a 2.25-MHz A-mode transducer.

In the past year several transducers have become available for needle biopsy using real time. Such transducers are either linear array or sector scanners. When a linear array aspiration system is used, some of the small transducers at the center of the linear array are removed and the needle is passed through this central slot. The obliquity can be varied by about 20°; needle visualization is easier when the needle enters at an oblique angle than when the axis is parallel to the ultrasound beam.

We have found with some practice that we can visualize a 22-gauge needle throughout its course with a 3.5-MHz linear array slotted transducer. Provided the needle tract lies directly in the beam path, one is able to see the passage of the needle; the larger the needle, the easier it is to see. Slotted transducers require the use of a very long needle, since the transducer itself adds about 4 cm to the distance from the skin surface. This is about double the extra distance that is needed if one uses an A-mode or B-scan aspiration transducer. A variant of the linear array aspiration transducer is now in use in the operating room; in this system there is a small cleft between the two components of the linear array. It is not as easy to trace the needle along its course with an operating room linear array, but the extra needle distance required is much less, so such a system may be easier to use.

Aspiration transducers for mechanical sector scanners have only recently been introduced. With these attachments, the needle enters the skin from an approximately 20° angle at a point lateral to the transducer. These systems are a little more cumbersome to use because of the increased needle insertion obliquity, but visualization of the needle appears to be of similar quality to that obtained with a linear array system. Sector scanner attachments are preferred for access to areas in the upper abdomen between ribs. We use such an attachment extensively in the investigation and placement of catheters within the biliary tract.

It is usually possible to see when the needle tip lies within a mass with modern real-time attachments. A useful method of confirming the biopsy site is to inject a small amount of air through the needle at the terminal pass. An echogenic spot is created within the mass if the location of the needle tip is correct [8].

There is no question that mass biopsy has made a major difference to the economic workup of patients with possible carcinoma of the pancreas. Mitty et al. [10] showed that fine-needle aspiration biopsy of the pancreas had an accuracy of about 85%–88%, sensitivity of 86%, and a specificity of 100% in 53 patients. Thirty laparotomies were avoided in 37 patients with positive biopsies, which they estimate to have saved about $170 000 in patient management. Similar results have been obtained from other series of mass biopsies, particularly in the pancreas and kidney.

Adequate percutaneous mass biopsy can only be performed if an expert cytopathologist is available. Cytopathology is a difficult art which requires a great deal of experience. We find it advantageous for the cytopathologist to be in the room at the time biopsy is performed so that he can analyze the frozen section to be certain that an adequate tissue specimen has been obtained. If he is not satisfied, we make repeated attempts until an adequate biopsy is obtained. Repeated passes with a 22-gauge or larger needle with a cutting technique are employed. The Rotex screw biopsy needle is often helpful if the 22-gauge Chiba, Greene, Madayag, or tumor biopsy needle has been ineffective. The Rotex screw biopsy needle has a 19-gauge outer lumen, but we have used it without complication in several examples of carcinoma of the pancreas.

Complications of aspiration techniques hardly ever occur, but a few have been recorded: pancreatitis with subsequent death [4], peritonitis, and two examples of tumor development in the biopsy tract [5, 7]. The complication rate is minute considering that thousands of biopsies have been performed. In one series of over 1000 biopsies, only two small incidental hematomas were found as complications [6]. Contraindications are almost nonexistent, but a severe hemorrhagic diathesis would be a reason for caution and it would be unwise to puncture a a possible pheochromacytoma. Pancreatitis, previously considered a contraindication, is now investigated with aspiration biopsy if the nature of the infecting bacteria is unknown. No evidence of fistula formation following the biopsy of pancreatitis or related lesions such as pancreatic pseudocysts has been found.

References

1. Barbaric ZL, MacIntosh PK (1981) Periureteral thin-needle aspiration biopsy. Urol Radiol 2:181–185
2. Berkowitz RS, Leavitt T, Knapp RC (1978) Ultrasound-directed percutaneous aspiration biopsy of periaortic lymph nodes in recurrence of cervical carcinoma. Am J Obstet Gynecol 131:906
3. Brinkley AB (1982) Mesenteric vascular gas secondary to ischemic bowel in transmesenteric hernia. Radiology 143:573
4. Evans WK, Chia SH, McLoughlin MJ, et al. (1981) Fatal necrotizing pancreatitis following needle aspiration biopsy of the pancreas. Radiology 141:61–62
5. Gibbons RP, Bush WH, Burnett LL (1977) Needle tract seeding following aspiration of renal cell carcinoma. J Urol 118:865–867
6. Holm HH, Pederson JF, Kristensen JK, et al. (1975) Ultrasonically guided percutaneous puncture. Radiol Clin North Am 13:493–503
7. Kim WS, Barth KH, Zimmer M (1982) Seeding of pancreatic carcinoma along the transhepatic catheter tract. Radiology 143:427–428
8. Lee TG, Knochel JQ (1982) Air as an ultrasound contrast marker for accurate determination of needle placement. Radiology 143:787–788
9. Mendley SJD, Wuilfsohn A, Efremidis SC, Mitty HA, Brendler H (1982) Lymphography and percutaneous lymph node biopsy in clinically localized carcinoma of the prostate. J Urol 127:695–698
10. Mitty HA, Efremidis SC, Yeh NC (1981) Inpact of fine-needle biopsy on management of patients with carcinoma of the pancreas. AJR 137:1119–1121
11. Wittenberg J, Mueller PR, Ferrucci JT et al. (1982) Percutaneous core biopsy of abdominal tumors using 22 gauge needles: Further observations. AJR 139:75–80
12. Yeh HC (1981) Percutaneous fine needle aspiration biopsy of intra-abdominal lesions with ultrasound guidance. Am J Gastroenterol 75:148–152

Percutaneous Nephrostomy in Obstructive Uropathy

R. Günther and P. Alken

Institut für Klinische Strahlenkunde, Universität Mainz, Langenbeckstrasse 1, 6500 Mainz, FRG

Since the original description by Goodwin in 1955, percutaneous nephrostomy (PNS) has assumed an important role in the management of obstructive uropathy. It was initially devised as an alternative to operative nephrostomy, but has now completely replaced the latter, for the following good reasons:

1. It can be done under local anesthesia.
2. It provides effective urinary drainage.
3. It carries an acceptable risk, with low morbidity and practically no mortality.

Percutaneous nephrostomy provides supravesical urinary diversion, as well as access for various endourologic manipulations of diagnostic or therapeutic nature. Therapeutic applications of percutaneous nephrostomy are:

1. Decompression in postrenal obstruction
2. Diversion in urinary fistulas
3. Endourologic manipulations

Technique

Basically there are two types of puncture technique for PNS, the Seldinger (catheter over guide wire) technique and the trocar technique.
The Seldinger technique uses a guide wire for catheter insertion [4, 9] whereas the trocar cannula permits direct introduction of a large-bore drainage tube without guide wire and further dilatation [7]. In an obstructed pyelocaliceal system the two techniques give identical results. In the absence of dilatation, however, fine-needle puncture and subsequent catheter insertion by the Seldinger technique seems to be more advantageous. The method used by us is depicted in Fig. 1. The fine-needle technique has the following advantages:

1. It permits several puncture attempts without major damage to the kidney.
2. Puncture of the nondilated pyelocaliceal system is facilitated.

The preferred catheter for initial decompression is a 5F PVC or polyethylene catheter. If pus or thick fluid must be drained an 8- to 10F catheter is used (Fig. 2).

Renal Localization

The methods available for localization of the kidney are (a) ultrasound, (b) fluoroscopy, and (c) computed tomography (CT). CT is basically unnecessary for localization of the kidney. The combination of real-time ultrasound guided puncture and fluoroscopic catheter placement can in our opinion not be bettered. In the absence of dilatation, additional intravenous contrast medi-

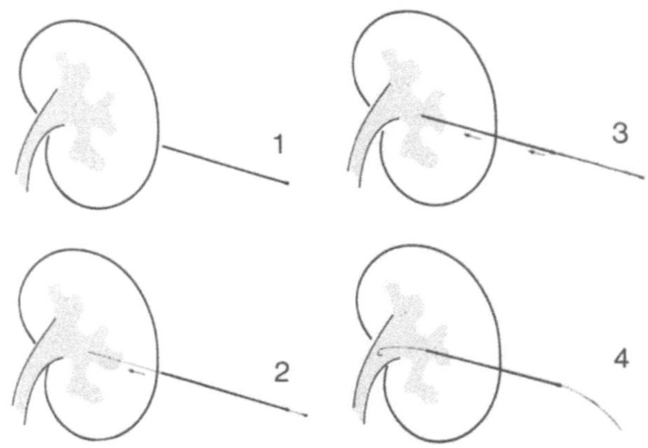

Fig. 1. The fine needle puncture technique of PNS. *1* Advancement of a short cannula (length 12 cm, OD 1.3 mm) to the perirenal space. *2* Long fine needle (length 21 cm, OD 0.7 mm) inserted through the cannula for puncture of the renal collecting system. *3* Following successful puncture, advancement of the shorter but larger bore outer cannula into the renal pelvis. *4* Replacement of the fine needle by a J guide wire (OD 1.0 mm) over which the drainage catheter is inserted

Radiology Today 2. Ed. by F. H. W. Heuck and M. W. Donner

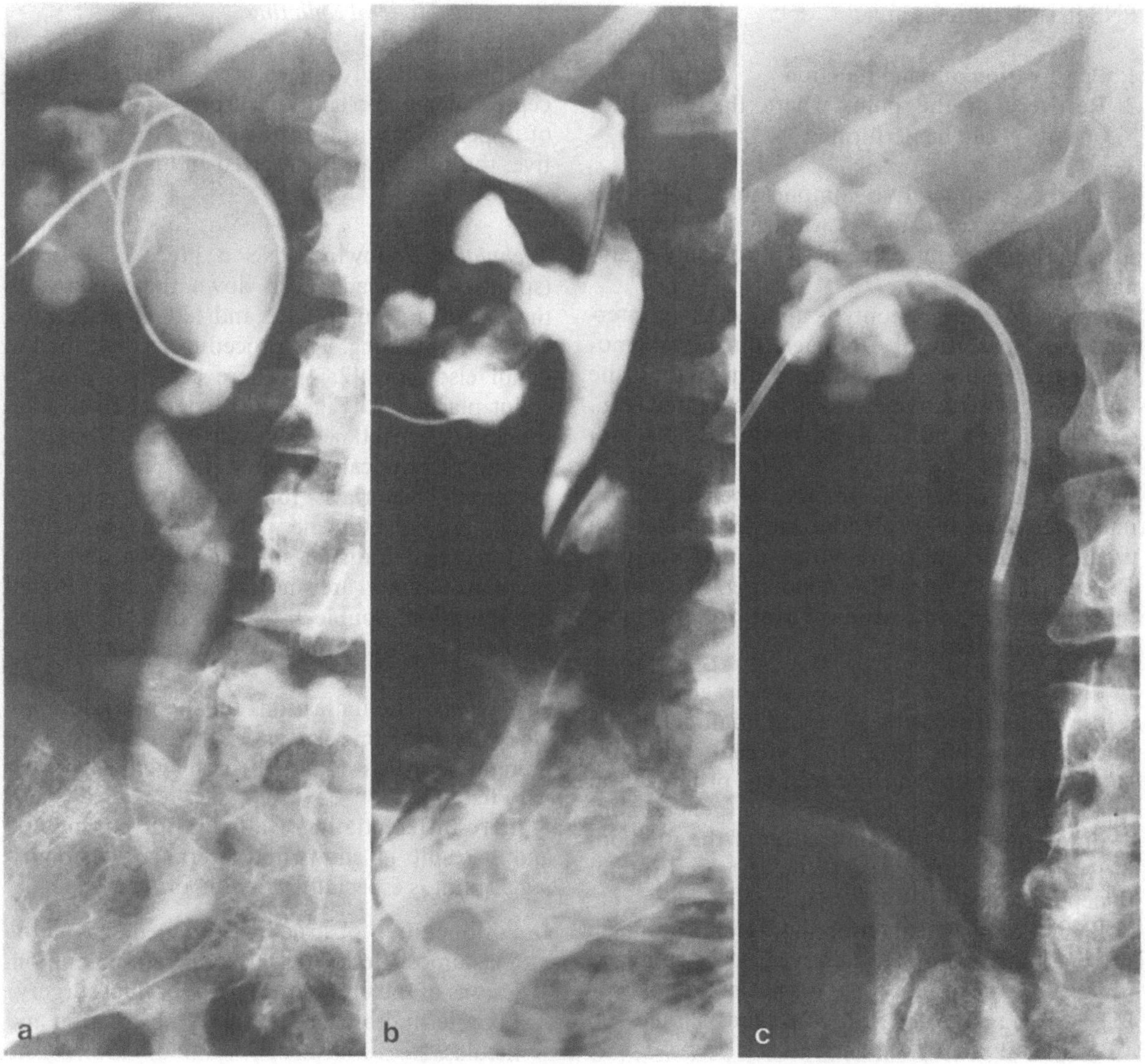

Fig. 2a–c. Possibilities of catheter placement in PNS. **a** Renal pelvis; **b** upper calix; **c** proximal ureter

um is administered for visualization of the pyelocaliceal system.

Patient Position

A variety of positions have been advocated for PNS in the literature, including prone, supine, lateral and supine oblique. The prone position is the one mostly employed, but if this is not tolerated by the patient the supine oblique position is used.

Puncture Success and Complications

Successful puncture can be achieved in more than 96% of cases irrespective of the method used (ultrasound or fluoroscopy). The rate of major complications amounts to 4%, bleeding being the main problem. In our series of more than 500 PNS procedures no deaths occurred.

Decompression in Postrenal Obstruction

Percutaneous nephrostomy can be applied as an emergency, intermediate, or palliative procedure. The original function of PNS was as an emergency decompression for severely ill patients with postrenal obstruction complicated by fever, septicemia, and uremia, which were the classic indications for operative nephrostomy. The aims of

PNS in such patients are:

1. Preservation of renal function
2. Recovery to the point where the definitive operation can be performed

Similarly, postoperative complications following upper urinary tract surgery (obstruction, leakage, urinoma) may require urgent nephrostomy drainage.
Percutaneous nephrostomy is applied as an intermediate measure for drainage during chemotherapy or radiotherapy, during which time the underlying obstructive disease can be treated (e.g., Crohn's disease, tuberculosis, Hodgkin's disease) [4].
In advanced pelvic malignancy, when operative intervention or surgical drainage techniques are unjustified or even contraindicated, PNS can preserve renal function for the remaining life span. In this connection, some words of caution concerning PNS seem justified:

1. The simplicity of PNS may encourage its overuse in patients with advanced malignant disease. However, PNS (or internal splinting) should not result in unnecessary prolongation of life. Intractable pains and poor general condition preclude the application of the method. Death in uremia would be more merciful than nephrostomy.
2. PNS is most valuable for short-term drainage. Long-term drainage, however, may result in chronic infection, stone formation, and progressive renal deterioration, and should be avoided if at all possible.

Management of Urinary Fistulas

Urinary fistulas due to intraoperative lesions or postoperative complications or secondary to a tumor can be managed percutaneously, either by external drainage or ureteral splinting. Small fistulas may dry up, but large fistulas usually require extensive operative reconstruction or, in inoperable cases, transrenal ureteral occlusion.

Endourologic Manipulations

Apart from drainage in obstruction and urinary fistulas, PNS offers a variety of catheter manipulations, the more important of which are discussed below.

Antegrade Ureteral Splinting

The cystoscopically placed ureteral splint is an accepted means for temporary or permanent relief of upper urinary tract obstruction. As an alternative, the splint can be inserted in antegrade fashion.

Technique. Following PNS a piece of catheter (splint/stent) is advanced down the ureter with the aid of a J guide wire and left in place after correct positioning. The procedure is described in detail elsewhere [2, 4]. There are two forms of splint placement (Fig. 3): (a) external fixation at the skin or subcutaneously and (b) indwelling.
In view of physical and biological properties, the preferred materials for short-term drainage splints are polyethylene, polyurethane, and PVC; for long-term drainage, silicone, Teflon, and polyurethane splints are more appropriate. Pigtail configuration, double-J, or Gibbon's splints may be useful to prevent migration or dislocation.

Indications. The indications for the procedure are generally the same as for PNS: (a) diversion in ureteral obstruction and (b) management of urinary fistulas.
A more differentiating evaluation of the method and its results [4] shows that internal diversion using a splint is especially valuable in:

1. Postoperative obstruction (e.g., edema at the anastomosis following ureteral reimplantation, lesions of the ureter during abdominal surgery)
2. Long-term drainage in urinary obstruction and fistulas.

In contrast to external urinary diversion, internal drainage by splinting has the following advantages:

1. No need for an external appliance
2. Lower infection rate

Complications. There are only minor complications in ureteral splinting, such as dislocation, incrustation, bending, and insufficient drainage. Infection is not uncommon in long-term drainage.

Percutaneous Catheter Extraction

Percutaneous nephrostomy enables management of complications caused by the procedure itself. If unsuitable catheter material is used a nephrostomy catheter can tear loose, and percutaneous retrieval is then the method of choice (Fig. 4). Simi-

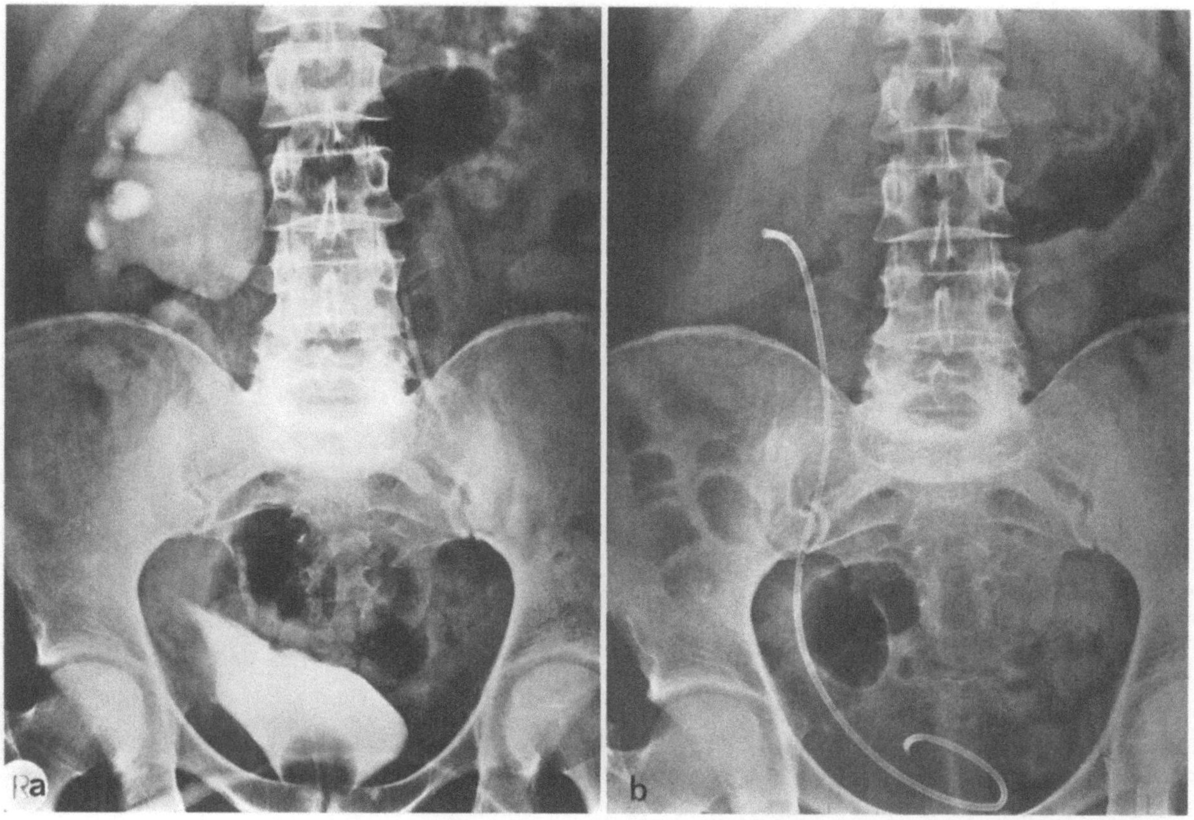

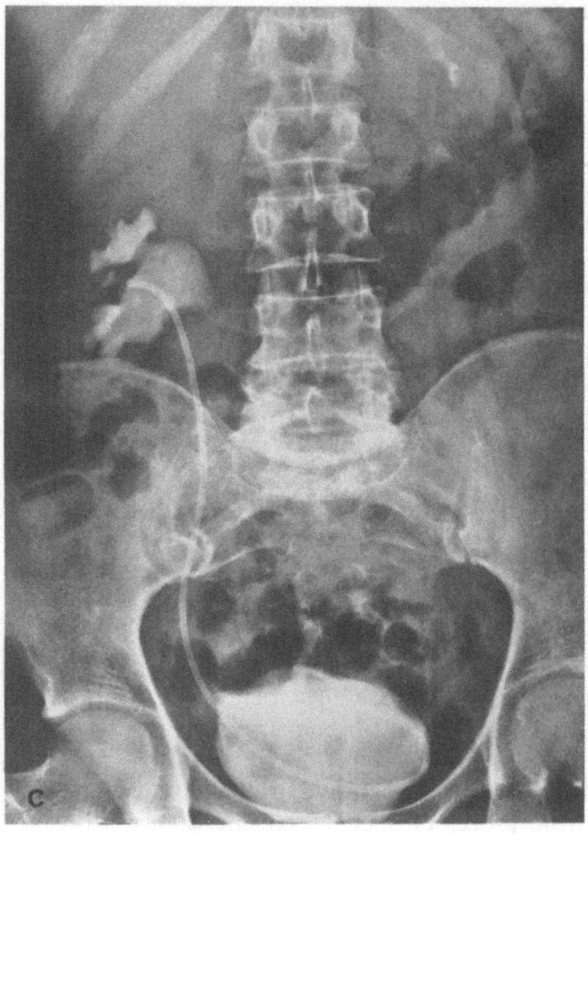

Fig. 3a–c. Antegrade ureteral splinting (indwelling splint) in postoperative stenosis following psoas-hitch-plasty. **a** Postoperative intravenous urogram showing obstruction on the right side. **b** Plain film of the antegrade inserted indwelling splint. **c** Intravenous urogram 5 months later confirms patency of the splint

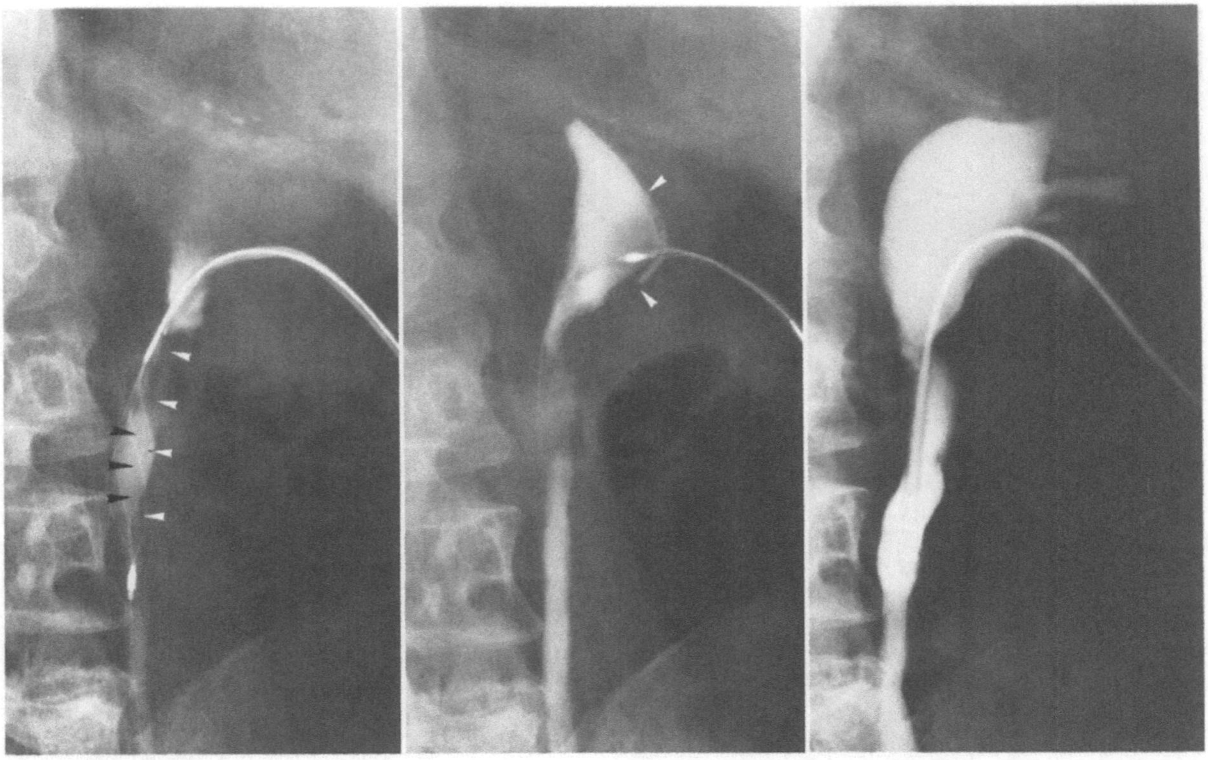

Fig. 4. Transrenal extraction of a broken nephrostomy tube. *Left:* Insertion of a Dormia basket for extraction of the nonradiopaque nephrostomy tube (*arrows*). *Middle:* Nephrostomy tube during retrieval. *Right:* Reinsertion of a nephrostomy tube after successful extraction

larly, obstructed internal splints may be removed by this approach if cystoscopy fails.

Following PNS a 9F Teflon catheter sleeve (length 20 cm) is inserted into the renal pelvis. The instrument for extraction is either a Dormia basket or a foreign-body-grasping forceps. The grasping forceps must be handled very cautiously to avoid perforation. To date no complications have been encountered as a consequence of this manipulation.

Percutaneous Ureteral Dilatation

Just as in percutaneous angioplasty, ureteral dilatation is performed using a Grüntzig balloon catheter via the transrenal approach. Indications are postoperative stenoses or chronic fibrotic strictures. While early postoperative stenoses may respond very well, fibrotic strictures are less suitable. Particularly unfavorable are long post-irradiation or postoperative strictures, as well as extrinsic processes such as retroperitoneal fibrosis [8].

Percutaneous Stone Manipulation

The percutaneous approach to the kidney allows stone manipulation without operation. The principal techniques are displacement, dissolution, extraction, mechanical fragmentation, and disintegration by ultrasound.

Dissolution. Stones amenable to dissolution by alkalinizing solution are urate and cystine calculi. Additional solvents for cystine calculi are acetylcysteine and Tham-E. Stones containing struvite and apatite can be dissolved by organic acids (Renacidin). If ureteral obstruction is present a double nephrostomy or U-loop nephrostomy is advisable. Close monitoring of creatinine and serum electrolytes is mandatory. Dissolution of stones may take from 10 to 30 days [6, 11].

Extraction. Stones not larger than the tube caliber can be extracted percutaneously with the aid of a Dormia basket, a snare or Randall forceps. A prerequisite is dilatation of the tract up to as much as 26F, depending on stone size. A steerable catheter may help to entrap the stones. No serious complications have been encountered by us or others [1, 3, 6].

Ultrasound Litholapaxy. Following PNS the tract is widened with a set of specially designed metal or Teflon dilators up to 27F. Initially, dilatation of the tract was performed in several sessions, but with increasing experience, dilatation and stone extraction are now carried out in one session. The method is thus an attractive alternative to operation (Fig. 5) [1].

Indications. General indications are stones in the upper urinary tract (renal collecting system, upper ureter):

1. Solitary stones in ideal position for extraction
2. Postoperative residual stones
3. Stones in patients with high surgical risk
4. Stones in patients with multiple previous operations; each additional operation increases the risk of loss of a kidney

Complications. The complication rate is low. In our series of more than 60 patients, bleeding was observed in two cases and treated conservatively. Further complications were one case each of pyelonephritis, extravasation, broken nephrostomy tube, and development of subpelvic stenosis. In view of the diversity of techniques the question arises of which method to use for which calculus. Our decision is influenced by safety, practicability, position and composition of the stone, and the time required for the procedure. Therefore dissolution is applied to readily dissolvable stones (urate, cystine). It should be noted, however, that the usual treatment for urate calculi without obstruction is peroral litholysis. In struvite or apatite stones an attempt at dissolution may be made for a reasonable period of time (2 weeks). The management of other stones depends on their size: stones up to the caliber of the nephrostomy tube are extracted, larger stones are disintegrated by ultrasound.

Transrenal Ureteral Occlusion

Transrenal ureteral occlusion is a new procedure for watertight closure of the ureter as a palliative measure in tumor patients [5].

Technique. Our original technique was embolization of the ureter, using the tissue adhesive butyl-2-cyanoacrylate and additional steel coil occlusion. This method proved to be effective for short-term occlusion, but in the long run 50% of the ureters became patent again. For this reason, ureteral occlusion using a detachable balloon was developed. A small rubber balloon filled with activated silicone is released in the distal ureter and reliably occludes the ureter if subsequent permanent external drainage is established (Fig. 6).

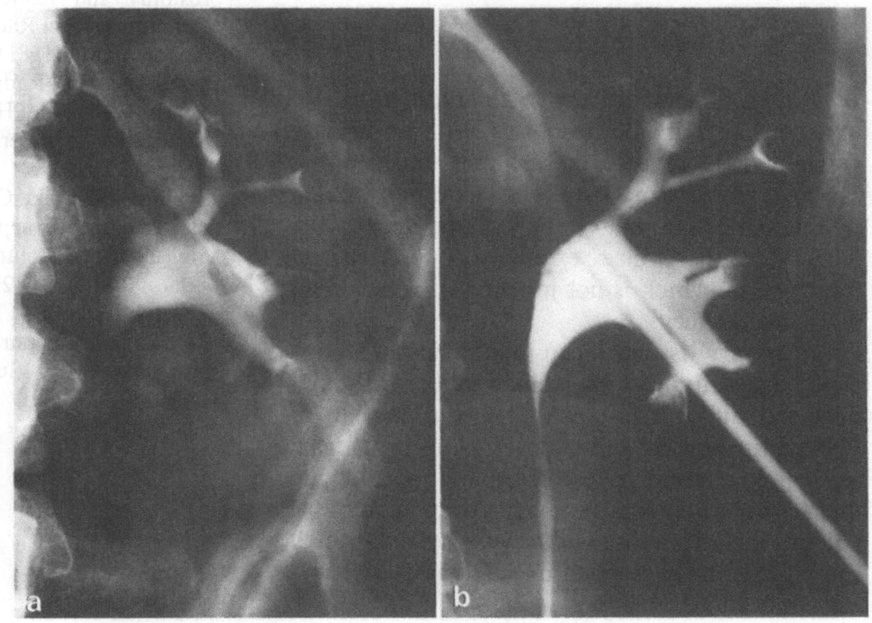

Fig. 5a, b. Percutaneous extraction of a stone from the renal pelvis: dilatation of the nephrostomy tract and stone extraction in one session. Hospital stay 4 days. **a** Intravenous urogram showing stone in the renal pelvis. **b** Following successful extraction of the stone, temporary reinsertion of a nephrostomy tube

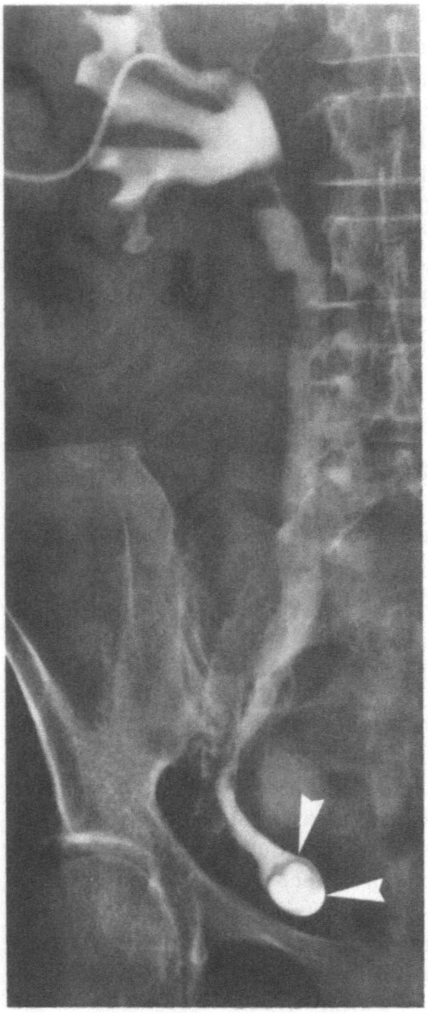

Fig. 6. Transrenal ureteral occlusion with a detachable balloon (*arrows*) filled with silicone. Indication: large vesicovaginal fistula due to local recurrence of a bladder tumor (69-year-old patient)

Indications. There are two main indications for transrenal ureteral occlusion: (a) a large urinary fistula and (b) severe dysuria in advanced pelvic cancer. Small urinary fistulas may be well treated by external or internal drainage; large urinary fistulas usually require extensive operative reconstruction, which is not justified in widespread pelvic malignancy.

Large urinary fistulas mean total urinary incontinence, a condition which is intolerable for the patient and difficult to treat. The combination of PNS and transrenal ureteral occlusion provides a reasonable alternative for these patients, allowing them a dignified life. Another group of tumour patients includes those with severe dysuria which can be effectively stopped by interruption of urinary flow into the bladder.

Summary

Percutaneous nephrostomy enables a variety of interventional procedures in the urinary tract. While most are temporary or palliative measures, some are curative, replacing operative intervention in some instances.

References

1. Alken P, Hutschenreiter G, Günther R, Marberger M (1981) Percutaneous stone manipulation. J Urol 125:463–466
2. Bigongiari LR, Lee KR, Moffat RE, Mebust WK, Foret J, Weigel J (1977) Percutaneous ureteral stent placement for stricture management and internal urinary drainage. AJR 133:865–868
3. Fernström I, Johannsson B (1982) Percutaneous extraction of renal calculi. Front Eur Radiol 1:1–24

3a. Goodwin WE, Casey WC, Woolf W (1955) Percutaneous trocar (needle) nephrostomy in hydronephrosis. JAMA 157, 891–894

4. Günther R, Alken P (1982) Percutaneous nephrostomy and endourologic manipulations. Front Eur Radiol 1:26–49
5. Günther R, Klose K, Alken P (1982) Transrenal ureteral occlusion using a detachable balloon. Radiology 142:521–523
6. Newhouse JH, Pfister RC (1981) Therapy for renal calculi via percutaneous nephrostomy. Dissolution and extraction. Urol Radiol 2:165–170
7. Pfister RC, Newhouse JH (1979) Interventional percutaneous pyeloureteral techniques. II. Percutaneous nephrostomy and other procedures. Radiol Clin North Am 17:351–363
8. Pollack HM, Banner MP (1981) Percutaneous nephrostomy and related pyeloureteral manipulative techniques. Urol Radiol 2:147–154
9. Saxton HM (1981) Percutaneous nephrostomy-technique. Urol Radiol 2:131–139
10. Smith RF, Lange PH, Miller RP, Reinke DB (1979) Controlled ureteral meatotomy. J Urol 121:587–589
11. Spataro RF, Linke CA, Barbaric ZL (1979) The use of percutaneous nephrostomy and urinary alkalizing in the dissolution of obstructing uric acid stones. Radiology 129:629–632
12. Zegel HG, Pollack HM, Bauner MP, et al. (1981) Percutaneous nephrostomy: comparison of sonographic and fluoroscopic guidance. AJR 137:925–927

Cardiovascular Radiology

Interventional Radiology: Overview

R. I. White, Jr.

Department of Radiology and Radiological Science, The Johns Hopkins Medical Institutions, 601 N. Broadway, Baltimore, MD 21205, USA

Introduction

Adaptation of cardiovascular catheters for therapeutic purposes has become known as interventional radiology. In recent years this subspeciality has continued its steady expansion. These techniques are just as applicable outside the cardiovascular system as within it.

Interventional radiology can be divided conveniently into four areas; percutaneous transluminal angioplasty (PTA), embolotherapy, drainage techniques, and chemotherapy. This brief review will highlight some of the advances in each area in recent years.

Percutaneous Transluminal Angioplasty

Since 1977, PTA has been reintroduced into the United States. Largely through the efforts of our European colleagues in preserving and perfecting the technique, North American angiographers took it up in earnest in late 1977. Reports of long-term follow-ups of patients after iliac, femoral, and renal angioplasty have been published [8, 16, 21, 25, 30, 31, 33, 39, 41, 42]. Despite the learning curves in many institutions, the results for localized stenoses and short occlusions compare favorably with those of surgery (Fig. 1). Recurrence rates are higher for femoral and popliteal stenosis than for iliac stenosis. Patients with restenosis can be redilated successfully in most instances.

New applications of PTA include dilatation of visceral artery stenoses, a wide variety of postgraft stenoses. biliary-intestinal strictures, esophageal, rectal, and urethral strictures, and even ureteral-pelvis junction obstruction [17, 28, 29, 36, 37, 40, 46]. Successful neurovascular applications of PTA include fibromuscular stenoses of the carotid artery and atherosclerotic and postinflammatory (Takayasu's) subclavian artery stenoses. Renal neurofibromatosis, renal artery stenosis due to atherosclerotic orifice plaques extending into the aorta, and secondary strictures due to iatrogenic injury of the biliary tract have not responded well to dilatation [17, 28, 29, 36, 37, 40, 46].

Coronary artery angioplasty is increasingly applied to focal stenoses in the proximal right coronary artery or left anterior descending branch of the left coronary artery [26, 27]. Noncoronary applications in congenital heart disease have included successful dilatation of valvar pulmonic stenosis and coarctation restenosis [22, 23]. Crucial to the acceptance of the technique will be the additional reporting of long-term (5-year) follow-ups. The original arguments for PTA are still valid now; it is a procedure which offers a very acceptable chance of success, has very little morbidity and almost no mortality, does not preclude surgery if technically unsuccessful, and can be repeated in most instances if restenosis recurs.

Embolotherapy

Although Table I was first published 2 years ago, it is still useful with the additional information concerning ethanol and contrast material [10, 12]. Intravascular ethanol has emerged as the latest embolic agent with promise for ablating renal tumors and esophageal varices following percutaneous coronary vein introduction. It may have equally devastating results when applied in pelvic, visceral, or neurovascular circulations. Necrosis after ethanol embolization arises through red-cell sludging in small arteries, spasm and disruption of endothelial membranes. Recently, contrast material ablation of parathyroid adenomas has been reported by Doppman [10]. By wedging a small catheter in the artery feeding the adenoma and injecting large amounts of contrast material, dense staining and necrosis of the gland are produced. Fine-particle polyvinyl alcohol (Ivalon) 250–1000 μm in diameter, has be-

Radiology Today 2. Ed. by F. H. W. Heuck and M. W. Donner

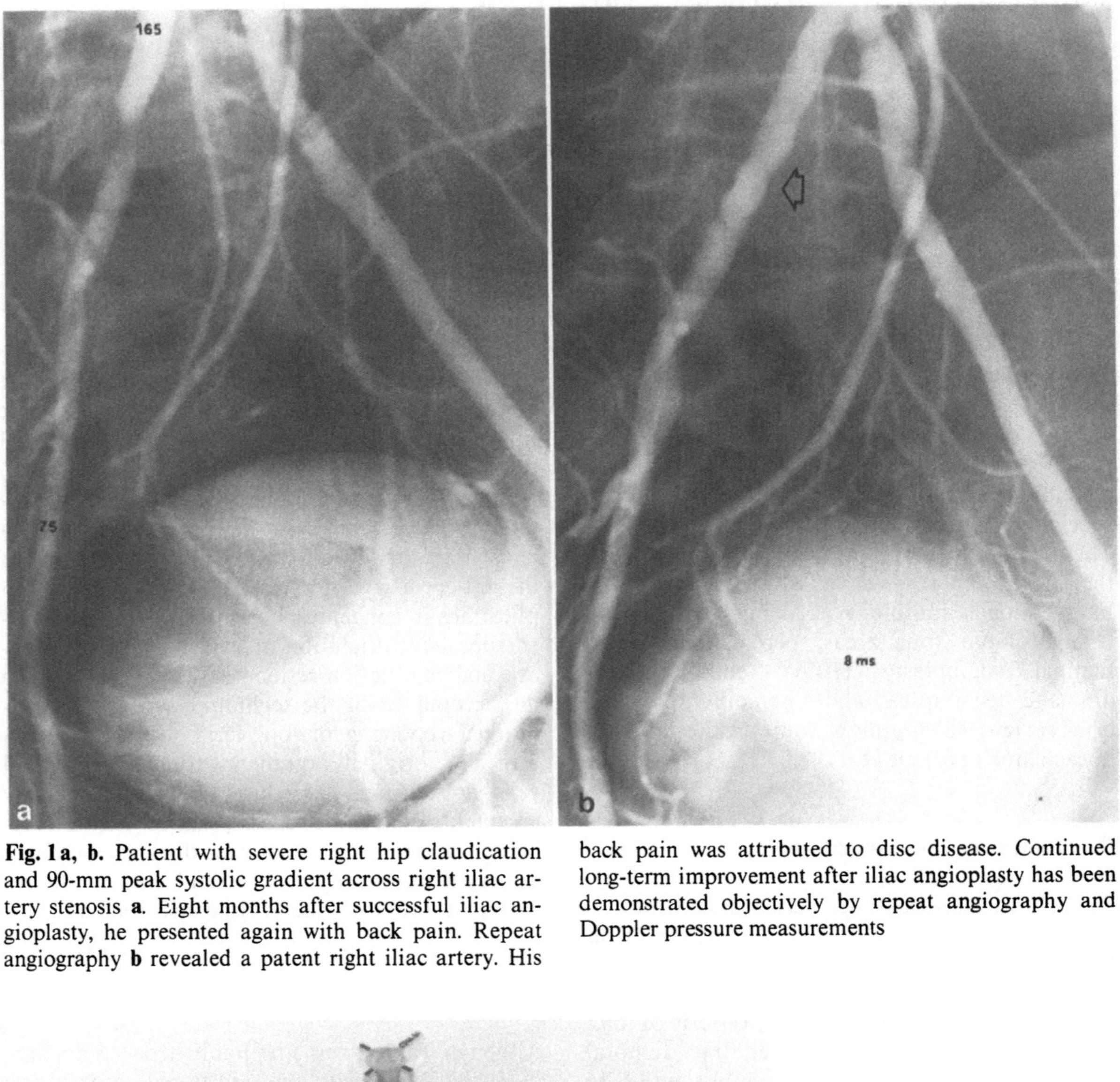

Fig. 1 a, b. Patient with severe right hip claudication and 90-mm peak systolic gradient across right iliac artery stenosis **a**. Eight months after successful iliac angioplasty, he presented again with back pain. Repeat angiography **b** revealed a patent right iliac artery. His back pain was attributed to disc disease. Continued long-term improvement after iliac angioplasty has been demonstrated objectively by repeat angiography and Doppler pressure measurements

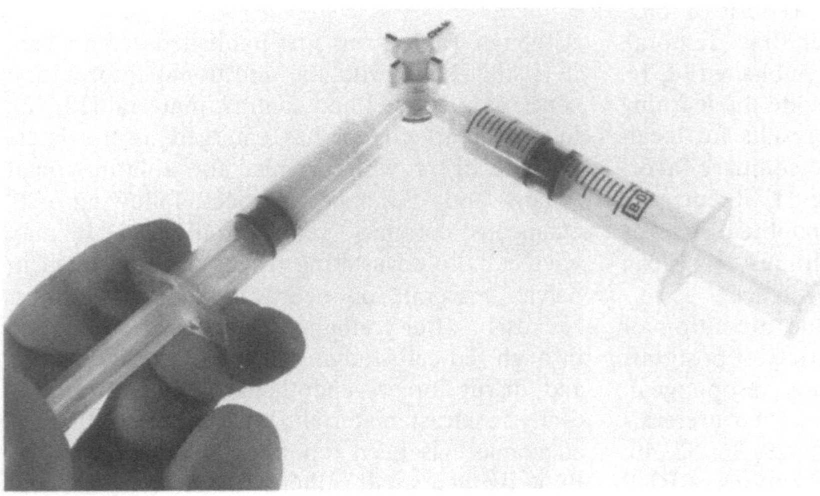

Fig. 2. Technique for suspending polyvinyl alcohol (Ivalon) particles in dilute contrast medium. Particles varying between 250 and 1000 μm in diameter are placed in dilute contrast medium and injected back and forth through a three-way stopcock. This serves to break up the surface tension of the particles and achieves a good suspension before injecting them into the subject. These particles provide excellent palliation of primary and secondary hepatic neoplasms and also of congenital systemic AVMS

Table 1. The properties and uses of materials employed in embolization techniques (adapted from White [43])

Material	Inflammation	Size of particle	Application
Autologous clot	Minimal	Variable	Historical
Gelfoam	Moderate: self limited	Large particles (1 – 3 mm)	Hemorrhage, preoperative neoplasms
Oxycel	Moderate: self limited	Variable	Difficult to use consistently
Avitene	Moderate: self limited	Thin slurry	Devascularization of head and neck neoplasms, renal neoplasms, contraindicated in AVMs
Ivalon	Minimal	250 – 1000 μm particles	Particles helpful for distal devascularization of AVMs and neoplasms
Coils	Minimal	Variable: 3 mm, 5 mm, 8 mm diameter	Preoperative neoplasms, hemorrhage
Balloons	Minimal	1 – 8 mm silicone 1 – 12 mm latex	Preoperative devascularization of neoplasms, hemorrhage, posttraumatic fistulas, pulmonary arteriovenous malformations, and varicocele
Isobutyl cyanoacrylate	Mild to moderate	Liquid	Preoperative devascularization of neoplasms, control of hemorrhage, AVMs
Liquid silicone	Minimal	Liquid	Preoperative devascularization of neoplasms of AVMs or devascularization of organs
Ethanol	Mild to moderate	Liquid	Renal ablation and esophageal varices
Contrast media	Mild to moderate	Liquid	Ablation of adrenal hyperplasia, parathyroid, adenoma

AVM, arteriovenous malformation

come an excellent agent for devascularizing primary or secondary liver tumors and palliating arteriovenous malformations (AVMs) [6, 34]. Particles are suspended in dilute contrast material by injecting them back and forth through a three-way stopcock (Fig. 2).

There is still a need for the development of safe and effective techniques for obliterating the matrix of congenital AVMs [4, 7]. Injection of dilutions of Bucrylate with Pantopaque through microballoon perfusion catheters appears to be the leading technique for palliating neurovascular congenital AVMs. AVMs in areas other than the head are so rare that it is difficult for any one institution to develop significant experience.

The success at M.D. Anderson Hospital, using a combination of intra-arterial chemotherapy and Ivalon embolization for treatment of metastatic adenocarcinoma of the colon, has stimulated a great deal of interest [6, 34]. Median survival of patients with metastatic adenocarcinoma of the liver has been extended from 5 to 15 months. It is quite likely that these techniques will be used increasingly by other institutions over the next several years.

Finally, older embolization techniques are being simplified. Among these is the Gianturco-Anderson-Wallace coil, which now comes in three sizes and is easily introduced through polyethylene catheters [7]. Detachable balloon techniques are also being simplified [3, 9, 44, 45], with the standardization of introducer catheters and the development of a disposable coiling chamber and coaxial valve. Detachable balloons offer unique advantages over other embolization techniques for the treatment of traumatic fistulas, pulmonary arteriovenous malformations (PAVMs), and varicoceles (Fig. 3).

Drainage Techniques

Biliary, urinary tract, and abscess drainage are among the most rapidly expanding techniques.

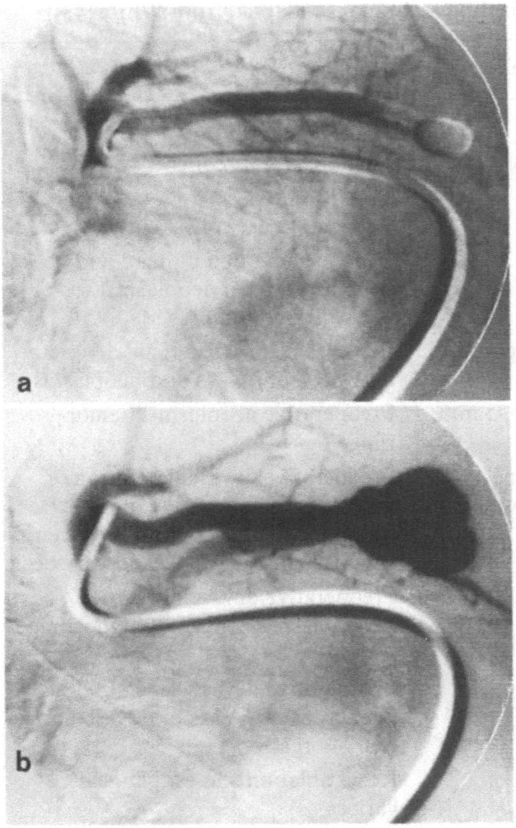

Fig. 3 a, b. Intra-arterial digital subtraction angiograms during occlusion of a right upper lobe PAVM. A large pulmonary artery branch is noted entering the PAVM (**a**). In **b**, a detachable silicone balloon has been flow-directed through the introducer catheter and a test inflation demonstrates excellent position beyond all normal branches to the lung. The balloon is still attached to its catheter and it is detached only after demonstrating complete occlusion and satisfactory position

They are quite successful, but complications are being recognized with increasing frequency [15, 19, 32]. With biliary drainage techniques, appropriate antibiotics are critical to avoid septic complications. Long-term infectious complications of biliary stenting are almost inevitable and require a thorough understanding of tube management. Abscess drainage and biliary stenting require close patient follow-up to detect complications. These techniques are generally replacing surgical drainage procedures, particularly in poor-risk patients.

Biliary endoprostheses are still associated with long-term obstruction due to biliary encrustation [18], but for short-term management or use in uncooperative patients they are a reasonable alternative to catheter drainage.

Once catheter drainage is instituted in the biliary or urinary tract, a whole host of retrieval techniques for stones, intracatheter radiotherapy for treatment of neoplastic strictures, and balloon dilatation for benign strictures are possible (Fig. 4) [1, 5]. It is likely that developments in these areas will continue in the future.

Chemotherapy

Intra-arterial vasopressin treatment of upper and lower gastrointestinal bleeding was the model for the development of interventional radiology. While vasopressin therapy has continued value for management of gastrointestinal bleeding, the overall incidence of patients with gastrointestinal bleeding has decreased due to the judicious use of cimetidine and antacids in stressed medical and postoperative patients.

Use of intra-arterial chemotherapy for treatment of liver, pelvis, and bone neoplasms continues to increase. Whether the results of repeated percutaneous catheterization for sequential chemotherapy warrants the fairly high patient complication rates and radiologist radiation doses is still debatable. The surgical introduction of hepatic catheters and subcutaneous pumps as advocated by Ensminger has appeal. By this technique chemotherapy can be administered repeatedly without having to recatheterize or hospitalize the patient [13]. If hepatic dearterialization of metastases by fine-particle Ivalon embolization is proven as efficacious as reported by Chuang and Wallace and Patt et al. [6, 34]. I believe that it will replace the more tedious techniques of repeated percutaneous catheterization for serial chemotherapy (Fig. 5).

Intravascular use of thrombolytic agents like streptokinase (SK) is a remarkable rediscovery of the past 2 years [11, 13, 24, 38]. SK is administered in high doses directly into the coronary artery (2–4000 units/min) for acute coronary artery thrombosis and in low doses intraclot (5–10000 units/h) for peripheral arterial occlusion. There are many exciting questions left unanswered. Will ischemic areas surrounding a myocardial infarction survive once the circulation is open? What percentage of chronic thrombi resolve with SK? Intuitively, thrombus formation occurs superimposed on stenosis in the peripheral circulation or spasm plus stenosis in the coronary circulation. Once the thrombus is lysed, PTA or surgical bypass should be performed soon in order to prevent reocclusion. The whole dilemma of

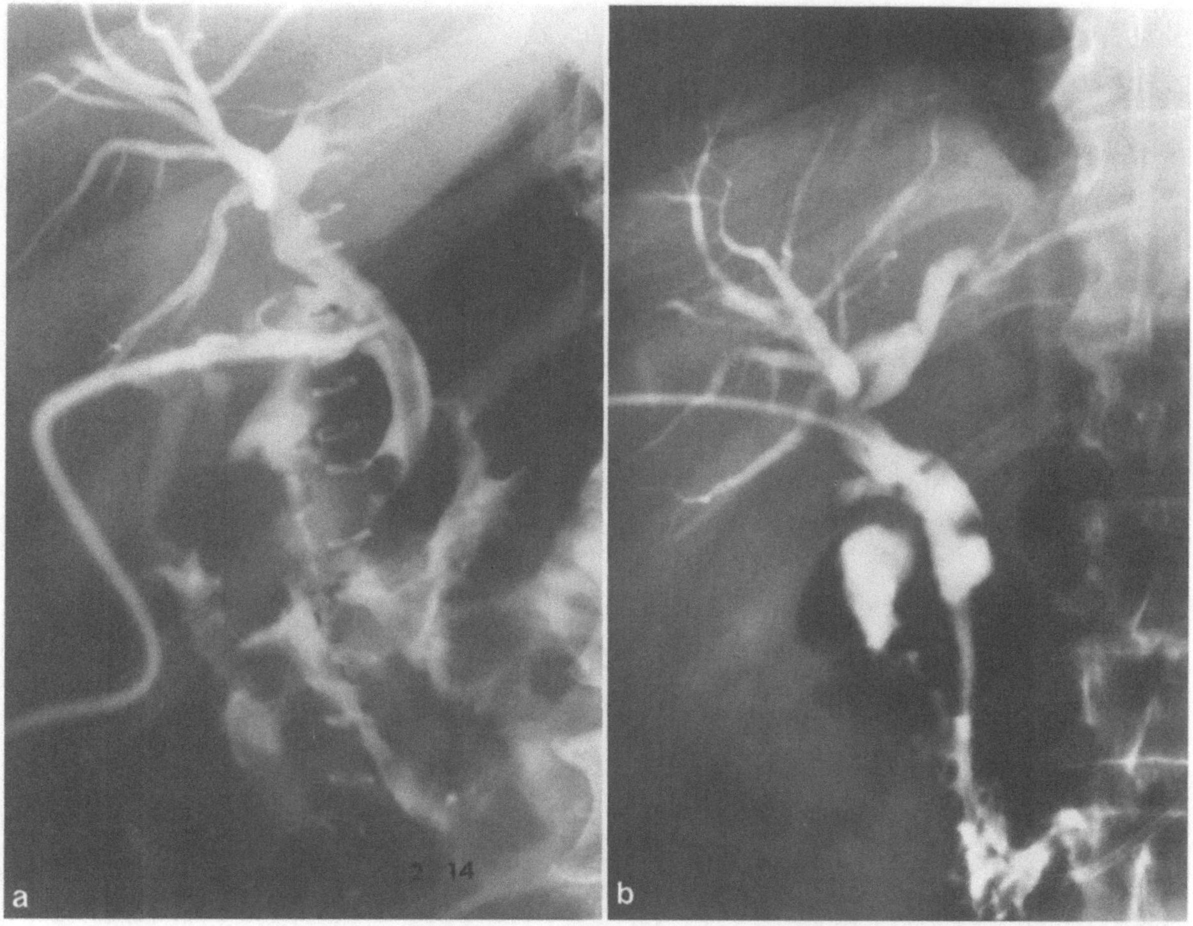

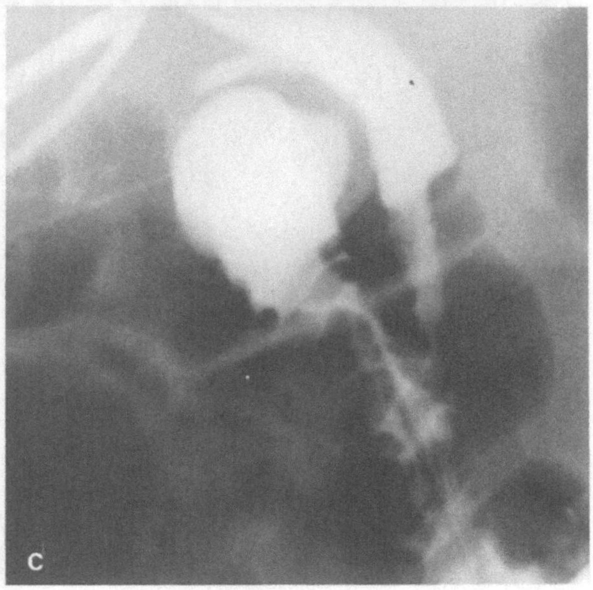

Fig. 4a–c. After two operations to remove a common duct stone, this middle-aged man was transferred to our hospital for further therapy **a**. The T-tube cholangiogram reveals paraduodenal extravasation (abscess formation) and a retained stone in the common and cystic ducts. The patient was drained externally via a percutaneously placed new intrahepatic stent and the T tube was removed. A retroperitoneal abscess was also drained. Four months later (**b**) a cholangiogram revealed two common duct stones and a stricture of the distal common duct. The patient was discharged. On an outpatient basis, the common duct stones were retrieved percutaneously with a basket and the stricture dilated with an 8-mm angioplasty balloon. Dilatations were performed in three occasions and a final cholangiogram (**c**) with a modified pediatric feeding tube proximal to the strictured distal common duct demonstrates a duct of acceptable caliber. The feeding tube was removed and the patient has remained asymptomatic for 2 years. Kadir et al. [19]

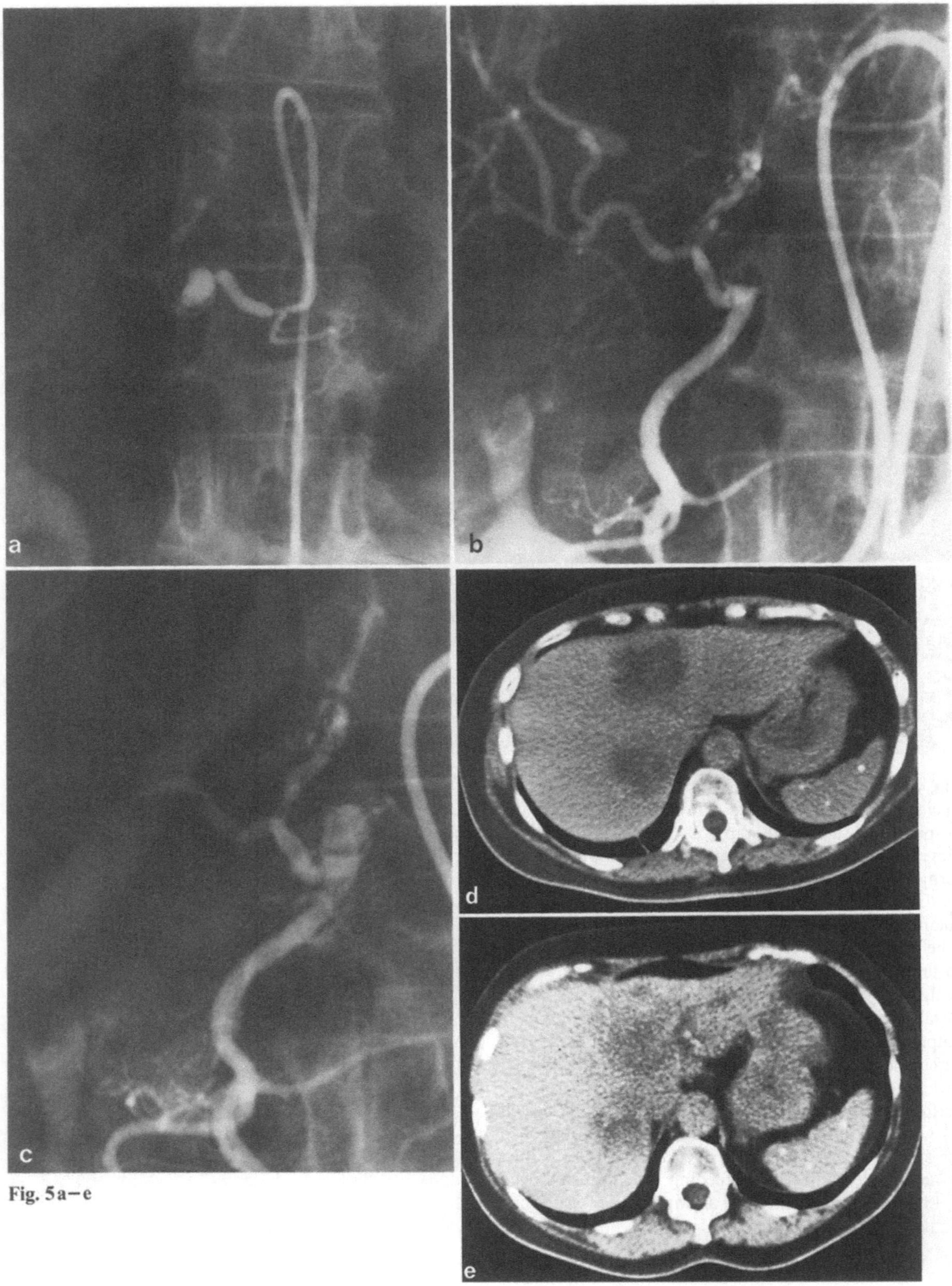

Fig. 5a–e

how to or whether to administer heparin in conjunction with thrombolytics is still open to question in the peripheral circulation.

Conclusion

One measure of the interest in and success of interventional radiology is the publication of four recent textbooks on the subject [1, 14, 20, 35]. Still to be resolved are the tough political issue of whether these techniques should be divided among radiology subspecialities by system (gastrointestinal, genitourinary, skeletal) or whether they should remain in the hands of the cardiovascular radiologist, who is often the one most experienced in needle, guide-wire, and catheter techniques. Interventional radiology is much like nuclear medicine in that it represents a collection of techniques requiring the same instrumentation and also requiring specialized training and expertise. It seems that the transition from cardiovascular radiology to cardiovascular-interventional radiology is a natural one, since the same techniques can be applied equally well to vascular and nonvascular problems.

References

1. Athanasoulis CA, Greene RE, et al. (1982) Interventional radiology. Saunders, Philadelphia
2. Bank WO, Kerber CW, et al. (1981) Treatment of intracerebral arteriovenous malformation with isobutyl 2-cyanoacrylate: initial clinical experience. Radiology 139:609–616
3. Barth KH, White RI Jr, et al. (1982) Embolotherapy of pulmonary arteriovenous malformations with detachable balloons. Radiology 142:599–606
4. Berenstein A, Kricheff I (1979) Catheter and material selection for transarterial embolization. Radiology 132:631–639

Fig. 5a–e. Selective hepatic arteriogram following short course of intra-arterial chemotherapy for metastatic colon carcinoma (**a**); the hepatic artery is occluded and a false aneurysm is present. The inferior pancreaticoduodenal arcades were catheterized in order to gain access to the gastroduodenal artery (**b, c**). Embolotherapy with Ivalon particles (250–500 μm) provided remission of symptoms. Computed tomographic scans before and 6 months after embolization show stabilization of liver metastasis (no growth) and calcification around the borders of the metastases (**d, e**)

5. Burhenne HJ (1980) Percutaneous extraction of retumed biliary tract stones: 661 patients. AJR 134:881–898
6. Chuang VP, Wallace S (1980) Current status of transcatheter management of neoplasms. Cardiovasc Intervent Radiol 3:256–257
7. Chuang VP, Wallace S, et al. (1980) A new improved coil for tapered-tip catheter for arterial occlusion. Radiology 135:507
8. Colapinto RF, Harries-Jones EP, et al. (1980) Percutaneous transluminal dilatation and recanalization in the treatment of peripheral vascular disease. Radiology 135:583–587
9. Debrun G, Lacour P, et al. (1981) Treatment of 54 traumatic carotid-cavernous fistulas. J Neurosurg 55:678–692
10. Doppman JL (1980) The treatment of hyperparathyroidism by transcatheter techniques. Cardiovasc Intervent Radiol 3:268–281
11. Dotter CT, Rösch J, et al. (1974) Selective clot lysis with low dose streptokinase. Radiology 111:31–37
12. Ellman RA, Parkhill BJ, et al. (1981) Ablation of renal tumors with absolute ethanol: a new technique. Radiology 141:619–626
13. Ensminger W, Niederhuber J, et al. (1981) Totally implanted drug delivery system for hepatic arterial chemotherapy. Cancer Treat Rep 65:393–400
14. Fenucci JT Jr, Wittenberg J (1981) Interventional radiology of the abdomen. Williams & Wilkens, Baltimore
15. Gerzof SG, Robbins AH, et al. (1981) Percutaneous catheter drainage of abdominal abscesses. A five-year experience. N Engl J Med 305:653–656
16. Greenfield AJ (1980) Femoral, popliteal, and tibial arteries: percutaneous transluminal angioplasty. AJR 135:927–935
17. Hasso AN, Bird CR, et al. (1981) Fibromuscular dysplasia of the internal carotid artery: percutaneous transluminal angioplasty. AJR 136:955–960
18. Hoevels J, Ihse I (1979) Percutaneous transhepatic insertion of a permanent endoprosthesis in the extrahepatic bile ducts. Gastrointest Radiol 4:367–377
19. Kadir S, Baassiri A, et al. (1982) Percutaneous biliary drainage in the management of biliary sepsis. AJR 138:25–29
20. Kadir S, Kaufman SL, et al. (1982) Selected techniques in interventional radiology. Saunders, Philadelphia
21. Kadir S, Smith GW, et al. (1982) Percutaneous transluminal angioplasty as an adjunct to the surgical management of peripheral vascular disease. Ann. Surg. 195:786–795
22. Kan JS, White RI, et al. (1982) Treatment of coarctation restenosis by percutaneous transluminal angioplasty (PTA) (abstr.) Circulation 66 (Supp II) II–360
23. Kan JS, White RI, et al. (1982) Balloon valvuloplasty for the treatment of pulmonary valvular stenosis. NESM 307:540–542

24. Katzen BT, van Breda A (1981) Low dose streptokinase in treatment of arterial occlusions. AJR 136:1171–1178
25. Kaufman SL, Barth KH, et al. (1982) Hemodynamic measurements in the evaluation and follow-up of transluminal angioplasty of the iliac and femoral arteries. Radiology 142:329–336
26. Kent KM, Bonow RO, et al. (1982) Improved myocardial function during exercise after successful percutaneous transluminal coronary angioplasty. N Engl J Med 306:441–446
27. Levy RI, Mock MB, et al. (1981) Percutaneous transluminal coronary angioplasty – a status report. N Engl J Med 305:399–400 (editorial)
28. Mahaler F, Probst P, et al. (1982) Lasting improvement of renovascular hypertension by transluminal dilatation of atherosclerotic and nonatherosclerotic renal artery stenoses. A follow-up study. Circulation 65:611–617
29. Martin EC, Diamond NC, et al. (1980) Percutaneous transluminal angioplasty in nonatherosclerotic disease. Radiology 135:27–33
30. Martin EC, Fankuchen GI, et al. (1981) Angioplasty for femoral artery occlusions: comparison with surgery. AJR 137:915–919
31. Motarjeme A, Keifer JW, et al. (1980) Percutaneous transluminal angioplasty of the iliac arteries: 66 experiences. AJR 135:937–944
32. Mueller PR, van Sonnenberg E, et al. (1982) Percutaneous biliary drainage: technical and catheter related problems in 200 procedures. AJR 138:17–23
33. Neiman HL, Brandt TD, et al. (1981) Percutaneous transluminal angioplasty. Arch Surg 116:821–828
34. Patt YZ, Wallace S, et al. (1981) The palliative role of hepatic arterial infusion and arterial occlusion in colorectal carcinoma metastatic to the liver. Lancet 1:349–351
35. Ring EJ, McClean G (1982) Interventional radiology principles and techniques. Little Brown, New York
36. Russinovich NAE, Lloyd LK, et al. (1980) Balloon dilatation of urethral strictures. Urol Radiol 2:33–37
37. Schwarten DE, Yune HY, et al. (1980) Clinical experience with percutaneous transluminal angioplasty (PTA) of stenotic renal arteries. Radiology 135:601–604
38. Sharma GVRK, Cella G, et al. (1982) Thrombolytic therapy. N Engl J Med 306:1268–1276
39. Spence RK, Freiman DB, et al. (1981) Long-term results of transluminal angioplasty of the iliac and femoral arteries. Arch Surg 116:1377–1386
40. Tegtmeyer CJ, Teates CD, et al. (1981) Percutaneous transluminal angioplasty in patients with renal artery stenosis. Radiology 140:323–330
41. Turcotte JK, Lu CT, et al. (1981) Role of transluminal angioplasty in limb salvage and claudication. J Surg Res 30:428–434
42. Waltman AC (1980) Percutaneous transluminal angioplasty: iliac and deep femoral arteries. AJR 135:921–925
43. White RI Jr (1981) Interventional radiology: overview. In: Donner MW, Heuck FHW (eds) Radiology today 1. Springer, Berlin Heidelberg New York, pp 50–58
44. White RI Jr (1982) Nontapered introducer catheters for embolotherapy. AJR 139:620–622
45. White RI Jr, Kaufman SL, et al. (1981) Occlusion of varicoceles with detachable balloons. Radiology 139:327–334
46. Zajko AB, McClean GK, et al. (1981) Percutaneous puncture of venous bypass grafts for transluminal angioplasty. AJR 137:799–802

Application of Embolotherapy with Detachable Balloons

K. H. Barth, S. L. Kaufman, and R. I. White, Jr.

Georgetown University Hospital, 3800 Reservoir Road, N.W., Washington, DC 20007, USA

Therapeutic angiographers are now familiar with a variety of embolization techniques, each adapted to specific needs. For example, preoperative or palliative tumor embolization fulfills a totally different purpose than embolization of a bleeding artery. In the first instance the technique of choice produces complete tissue ischemia, in the second instance a limited arterial occlusion is required and tissue loss is a complicating effect.

Detachable balloon embolization provides a strictly localized vascular occlusion similar to surgical ligation. Detachable balloons have certain unique characteristics which set them apart from all other clinically applicable agents. As inflatable devices they are blood flow directable, and since they are attached to a catheter their placement can be corrected if found unsuitable upon test occlusion. Generally the best way to deliver the balloon to the site of embolization is injection of the balloon catheter through the introducer catheter. Some stiffer balloon catheters can be threaded through large-caliber introducer catheters, as in Debrun's system [3].

Several detachable balloon systems are available, all employing introducer catheters and a thin coaxial balloon-bearing catheter [1, 3–5]. In one particular system, with which we have gained most of our experience, the balloon detachment is accomplished by pulling the balloon catheter out of the occlusive balloon cuff [1]. Other systems use a second coaxial catheter over the balloon-bearing catheter to push the balloon off [3–5]. Among these the system introduced by Debrun is probably the best known [3]. Balloons are made of either silicone or latex. Latex balloons allow expansion up to about 1.5 times that of silicone balloons. On the other hand, Latex appears to be more thrombogenic and is not proven to be an inert long-term implant material like silicone. Membrane characteristics of Latex and silicone differ, the latter being a semipermeable membrane and the former a fine lattice. Consequently, occlusive silicone balloons can be expanded with fluid permanently, provided the fluid is isosmolar to blood. Latex balloons will leak their fluid contents gradually over a period of weeks and deflate. By this time the occlusion may be permanent due to thrombus surrounding the latex balloon. To guarantee lasting balloon expansion, latex balloons can be filled with a solidifying liquid such as silicone.

The small-size silicone balloon with "pull-out" detachment has a uninflated diameter of 1 mm and a maximum inflated diameter of 4 mm. A second larger silicone balloon has an outer diameter of 2 mm and expands up to 9 mm [2]. The former can be injected through a catheter with a 1.3 mm (0.042–in.) lumen, whereas the latter requires a lumen of almost 3 mm. Catheters suitable for small-balloon (1-mm diameter) embolization include most nontapered, high-torque, precurved, selective catheters (Torcon catheters, Cook Inc., Bloomington, Ind., USA) introduced through a femoral sheath. Also available are 5F nontapered catheters with adequate inner lumens (Formocath, Becton, Dickinson Inc., Rutherford, N.J., USA).

Based on our experience, detachable balloon embolization appears most appropriate for the following applications:

Head and Neck

1. Carotid cavernous and vertebral basilar fistulas
2. Inoperable aneurysms
3. Preoperative embolization of vascular neoplasms in order to limit the degree of particulate embolization

Chest

1. Pulmonary arteriovenous malformations
2. Bronchopulmonary fistulas

Radiology Today 2. Ed. by F. H. W. Heuck and M. W. Donner

Abdomen
1. Hematobilia
2. False aneurysms of hepatic, splenic, and pancreatic circulation
3. Preoperative embolization of hepatic artery branches before segmental resection
4. Exclusion of right or left hepatic artery or gastroduodenal artery for hepatic chemotherapy infusion

Kidney
1. Any traumatic bleeding
2. Arteriovenous fistulas

Retroperitoneum and Pelvis
1. False aneurysms
2. Spermatic vein for varices

Extremities
Traumatic fistulas or aneurysms

In the head and neck region, occlusion of a carotid cavernous fistula represents a most rewarding procedure, considering the surgical alternatives. Frequently no intracranial contrast filling is seen on the ipsilateral carotid arteriogram (Figs. 1, 2). In this instance the patient has already demonstrated whether or not he is able to tolerate the loss of unilateral carotid flow. Otherwise competent cross-circulation needs to be demonstrated to assess the risk involved in inadvertent carotid occlusion during balloon embolization. The goal of embolization is placement of the occluding balloon directly into the fistula, avoiding occlusion of the cavernous sinus (Fig. 3). Sometimes more than one balloon may be required to occlude the fistula completely. The risk of multiple embolizing balloons is obviously cavernous sinus thrombosis, which may aggravate the patient's preexisting symptoms. The introducer catheter should be left within the common carotid artery to avoid spasm of the internal carotid artery, which can inhibit balloon advancement.

Spherical latex balloons designed by Debrun are suitable for embolization of intracranial aneurysms [3]. Their purpose is to fill the aneurysmal pouch and exclude arterial pressure on its walls.

For preoperative embolization of head and neck tumors, the balloon may serve as a proximal point occlusion to interrupt a larger feeder artery selectively, avoiding the risk of particle embolization into intracranial branches [1].

Pulmonary arteriovenous malformations (PAVMs) have in our experience been very suitable

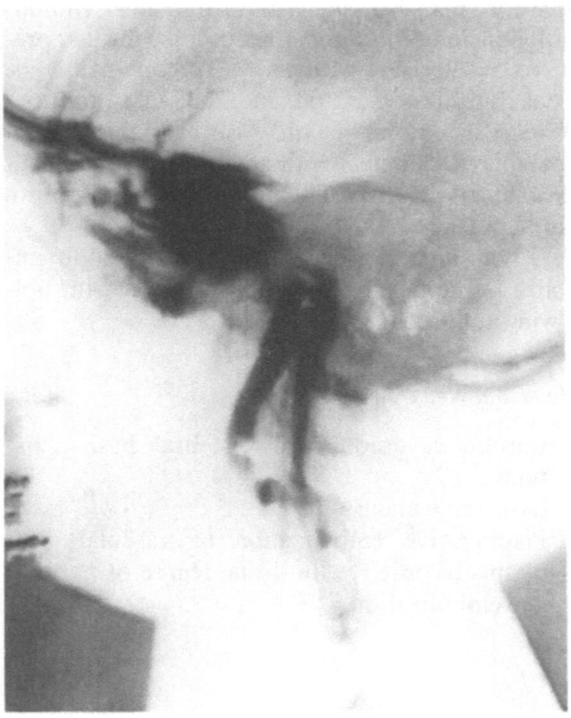

Fig. 1. A 42-year-old woman with right carotid cavernous fistula. No intracranial flow from ipsilateral internal carotid artery

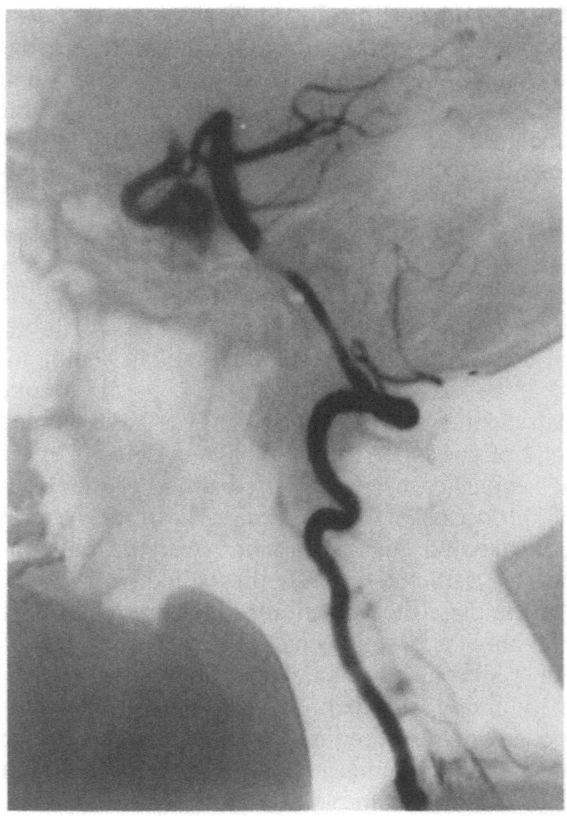

Fig. 2. Vertebral arteriogram demonstrating retrograde flow in cavernous portion of carotid artery towards fistula and also localizing the point of fistula proximal to the S-loop of the cavernous portion of the carotid artery

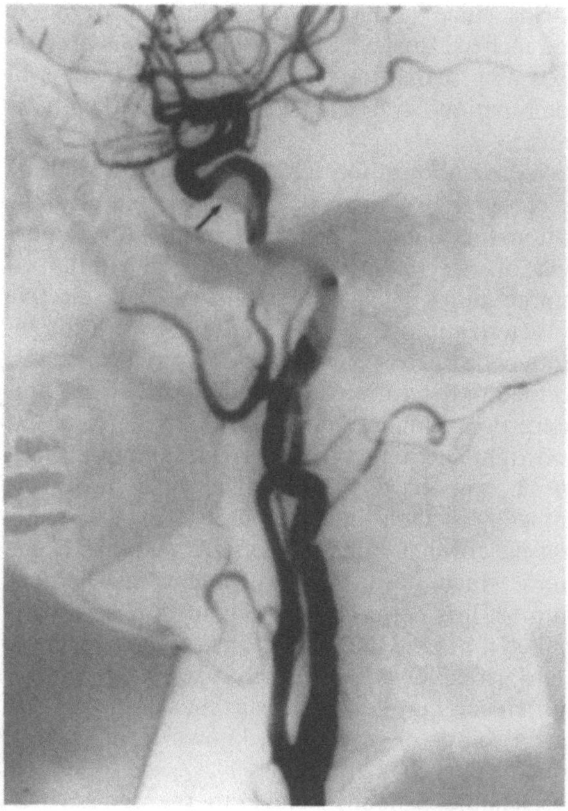

Fig. 3. Following balloon embolization into the fistula (*arrow*). Intracranial carotid blood flow returned

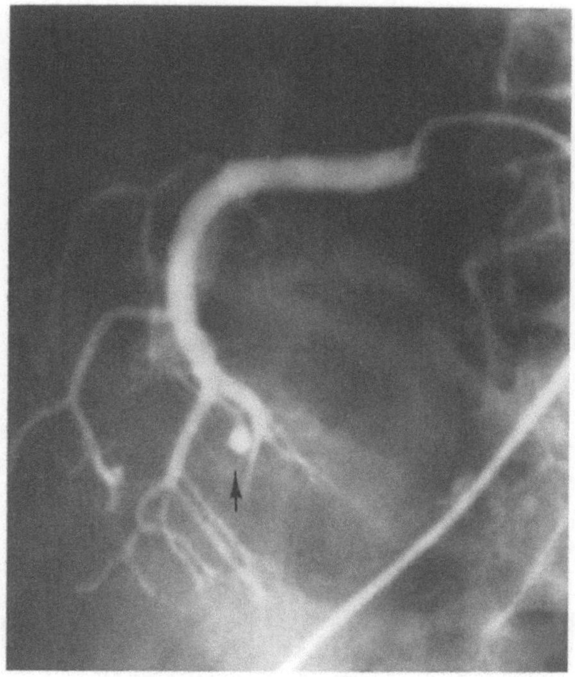

Fig. 4. A 65-year-old man with pelvic kidney and AV fistula following retrograde instrumentation. The AV communication is marked by bulbous ectasia of the renal vein (*arrow*)

targets for balloon embolization [6]. Their anatomic characteristics set them apart from systemic AVMs. Most frequently a single pulmonary artery feeder is present with a larger-caliber AV fistula. The caliber of the fistula may require the largest available detachable balloons and a 9F introducer catheter. As a pathfinder a Swan-Ganz catheter is introduced coaxially through the 9F introducer catheter. If the diameter of the fistula exceeds 9 mm, the largest available silicone balloon is too small and a latex balloon must be substituted. The largest Debrun-type latex balloon expands up to 12 mm. In the presence of multiple PAVMs the goal of embolization is to occlude the largest shunts and establish a satisfactory blood oxygen saturation. Severe cyanosis is the most frequent presenting symptom; much less frequent is hemoptysis.

In the abdomen, point sources of bleeding in the hepatosplenic arteries are suitable for balloon embolization. Exclusion of a common hepatic artery branch may at times be desirable for a patient undergoing hepatic artery chemotherapy infusion. Since the gastroduodenal mucosa is vulnerable to certain cytostatic drugs its perfusion should be avoided. If the hepatic bifurcation is in close proximity to the gastroduodenal artery or if the infusion catheter cannot be positioned in the proper hepatic artery, the gastroduodenal artery origin can be occluded safely provided the remaining gastric circulation is intact. Alternatively, the origin of one hepatic artery, can be occluded, relying on intrahepatic collateralization for the occluded branch. Before considering any distal hepatic artery occlusion one should confirm patency of the portal system to avoid acute liver ischemia.

Benign renal arterial bleeding is an ideal case for balloon embolotherapy, whose selectivity enables sparing of normal arteries, thus avoiding tissue loss inevitably connected to more widespread embolization with particles or coils. High-flow AV fistulas are most favorable targets for the flow-directable balloon (Fig. 4). Frequently the balloon will travel through the fistula on initial injection and can then be detached directly within the fistula after pullback (Fig. 5).

In the retroperitoneal area, in the pelvis, and in the upper and lower extremities balloons may be used equally well for embolization of post-traumatic aneurysms or AV fistulas. Balloon embolization should not be considered definitive for

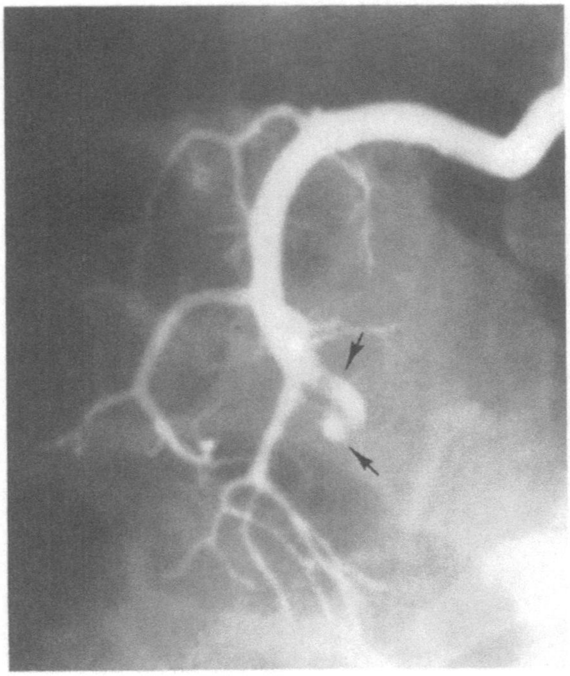

Fig. 5. Balloon embolized directly into fistula communication (*arrows*)

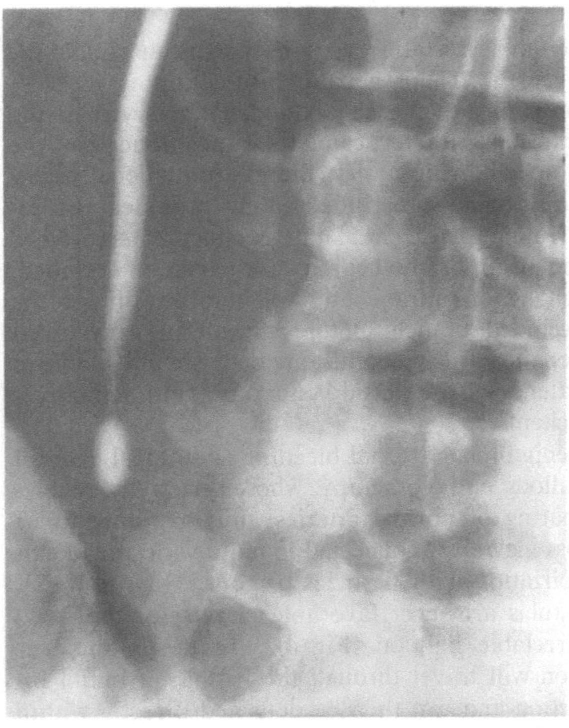

Fig. 6. A 28-year-old man with bilateral varicocele and internal spermatic vein insufficiency. Balloon before detachment occluding the distal right spermatic vein

AVMs, since the nidus of those lesions can never be reached. However, like coils, balloons may be used as proximal occluders of arterial feeders in combination with distal small-particle embolization.

Balloon embolization for treatment of varicocele is considered similar in effect to a surgical ligation [6]. Balloon occlusion in the distal portion of the internal spermatic vein similar to suprainguinal ligation starts with selective catheterization of the spermatic vein with the introducer catheter. Careful venography is then performed to determine the most suitable site of embolization. In many instances insufficiency of left and right spermatic veins is found and both need to be embolized (Fig. 6). The balloon-bearing catheter is then injected and most frequently travels down to the level of the inguinal canal, from which position readjustment can be performed. It is not necessary to place the introducer catheter beyond the first 2 cm of the spermatic vein orifice. Overlooked right spermatic vein insufficiency may lead to recurrence. Another frequent source of recurrence, known from surgical treatment, is collateral veins.

Detachable balloons belong in the armamentarium of therapeutically oriented angiographers for use in the indications described, where flow directability of the embolizing agents, point occlusion, and correctability of the occlusion are advantageous for optimal therapeutic results.

References

1. Barth KH, Kuman AJ, Kaufman L, White RI (1980) Therapeutische Embolisationen im extrakraniellen Kopf- und Halsbereich mit einem neuen System abstoßbarer Silikonballone. RoFo 133/4:409–415
2. Barth KH, White RI Jr, Kaufman SL, Terry PB, Roland JM (1982) Embolotherapy of pulmonary arteriovenous malformations with detachable balloons. Radiology 142:599–606
3. Debrun G, Lacour P, Caron PJ, Hurth M, Comoy J, Keravel Y (1978) Detachable balloon and calibrated-leak balloon techniques in the treatment of cerebral vascular lesions. J Neurosurg 49:635–649
4. Hieshima GB, Grinnell VS, Mehringer MC (1981) A detachable balloon for therapeutic transcatheter. Radiology 138:227–228
5. Taki W, Handa H, Yamagata S, Matsuda I, Yonekawa Y, Iwata H, Ikada Y (1979) Embolization and superselective angiography by means of balloon catheters. Surg Neurol 12:7–14
6. White RI, Kaufman SL, Barth KH, Kadir S, Symth JW, Walsh PC (1981) Occlusion of varicoceles with detachable balloons. Radiology 139:327–334

Angiography and Embolization of Bronchial Arteries

W. Reichardt

Katharinenhospital, Zentrum für Radiologie, Radiologisches Institut, Kriegsbergstrasse 60, 7000 Stuttgart, FRG

During the past 10 years there have been a few reports in the English-language literature on massive hemoptysis treated by transcatheter embolization of the bronchial or intercostal arteries [4, 6, 10, 11]. The reports are based on one to seven case histories each, and these numbers indicate that the method is not very common and not widespread in its use. More experience with 39–104 treated patients is reported from France by Remy et al. [8] and from Russia by Rabkin et al. [7]. The intention of this contribution is to emphasize that bronchial and intercostal arteriography and embolization of the arteries in patients with massive hemoptysis is worthwhile in selected cases.

Most acute hemoptysis is small in volume and will stop spontaneously. When it is massive and unremitting, however, airway obstruction and shock may be life threatening. In patients with massive hemoptysis, bronchoscopy for identification of the bleeding bronchial orifice and pulmonary resection without further diagnostic studies is the treatment of choice [5, 11].

Embolization of the bronchial and/or intercostal arteries is only indicated if there are temporary or permanent contraindications to surgical intervention.

The usual definition of massive and life-threatening hemoptysis is bleeding at a rate of 600 ml/24 h period. However, the mortality for pulmonary hemorrhage is more closely related to the severity of airway obstruction than to the amount of blood lost [3]. A surge of 200–300 ml blood is dangerous, especially in patients with underlying chronic pulmonary disease, and the definition cannot be applied strictly.

Arteriography is a poor method of obtaining direct evidence of the site of bleeding. Rabkin et al. [7] found extravasation of contrast medium only in 6.3% of patients with hemoptysis. Usually only hypervascularity, wide tortuous arteries, and arterioarterial bronchopulmonary shunts are found defining a possible or probable site of bleeding (Fig. 1) [1, 7].

These findings are common in chronic inflammatory pulmonary disease, bronchiectases, abscess formation, and old tuberculosis. In bilateral disease it is as a rule impossible to determine the site of bleeding by angiography (Fig. 2). When there are pleural adhesions, not only bronchopulmonary but also intercostopulmonary arterioarterial shunts are found (Fig. 1 a).

Performing angiography, we always try to examine all the bronchial arteries. The anatomy of the bronchial arteries varies widely but three combinations occur most frequently [1]. All the arteries arise from the descending aorta opposite the vertebrae T5-6 or at the right from the high intercostal arteries: (a) one artery on the left and one on the right, (b) two arteries on the left and one on the right, or (c) one common trunk and one left and one right artery. The most common situation is one right and two left arteries, the former arising from the first right intercostal and usually called the intercostobronchial trunk and the latter arising ventrally from the aorta. In about 23% of patients Botenga found aberrant arteries from the subclavian, the internal mammary, the pericardiophrenic, and others [1].

Prior to an embolization procedure it is mandatory to obtain a selective angiogram of good quality to determine if there are any branches to the spinal cord. If this is the case embolization is contraindicated, as spinal cord infarction may occur. However, spinal cord infarction and paraplegia after embolization has been reported even when no spinal branches were observed on preliminary arteriography [10].

Since July 1980 we have performed bronchial arteriography and embolization in eight patients with massive hemoptysis in whom surgical treatment was contraindicated (Figs. 3, 4). The diagnoses were bilateral tuberculosis in three patients (including one also with aspergilloma),

Radiology Today 2. Ed. by F. H. W. Heuck and M. W. Donner

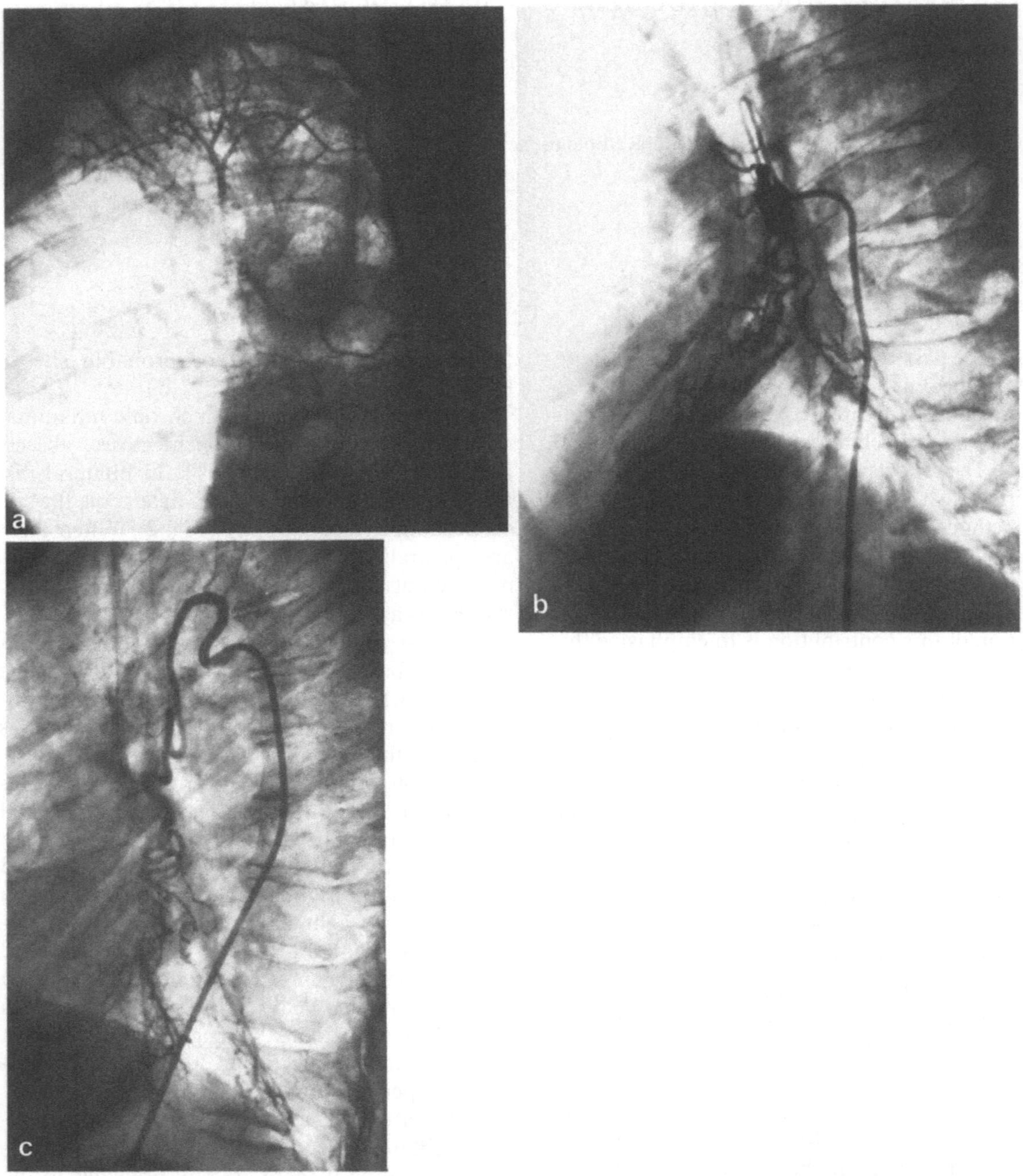

Fig. 1a–c. Angiographic findings in patients with chronic inflammatory pulmonary disease and hemoptysis. **a** Pleural adhesions. Hypervascularity and intercostopulmonary arterioarterial shunts. **b** Bronchiectases of the middle lobe. Excessive hypervascularity and widened tortuous bronchial artery. **c** Chronic bronchitis. Widened bronchial artery and bronchopulmonary arterioarterial shunts

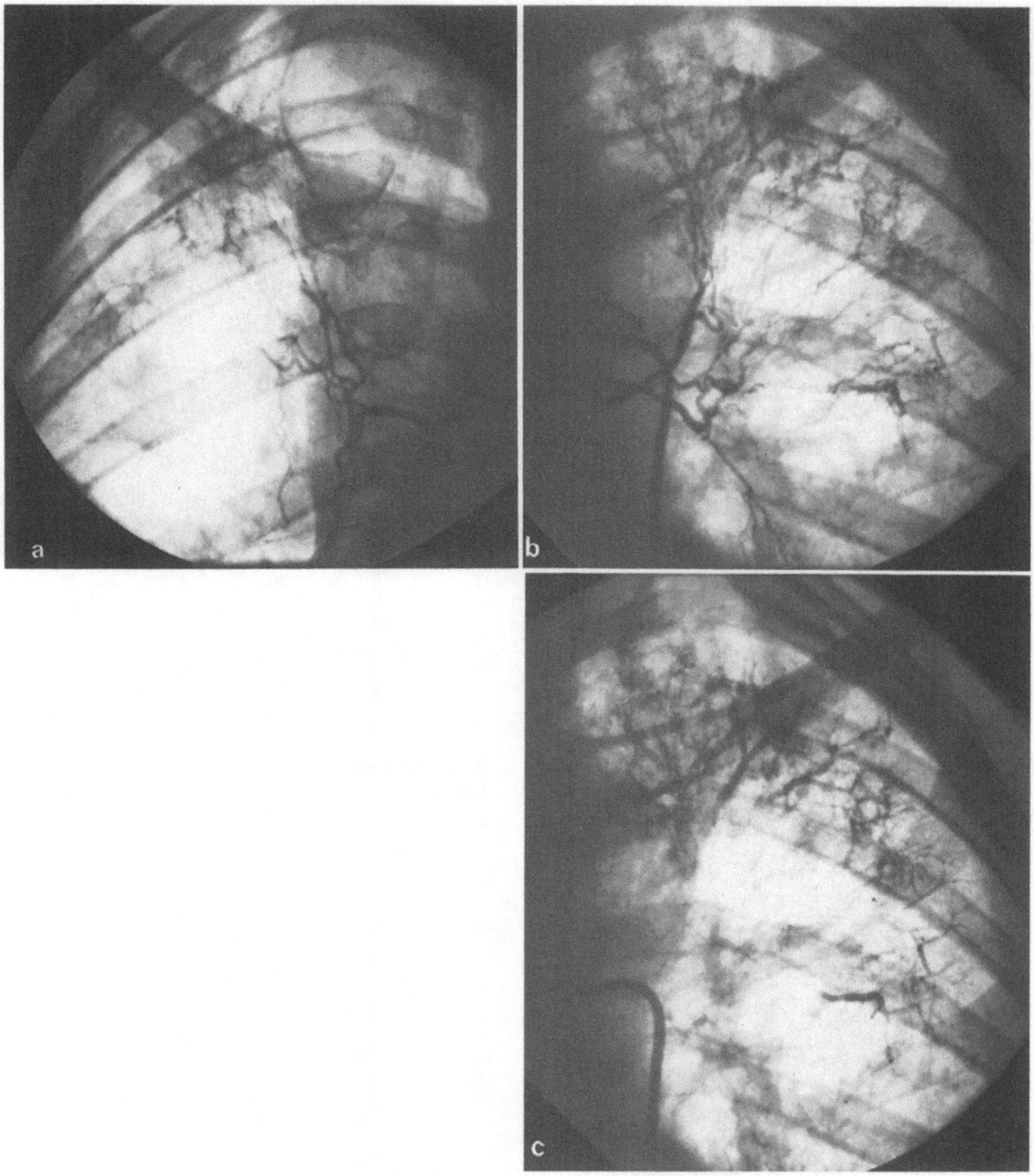

Fig. 2a–c. Patient with old bilateral tuberculosis. At the time of angiography, bleeding from the right upper lobe. **a** Right bronchial artery. **b** Left bronchial artery, early phase. **c** Late phase. Bilateral hypervascularity and bronchopulmonary arterioarterial shunting, left more than right

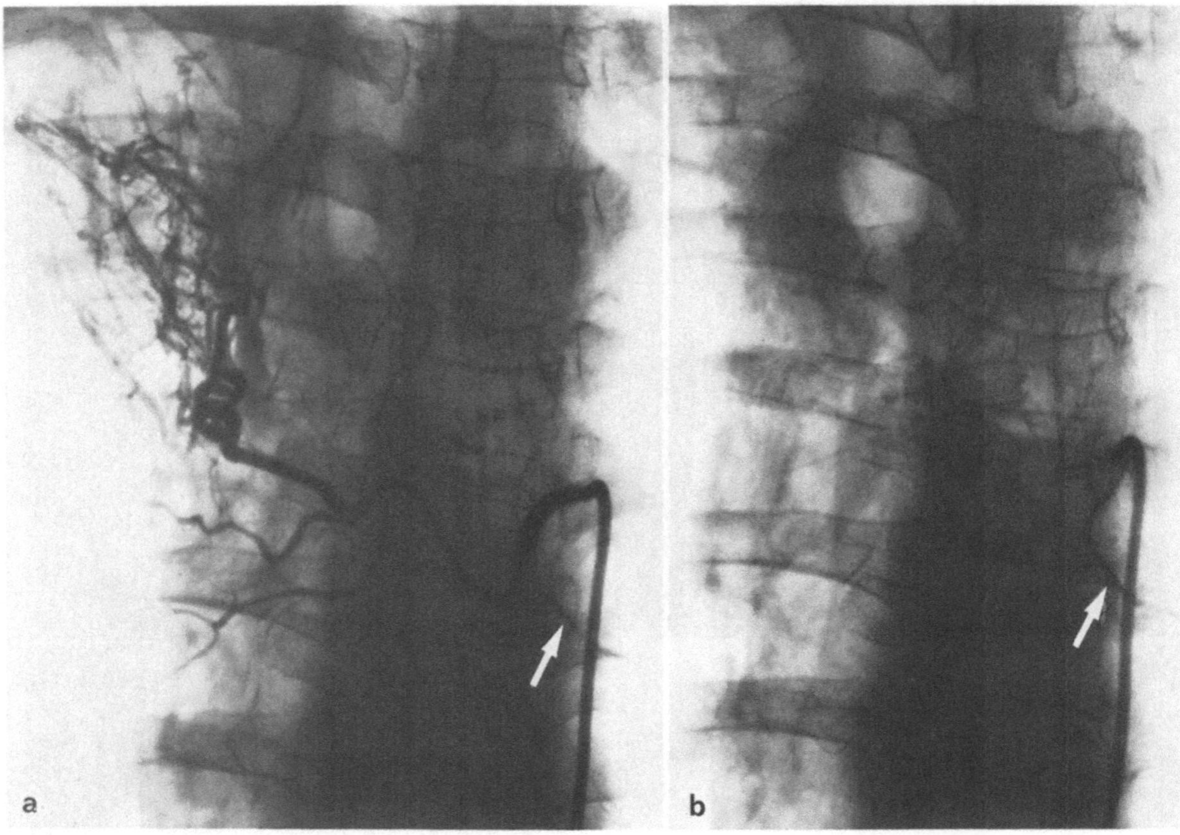

Fig. 3a, b. Angiography in a 41-year-old patient with old bilateral tuberculosis, bleeding from the right upper lobe. **a** Bronchial artery. Excessive hypervascularity and bronchopulmonary arterioarterial shunting. **b** After embolization only a small branch to the left is visible (→)

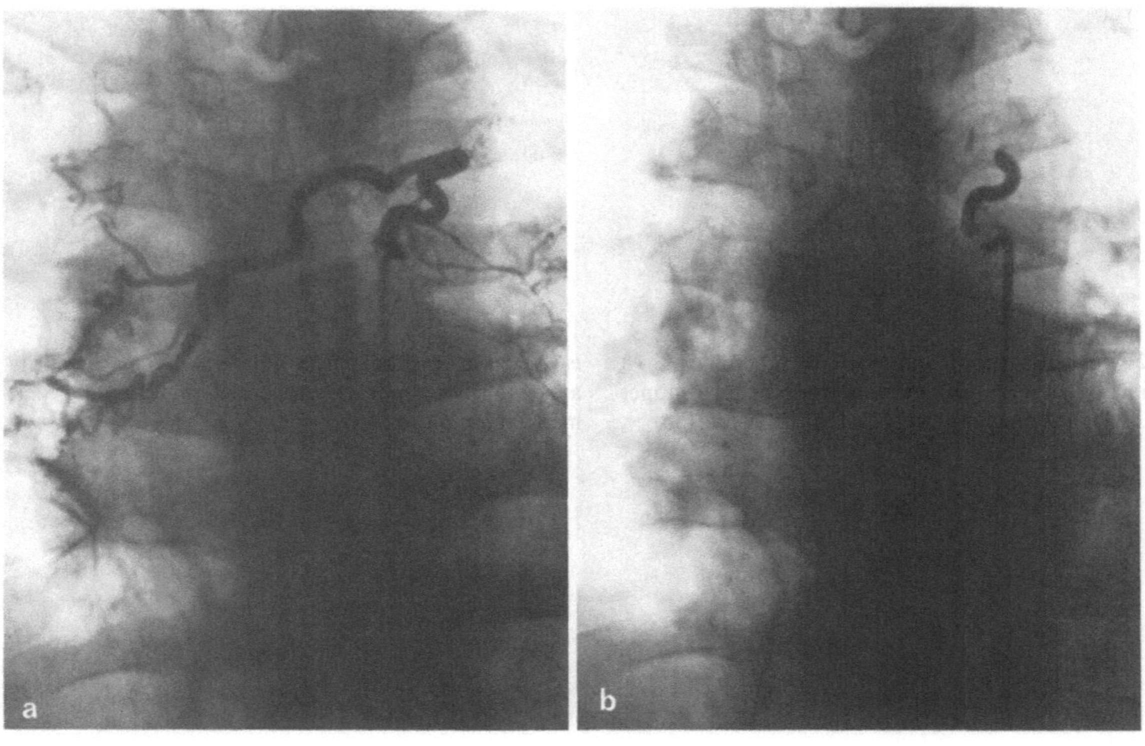

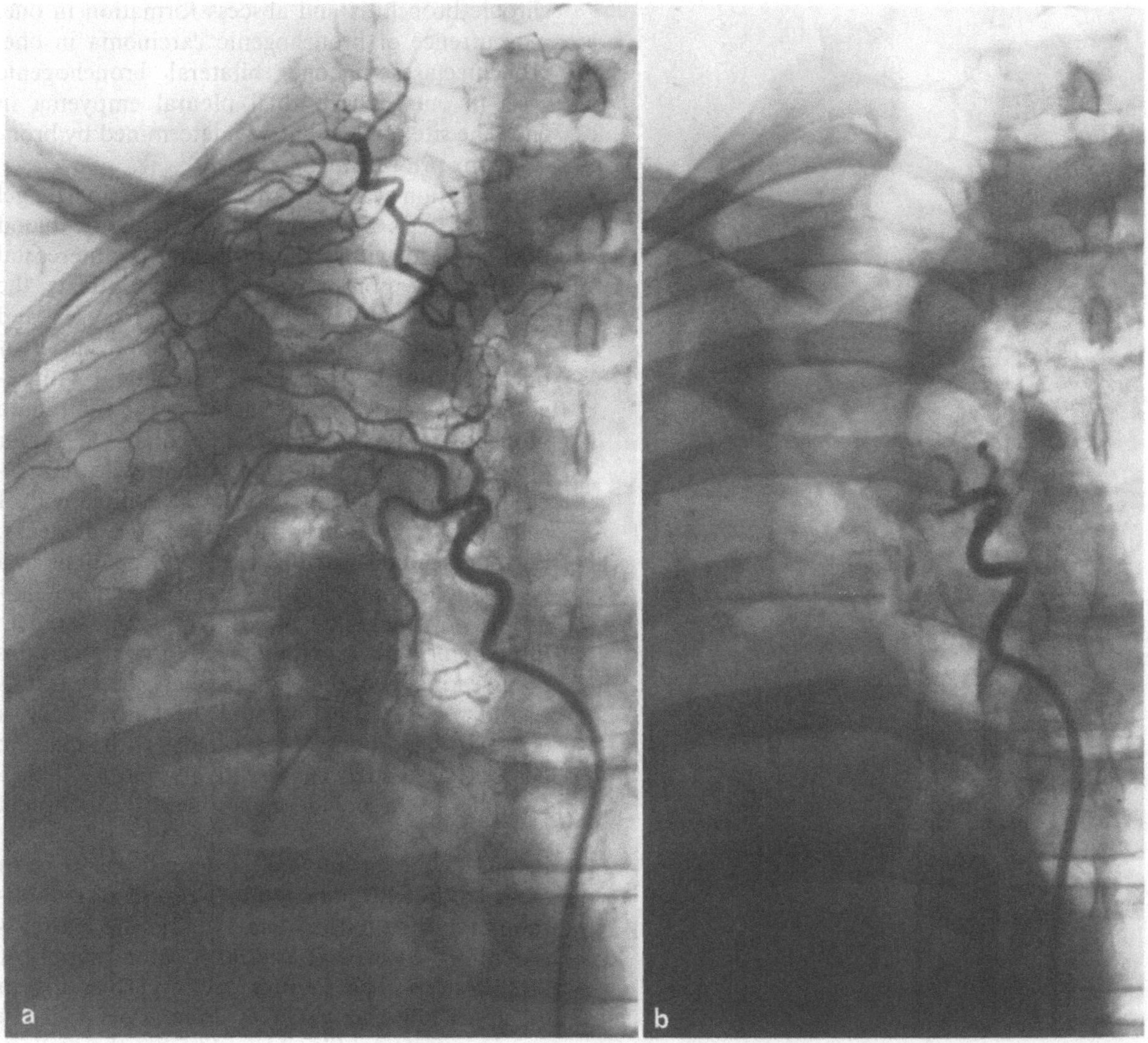

Fig. 5a, b. Angiography in a 53-year-old patient, right upper lobe lobectomy performed because of bronchogenic carcinoma, recurring in the right main bronchus; bleeding. **a** Bronchial artery. Moderate staining of the tumor recurrence. No extravasation of contrast medium. **b** After embolization

Fig. 4a, b. Angiography in a 43-year-old patient with bilateral cysts and chronic infections, bleeding from the right lower lobe. **a** Common trunk of the bronchial arteries. The right one is widened and tortuous. Bronchopulmonary arterioarterial shunts in the wall of the cysts. **b** After embolization

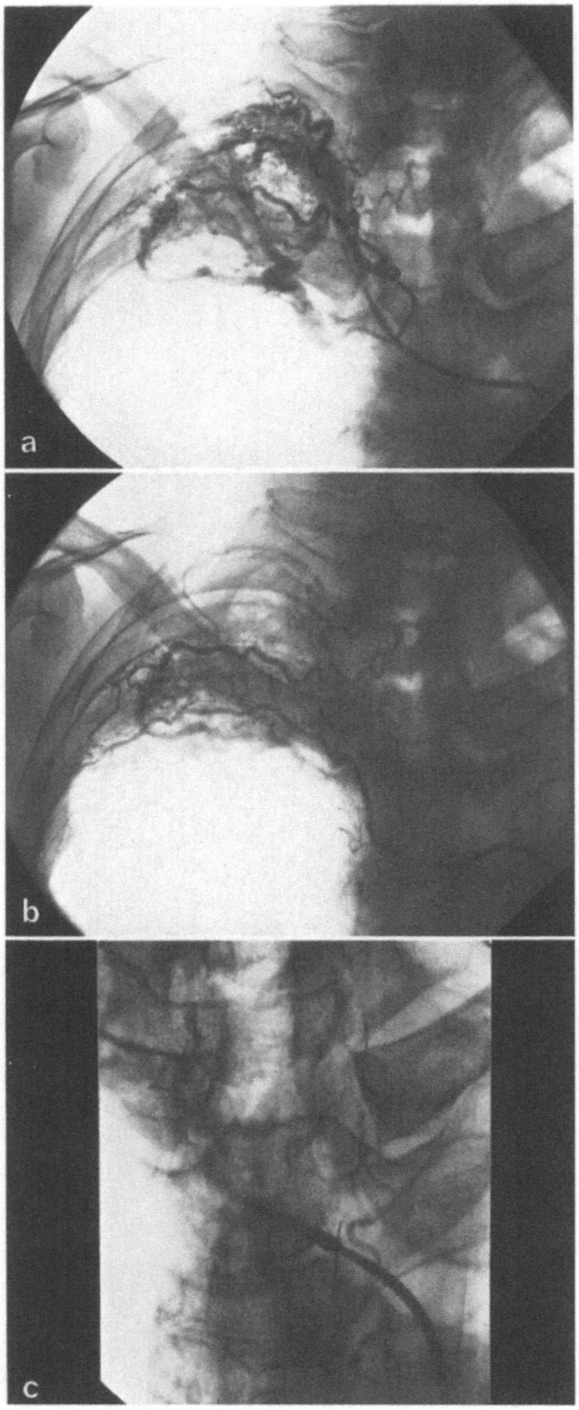

Fig. 6. a–c. Angiography in a 73-year-old patient with old bilateral tuberculosis and aspergilloma of a cavity in the right upper lobe. **a, b** Right cranial intercostal arteries. Excessive vascularity in the wall of the cavity. **c** Intercostal trunk after embolization

chronic bronchitis and abscess formation in one, reoccurrence of bronchogenic carcinoma in one, bronchiectases in one, bilateral bronchogenic cysts in one, and residual pleural empyema in one. The site of bleeding was determined by bronchoscopy prior to angiography.

Embolization was performed by injection of gel foam particles 5 × 2 mm in size until the blood flow stopped within the bronchial or intercostal arteries, as appropriate. In seven patients the acute bleeding stopped after embolization, and four had no further bleeding during an observation period of 1–23 months. The patient with recurrent bronchogenic carcinoma of the right main bronchus (Fig. 5) rebled and died of tumor growth in the trachea. One patient who had reoccurring purulent infections and complained of spitting blood was hospitalized for several weeks, but no bleeding was observed. One patient had recurring hemoptysis after 4 months, and one failure to stop the acute bleeding was registered in the patient with aspergilloma. No complications occurred in any of the eight patients. These results should be seen against the background of a 60%–80% mortality in patients with massive hemoptysis treated conservatively and 19%–30% mortality in those undergoing operative treatment [2, 5, 7, 9].

Patients with intracavitary aspergilloma (Fig. 6) are a group with poor primary results of embolization reported in the literature [2]. The reason is probably the excessive arterial collateral supply of these lesions. The cavities occur particularly in the upper lobes, at which level the cavity wall can receive a systemic blood supply from the axillary and the subclavian arteries via pleural adhesions. There are the internal and external mammary arteries, the thyrocervical trunk, the costocervical trunk, and more. Embolization of all the supplying arteries is difficult or impossible.

Conclusion

Embolization of bronchial arteries is a successfull method for arresting the bleeding in life-threatening hemoptysis in patients in whom pulmonary resection is contraindicated. The long-term results depend on the underlying disease. If arterial supply to the spinal cord is demonstrated by angiography, embolization is contraindicated. However, the possibility of spinal cord lesions following embolization cannot safely be discounted when no arteries to the spinal cord are visualized.

References

1. Botenga ASJ (1970) Selective bronchial and intercostal arteriography. Steufert Kroese, Leiden
2. Crocco JA, Rooney JJ, Fankushen DS, et al. (1968) Massive hemoptysis. Arch Intern Med 121:495–498
3. Garzon AA, Ceruti M, Gourin A, et al. (1970) Pulmonary resection for massive hemoptysis. Surgery 67:633–638
4. Harley JD, Killien FC, Peck AC (1977) Massive hemoptysis controlled by transcatheter embolization of the bronchial arteries. AJR 128:302–304
5. McCollum WB, Mattox KL, Guinn GA, Beall AC Jr (1975) Immediate operative treatment for massive hemoptysis. Chest 67:152–155
6. Prioleau WH, Vujic I, Parker EF, Voegele LD, Hairston P (1980) Control of hemoptysis by bronchial artery embolization. Chest 78:878–880
7. Rabkin IC, Perelman MI, Birjukov JV, Gotman LN, Ambrozaitis RK (1980) Die angiographische Diagnostik und Katheterembolisation bei Lungenblutungen. Radiol Diagn (Berl) 22:309–315
8. Remy J, Arnaud A, Fardou H, Giraud R, Voisin C (1977) Treatment of hemoptysis by embolization of bronchial arteries. Radiology 122:33–37
9. Thoms NW, Wilson RF, Puro HE, et al. (1972) Life-threatening hemoptysis in primary lung abscess. Ann Thorac Surg 14:347–358
10. Vujic I, Pyle R, Parker E, Mithoefer J (1980) Control of massive hemoptysis by embolization of intercostal arteries. Radiology 137:617–620
11. Wholey MH, Chamoro HA, Rao G, Ford WB, Miller WH (1976) Bronchial artery embolization for massive hemoptysis. JAMA 236:2501–2504

Long-Term Results of Percutaneous Transluminal Angioplasty

E. Zeitler

Radiologisches Zentrum, Abteilung Diagnostik, Klinikum Nürnberg, Flurstrasse 17, 8500 Nürnberg, FRG

Introduction

The technique of percutaneous transluminal angioplasty (PTA), first described by Dotter and Judkins [3] in 1964, has been considerably modified by the development of double-lumen balloon catheters by Grüntzig and Hopff [6]. This therapeutic approach, primarily developed for the dilatation of arterial stenoses and for recanalization of arterial occlusions in pelvic and lower extremity arteries, has been able to be applied more widely since the development of the Grüntzig [4] balloon catheter technique. Coronary artery stenoses [5, 7, 12], renal artery stenoses [8, 9, 15], and obstructive lesions in major branches of the aortic arch [1, 10, 11] have now become accessible. While many reports of preliminary results have been published [2, 16–18, 20], the number of studies with long-term results remains small [13, 14, 16, 20].

Previous reports have indicated that the use of platelet aggregation inhibitors before and after PTA considerably reduces the rate of rethrombosis in the first 10 days after the procedure [4, 10]. Furthermore, several studies [4, 13, 20] confirm that long-term anticoagulant therapy results in improved patency rates over several years.

At a symposium in Nürnberg on 13th–15th May 1982, the results obtained to date in various institutions were discussed. In this way a collective of more than 5000 cases was assembled to clarify the efficacy of PTA under present conditions.

Materials and Methods

Only symptomatic patients with angiographically and hemodynamically demonstrated obstructive arterial lesions were included.

In total, 2808 obstructive lesions of the femoral and popliteal arteries (1540 stenoses, 1268 occlusions) and 2364 obstructions of the iliac arteries (2264 stenoses, 100 occlusions) were embraced by the study.

Only cases involving treatment using the balloon catheter technique were accepted. Included are cases in which the first passage of the obstruction was obtained with a 7F or 9F polyethylene or single Teflon catheter or with a balloon catheter. In each case, definitive dilatation was attempted with a balloon catheter.

Primary success was defined as angiographic, hemodynamically confirmed improvement in arterial perfusion. Hemodynamic status was monitored by measurements of peripheral pulse and Doppler arterial pressure. A decrease of at least 20 mm Hg in the difference between systolic arm pressures and those at the ankle, or an increase in the Doppler quotient (systolic blood pressure at the ankle over systolic brachial artery pressure) of more than 0.2 was considered a positive result.

Clinical improvement, manifested by improvement in pain-free walking range at a defined pace or on a treadmill, relief of rest pain, and healing of gangrene, was also taken into consideration in judging positive results. However, clinical criteria were never used exclusively. On the other hand, in cases of two- or three-level obstruction, ankle pressures alone could not be used to judge a therapeutic success of a given procedure.

Most of the investigating teams employed platelet aggregation inhibitors, both before and after dilatation, as an adjunct to PTA. The procedure was conducted under local anesthesia in all centers, but additional medication provided varied with the institution. In one center no adjunct drug therapy was recommended, and in two groups anticoagulant therapy was initiated only later.

Follow-up examinations were conducted at 3, 6, 9, and 12 months after hospital discharge and then annually for 4 more years.

From the 5172 treated cases followed up for 2–5 years, it has become obvious that the greatest number of recurrences appear in the first 6

Radiology Today 2. Ed. by F. H. W. Heuck and M. W. Donner

months. Patency rates did not diminish significantly between 2 and 5 years. The long-term success rate at those centers without adjunct anticoagulant therapy remained lower over the years, and conversely those groups instituting anticoagulation had clearly better results than average over the long term. These differences cannot be construed as statistically significant, however, since no randomized study was conducted and since patient selection and indications were not completely uniform from one center to another.

In order to obtain the most objective judgement of the efficacy of PTA, the results were formulated as a "cure rate," defined as follows:

Primary success (e.g., 0.93) × patency rate (e.g., 63%) = cure rate (e.g., 58.6%)

With this definition and under the conditions defined above, 2- to 5-year cure rates of 61% in 2101 femoropopliteal obliterations and 75% in 1082 iliac artery stenoses were obtained. A cure rate of 25% was found in the 100 iliac occlusions treated.

Similarly assembled long-term results after dilatation of renal artery stenoses in 792 patients showed a significant difference in efficacy between patients with fibromuscular dysplasia (78%) and those with atherosclerotic stenoses (57%).

The reported frequency of complications requiring surgery is comparable to previously published figures of under 2%. No deaths were reported during the procedure itself. However, a 10-day mortality of 0.2% after PTA has been observed, primarily from myocardial infarct, cardiac insufficiency, or pulmonary emboli.

Discussion

The assembled results indicate that the prognosis depends on the type of obstruction. The patency and success rate in femoropopliteal stenoses or occlusions shorter than 3 cm are significantly better than those in femoropopliteal occlusions longer than 12 cm.

The influence of clinical stage as classified by Fontaine (II = claudication; III = rest pain; IV = gangrene) and adjunct medical therapy remain problems for further study.

The only study with follow-up controls after PTA using the original Dotter method or with single Teflon catheter, involving 81 patients treated for claudication (Fig. 1), shows that femoropopliteal occlusions longer than 12 cm present no indication for PTA. The only exception to this may be in cases of limb salvage in poor surgical candidates. Additionally, comparison of results shows that patency rate and cure rate have been improved considerably since the introduction of Grüntzig's balloon catheter technique, leading to good long-term results in iliac and femoral stenoses and short femoropopliteal occlusions.

The long-term results of the cooperative study confirm the special advantages of PTA when used for optimal indications. The length of hospital stay is decreased, and risks related to the procedure are low. Data have yet to be obtained on results in coronary and supra-aortic arteries and in other areas where the indications have not yet been defined.

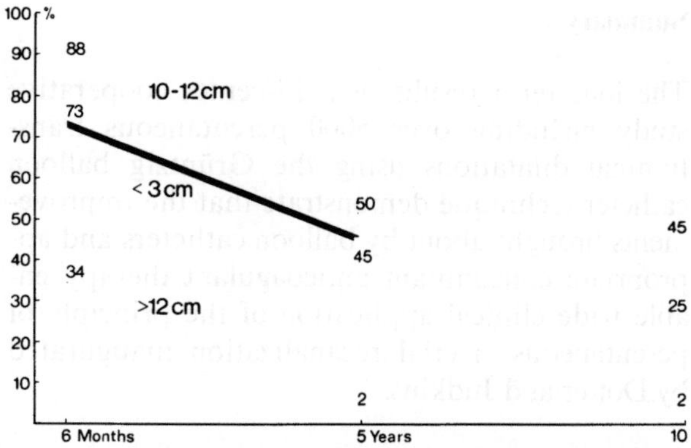

Fig. 1. Patency rate after good primary result of PTA in patients with femoropopliteal obliterations (with and without Anticoagulation + Commatin)

Table 1. Long-term results after PTA

Condition	*n*	Two-to-five-year cure rate (%)	Two-to-four-year normalization/improvement in blood pressure (%)
Femoropopliteal obliteration	2101	61	–
Iliac artery stenosis	1082	75	–
Renal artery stenosis	792	–	
Fibromuscular dysplasia		–	78
Atherosclerosis		–	57

Summary

The long-term results of a 14-center cooperative study including over 5000 percutaneous transluminal dilatations using the Grüntzig balloon catheter technique demonstrate that the improvements brought about by balloon catheters and appropriate concomitant anticoagulant therapy enable wide clinical application of the principle of percutaneous arterial recanalization inaugurated by Dotter and Judkins.

References

1. Colapinto RF, Harries-Jones EP, Johnson KW (1980) Percutaneous transluminal dilatation and recanalization in the treatment of peripheral vascular disease. Radiology 135:583–587
2. Dotter CT (1978) Transluminal angioplasty – pathologic basis. In: Zeitler E, Grüntzig A, Schoop W (eds) Percutaneous vascular recanalization. Springer, Berlin Heidelberg New York 3–12
3. Dotter CT, Judkins MP (1964) Transluminal treatment of arteriosclerotic obstruction: description of a new technic and a preliminary report of its application. Circulation 30:654–670
4. Grüntzig A (1977) Die perkutane transluminale Rekanalisation chronischer Arterienverschlüsse mit einer neuen Dilatationstechnik. Witzstrock, Baden-Baden
5. Grüntzig A (1978) Transluminal dilatation of coronary artery stenoses. Lancet 1:263
6. Grüntzig A, Hopff H (1974) Perkutane Rekanalisation chronischer arterieller Verschlüsse mit einem neuen Dilatationskatheter. Dtsch Med Wschr 99:2502–2505
7. Kaltenbach M (1981) Coronary dilatation. Fourth Symposium on Coronary Heart Disease, Springer, Berlin Heidelberg New York
8. Kuhlmann U, Grüntzig A, Vetter W, Furrer J, Lütolf U, Siegenthaler W (1978) Renovaskuläre Hypertonie: Therapie durch perkutane transluminale Dilatation von Nierenarterienstenosen. Schweiz Med Wochenschr 108 [Suppl 47]: 1847–1859
9. Mahler F, Krneta A, Haertel M (1979) Treatment of renovascular hypertension by transluminal renal artery dilatation. Ann Intern Med 90:56–57
10. Mathias K, Schlosser V, Reinke M (1980) Katheterrekanalisation eines Subclaviaverschlusses. ROFO 132 [Suppl 3]:346–347
11. Motarjeme A, Keifer JW, Zuska AJ (1981) Percutaneous transluminal angioplasty as a complement to surgery. Radiology 141:341–346
12. Myler RK, Stertzer SH, Wallsh E, Bruno MS (1982) Transluminal coronary angioplasty: Results, complications, follow-up, and considerations of extension of indications. An analysis of 409 procedures. In: Kaltenbach M, Grüntzig A, Rentrop K, Bussmann, W-D (eds) Transluminal Coronary Angioplasty and Intracoronary Thrombolysis. Springer, Berlin Heidelberg New York 6–10
13. Schmidtke I, Zeitler W, Schoop W (1975) Langzeitergebnisse der perkutanen Katheterbehandlung (Dotter-Technik) bei femoropoplitealen Arterienverschlüssen im Stadium II. Vasa 4:210
14. Schmidtke I, Zeitler E, Schoop W (1978) Spätergebnisse (5–8 Jahre) der perkutanen Katheterbehandlung (Dotter-Technik) bei femoropoplitealen Arterienverschlüssen. Vasa 7:4–15
15. Schwarten DE, Yune HY, Klatte EC, Grim CE, Weinberger MH (1980) Clinical experience with percutaneous transluminal angioplasty (PTA) of stenotic renal arteries. Radiology 135:601–604
16. Wierny L, Plass R, Porstmann W (1974) Long-term results in 100 consecutive patients treated by transluminal angioplasty. Radiology 112:543–548
17. Zeitler E (1980) Percutaneous dilatation and recanalization of iliac and femoral arteries. Cardiovasc Intervent Radiol 3:207–212
18. Zeitler E, Schoop W, Zahnow W (1971) The treatment of occlusive arterial disease by transluminal catheter angioplasty. Radiology 99:19–26
19. Zeitler E, Reichold J, Schoop W, Loew D (1973) Einfluß von Acetylsalicylsäure auf das Frühergebnis nach perkutaner Rekanalisation arterieller Obliterationen nach Dotter. Dtsch Med Wochenschr 98:1285–1288
20. Zeitler E, Grüntzig A, Schoop W (1978) Percutaneous vascular recanalization. Springer, Berlin Heidelberg New York

Percutaneous Transluminal Renal Angioplasty: Clinical and Angiographic Follow-up Results

I. Obrez, S. Šimunić, E. Baretić-Kolar, M. Šurlan, R. Gürtl, M. Klenkar, S. Kaplan-Pavlovič, and I. Fudurić-Winter

Institute of Roentgenology, University Clinical Center, Ljubljana, Yugoslavia

Since the first percutaneous transluminal renal angioplasty (PTRA) by balloon catheter was performed in 1978 for treatment of renovascular hypertension [1], more than 1000 patients have been treated by this method throughout the world.

The purpose of this communication is to present our own clinical and angiographic follow-up results of PTRA and to compare them with the results of other authors [1].

Material and Methods

Sixty-two patients, 41 males and 21 females, aged from 20 to 67 years, were treated by PTRA between December 1979 and May 1982 for relief of renovascular hypertension. All patients were followed-up clinically and angiographically for 2–30 months (mean 11 months).

The PTRA protocol included general clinical background with classification of hypertension, as well as evaluation of response to medical and/or surgical therapy for each patient. Informed consent was obtained. Prior to PTRA, a set of standard diagnostic tests was utilized, e.g., renal function tests, sequential i.v. urography, renal isotope studies, renin assay, renal angiography, and measurement of pressure gradient. Patients were premedicated for the 3 days prior to the procedure with aspirin (1.5 g/day) and dipiridamole (225 mg/day).

The transfemoral or transaxillary approach was used for introduction of catheters. In the majority of patients, double-lumen balloon catheters (7F, short tip, straight or curved, balloon diameter 4–6 mm) were utilized for angioplasty. In tight stenoses, however, a coaxial balloon catheter system was preferred.

During the procedure, the vascular surgical team was on standby. Immediate results of PTRA were assessed by measurement of pressure gradient, renal angiography, blood pressure measurements (hourly for 24 h), renal function tests, and isotope studies.

Following the procedure, patients were transferred to the intensive care unit for 24 h. The same medication was continued for 6 days. Clinical follow-up controls were scheduled at 1, 3, 6, 9, and 12 months after PTRA and then every 6 months. The effect on blood pressure was determined, and the necessary tests, including renal function tests, isotope studies, renin assay, renal angiography, and measurement of pressure gradient, were performed according to the clinical result.

Results

Based on the technical success of PTRA and its effect on blood pressure, patients are divided into three groups:

1. "Cured": patient is normotensive (150/95 mm Hg or less) without hypertensive therapy.
2. "Improved": patient is either normotensive with basic antihypertensive therapy or has a drop of diastolic blood pressure of at least 10%.
3. "Failed": no change in blood pressure.

The overall follow-up results in our series are presented in Table 1.

The best clinical results were obtained in patients with fibromuscular dysplasia (FMD), followed by those with atherosclerosis of the renal arteries (AS) and finally by those with lesions of the miscellaneous group (MISC).

[1] Drs. T.A. Sos of New York, C.B. Puijlaert of Utrecht, R. M. Paolini of São Paulo, and E. Zeitler of Nürnberg kindly made their PTRA follow-up results available

Radiology Today 2. Ed. by F. H. W. Heuck and M. W. Donner

Table 1. Overall results on PTRA follow-up in 62 patients

	FMD	AS	MISC
No. of patients	18	39	5
Technical success	14	32	1
Cured and improved	86%	62%	20%

Table 2. Immediate and follow-up results of PTRA in FMD

	Technical failure	Cured *n* (%)	Improved *n* (%)	Failed *n* (%)
Immediate	4	7 (46.6)	6 (40)[a]	1 (13.4)
Follow-up		7 (46.6)	6 (40)	1 (13.4)

[a] Including one patient with bilateral FMD scheduled for contralateral PTRA and one patient with only one kidney

The accumulated experience of other authors demonstrates similar differences in the success rate of PTRA in vascular lesions of various etiologies. It seems appropriate, therefore, to evaluate the follow-up results of PTRA in each etiologic group separately.

Fibromuscular Dysplasia

The immediate and follow-up results of PTRA in FMD are listed in Table 2. There were 19 attempts in 18 patients (12 female, 6 male, mean age 36 years). Included are three patients with bilateral disease and one patient with only one kidney (Fig. 1) The best clinical results were obtained in patients having unilateral or bilateral focal lesion in the middle or distal third of the renal artery. Following PTRA, six of the seven patients who became normotensive did so within 48 h. All of them remained normotensive during the observation period (2–26 months, mean 11 months). Depending on the extent of FMD, moderate to significant clinical improvement was noted in the majority of patients having multifocal extra- and intrarenal lesions (Fig. 1).
Technical failures occurred in patients with advanced FMD in whom the passage of a guide wire and/or balloon catheter through the lesions was not possible. For comparison, the follow-up results of PTRA in FMD obtained by Drs. Sos, Puijlaert, and Paolini are presented in Table 3.

Atherosclerotic Stenosis

The immediate and follow-up results for the entire AS group are shown in Table 4. There were 41 attempts in 39 patients (female 9, male 30, mean age 50 years). Included are two patients with ostial stenosis (both failures), three with multifocal bilateral lesions, and four with shrunken kidneys.
Follow-up was for 2–30 months (18 patients over 12 months). Four of eight patients initially normotensive remained so for 12–30 months after PTRA (Fig. 2). Four patients in whom good clinical results were obtained immediately following PTRA became gradually hypertensive after 12 months due to restenosis and required basic antihypertensive medication. Also, three patients from the improved group were classified as failures 10–12 months after PTRA. In one of them, the procedure was repeated 22 months after the first PTRA with subsequent clinical improvement. In the four patients with shrunken kidneys there was no blood pressure benefit but the renal function improved. Again, for comparison, the follow-up results of PTRA in AS obtained by Drs. Sos, Puijlaert, and Paolini are presented in Table 5.

Table 3. PTRA in FMD: comparative results

Author (follow-up in months)	*n*	Cured	Improved	Failed
Sos (New York) (4–40, mean 16)	27	60%	33%	7%
Puijlaert (Utrecht) (6 and longer)	26	95%		5%
Paolini (São Paulo) (8–12)	21	60%	26%	14%
Our study (2–30, mean 11)	14	47%	40%	13%
Cured and improved			86%–95%	

Table 4. Immediate and follow-up results of PTRA in AS

	Technical failure	Cured *n* (%)	Improved *n* (%)	Failed *n* (%)
Immediate	7	8 (23.5)	15 (44.1)	9 (32.4)
Follow-up		4 (12.5)	16 (50)	12 (37.5)
Cured and improved			62%	

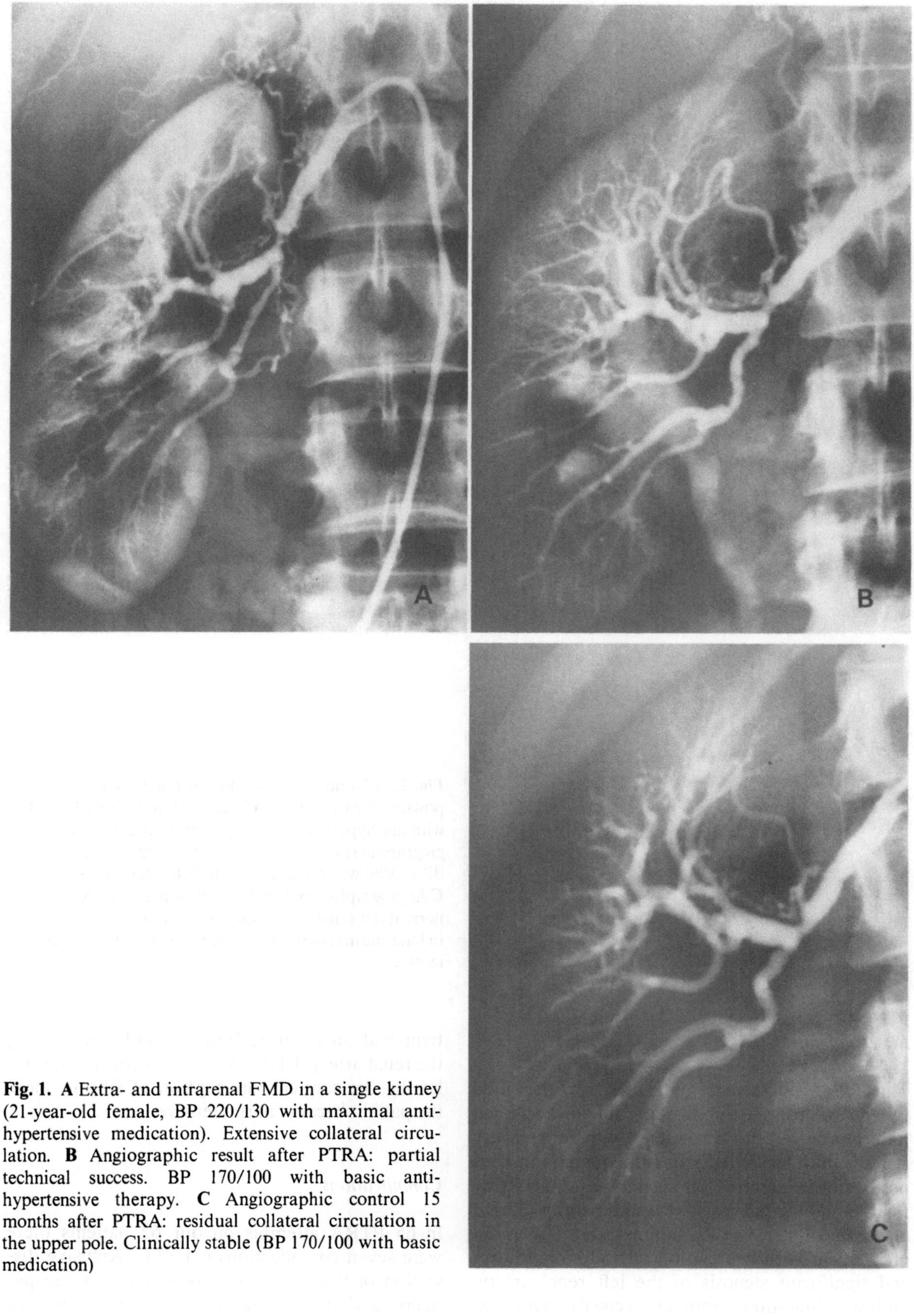

Fig. 1. A Extra- and intrarenal FMD in a single kidney (21-year-old female, BP 220/130 with maximal antihypertensive medication). Extensive collateral circulation. **B** Angiographic result after PTRA: partial technical success. BP 170/100 with basic antihypertensive therapy. **C** Angiographic control 15 months after PTRA: residual collateral circulation in the upper pole. Clinically stable (BP 170/100 with basic medication)

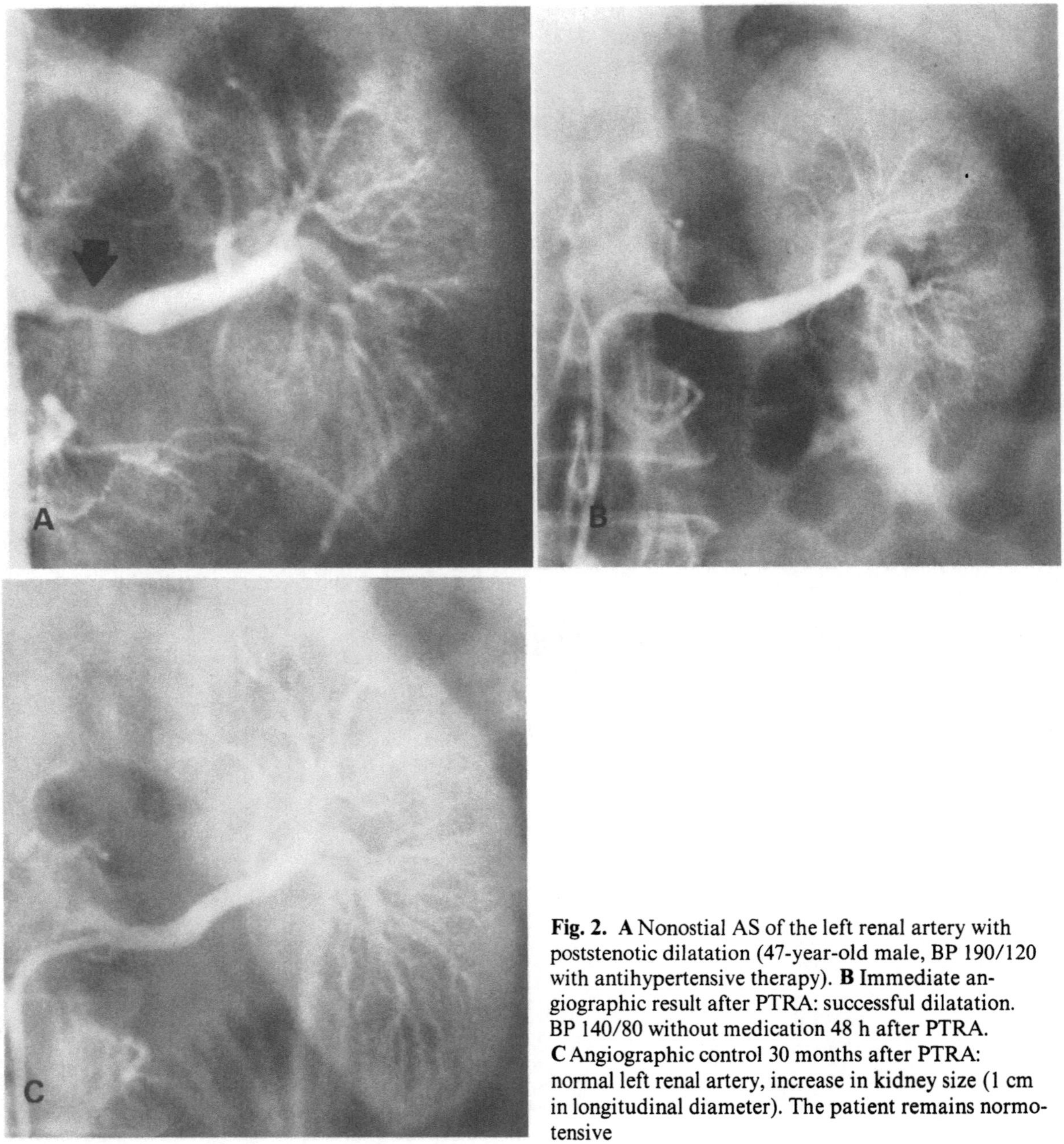

Fig. 2. **A** Nonostial AS of the left renal artery with poststenotic dilatation (47-year-old male, BP 190/120 with antihypertensive therapy). **B** Immediate angiographic result after PTRA: successful dilatation. BP 140/80 without medication 48 h after PTRA. **C** Angiographic control 30 months after PTRA: normal left renal artery, increase in kidney size (1 cm in longitudinal diameter). The patient remains normotensive

Miscellaneous

The follow-up results of PTRA in the miscellaneous group are shown in Table 6. Technical failure occurred in two patients with renal artery stenosis in transplanted kidneys. One patient with postoperative stenosis of the native renal artery (end-to-end anastomosis) was successfully dilated and is normotensive 17 months after PTRA. In one patient with coarctation of abdominal aorta and significant stenosis of the left renal artery, multiple dilatations were unsuccessful. One patient had an extrinsic fibrous band compressing the renal artery. PTRA was not successful, but following the surgical interruption of fibrous band the patient became normotensive.

Complications

In 65 PTRA attempts on our 62 patients there were seven complications (11.3%). Occlusive dissection of the renal artery occurred in three patients, and despite surgical intervention two of

Table 5. PTRA in AS: comparative results

Author (follow-up in months)	*n*	Cured (%)	Improved (%)	Failed (%)
Sos (New York) (4–40, mean 16)				
Unilateral				
Nonostial stenosis	16	31	56	13
Ostial stenosis	5	0	0	100
Occlusion	5	20	0	80
Bilateral	21	10	5	85
Puijlaert (Utrecht) (6 and longer)	52	52		48
Paolini (São Paulo) (8–12)	30	41	41	18

Table 6. Follow-up results of PTRA in the miscellaneous group

Type of lesion	*n*	Cured	Improved	Failed
Renal transplant stenosis	2			2
Postoperative stenosis of native renal artery	1	1		
Perivascular sclerosis	1			1
Extrinsic band	1			1
Total	5	1 (20%)		4 (80%)

them eventually required nephrectomy. Following surgery, one patient became normotensive. There were two minor segmental infarctions and two transient increases in blood pressure.

The incidence of complications after PTRA in the literature is 10%–17%, with no deaths reported. The range of complications is as follows:

Major
Occlusive dissection of renal artery
Thrombosis of renal artery
Rupture and/or perforation of renal artery
Retroperitoneal hematoma
Major segmental infarction
Renal failure
Distal embolization
Axillary hematoma (Neurological deficit)

Minor
Nonocclusive dissection
Minor segmental infarction
Spasm of renal arteries
Hematoma at puncture site
Transient hyper- or hypotension

Discussion

Simultaneously with the growing experience, standardization of the protocol and techniques of PTRA is under way [2, 3, 4–7]. Close collaboration with nephrologists and vascular surgeons is essential. Different opinions still exist regarding the medication of patients before and after PTRA; further studies are needed to find the optimal solution to this problem.

Significant differences in the success rate of PTRA within and between the various etiologic groups underline the need for a proper selection of patients.

Compared to other groups, hypertensive patients with FMD are relatively homogeneous: females predominate, the patients are usually younger (mean age 35 years in our series), and there are no or few associated medical problems. Also, our follow-up results indicate that the therapeutic effect of PTRA has a tendency to remain stable in FMD. On the other hand, the hypertensive AS patients are much less homogeneous: age, type, and distribution of lesions as well as associated renal and extrarenal disease may influence the angioplastic procedure and the therapeutic result.

Breaking down the follow-up results into subgroups, Sos (personal communication, 1982) has shown that there are significant differences in the success rate of PTRA in unilateral nonostial or ostial AS and occlusion of the renal artery. Also, in bilateral lesions, the success rate depends on technical success of PTRA (unilateral, bilateral), on distribution and type of lesions, and on associated disease (shrunken kidney, aortic aneurysm, etc.).

Puijlaert (personal communication, 1982) has analyzed the influence of age on the success rate of PTRA in AS: 55% of 30 hypertensive patients under 55 years of age were cured or improved, and only 45% of 22 patients aged over 55 years benefited from the procedure. It is evident from our follow-up results that the natural progression of AS may compromise the therapeutic effects of PTRA in a relatively short period of time.

Zeitler (personal communication, 1982) has collected the follow-up results of PTRA in 792 patients from several centers: overall, 78% of FMD patients and 57% of AS patients were cured or improved.

In our angiographic follow-up studies, further changes of arterial lumen were noted at the site of dilatation. In successful cases, poststenotic dilatation of the artery and collateral circulation regressed completely. Also, a moderate enlargement of the kidney was observed (up to 1 cm in length).

In the miscellaneous group, PTRA was performed mostly in patients with postoperative stenosis of the renal artery (renal transplants and native renal artery), secondly in renal venous grafts, postirradiation stenosis, and stenosis caused by arteritis. Further experience is needed for adequate follow-up evaluation in this group of patients.

Today, after 4 years experience in more than 1000 patients, it can be stated that PTRA is an effective alternative to medical and surgical treatment of renovascular hypertension.

References

1. Grüntzig A, Kuhlman U, Vetter W, et al. (1978) Treatment of renovascular hypertension with percutaneous transluminal dilatation of a renal artery stenosis. Lancet 1:801–802
2. Puijlaert CB (1979) Preliminary report on dilatation of renal artery stenosis in hypertension with the aid of a balloon catheter. J Belge Radiol 62:345–355
3. Richter EI, Grüntzig A, Ingrisch H, et al. (1980) Percutaneous dilatation of renal artery stenoses. Ann Radiol (Paris) 23:275–278
4. Schwarten DE, Yune HY, Klatte EC, et al. (1980) Clinical experience with percutaneous transluminal angioplasty (PTA) of stenotic renal arteries. Radiology 135:601–604
5. Sörensen R, Grüntzig A, Apitzsch E, et al. (1979) Transluminale Angioplastie von Nierenarterinstenosen zur Behandlung des renalen Hochdrucks. RoFo 131:575–580
6. Tegtmeyer CJ, Dyer R, Teates CD, et al. (1980) Percutaneous transluminal dilatation of the renal arteries. Techniques and results. Radiology 135:589–599
7. Tegtmeyer CJ, Teates CD, Crigler N (1981) Percutaneous transluminal angioplasty in patients with renal artery stenosis. Follow-up studies. Radiology 140:323–330

Radiology of Lymphatic System

Diagnostic Radiology of Lymph Node Disease

W. A. Fuchs

Institut für Diagnostische Radiologie, Universität Bern, Inselspital, 3010 Bern, Switzerland

The radiological evaluation of malignant lymph node disease is currently being transformed due to the development of noninvasive cross-sectional imaging techniques, i.e., sonography and, particularly, computed tomography.

Pelvis and Abdomen

In the pelvic and abdominal areas, lymphography, frequently used in combination with cavography and urography, has for the past 20 years been the classical radiological method of detecting malignant spread to lymph nodes. Because of the great clinical experience gained with this investigation technique, it still represents the "gold standard" against which the newer imaging techniques should be measured.

Lymphography

Because of its high degree of spatial resolution lymphography is able to detect macroscopic tumor foci within lymph nodes. Characteristic lymphographic findings in *metastatic spread of epithelial neoplasms* include [5]:

- Filling defects of 5–10 mm minimal diameter impervious to contrast material, due to malignant tissue in normal-sized or moderately enlarged regional lymph nodes.
- Obstruction of the lymphatic circulation by malignant infiltration, leading to contrast filling of collateral lymphatics.

In *Hodgkin's disease* and *non-Hodgkin's lymphoma* the internal architecture of the lymph nodes is altered and they are moderately to grossly enlarged. Obstruction of lymph flow is rare and mostly occurs after radiotherapy. It must be stressed that there are no lymphographic patterns pathognomonic of any specific disease. Both acute and chronic inflammation, as well as reactive hyperplasia or even fibrolipomatosis, may produce structural alterations similar to those in metastatic disease and malignant lymphoma. False-positive lymphographic diagnosis may thus arise.

Topographic anatomy enables lymphography to visualize only the external and common iliac and the aortic lymph nodes. Most of the internal iliac nodes and some of the upper aortic nodes, but most notably the visceral pelvic nodes and nodes within the mesentery, the hilus of the liver, and the spleen are not amenable to diagnosis by lymphography. Consequently, the possibility of false-negative lymphographic findings has to be taken into consideration. In addition, false-negative lymphograms may also result from microscopic tumor involvement.

Sonography

Enlarged infradiaphragmatic lymph nodes of more than 3 cm in diameter may be visualized by sonography [2, 3, 13, 15]. In such cases the contours of both the abdominal aorta and the inferior vena cava may be obliterated. Ultrasound-guided biopsy of a lymphomatous mass is readily achieved, with conclusive results in about two-thirds of cases. Considerable difficulties in the performance of sonographic investigations may occur when loops of bowel and folds of mesentery cover the lumbar region, particularly in obese patients. For this reason diagnostic limitations are imposed on sonography in about one-third of cases.

Computed Tomography

Computed tomography (CT) consistently demonstrates enlarged lymph nodes of any localization

Radiology Today 2. Ed. by F. H. W. Heuck and M. W. Donner

[7, 9, 20]. Lymph nodes measuring more than 10–15 mm in transverse diameter are generally regarded to be abnormal. Asymmetrical size and configuration of corresponding lymph nodes within regional lymph node groups are additional diagnostic signs of abnormality.

Conclusive analysis of the accuracy of radiological imaging methods must be based solely on histological findings in lymph nodes obtained at surgical exploration, not on corroboration by other imaging procedures or on the basis of clinical data. The relative diagnostic accuracy of lymphography and CT has been investigated at our institution for the pelvic and abdominal regions:

Overall accuracy = *true positives* + *true negatives*
total number of patients
Sensitivity (true-positive rate) = proportion of true-positive diagnoses in patients with histopathologically positive findings
Specificity (true-negative rate) = proportion of true-negative diagnoses in patients with histopathologically negative findings
False-positive rate = proportion of false-positive diagnoses in patients with histopathologically negative findings
False-negative rate = proportion of false-negative diagnoses in patients with histopathologically positive findings

All results were verified by staging lymphadenectomy.

In 44 patients, histopathologically proven *carcinoma of the urinary bladder* was investigated by CT [18]. In addition, lymphography was performed in 29 of these patients. The evaluation of lymph nodes by CT was accurate in 39 of 44 patients (89.5%), whereas the overall accuracy rate of lymphography was only 72.5%. The sensitivity in detection of malignant lymph node involvement was 85% for CT but only 46% for lymphography. On the other hand, the specificity was lower for CT (85%) than for lymphography (94%).

In 30 patients with *nonseminomatous testicular tumors*, the diagnostic results of lymphography and CT were verified by therapeutic radical lymphadenectomy. For lymphography the overall accuracy rate was 80% with a true-positive rate (sensitivity) of 78% and a true-negative rate (specificity) of 81%. CT had an overall accuracy rate of 83% with a low sensitivity of 44%, i.e., a relatively high rate of positive CT diagnoses in histopathologically negative lymph nodes. Negative CT findings in histopathologically tumorous lymph nodes were quite rare, specificity being 86%.

The relative value of lymphography and CT for the *N-staging of epithelial neoplasms* may be summed up as follows: Bulky metastatic disease may easily be identified by either CT or lymphography. Negative lymphographic findings do not exclude metastatic disease in a high proportion of cases. This diagnostic drawback may readily be explained by the fact that lymphography does not completely visualize the regional lymph nodes of primary malignancy. In addition, small metastatic foci within lymph nodes are not visualized by lymphography. On the other hand, a positive lymphogram is diagnostic since the true-negative rate is high. Negative CT findings are highly suggestive of negative lymph node involvement, whereas marginal lymph node enlargement does not necessarily indicate malignant metastatic spread to regional lymph nodes.

CT-guided needle biopsy may provide conclusive diagnostic results for the detection of malignant metastatic spread to regional lymph nodes in about two-thirds of cases. However, retroperitoneal lymphadenectomy remains an important method for accurate staging.

In *Hodgkin's disease* and *non-Hodgkin's lymphoma*, infradiaphragmatic nodal presentation is visualized by CT without any topographical limitations [1, 4, 10].

In order to evaluate the diagnostic accuracy of CT and lymphography in *Hodgkin's disease*, 52 patients were investigated by lymphography and then underwent staging laparotomy. The overall accuracy rate was 82.5%. The sensitivity (true-positive rate) of lymphography was 46%, whereas the specificity (true-negative rate) was 95%. False-negative lymphographic findings may occur due to nonvisualization of pathological lymph nodes, and lymphographic overdiagnosis of malignancy may be possible because lymphographic patterns of reactive lymph node disease can simulate Hodgkin's disease.

Another group of 32 patients was recently investigated by CT and then underwent staging laparatomy. The overall accuracy of 75% was somewhat lower than that of lymphography observed in the first group of patients whereas both sensitivity (45%) and specificity (90%) were about the same for the two investigation techniques in the two separate patient groups.

The *diagnostic performance of CT* is limited by the possibility of false-negative evaluation of nonspecifically enlarged lymph nodes as tumorous. On the other hand, nonenlargement of lymph nodes at CT generally excludes nodal presentation of Hodgkin's disease, since the true-negative rate (specificity) of CT is about 90%.

Mediastinum

In the mediastinum, CT has challenged the value of conventional radiology in the diagnosis of malignant lymph node disease [6, 12].

On CT, mediastinal lymph nodes [8] are generally considered to be abnormal when the solid rounded or oval mass lesion exceeds 10 mm in diameter [14]. Malignancy is also diagnosed if a conglomerate mass of nodes extends into the mediastinal fat or invades the mediastinal vessels. The diagnosis of lymphadenopathy of the bronchopulmonary (hilar) lymph nodes is based upon enlargement of nonvascular hilar structures and distortion or obstruction of normal bronchi [11, 19].

The malignant involvement of a total of 25 mediastinal lymph nodes was investigated by histopathology in 12 patients with *bronchogenic carcinoma* in order to compare prospectively the diagnostic performances of conventional and computed tomography.

The diagnostic results of CT were clearly superior, the true-positive rate (sensitivity) being 96%. False-positive results on CT did however, occur in five cases. In addition, the diagnostic performance of inclined frontal tomography (IFT) was superior to posterior oblique tomography (POT) with regard to the detection of mediastinal lymphadenopathy, the sensitivity of IFT being 76%, that of POT 56%. This difference is mainly due to the better identification of paratracheal and subcarinal lymphadenopathies by IFT. The specificity (true-negative rate) of the three tomographic methods cannot be conclusively quantitated in this study, since normal-sized lymph nodes were not routinely removed for histological investigation. However, the false-negative rate of CT is clearly more favorable than that of conventional tomography.

The diagnostic value of *CT for the N-staging of bronchogenic carcinoma* was investigated in a retrospective study of 135 cases. The regional lymph nodes were investigated histopathologically by exploratory thoracotomy or postmortem studies in 87 cases [16]. The overall accuracy rate of N-staging was about 82%. The true-positive rate (sensitivity) of CT for N-staging was 93.5%, 62 of 64 examinations actually being positive. On the other hand, the true-negative rate, (specificity) was only 73%, because 17 of 23 examinations were correctly negative. In other words, overstaging was much more common then understaging. The figures of the true-negative rate (sensitivity) must, however, be reduced, since systematic histopathological analysis of the mediastinal and bronchopulmonary lymph nodes was not performed.

From these results it may be concluded that nonenlargement of lymph nodes at CT examination usually signifies operability of bronchogenic neoplasm, avoiding further preoperative N-staging procedures. The diagnostic value of enlarged lymph nodes as demonstrated by CT is limited because of the possibility of inflammatory reactive nontumorous lymph node enlargement. However, massive nodal enlargement to more than 15 mm in diameter usually indicates malignant metastatic spread and inoperability, whereas the presence of smaller nodes necessitates further staging procedures, such as mediastinoscopy and exploratory thoracotomy, to evaluate operability. Finally, it is of interest that the overall accuracy of T-staging of bronchogenic carcinoma by CT was 89.5% and that of M-staging 92% in this series.

CT for staging of Hodgkin's disease was evaluated in a series of 65 nontreated patients with supradiaphragmatic presentation [17]. Enlargement of mediastinal lymph nodes to more than 10 mm diameter, considered to represent nodal involvement, was observed in 58 cases (89%). Anterior mediastinal (78%) and paratracheal (74%) nodes were most frequently enlarged; bronchopulmonary (26%), subcarinal (25%), posterior mediastinal (11%), and pericardial (15%) nodes were less frequently abnormal. *Extranodal involvement* of Hodgkin's disease was observed in the pleural cavity in 26%, in the thoracic wall in 15%, in lung parenchyma in 29%, and in bone in 24.5%. Pericardial infiltration was present in 7.5%. Verification of the pathological findings in this series was based on biopsy at mediastinoscopy and on the impact of tumor-specific treatment.

These results clearly demonstrate the obvious value of CT in localizing the various lymph node groups affected by malignant disease. The visualization of direct or metastatic involvement of extranodal sites, particularly the thoracic wall, the pericardium, and bone structures, provides detailed information for accurate staging and treatment planning of the disease.

Conclusions

In *epithelial tumors,* nonenlargement of regional lymph nodes as demonstrated by CT generally indicates operability; massively enlarged lymph nodes on CT indicate the presence of malignant metastases. Moderate nodal enlargement is nonspecific and calls for histopathological investigation by biopsy or operative lymphadenectomy. In addition to N-staging, CT provides extremely valuable information about the full topographic extent of malignant disease. It facilitates T-staging by demonstrating both the location and size of the primary tumor as well as its extension into the adjacent structures and organs. Distant metastatic spread (M-staging), i.e., involvement of liver, lung, bone, brain, or adrenal glands, is readily demonstrated by CT.

In *malignant lymphoma,* CT enables evaluation of the overall distribution of lymph node involvement both above and below the diaphragm. Extranodal involvement of the bone and lungs is identified, and malignant infiltration of the spleen, liver, and other organs may be suspected.

For these reasons, lymphography is gradually being abandoned as a diagnostic tool for the diagnosis of infradiaphragmatic malignant lymph node disease, as is conventional tomography for the radiological evaluation of mediastinal lymph nodes.

References

1. Blackledge G, et al. (1980) Computed tomography (CT) in the staging of patient with Hodgkin's disease: a report on 136 patients. Clin Radiol 31:143
2. Brascho DJ, et al. (1977) The accuracy of retroperitoneal ultrasonography in Hodgkin's disease and non-Hodgkin's lymphoma. Radiology 125:485
3. Burney BT, et al. (1979) Ultrasound and computed tomography of the abdomen in the staging and management of testicular carcinoma. Radiology 132:415
4. Earl HM, et al. (1980) Computerised tomography (CT) abdominal scanning in Hodgkin's disease. Clin Radiol 31:149
5. Fuchs WA (1971) Neoplasms of epithelial origin. In: Angiography, 2nd ed. Little Brown, Boston, p 1369
6. Fuchs WA (1983) Malignant Metastatic Disease. Malignant Lymphoma. The Diagnostic Impact of Sonography and Computed Tomography on Lymphography. 3rd ed. Little, Brown and Company, Boston 2047
7. Heitzman ER (1981) Computed tomography of the thorax: current perspectives. AJR 136:2
8. Husband JE, et al. (1980) The role of abdominal computed tomography in the management of testicular tumours. Comput Tomogr 4:1
9. Kubik S, et al. (1981) Topographische Anatomie des Mediastinums mit besonderer Berücksichtigung der Querschnittdiagnostik. Radiologe 21:310
10. Lackner K, et al. (1979) Computertomographischer Nachweis von Lymphknotenmetastasen bei malignen Hodentumoren. Ein Vergleich der Ergebnisse von Lymphographie und Computertomographie. RoFO 130:636
11. Lackner K, et al. (1980) Wertigkeit der Computertomographie bei der Stadieneinteilung primärer Lymphknotenneoplasien. RoFO 132:21
12. Naidich DP, et al. (1981) Computed tomography of the pulmonary hila: 2. abnormal anatomy. J Comput Assist Tomogr 5:468
13. Osborne DR, et al. (1982) Comparison of plain radiography, conventional tomography, and computed tomography in detecting intrathoracic lymph node metastases from lung carcinoma. Radiology 142:157
14. Rochester D, et al. (1977) Ultrasound in the staging of lymphoma. Radiology 124:483
15. Schnyder PA, et al. (1981) CT of the pretracheal retrocaval space. AJR 136:303
16. Triller J, et al. (1980) Abdominelle Sonographie, Lymphknoten. Thieme, Stuttgart
17. Vock P, et al. (1981) Die Computertomographie zur Stadieneinteilung des Bronchuskarzinoms. RoFO 134:131
18. Vock P, et al. (1981) Die thorakale Computertomographie beim Lymphoma malignum Hodgkin. Computertomographie 1:68
19. Vock P, et al. (1982) Computed Tomography in Staging of Carcinoma of the Urinary Bladder. Br J Urol 54:158
20. Webb WR, et al. (1981) Computed tomography of the abnormal pulmonary hilum. J Comput Assist Tomogr 5:485
21. Zelch MG, et al. (1979) Clinical comparison of computed tomography and lymphangiography for detection of retroperitoneal lymphadenopathy. Radiol Clin North Am 17:157

Lymphography with the Water-Soluble Contrast Medium Iotasul

V. Taenzer

Abteilung für Röntgen-Diagnostik, Krankenhaus Moabit, Berlin-Tiergarten, Turmstrasse 21, 1000 Berlin 21, FRG

At the present time, radiography of the lymphatic system is carried out with the oily contrast medium Lipiodol, which is injected into the lymphatic vessels directly after they have been surgically exposed. Conventional, water-soluble contrast media are unsuitable for lymphography. Rapid diffusion of the hypertonic solutions of their salts through the loose endothelia of the lymphatic vessel wall into the surrounding tissue leads to blurring and loss of contrast, which are intensified still more by dilution with lymph. Consequently, X-ray visualization of peripheral lymphatic structures is only possible to an inadequate extent, and not at all in the case of central lymphatic structures. Inter alia, the rate of diffusion is influenced by concentration and molecular size. *Indirect* lymphography by nonspecific administration of contrast medium, e.g., intracutaneously or into organs, is not possible with conventional, water-soluble contrast agents.

Even in the age of computed tomography, the desire still exists to have a lymphographic agent which enables X-ray visualization of lymphatic vessels and lymph nodes, quickly and reproducibly, by an indirect route. Iotasul is a new, water-soluble, nonionic, dimeric contrast medium for lymphography. It is distinguished by great molecular size and low osmotic pressure, which guarantee it a sufficiently long residence time in the lymphatic system. Furthermore, molecular size is apparently increased due to association of the individual molecules. Moreover, residence time is prolonged by inclusion of certain additives in the formulation of the contrast medium. The iodine content is 300 mg/ml.

In 1981, Siefert et al. [8] reported on the properties of iotasul, which differ from those of other contrast media, and on initial preclinical experience with this compound.

When it comes in contact with body fluids, the aqueous solution of this nonionic compound separates into two components with different degrees of molecular association. Like conventional contrast media, iotasul is eliminated by the kidneys. In experiments in the dog, blood concentration rises quickly after intralymphatic administration. This persists to the end of infusion and thereafter blood concentration decreases with a biological half-life of 1 h. In the main, elimination in the urine has been completed after 24 h. Iotasul is distinguished by low acute toxicity. The LD_{50} in rats, mice, and dogs exceeds 11–14 g iodine/kg and is thus in the order of magnitude of that for urographic contrast media.

Preclinical Animal Studies

Several reports are available on the results of direct and indirect lymphography in animal experiments [1–3, 6–10]. Other research teams have verified the excellent, initial results obtained by Siefert et al. [8] in dogs, pigs, and monkeys.

Direct Lymphography

In the case of direct lymphography by administration of the contrast medium into lymphatic vessels or lymph nodes, iotasul has no or only a negligible tendency to pass through the lymphatic vessel wall. Any lymph flowing behind has no influence on the density of contrast.

Thus the preconditions for sufficiently complete filling of lymphatic vessels are fulfilled. In comparison X-ray visualization as good as that with Lipiodol, as regards both recognition of contrast and sharpness of detail, can be achieved. This holds both for the lymphatic vessels and lymph nodes of the pelvic and para-aortic regions and for the thoracic duct, of which complete X-ray visualization up to the junction with the venous system is obtained, but only after the contrast medium has passed through several groups

Radiology Today 2. Ed. by F. H. W. Heuck and M. W. Donner

of lymph nodes. Opacification of the lymphatic system persists for 30–45 min after the end of contrast medium infusion.

Indirect Lymphography

Using iotasul, it is for the first time possible in animal experiments to obtain from indirect (intracutaneous, submucous, or parenchymal) administration of the contrast medium lymphograms of the excellent quality known from direct lymphography with iotasul or Lipiodol. Interdigital, intracutaneous perfusion of iotasul into the hindpaws of dogs, pigs and monkeys quickly produces a diagnostically informative image of the retroperitoneal lymphatic system and thoracic duct, which can be repeated at no great expense and as often as necessary. For this, administration of 5–10 ml contrast medium at an infusion rate of 5–15 ml/h has proved to be suitable. After intracutaneous perfusion of iotasul, visualization of lymph node architecture similar to that after administration of Lipiodol is achieved. X-ray visualization of the lymphatic system is quicker after indirect perfusion of iotasul, and contrast is just as good as or even better than that obtained after intralymphatic injection [1]. Perfusion of contrast medium from several puncture sites simultaneously increases the probability that opacification of the lymphatic system will be satisfactory.

Successful intradermal perfusions of iotasul in animals have been performed on the back of the hind- and forepaws, the neck, the eyelid [3, 10], and the mammary gland [6, 7].

Indirect lymphography in animals has been successful after submucous administration of iotasul via the rectum. For this route, Grabbe [2] reports opacification of efferent, regional lymph vessels of a quality not achieved before. Siefert et al. [6–8] succeeded in obtaining good visualization of the efferent lymph vessels of vagina, urinary bladder, and stomach. Studies are available on successful, indirect lymphographic procedures by injection of iotasul into parenchymatous organs and perfusion of testis and prostate gland [6–8].

Clinical Investigations in Humans

Information on experience with iotasul in humans has been sparse. Apitzsch et al. [1] performed individual, successful lymphographic procedures by pernodal administration in patients with malignant systemic diseases. Individual observations by Wenzel-Hora [9, 10] on indirect lymphographic procedures of the arm are available. Partsch, Vienna, reported at the 7th International Congress of Angiologists in Berlin on his experiences with iotasul in patients with lymphedema. I report now on my own experiences, gained with direct and indirect lymphographic procedures in over 40 patients aged between 18 and 88 years.

Direct Lymphography

Direct lymphography was performed with iotasul in 16 patients in whom the indication for caudal lymphography was a malignant disease. Intralymphatic administration of the contrast medium was carried out by the well-known technique, using doses of 7–14 ml and mechanically constant injection rates of 5.6, 14.0, and 28.0 ml/h. The 14 ml/h rate proved to be the most suitable. In some of the patients, the investigation was con-

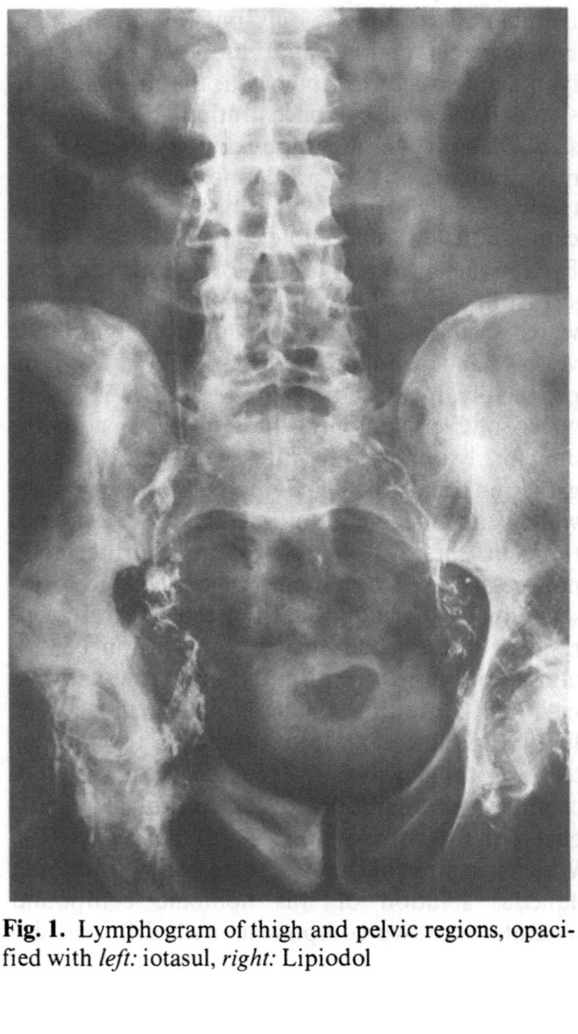

Fig. 1. Lymphogram of thigh and pelvic regions, opacified with *left:* iotasul, *right:* Lipiodol

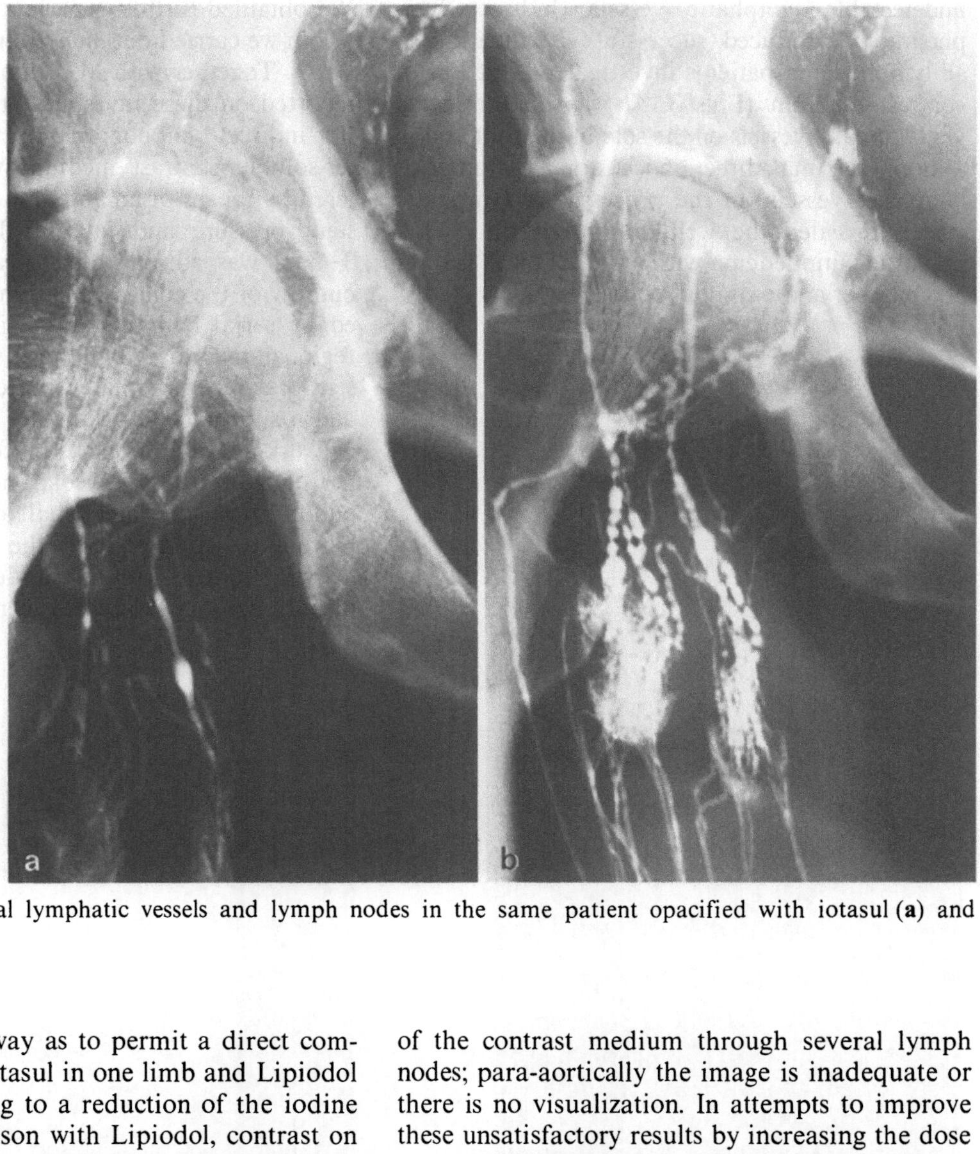

Fig. 2. Right inguinal lymphatic vessels and lymph nodes in the same patient opacified with iotasul (**a**) and Lipiodol (**b**)

ducted in such a way as to permit a direct comparison between iotasul in one limb and Lipiodol in the other. Owing to a reduction of the iodine content in comparison with Lipiodol, contrast on the iotasul side is somewhat slighter but nevertheless good (Fig. 1). In other patients, an investigation of both lower limbs was conducted with iotasul immediately before conventional lymphography with Lipiodol. To a large extent, the results of animal experiments can be confirmed: X-ray morphological visualization of lymphatic vessels and lymph nodes is obtained after administration of iotasul in the limbs and true pelvis in the manner known from Lipiodol.

Afferent and efferent lymph vessels can be differentiated, as with Lipiodol (Fig. 2a, b). The well-known lymph node pattern, with a fibrolipomatous defect in the inguinal lymph node in the example here, is clearly visible. However, in contrast to lymphography with Lipiodol and the results of animal experiments with iotasul, density of contrast decreases in the patient after passage of the contrast medium through several lymph nodes; para-aortically the image is inadequate or there is no visualization. In attempts to improve these unsatisfactory results by increasing the dose or rate of injection, the contrast medium escaped from the lymphatic vessels. Our most recent investigations show that by modification of additives to the contrast medium, extravasation is eliminated and proximal, para-aortic opacification is improved. Nevertheless, on the basis of our initial experiences with the limited quantities of contrast medium available it is not yet possible to come to definite conclusions in this respect.

Indirect Lymphography

We performed indirect lymphographic investigations in 6 patients with lymphedema in whom, despite ample experience on the part of the investigator, direct lymphography was no longer, feasible because of marked dermal backflow and undetectable lymphatic vessels. Indirect lymphography produced successful visualization in all lymphedema patients investigated. Outflow of contrast medium (Figs. 3, 4) was demonstrated via lymphatic vessels on the sole of the foot and in a more proximal direction via dorsal or anterior lymphatic vessels. In the process, the lymphatic vessels revealed the well-known criteria of hypoplastic lymphedema with a reduction in caliber and number and a sinuous course.

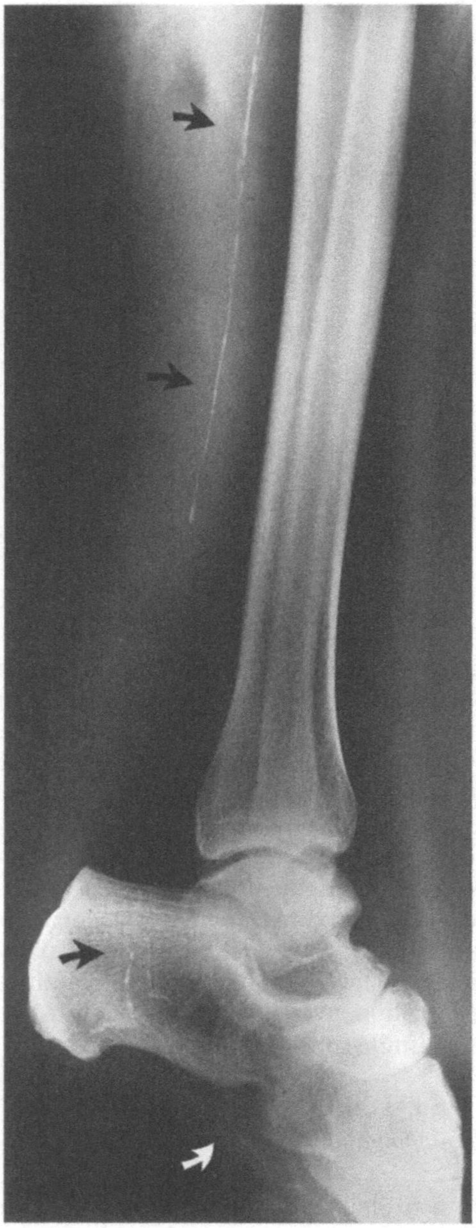

Fig. 3. Indirect lymphogram with iotasul in lymphedema. Lymphatic drainage via sole of foot (*arrow*)

We obtained further experience in 22 patients in whom we carried out *indirect lymphography of the breast.* Together with M. Schmidt, I have already reported on these investigations elsewhere [4, 5]. For indirect lymphography of the breast, the water-soluble contrast medium was also administered by means of an automatic injector at a constant pressure and rate of flow. The dose of 3–5 ml was administered at a rate of 14 ml/h, outflow of the contrast medium being documented by serial lymphograms. Zinser describes the regional, mammary lymphatic system, which consists of a subepidermally located papillary plexus and a subcutaneous plexus. A particularly dense network of lymph tracts is preformed in the manner of Sappey's "subareolar plexus." Lymphatic outflow from the lateral half of the breast takes place at a lymph node on the edge of the major pectoral muscle (Sorgius node), proceeding via lateral, axillary nodes to central axillary and

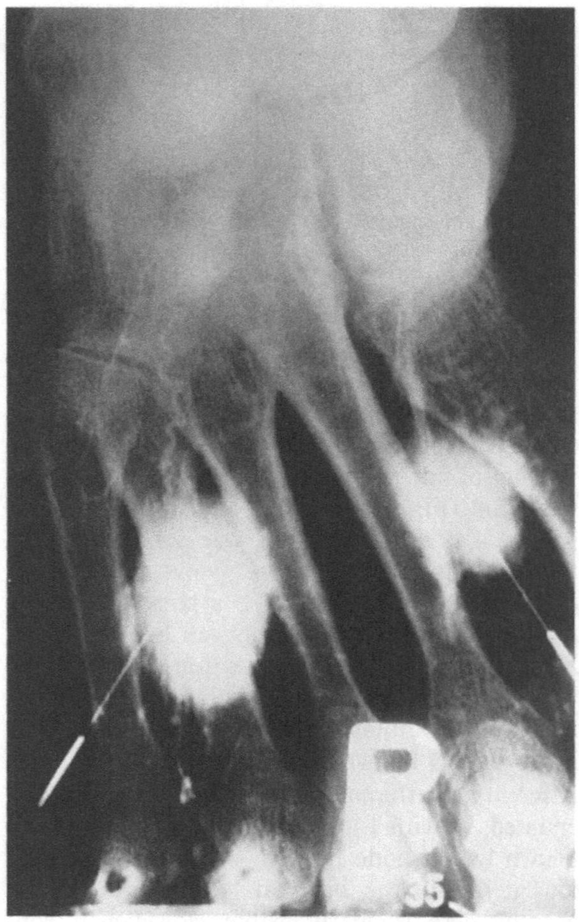

Fig. 4. Indirect lymphogram with iotasul in hypoplastic lymphedema

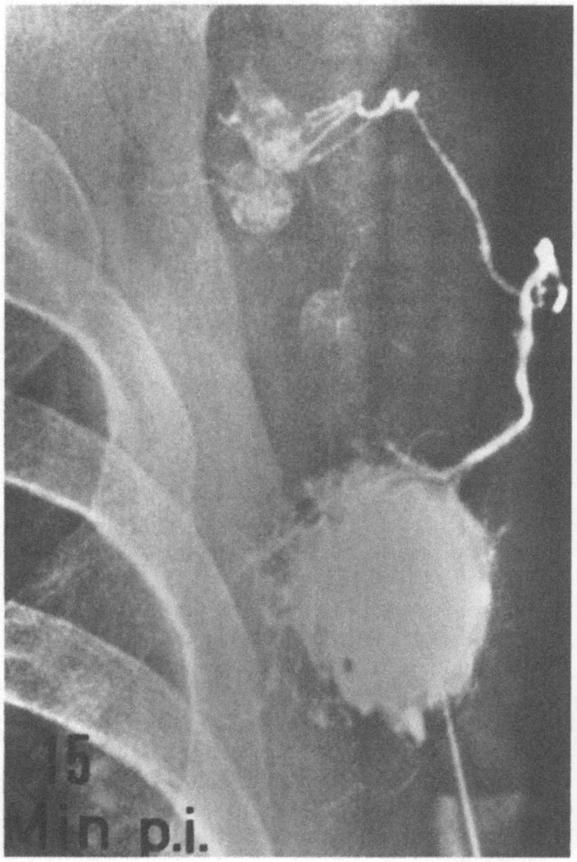

Fig. 5. Indirect lymphogram of breast (normal findings) with visualization of subareolar plexus. Lymphatic drainage in axillary direction

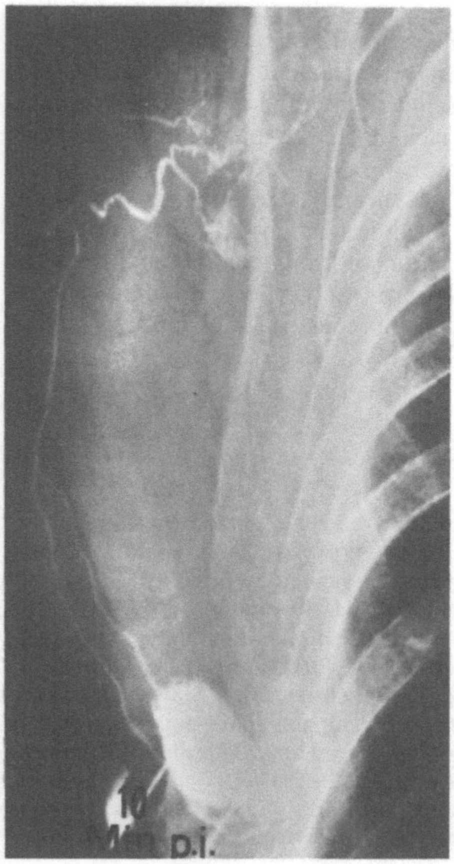

Fig. 6. Indirect lymphogram of breast with efferent tracts, caudopectoral lymph nodes with filling defects

subclavicular apical nodes. Lymphatic drainage of the medial half of the breast takes place via substernal lymph tracts.

With indirect lymphography of the breast there is opacification of the subareolar plexus after as little as a few minutes. Lymphatic drainage at the axilla is also visible early (Fig. 5). Pathological lymphograms included the typical radiological signs of metastasis well known from lymphography with Lipiodol, such as abruptly terminating and congested lymphatic vessels or filling defects (Fig. 6). An angiogram permitting good diagnostic evaluation was obtained in all 22 patients after intracutaneous administration of iotasul. Opacification of lymph nodes, varying in quality, was successful in 14 of the patients.

Side Effects

During indirect lymphography an interstitial depot of contrast medium is formed at the site of perfusion, sometimes urticarial and sometimes bullous. There are no subjective complaints and the depot quickly resolves after the end of perfusion. General side effects were not observed in any patient. Not even in electron microscopic examinations of the lymphatic system and other organs, in particular the kidney, which is responsible for elimination, Wenzel-Hora [9] detected any changes.

Conclusions

Direct lymphography with iotasul does not yet fulfill all the expectations aroused by the results of animal experiments, probably due to the greater length of the human lymphatic system associated with a longer injection time. We can expect optimization of radiological results on the basis of improvements in the formulation of the contrast medium. Indirect lymphography with iotasul is successful in the case of lymphedema, and makes diagnostically accessible areas of lymphatic drainage of which no visualization has previously been possible, e.g., in the breast. Advantages of indirect lymphography with iotasul are: (a) the lack of need to inject a dye, and therefore of risk of an allergic reaction to it; (b) the avoidance of surgical exposure of lymphatic vessels and local damage to the lymphatic system due to a reaction with oily contrast medium; and (c) the absence of the risk of embolism. The investigation can be repeated simply and quickly.

References

1. Apitzsch DE, Kroll HU, Zühlke HV (1981) Indirect caudal lymphography using a new water-soluble contrast agent – animal experimental studies in pigs. Lymphology 14:95–100
2. Grabbe E (1981) Indirekte Rektumlymphographie. Tierexperimentelle Erfahrungen. RoFo 135:98–102
3. Grüntzig J, Wenzel-Hora BJ, Siefert HM (1982) Die indirekte Lymphographie am Auge und im Gesichts-Hals-Bereich mit Iotasul im Tierexperiment. RoFo 136:592–594
4. Schmidt M, Taenzer V (1981) Indirekte Mamma-Lymphographie mit dem neuen wasserlöslichen Kontrastmittel Iotasul. 15. Internat. Congr. of Radiology in Brussels, abstract
5. Schmidt M, Taenzer V (1982) Indirekte Mammalymphographie. RoFo 136:359–498
6. Siefert HM, Mützel W, Schöbel C, et al. (1980) Iotasul, a water-soluble contrast agent for direct and indirect lymphography. Results of preclinical investigations. Lymphology 13:150–157
7. Siefert HM, Wenzel-Hora BI, Sigmund F (1981) Indirekte Lymphographie mit Iotasul. 15. Internat. Congr. of Radiology in Brussels, abstract
8. Siefert HM, Miklautz H, Mützel W, et al. (1981) Iotasul, a water-soluble contrast agent for direct and indirect lymphography: preclinical results. In: Donner MW, Heuck FHW (eds) Radiology today 1. Springer, Berlin Heidelberg New York
9. Wenzel-Hora BI, Kalbas B, Siefert HM et al. (1981) Iotasul, a water-soluble (non-oily) contrast medium for direct and indirect lymphography. Radiological and morphological investigations in dogs. Lymphology 14:101–112
10. Wenzel-Hora BI, Siefert HM, Grüntzig J (1982) Animal experimental studies of indirect lymphography of the eye, face and neck regions using iotasul. Lymphology 15:32–35
11. Partsch HB, Urbanek WA (1983) Differential diagnosis of lymphedema after indirect lymphography with itosul. Lymphology 16:12–18
12. Zinser HK (1972) Mammakarzinom und Differentialdiagnose. Thieme, Stuttgart

Chest Radiology

Computed Tomography of Mediastinal Tumors: Overview

J. Lissner and B. Sommer

Radiologische Klinik und Poliklinik, Klinikum Grosshadern, Marchioninistrasse 15, 8000 München 70, FRG

Radiological examination of the mediastinum has been revolutionized within the past 6 years. The fast generation of computed tomography (CT) scanners, introduced in 1977, has been instrumental in this development. Before that time, conventional tomography, angiography, and to a certain extent pneumomediastinum were the standard diagnostic tools, in skillful hands giving excellent results in some spectacular cases. Today, however, the mediastinum is governed almost totally by CT. The plain thorax X-ray does have a role to play, but in many cases with strong evidence of pathology in the mediastinum it is followed by CT examination, since its differential diagnostic possibilities are poor.

Table 1 lists the primary and secondary tumors and similar pathological densities which we found in the mediastinum in the period of 1 year. We concentrate here on some interesting aspects of primary tumors.

Thymus tumors are usually well demarcated, often centrally necrotic, and have a pear-like shape with the peduncle attached to the sternum at the level of the second rib.

Table 1. CT of the mediastinum

Metastatic lesions	154
Esophageal tumors	24
Thymomas	38
Mediastinal tumors	47
Malignant lymphomas	7
Aneurysms	9
Anomalies	3
Hemorrhages	18
Bronchial carcinoma	104
Parathyroid adenomas	5
Abscesses	5
Neurinomas/Neuroblastomas	5
Total	469

Not all thymomas are histologically well defined. They can even bear a *close resemblance to Hodgkin's disease* or have a granulomatous pattern. The lesion shown in Fig. 1 was finally proved to be malignant thymoma.

Figure 2 shows a *malignant lymphoma* of the thymus. The tumor is necrotic with lymphocytic cells and no epithelial structures, and must therefore be classified as a T-cell lymphoma.

Thymomas are sometimes *totally cystic* with only a small border. This means that CT cannot make a reliable diagnosis even in these otherwise very characteristic lesions.

Thymomas can be *calcified* even when malignant. CT shows the different density but cannot assign the lesion to a histological type.

Myasthenia gravis is often (20%) combined with thymus hyperplasia. We know this from the era of pneumomediastinum, when it was most exceptional to find the hyperplasia, normally to be sought near and somewhat lateral to the pulmonary artery.

Primary teratomas, like thymomas, are necrotic in the center.

Neuroblastomas in childhood can be benign or malignant. Originally they are noninvoluted organ cells, e.g., from the suprarenal gland. They can grow or can decrease and vanish. No signs on CT or any other macropathological examination identify them; even histologically this can be difficult. CT can only describe the shape, contours, and density of such a lesion. They do not necessarily have their origin in the spinal cord, as was shown by Amipaque myelography in one 2-year-old child (Fig. 3).

The mammary lymph node chain is a hidden area on conventional X-ray, with metastatic enlargements hardly detectable. CT, however, can show for instance metastatic lymph node infiltration from a breast carcinoma with enlarged lymph nodes in the mammary group and in the right part of the ventral mediastinum. In one case of

Radiology Today 2. Ed. by F. H. W. Heuck and M. W. Donner

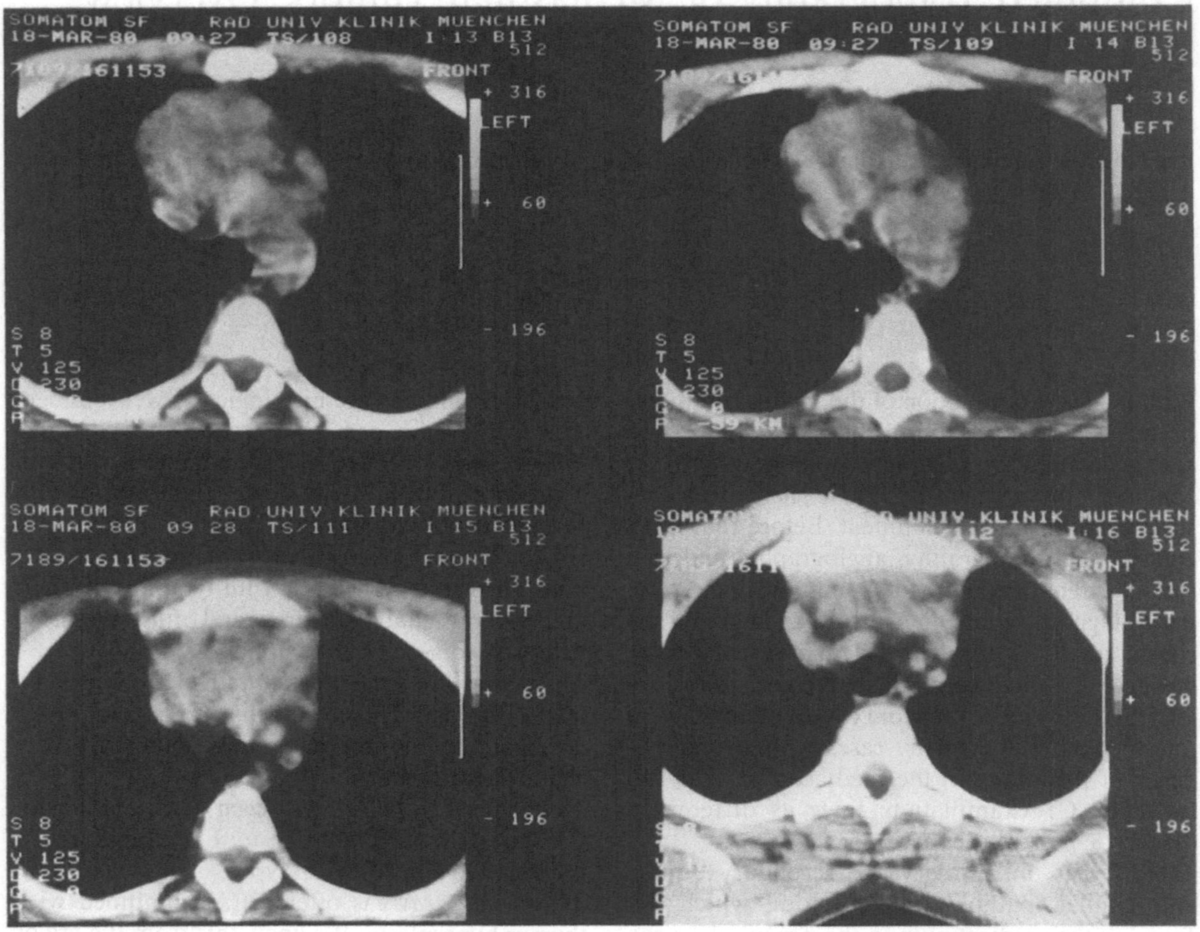

Fig. 1

neuroblastoma, metastasis into the mammary chain could be seen in the lateral view of the plain film, but only as an indifferent homogeneous shadow without any connection to a topographical area.

Esophageal lesions, whether malignant or benign, are an indication for CT, which can classify the extension or spread of a carcinoma and determine its proximity to the bronchus, pleura, and lung or can ascertain the density and shape of benign tumors.

A *cyst of the esophageal wall* has a density about that of water and a sharp contour, the latter also noted in the conventional barium swallow.

CT examination of an *esophageal carcinoma* shows the spread into peribronchial tissue, pleura, and necrotic areas, as shown in. The conventional tomogram shows the cavity in the apical segment of the lower lobe in connection with the bronchus. CT shows tumor expansion in axial section. Difficulties exist regarding lymph node infiltration in esophageal carcinoma, and we have to gather further experience.

Figure 4 shows an esophageal carcinoma. To the right of the esophagus there is a round dense area which cannot be related to the azygos vein, with some smaller dense areas in front of and below the carina. We thought of metastatic infiltration but none was found on surgery. Either it was too small to separate it from the tumor, or from the surgeon's compound.

On primary mediastinal tumors and CT it can be stated that the lesion can be described very precisely in a high percentage of cases, but accurate identification of origin and histology is only possible when the lesion has characteristic density and well-defined contours.

In addition to the problems of differentiation of primary mediastinal tumors, there are very similar *nonprimary* and even *nontumorous lesions.* Dif-

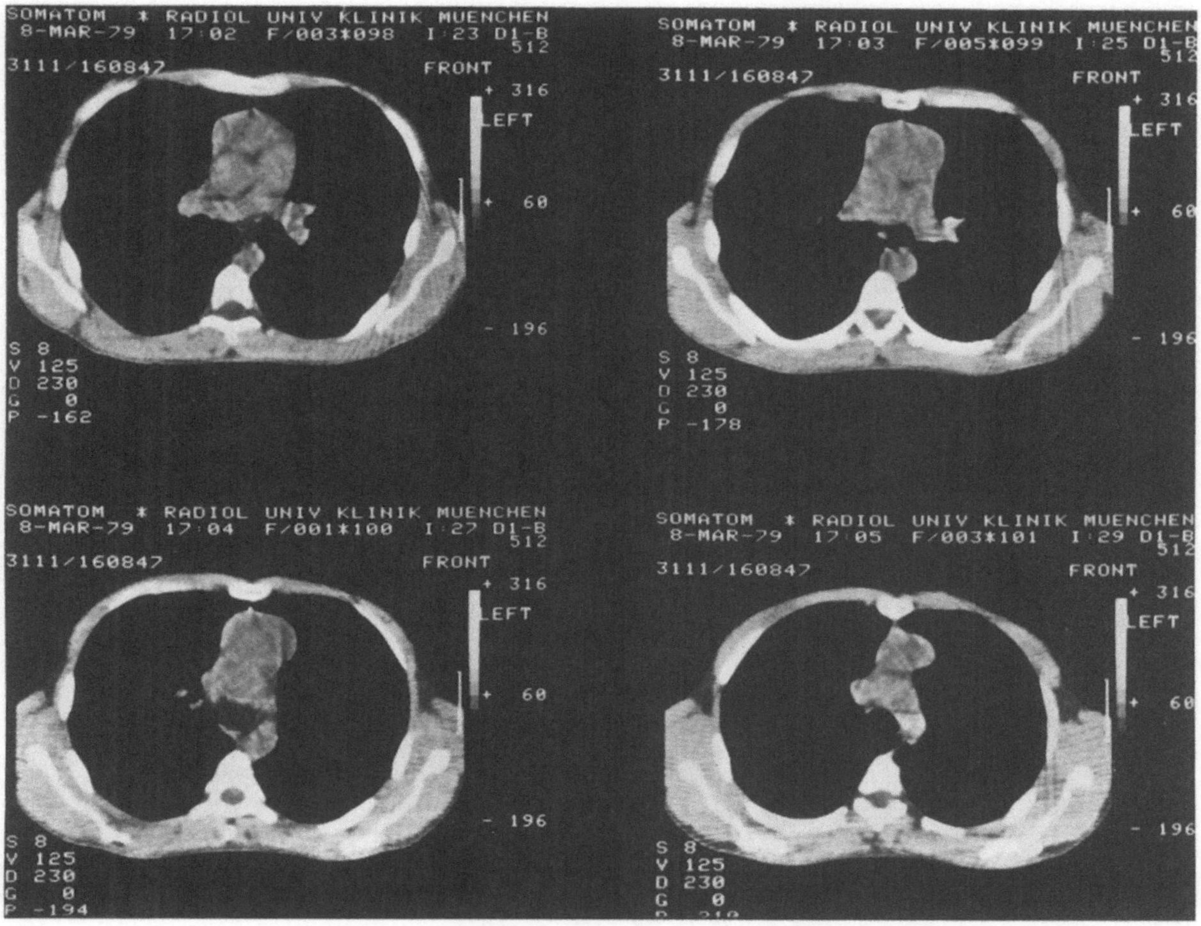

Fig. 2

ferential diagnostic possibilities of some importance are:

- Anomalies, especially of the vessels
- Post-traumatic and other abscesses
- Tumors of the bronchi, lipomas, and hemangiomas
- Hemorrhages

The *Hodgkin's-affected skeletal area (Biehler)* shows infiltration not only of bone but also of the surrounding soft tissue, which may produce a widening of the mediastinal shadow.

CT is also useful in cases of *tumor infiltration or tumor-like aneurysm in the heart.* Figure 5 shows a Hodgkin's disease with infiltration of the pericardium and left atrium. The patient suffered from severe dyspnea. After chemotherapy (de Vita) the atrial infiltration diminished, as could be seen 5 months later. An example of a tumor-like aneurysm is an *aneurysm of the sinus of Valsalva.*

Abscesses, benign intraluminal bronchial tumors, vessel anomalies, hemorrhages, and skeletal infiltrations all have in general some characteristic features, vessels especially after contrast medium enhancement. Differentiation from primary mediastinal tumors can at least to some extent be achieved.

Experience with CT in the localization of *parathyroid glands* is limited. The most common diagnostic procedures for localizing enlarged parathyroids are ultrasound (US), arteriography, and venous sampling.

Neither intrathoracic parathyroid adenomas in the anterior or posterior mediastinum nor retrotracheal or retroesophageal adenomas can be detected by US. Nodular goiters and cystic changes in goiters, especially if located dorsally, may cause diagnostic problems for US. To evalu-

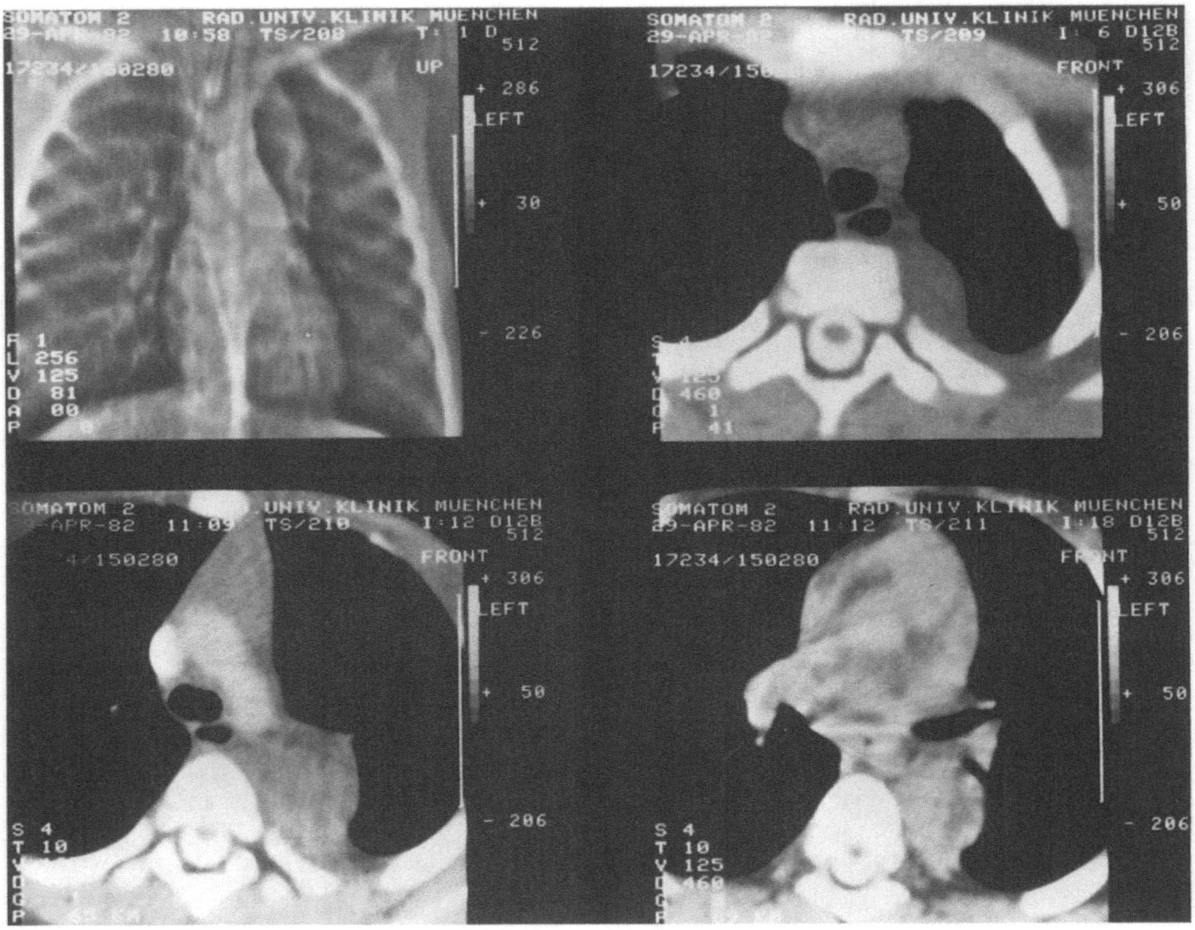
RAD.UNIV.KLINIK MUENCHEN
10:58 TS/208
UP
+ 286
LEFT
+ 30
- 226
SOMATOM 2 RAD.UNIV.KLINIK MUENCHEN
TS/209
FRONT
+ 306
LEFT
+ 50
- 206
MATOM 2 UNIV.KLINIK MUENCHEN
-APR-82 11:09 TS/210
4/150280
FRONT
+ 306
LEFT
+ 50
- 206
S 4
T 10
MATOM 2 RAD.UNIV.KL NIK MUENCHEN
29-APR-82 11:12 TS/211
17234/150280
+ 306
LEFT
+ 50
- 206
S 4
T 10
V 125
460

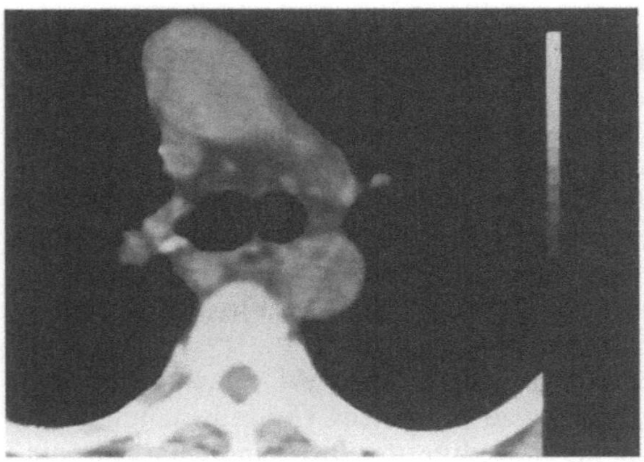

Fig. 4

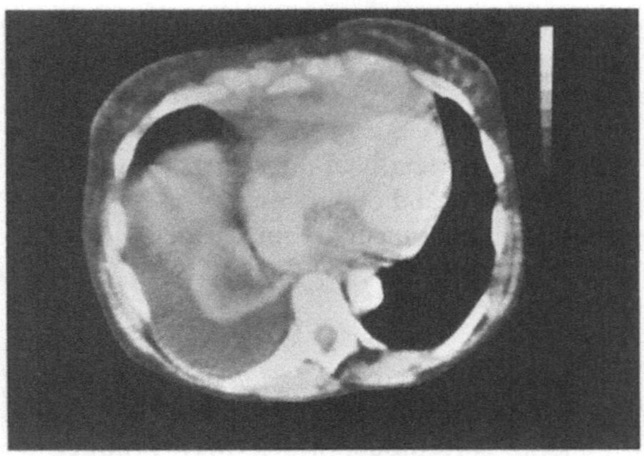

Fig. 5

Table 2. CT in mediastinal adenomas

CT findings	A		B		A + B	
	n	%	*n*	%	*n*	%
True positive	31	81	15	71	46	78
False negative	7	19	6	29	13	22
False positive	6	16	–	–	6	10

A, solitary adenomas ($n = 38$); *B*, multiple adenomas ($n = 21$)

ate the diagnostic accuracy of CT, Sommer and Fenzl performed CT studies on a group of patients with primary hyperparathyroidism. The CT scans were interpreted without knowledge of the US findings.

CT was performed in 45 patients in an attempt to localize parathyroid tumors preoperatively (Table 2). On subsequent surgery, 38 patients had solitary adenomas, seven patients had multiple hyperplastic glands, and a total of 59 enlarged glands were removed. Intraoperatively, eight adenomas were found in the mediastinum, three anterior and five posterior. Seven of the eight had been detected by CT.

The true-positive diagnostic rate of CT for all the enlarged glands was 78%, with a false-negative rate of 22%. Invasive angiographic techniques such as arteriography had venous sampling can be reduced considerably by utilization of CT. Preoperative angiography was also carried out.

On the basic of our experience we propose the following, *indications for CT* in primary hyperparathyroidism. A CT scan of the neck and mediastinum should be performed:

1. After questionable or normal findings in US
2. In patients with high operative risk
3. After unsuccessful surgical intervention or recurrence
4. Before any invasive angiographic procedure

The *consequences for surgery* are important:

– Reduction in operating time
– Fewer complications, especially in reintervention (scar tissue)
– Reduction in the number of reinterventions

There is a close connection between assessment of the *operability of bronchial carcinomas* and staging. Conventional X-ray methods tend to considerably underestimate the extent of the tumors into the mediastinum. Mediastinoscopy currently plays the main part in evaluation of mediastinal involvement, but the superior preoperative staging ability of CT has now been proved by the work of Sommer and other investigators.

In 60 of 89 bronchial carcinomas with preoperative CT, the CT findings could be compared with endoscopic or operative results. A correct CT judgement of T-stage was made in 95% of cases. CT overestimated the extension of the tumor in two cases and underestimated it in one case. CT has an important role in the assessment of the operability of T3 tumors, where there are numerous criteria to observe.

There are limitations to CT. For instance, although even small lymph nodes can be seen in the mediastinum, this does not necessarily mean safety of interpretation. Even rather small nodes can be infiltrated, but the probability of metastatic infiltration does grow with increasing size. A zone of incertainty seems to exist between 1 cm and 1.5 cm. We classified all lymph nodes larger than 1 cm as infiltrated. In 42 cases we could compare our assessment with endoscopic or operative findings; in 24 we had false-positive results and only in one a false-negative result. We feel that if there is a complete normal CT finding regarding lymph nodes, mediastinoscopy can be omitted.

Of 38 patients with thoracotomy still five in whom only trials did result. All of them had positive CT findings but were negative on mediastinoscopy. Confidence in CT findings has slowly grown, results like ours helping lead to a change of attitude among surgeons. We can summarize our views as follows:

1. It can be regarded as settled that CT is now the method of choice for detection of mediastinal tumors.
2. Differentiation from other space-occupying lesions is often made by the history, e.g., accident or previous medical treatment. Differentiation from vessel anomalies, aneurysms, and primary tumors in cases without relevant history may be more difficult, but contrast enhancement can be helpful.
3. Parathyroid adenomas in the mediastinum are a real hunting ground for radiologists with a keen interest in CT who have as colleagues surgeons specializing in parathyroid adenoma resection. This was the situation in our hospital and the result is Dr. Sommer's collection of cases, the largest in the world.
4. Lung cancer staging can be improved by CT, but whether or not exploratory thoracotomy is abandoned as a result depends on the confidence of surgeons in the CT findings.

Structural Analysis of Lung Tissue by Computed Tomography

O. H. Wegener

Strahleninstitut und Radiologische Klinik, Krankenanstalten Neuss, Lukaskrankenhaus, Akademisches Lehrkrankenhaus der Universität Düsseldorf, Preussenstrasse 84, 4040 Neuss, FRG

Introduction

In a complex and yet systematic manner, lung tissue is composed of blood vessels and interstices on one hand and the air space on the other. As a result of the great inherent tissue contrast, the structure appears to be sufficiently assessable even on a plain radiograph, and numerous investigators have developed diagnostic criteria for the film analysis of lung structure.

What additional information regarding lung structure can computed tomography provide? The characteristics of computed tomography are:

1. It enables transverse visualization of the lung without overshadowing. The criteria of structural analysis developed from plain radiographs can with limitations be applied to computed tomography.
2. Its spacial resolution is determined by the size of the volume element (matrix size, slice thickness) and is markedly lower than that of X-ray film.
3. It enables quantitative analysis, since the volume elements indicate a reproducible density value for the tissue volume they represent. That is why some attempts have been made to measure lung density by computed tomography [1, 2, 6, 9, 10].

In spite of the reduced spatial resolution capacity, structural alterations of the lung are often better shown or first discovered in the computed tomogram through their visualization in transverse section or through the higher density resolution [3–5, 8]. The structural analysis, however, remains qualitative; it supplements the findings obtained from the chest X-ray or conventional lung tomography. It also remains subjective, particularly since the visual impression at the monitor can be considerably influenced by changes of window width and level.

The quantitative possibilities of structural analysis of lung tissue will now be described. In this connection, a method has been developed which – free of subjective influences – enables automatic computer analysis.

How To Quantify Lung Structure

The X-ray density of a homogeneous object is given as a mean value in the computed tomogram, since the statistics of the photon flow and the imaging process itself result in a normal distribution of the density values. The standard deviation of this Gaussian curve, which is bell-shaped in the histogram, is at the same time the measure of the absorption resolution for the scanner (i.e., for the selected scan parameters). Broadening of the histographic curve, symmetrical and asymmetrical, is found with inhomogeneous objects. With objects of an ordered structure, such as the lung, an asymmetrical expansion is seen in the direction of higher density values.

The lowest density values represent the most inflated (ventrally situated) alveolar space (Fig. 1 b, c); this is followed, progressing up the density scale of the histogram, by the dorsally located alveolar space (Fig. 1 d) and then by mixed values with peripheral and central pulmonary vessels (Fig. 1 f). The asymmetry of the histogram, i.e. the lack of the normal distribution of density values of a healthy lung, renders it impossible to state the lung tissue density as mean value with standard deviation. It has not as yet been possible to find a precise mathematical description of the histogram of a healthy or diseased lung. Therefore we searched for a characterization of the lung histogram which would be as stable as possible but which could also be calculated automatically by computer. The following description has proven reliable [7] (Fig. 2):

Radiology Today 2. Ed. by F. H. W. Heuck and M. W. Donner

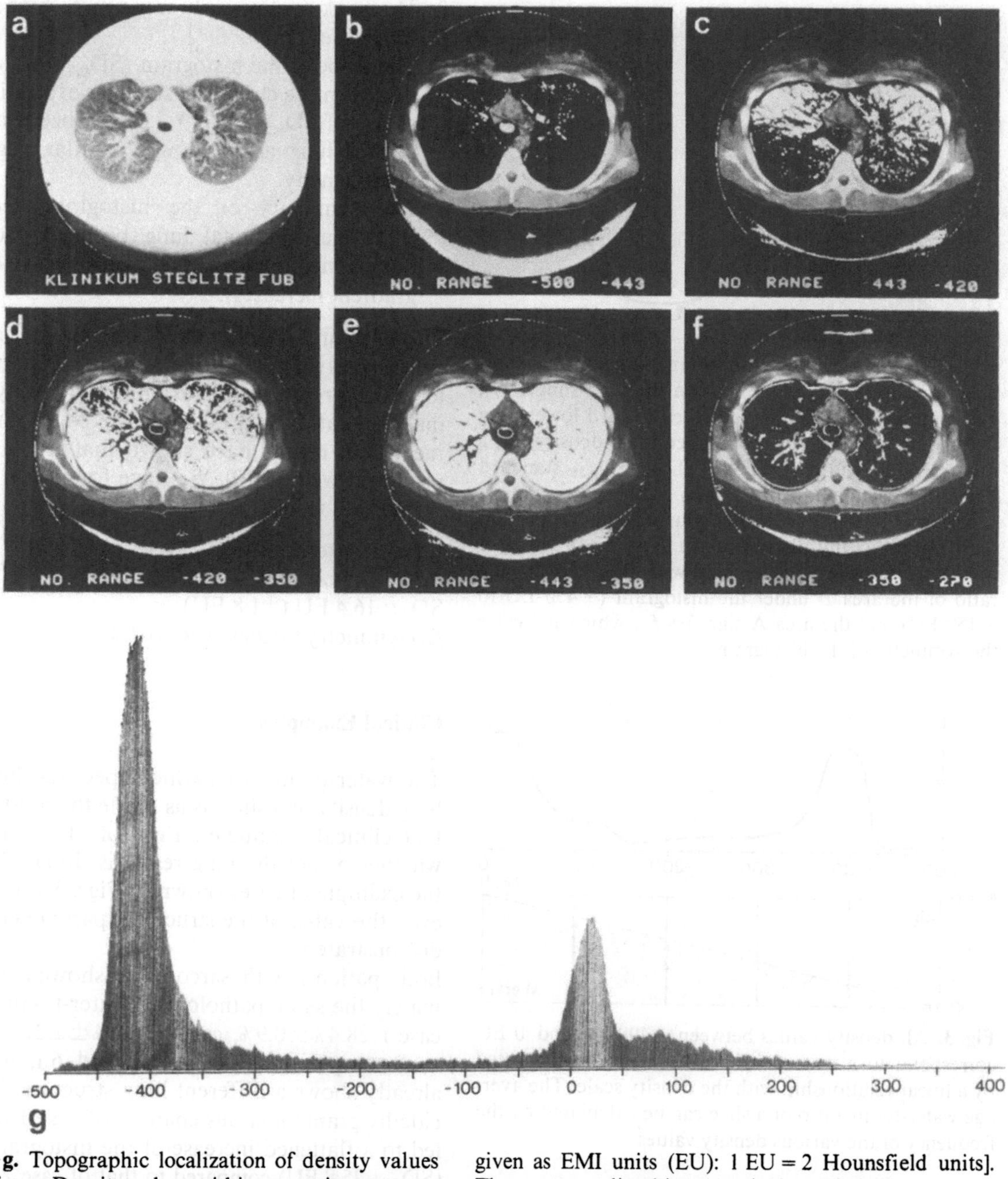

Fig. 1a–g. Topographic localization of density values of lung tissue. Density values within a certain range are shown in *white* (highlighting) [The density values are given as EMI units (EU): 1 EU = 2 Hounsfield units]. The corresponding histogram is shown below **g**

1. Location of the peak
2. Determination of the half- and quarter-value widths towards lower density values
3. Definition of the asymmetry of the histogram

The standard deviations ($SD_{0.5}$, $SD_{0.25}$) of a Gaussian curve A can be calculated from the half- and quarter-value widths (see Fig. 2), because in most cases the increase of the histogram to its peak resembles a Gaussian distribution. The ratio of the areas under the Gaussian curve A and under the histogram B [< 150 EMI units (EU): 1 EU = 2 HU] was defined as the measure of symmetry (symmetry factor f_{sy}: the smaller f_{sy}, the more asymmetrical the histogram). These histogram parameters can be determined automatically via a computer: smoothing of the histogram, peak search, determination of $SD_{0.5}$, $SD_{0.25}$, and f_{sy}. Knowledge of the global density of a lung

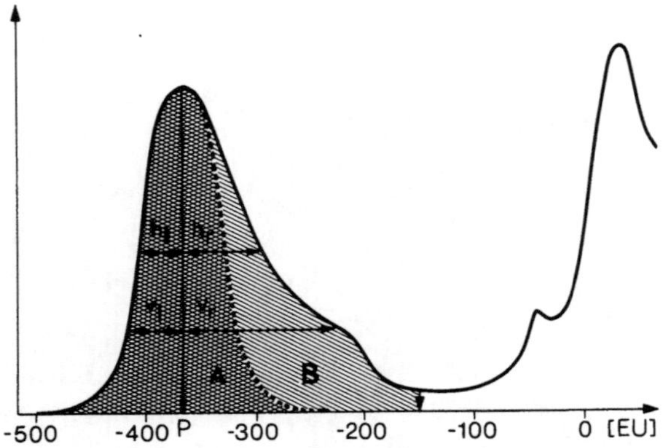

Fig. 2. Analysis of a lung histogram. *P* peak (most frequent density value, mode) within the lung range; $h_{l,r}$, half-value width (HVFW; left-sided toward lower lung density, right-sided toward higher lung density); $v_{l,r}$, quarter-value width (QVFW). $SD_{0.5}$, $SD_{0.25}$ standard deviations calculated from h_l or v_l. With $SD_{0.5} = SD_{0.25}$, a normal distribution can be assumed, marked within the diagram as the distribution *A*. The mean value of this distribution would coincide with the peak *P*. The ratio of the area *B* under the histogram (− 450 EU to − 150 EU) and the area A signifies f_{sy}, which indicates the symmetry of the histogram

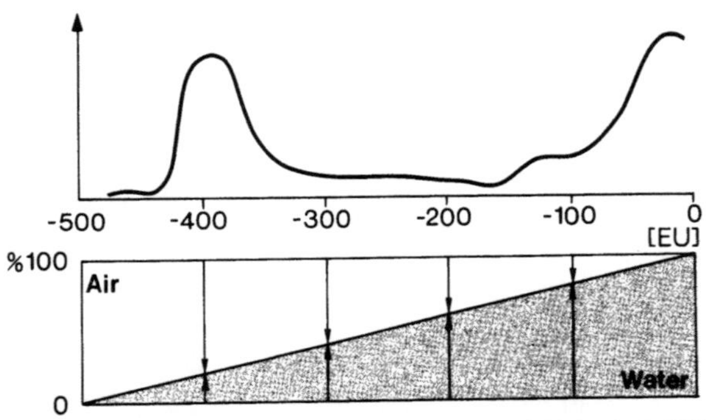

Fig. 3. All density values between − 499 EU and 0 EU correspond to a water-to-air ratio, which is connected by a linear relationship with the density scale. The average water-to-air ratio of a slice can be calculated by the frequency of the various density values

slice is of value for the structural analysis. It can be stated as global water-to-air ratio. It is calculated from the respective histogram by ascribing a water-air relationship to each negative density value (Fig. 3).

The interaction of the parameters presented here is clearly demonstrated from the example of a fractionated expiration of a normal lung (Fig. 4):

1. As expected, the global lung density of a layer increases from a water-air quotient of 18.4% to one of 39.9%.
2. The peak continuously wanders to higher density values.
3. The slope of the histogram ($SD_{0.5}$, $SD_{0.25}$) only flattens more clearly on stronger expiration (increase of $SD_{0.5}$, $SD_{0.25}$), i.e., the better aerated ventral lung areas show a similar degree of homogeneity.
4. The symmetry of the histogram decreases ($f_{sy}\downarrow$), i.e., the total lung becomes more inhomogeneous (here: the ventrodorsal density gradient increases).

The structural parameters of the lung thus depend considerably on the degree of inspiration. In order to achieve reproducible examinations, only maximal inspiration was taken as the condition to be measured; results have shown that it can be reproduced well [9, 10]. We have found the following normal values [7]:

Q_w (water-to-air ratio): 21.45% (±1.06%)
P_k (peak position): − 415.7 EU (±4.8 EU)
$SD_{0.5}$: 16.4 EU (±1.8 EU)
f_{sy} (symmetry factor): 0.74 ±0.04

Clinical Examples

The water-to-air ratio, which specifies the global lung density of a slice, is as a rule the most important clinical parameter. First of all, it indicates whether or not the lung really is diseased. Using the example of cases shown in Figs. 5 and 6, however, the value of the structural parameter can be demonstrated.

Both patients with sarcoidosis showed approximately the same pathological water-to-air ratio – case 1 28.4% ± 0.9%, case 2 28.6% ± 2.2%. The visual comparison in Figs. 5a and 6a, however, already shows a different lung structure. The decidedly granulomatous changes of case 1 in Fig. 5 led to a flattened increase of the histogram curve ($SD_{0.5}$: 25.8 EU) compared to that of case 2 ($SD_{0.5}$: 21.0 EU). In addition, the granulomatous changes effected a stronger asymmetry of the histogram curves than in case 2.

The water-to-air ratio indicates a global density value for the lung cut. Calculation of the same value can, however, be based on different histograms. Thus, dense bulky structures with overinflated surrounding lung areas can produce a water-to-air ratio resembling, e.g., a diffuse edema. The structural parameters ($SD_{0.5}$, f_{sy}, P_k), however, permit a clear differentiation: thus a narrow peak ($SD_{0.5}\downarrow$, $f_{sy}\uparrow$) signifies that the lung structure is homogeneous (Fig. 7), and the degree

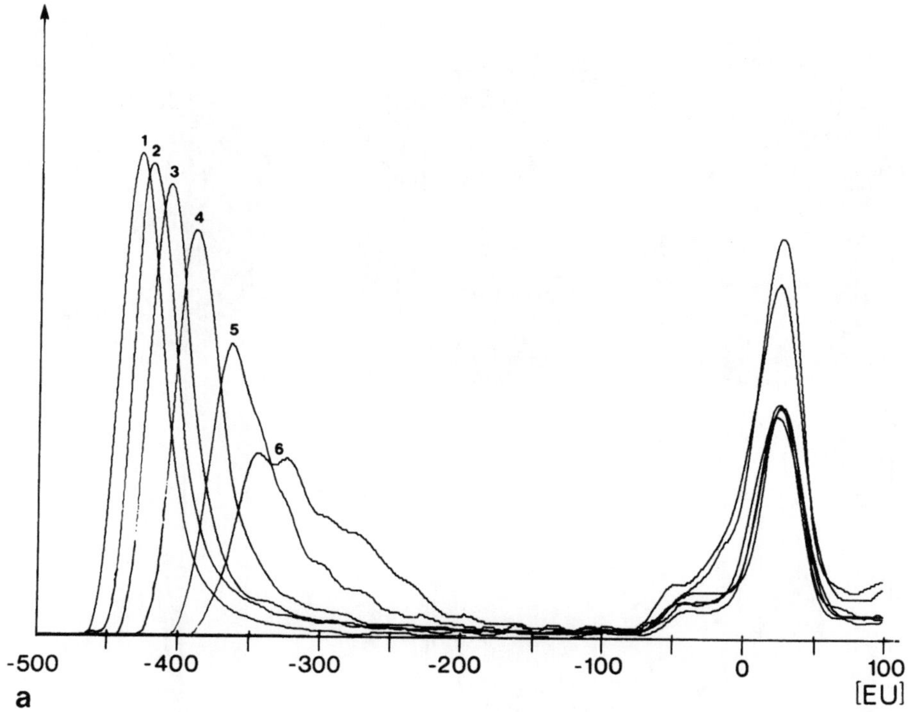

a

	peak position P_k	$SD_{0,50}$	$SD_{0,25}$	H_2O/air Ratio Q_w	f_{sy}	median
	EU	EU	EU			EU
max. Inspiration I	– 420,9	16,42	16,26	19,64	0,775	– 420,2
max. Inspiration II	– 426,9	14,98	13,89	18,42	0,806	– 427,0
Expiration – 500 ml	– 423,9	12,45	11,67	19,56	0,723	– 422,7
Expiration – 1000 ml	– 418,9	13,23	12,37	21,06	0,692	– 416,8
Expiration – 2000 ml	– 405,9	14,73	13,91	23,63	0,734	– 405,4
Expiration – 3000 ml	– 387,9	14,79	13,85	27,72	0,667	– 385,2
Expiration – 4200 ml	– 361,9	16,45	15,92	34,32	0,521	– 351,4
Expiration – 4700 ml (maximal)	– 342,9	16,82	18,20	39,90	0,351	– 316,2

b

Fig. 4a, b. The same lung slice in different states of inflation. **a** Histograms during *1*, maximal inspiration, *2*, expiration of 1000 ml, *3*, expiration of 2000 ml, *4*, expiration of 3000 ml, *5*, expiration of 4200 ml, *6*, maximal expiration (4700 ml). **b** Histographic parameters calculated by automatic analysis

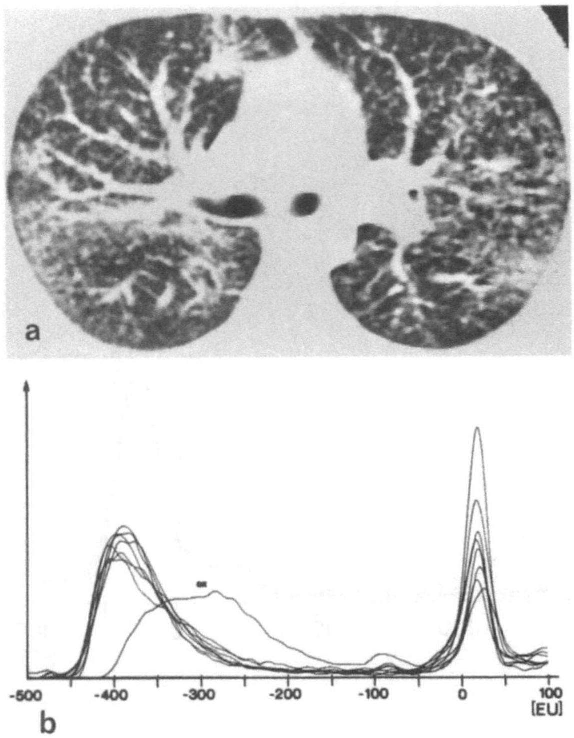

Fig. 5 a, b. *Case 1.* CT demonstrates clearly the granulomatous alterations of the lung (**a**). Automatic analysis of the histograms of various slices (**b**) yields the following mean parameters: Q_w, 28.4%; P_k, − 392.4 EU; $SD_{0.5}$: 25.8 EU; f_{sy}, 0.60

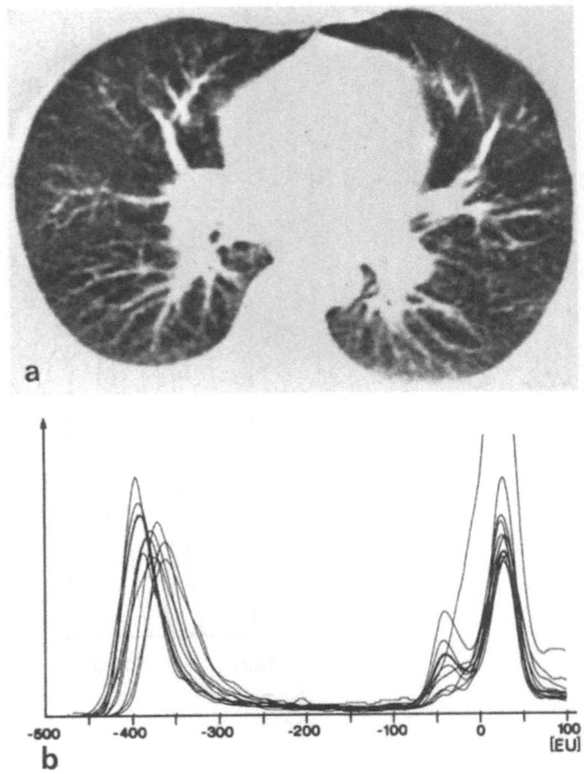

Fig. 6 a, b. *Case 2.* The CT image demonstration no abnormality of the lung tissue (**a**). Automatic analysis of histograms of various slices (**b**) shows the same pathological water-to-air ratio Q_w, 28.6%, but different structural parameters: P_k, − 382.9 EU; $SD_{0.5}$, 21.0 EU; f_{sy}, 0.72

of broadening ($SD_{0.5}\downarrow$, $f_{sy}\downarrow$) indicates the grade of inhomogeneity. As can be seen in Fig. 7, the increase of the histogram represents the essential parts of the lung periphery, so that a high $SD_{0.5}$ signifies an inhomogeneous lung periphery. The value $SD_{0.5}$ alone, however, leads to the false conclusion that a histogram can show a steep increase (Fig. 7d) but a very flat drop towards high density values. For this reason, the symmetry factor f_{sy} was introduced, which presupposes knowledge of the histogram peak.

The automatic assessment procedure was tested on more than 150 patients and over 1300 individual slices [7]. Calculation of the structural parameters presented here was also done successfully in very complicated histogram curves, some of which had multiple peaks. The results can be summarized as follows:

1. Because of the limited area fraction in the transverse section, very circumscribed lung alterations can escape the automatic histogram analysis.
2. General structure and density changes of the lung are detected even when the computed tomogram at the monitor appears normal.
3. The method is particularly suitable for the early diagnosis and follow-up control of interstitial lung diseases, e.g., lung fibrosis, sarcoidosis, hyperhydration, and heart congestion.
4. The described procedure appears to be suitable for obtaining an assessment of pneumoconioses which is free of subjective influences.
5. For reproducible results, however, the method requires maximal inspiration, i.e., good cooperation on the part of the patient.

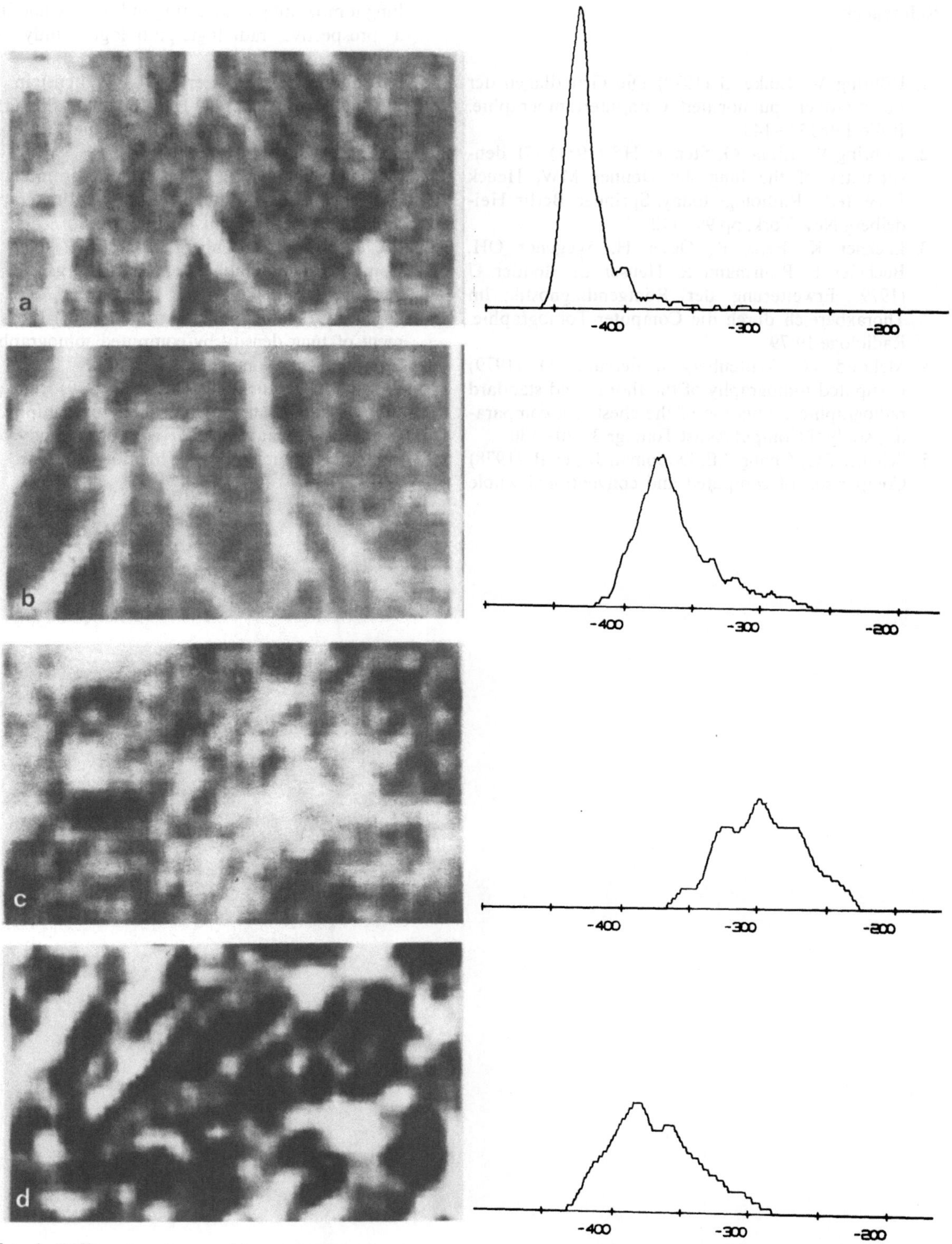

Fig. 7a–d. Different patterns of lung structure lead to certain constellations of histographic parameters. **a** Normal lung Q_w, 15,1%; P_k, − 432 EU; $SD_{0.5}$, 10.5 EU; f_{sy}: 0.95. **b** Pulmonary arterial hypertension Q_w, 27.7%; P_k, −377 EU; $SD_{0.5}$, 12.5 EU; f_{sy}: 0.95. **c** Pulmonary fibrosis Q_w, 40.7%; P_k, − 300 EU; $SD_{0.5}$, 29.5 EU; f_{sy}: 0.97. **d** Coarse miliary tuberculosis Q_w, 29.0%; P_k, − 385 EU; $SD_{0.5}$, 23.7 EU; f_{sy}: 0.61

References

1. Döhring W, Linke G (1979) Die Grundlagen der quantitativen pulmonalen Computertomographie. RoFo 130:133–143
2. Döhring W, Linke G, Stender HS (1981) CT densitometry of the lung. In: Donner MW, Heuck FHW (eds) Radiology today. Springer, Berlin Heidelberg New York, pp 99–112
3. Lackner K, Felix R, Oeser H, Wegener OH, Bücheler E, Buurmann R, Heuser L, Mödder U (1979) Erweiterung der Röntgendiagnostik im Thoraxbereich durch die Computer-Tomographie. Radiologe 19:79
4. McLoud TC, Wittenberg J, Ferrucci JT (1979) Computed tomography of the thorax and standard radiographic evaluation of the chest – a comparative study. J Comput Assist Tomogr 3:170–180
5. Schaner EG, Chang AE, Doppman JL, et al. (1978) Comparison of computed and conventional whole lung tomography in detecting pulmonary nodules – a prospective radiologic-pathologic study. AJR 131:51–54
6. Rosenblum LJ, Mauceri RA, Wellenstein DE, Bassano DA, Cohen WN, Heitzman ER (1978) Computed tomography of the lung. Radiology 129:521–524
7. Wegener OH (1979) Die Dichtebestimmung des Lungengewebes mittels Computertomographie. *Habilitationsschrift*, University of Berlin
8. Wegener OH, Gerstenberg E, Oeser H (1977) Die Computer-Tomographie der Thorax-Organe. Rontgenberichte 6:294
9. Wegener OH, Koeppe P, Oeser H (1978) Measurement of lung density by computed tomography. J Comput Assist Tomogr 2:263–273
10. Wegener OH, Koeppe P, Oeser H (1979) Lung density measurements by computed tomography. In: Gerhardt P, van Kaick G (eds) Total body computerized tomography. Thieme, Stuttgart, pp 32–39

Diffuse Lung Disease: How to Slice It

W. S. Rau

Abteilung Röntgendiagnostik, Klinikum der Albert-Ludwigs-Universität, Hugstetter Strasse 49, 7800 Freiburg, FRG

Radiographs of diffuse lung disease are often ambiguous. To get greater reliability, radiologic-pathologic correlations are necessary, but in contrast to other organs, there are difficulties. One cannot use the collapsed specimen: morphologic and roentgenologic examination require an organ reexpanded to its original size and gas content.

We use two methods for fixation of lung specimens: either hot formalin vapor [8] or liquid nitrogen [9]. The fixed lungs are cut in 1-cm slices and radiographs are taken with the mammography technique.

In the central slice of a normal lung, the arteries show a monopodial kind of branching and are accompanied by bronchi. Veins branch dichotomously and are directed toward the interlobular septa. Small ring figures of less than 0.5 mm in diameter represent the superimposed shadows of alveoli. If the vessels are filled with barium, the smaller branchings are also visible. Angiography of pulmonary arteries demonstrates the lobular organization of lung parenchyma. In contrast, bronchial arteries do not respect lobular borders [10].

Fluid Accumulation

In the beginning of pulmonary edema, there is an excess lymph flow. Only when the capacity of the lymph vessels is exceeded by a factor of 10 is the excess fluid retained in the interstitial tissue of the lung [13].

The first morphologic site of fluid accumulation is the loose connective tissue sheets around larger vessels and bronchi. The vessels are thicker, with ill-defined contours. Also the bronchial walls are broadened and hazy [6].

The second site of interstitial edema is the interlobular septa (Fig. 1). If the excess fluid fills and widens this compartment, and the septa are viewed laterally and not from the surface, Kerley's B lines will be recognized on the plain film.

If this compartment is also full to capacity, any further fluid will collect in the third site of interstitial edema, the interalveolar space. The ring figures of the alveoli are now very pronounced.

If the whole interstitial tissue is full of fluid, and if the underlying disease progresses, the fluid passes the alveolar wall and fills the lumen of the alveoli. While interstitial edema can only be di-

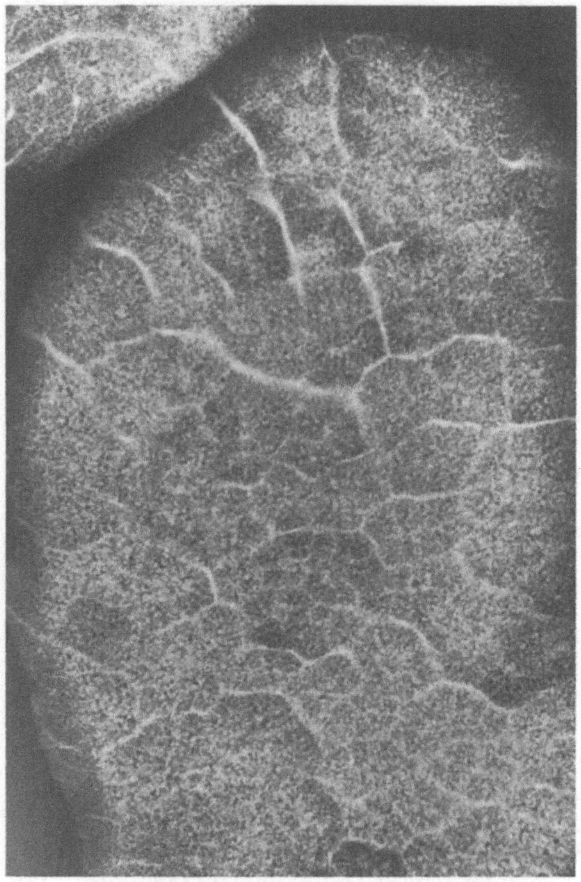

Fig. 1. Severe interstitial edema. The interlobular septa are broadened and there is a pronounced alveolar pattern due to broadened alveolar walls. Several alveoli are already filled with fluid

Radiology Today 2. Ed. by F. H. W. Heuck and M. W. Donner

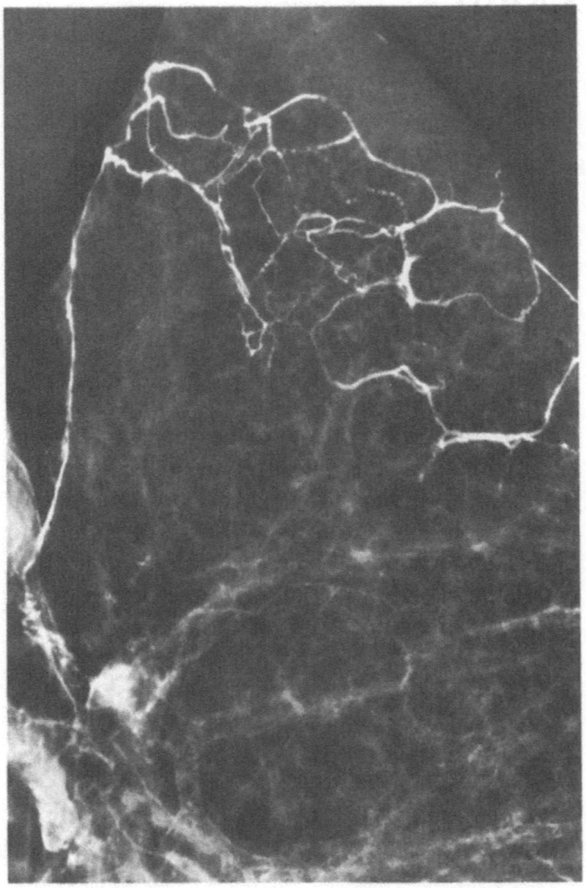

Fig. 2. Direct lymphography with barium sulfate. Large suppleural meshes of lymph vessels demarcate the interlobular septa on the surface of the lung. A large lymph vessels drains directly into a hilar lymph node

agnosed by radiographs or pulmonary function tests, alveolar edema can be detected by auscultation. If the fluid reaches larger bronchi, it is expectorated as frothy sputum, and you see an air bronchogram.

Sometimes the fluid accumulates only in the central parts of the lung, the periphery remaining free. This "butterfly shadow" is observed especially in renal or cardiac failure [2]. Several possible causes have been discussed. The most probable, we think, is different behavior of the lymph vessels in the superficial and deep lymph systems of the lung [4, 5, 14]. In contrast to Pennell and Bradshaw [7] we were able to demonstrate direct drainage from superficial lymph vessels to hilar lymph nodes. Figure 2 shows a lymphography with barium sulfate. Obviously, the flow resistance is lower and the pumping effect of respiratory movements is greater in the superficial lymph system, than in the central parts of the lung.

So far, we have considered hydrostatic edema. In edema with increased vascular permeability there are some peculiarities, the most important of which is the adult respiratory distress syndrome or shock lung. As an effect of the increased vascular permeability, the edema fluid has a high protein content and cannot pass the intact alveolar wall. Dilatation of alveolar septa is therefore much more distinct than in hydrostatic edema. The shadows of the enlarged alveolar walls are superimposed over everything else; Kerley's lines are not visible.

If in a case of shock lung the alveolar lumen is filled with fluid, this is always a sign of alveolar wall necrosis. The epithelium is not only functionally, but already morphologically damaged.

Attempts at tissue repair often produce no restitutio ad integrum, but a more or less progressive fibrosis [11]. If a plain film shows the reticular pattern of fibrosis, the patient will deteriorate. In this late phase of shock lung, respiratory insufficiency is also made worse by occlusion of alveolar capillaries. In a peripheral angiogram of normal pulmonary arteries, the vessels are filled down to the capillary bed. In contrast to that, Fig. 3 shows a respiratory distress syndrome in the stage of fibrosis. The vessels are reduced in number and diameter, and branchings are very rare.

Other kinds of fibrosis cause vascular obstruction too, but sometimes angiography allows differentiation. In a case of progressive systemic fibrosis, for example, the lobular vessels are enlarged and tortuous. Many capillaries are not perfused, but the number of branchings is reduced only slightly. Characteristically, there is proliferation of the intima in vessels with a diameter of 0.1–0.3 mm [12].

Emphysema

Another reason for reduction of capillaries is emphysema. Alveolar septa and the enclosed capillaries vanish. There are two types of emphysema. Figure 4 shows a *panacinar* emphysema, the type found in older patients or those with alpha-1-antitrypsin deficiency, without preceding bronchitis. All terminal air spaces are evenly dilated. The capillaries vanish in proportion to their septa [12]. In *centroacinar* emphysema, however, there are inflammatory changes due to chronic bronchitis. Focal inflammations produce stenoses of bronchioli, with consequent bulla formation, and stenosis of vessels, followed by the development of

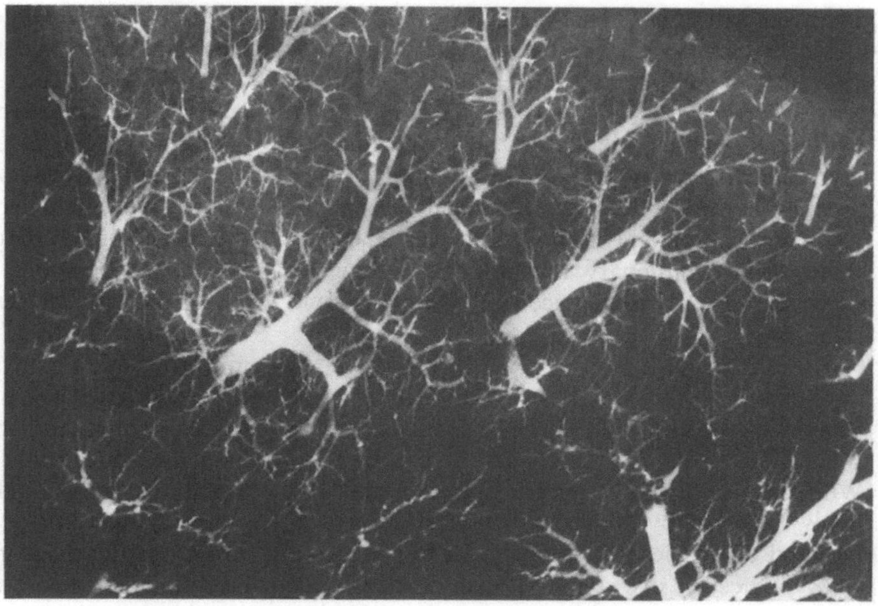

Fig. 3. Peripheral angiography of pulmonary arteries with barium sulfate. In the late phase of the adult respiratory distress syndrome, fibrosis reduces the number and the diameter of smaller vessels and capillaries

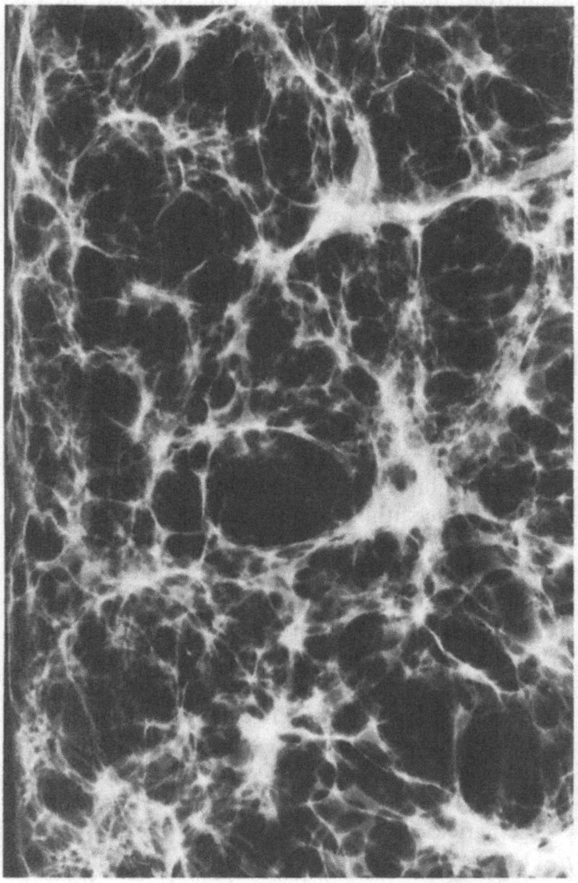

Fig. 4. Severe panacinar emphysema. Enlargement of the terminal air spaces up to 8 mm

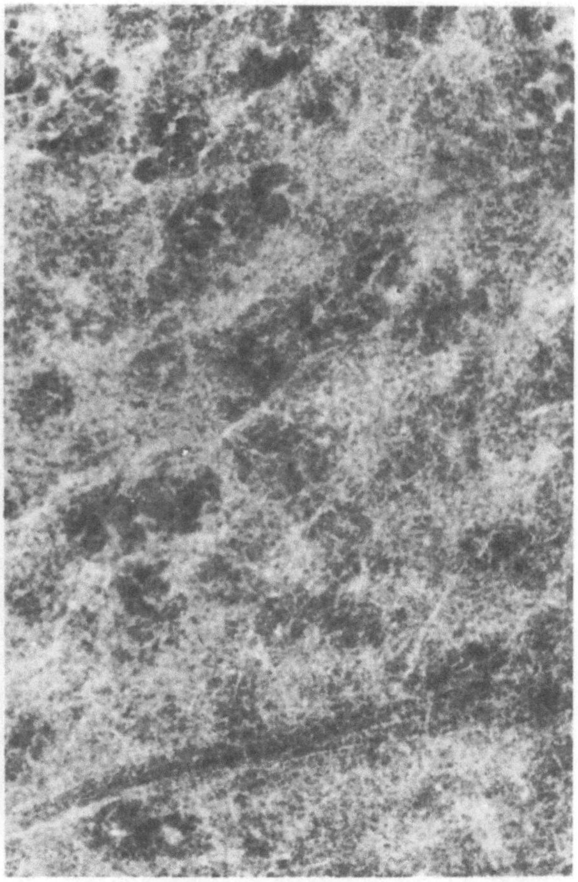

Fig. 5. Early centroacinar emphysema. The central parts of acini are hyperinflated, while the periphery is normal. The emphysematous spaces have uniform diameters of 3–4 mm

pulmonary hypertension. Angiography shows not only the inflammatory destruction of lung parenchyma [3], but also the rarefication of blood vessels.

It is even possible to demonstrate the beginning of centroacinar emphysema. All the small lucent areas in Fig. 5 are hyperinflated centers of acini whose bronchioli are narrowed or closed by inflammation. Pulmonary function tests show air trapping as a consequence of these multiple stenoses.

Fibrosis

While respiratory function in emphysema is definitely impaired by the reduction of alveolar surface and capillaries, the impairment in fibrosis is still a subject of discussion. The thickened septa are commonly assumed to increase the diffusion barrier. Morphometric measurements by Bignon et al. [1], however, demonstrate the outstanding importance of enlarged terminal air spaces and the reduction of alveolar surface in fibrosis too.

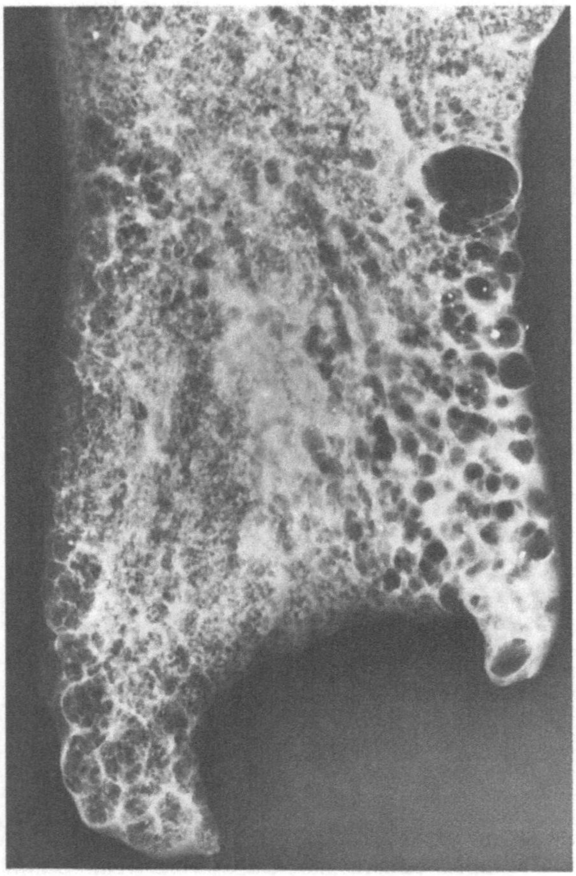

Fig. 6. Fibrosis due to an allergic reaction to budgerigar antigens. The terminal air spaces are enlarged and their walls are broadened

We tried to get such comparative measurements not only from microscopic sections, but also from radiographs (Fig. 6). A film moved in a straight line through a photometer yields an extinction curve. The regular arrangement of normal alveoli produces ring figures of about 330 μm in diameter by superimposition. The distance between periodic peaks in the extinction curve of a normal lung is also 330 μm. There are striking differences in fibrosis and emphysema. The distance between the peaks gives the diameter of the terminal air spaces, which are enlarged up to several millimeters. The altitude of the peaks is proportional to the membrane thickness, which is 10–20 times greater than normal.

Knowing the alveolar surface, the capillary surface, and the membrane thickness, it should be possible to calculate the maximal diffusion capacity of a lung [15].

Radiographs such as those shown here cannot be taken from the living patient, but do show the diagnostic value of a high-resolution technique. It is therefore important to improve the quality and resolution of chest films from the intensive care unit. We also hope that our postmortem radiographs will help us to a better understanding of the morphologic and pathophysiologic changes in the lung and lead to more reliable diagnosis.

References

1. Bignon J, Hem B, Molinier B (1975) Morphometric and angiographic studies in diffuse interstitial pulmonary fibrosis. In: Basset F, Georges R (eds) Alveolar interstitium of the lung. Pathological and physiological aspects. Karger, Basel, pp 141–160
2. Fleischner FG (1967) The butterfly pattern of acute pulmonary edema. Am J Cardiol 20:39–46
3. Heard BF (1959) Further observations on the pathology of pulmonary emphysema in chronic bronchitis. Thorax 14:58–70
4. Miller WS (1900) Das Lungenläppchen, seine Blut- und Lymphgefäße. Arch Anat Physiol Anat Abt 197–228
5. Miller WS (1947) The lung, 2nd edn. Thomas, Springfield
6. Ostendorf P, Birzle H, Vogel W, Mittermayer C (1975) Pulmonary radiographic abnormalities in shock. Radiology 115:257–263
7. Pennell TC, Bradshaw HH (1966) Anatomical study of the peripheral pulmonary lymphatics. J Thorac Surg 52:629–634

8. Rau WS, Mittermayer C (1980) Die röntgenologische Feinstruktur der Lunge. I. Volumenkontrollierte Fixierung isolierter Lungen mit Formalindampf. RoFo 133:233–239
9. Rau WS, Hauenstein K, Volk P, Mittermayer C (1980) Die röntgenologische Feinstruktur der Lunge. II. Gefrierhärtung isolierter Lungen in flüssigem Stickstoff. RoFo 133:400–405
10. Rau WS, Wybitul K, Tassinari A (1980) Die röntgenologische Feinstruktur der Lunge. III. Lobulus und Acinus. RoFo 133:571–577
11. Riede UN, Mittermayer C, Horn R, Friedburg H, Sandritter W (1980) Funktionelle Pathologie der menschlichen Schocklunge. Eine histologische, ultrastrukturelle und morphometrische Studie. Med Welt 31:491–501
12. Spencer H (1977) Pathology of the lung. Pergamon, Oxford New York Toronto Sydney Paris Frankfurt
13. Staub NC (1974) "State of the art" review. Pathogenesis of pulmonary edema. Am Rev Respir Dis 109:358–372
14. Trapnell DH (1963) The peripheral lymphatics of the lung. Br J Radiol 36:660–672
15. Weibel ER (1973) A simplified morphometric method for estimating diffusing capacity in normal and emphysematous lungs. Am Rev Respir Dis 107:579–588

Skeletal and Soft Tissue Radiology

Chondrosarcoma Variants

H. D. Dorfman

Department of Pathology, Sinai Hospital of Baltimore, Baltimore, MD 21215, USA

Malignant cartilage tumors may arise de novo in bone or they may be superimposed on preexisting benign cartilage tumors. The former are classified as primary chondrosarcomas and the latter as secondary. Also, chondrosarcomas may arise peripherally or centrally with relation to the bone and some may even arise extraskeletally. The common histologic features are that all are composed of cells that can produce hyaline cartilage matrix and that there is a tendency toward lobulation. Cartilage matrix undergoes calcification in characteristic patterns, producing telltale radiologic signs which aid diagnosis. The roentgenogram in cartilage tumors is also useful in that it provides clues as to the aggressiveness of the lesion, based on its size, pattern of bone destruction, and reactive bone formation.

The majority of chondrosarcomas (85%) arise de novo, only about 15% arising in association with enchondromatosis, multiple osteochondromas, Paget's disease, or fibrous dysplasia.

The location of a cartilage tumor is an important factor in determining the likelihood of malignancy. The more centrally or axially located a cartilage tumor is, the more likely it is to be malignant. Chondrosarcomas are more common in the pelvis, ribs, femur, humerus, sternum, and scapula. They are extremely rare in the short tubular bones of the hands and feet.

Age is also a determinant of malignancy. The more common varieties of low-grade (well-differentiated) neoplasms producing abundant hyaline cartilage matrix are seen mostly from middle age onwards, and are particularly uncommon under the age of 20. The highly malignant variant of dedifferentiated chondrosarcoma tends to occur in old age, however, and the rarer variants, clear cell and mesenchymal chondrosarcoma, are seen in relatively young patients.

Clinically, pain is the most common symptom of central chondrosarcomas; painless swelling over many months may signal the development of a peripheral chondrosarcoma. In the more borderline or low-grade chondrosarcomas, when the cytologic evidence of malignancy is questionable, the pathologist may find it necessary to rely on clinical (pain) or radiologic (size, permeation, cortical erosion, and thickening) features to arrive at a diagnostic conclusion.

Chondrosarcomas in general are slow-growing, tend to recur locally, and may implant in the soft tissue and grow into veins. The likelihood of hematogenous spread is closely correlated with the histologic grade, based on a scale of grades I to III, in increasing order of aggressiveness [5]. Sites of blood-borne metastases are lungs, liver, other bones, and brain. Spread to regional lymph nodes is very rare.

Fortunately, most chondrosarcomas (about 75%) are of grade I. These are the tumors which show the characteristic punctate or ring-like calcifications radiographically. In the young, it is important to distinguish chondrosarcomas from chondroblastic osteosarcomas, which have a much poorer prognosis. This distinction is made on histologic grounds.

Dedifferentiated chondrosarcoma is a variant which occurs almost exclusively in older individuals, and is relatively common [2, 10, 14, 15, 17]. About 10% of chondrosarcomas of the well-differentiated type can be expected to undergo this change. The high-grade anaplastic portion of these tumors usually shows a malignant fibrous histiocytoma pattern, but it may also assume the appearance of a fibrosarcoma or an osteosarcoma (Fig. 1). The prognosis is extremely bad, almost all patients dying of blood-borne metastases within 1–2 years in spite of radical surgical treatment. Radiographically, it is often possible to predict that this change has occurred when a highly destructive area develops in juxtaposition to a heavily calcified older lesion (Fig. 2). The distinction between this lesion and an infarct sarcoma may be difficult or impossible.

Radiology Today 2. Ed. by F. H. W. Heuck and M. W. Donner

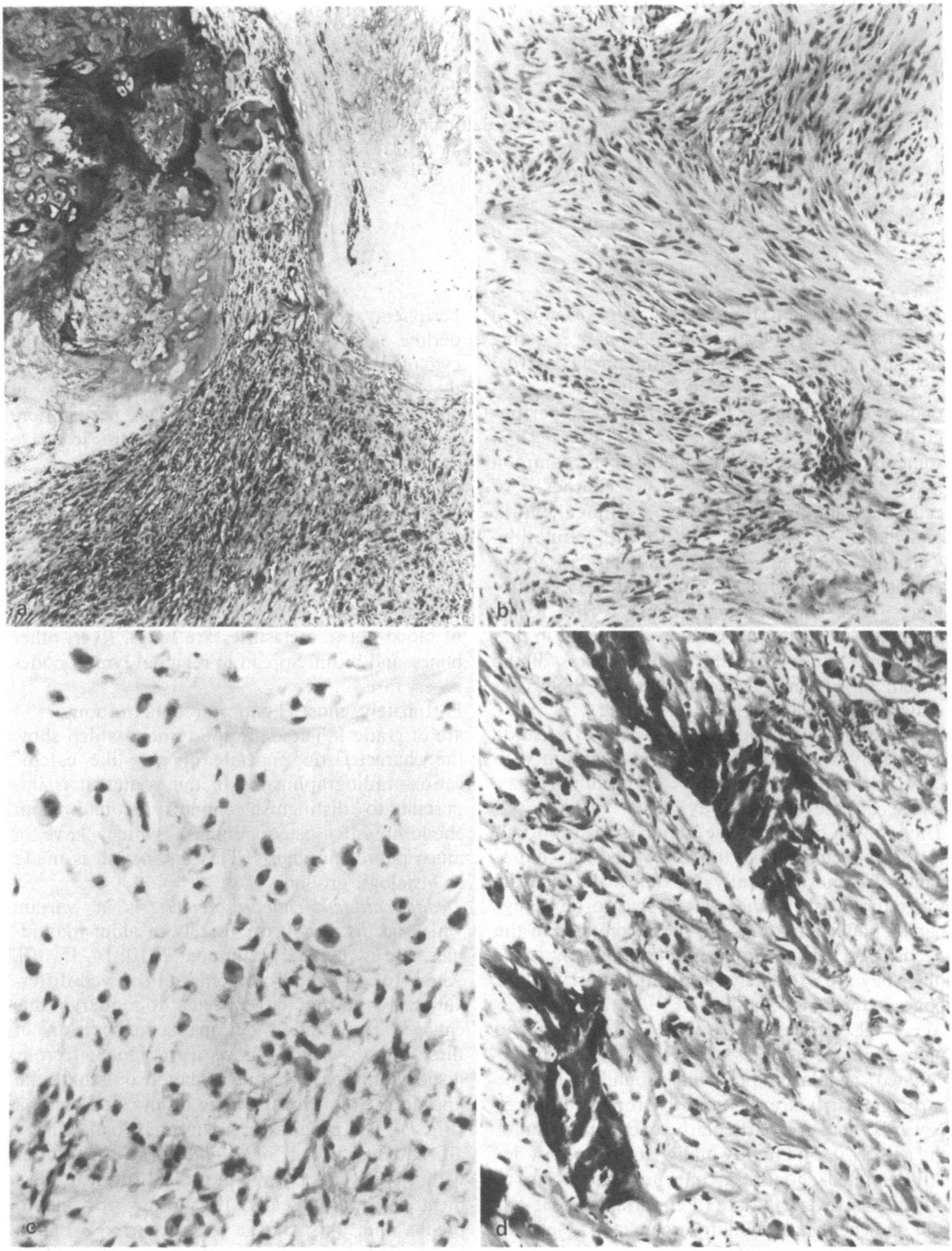

Fig. 1. a Dedifferentiated chondrosarcoma showing islands of conventional chondroid-producing tumor and focal calcification surrounded by highly anaplastic spindle cell sarcoma with pattern of malignant fibrous histiocytoma. × 120. **b** Spindle cell sarcomatous dedifferentiation in a low-grade chondrosarcoma (fibrosarcoma pattern). × 180. **c** Low-grade chondrosarcoma lobules adjacent to more anaplastic area in a dedifferentiated chondrosarcoma. × 250. **d** Osteosarcoma pattern in a dedifferentiated chondrosarcoma

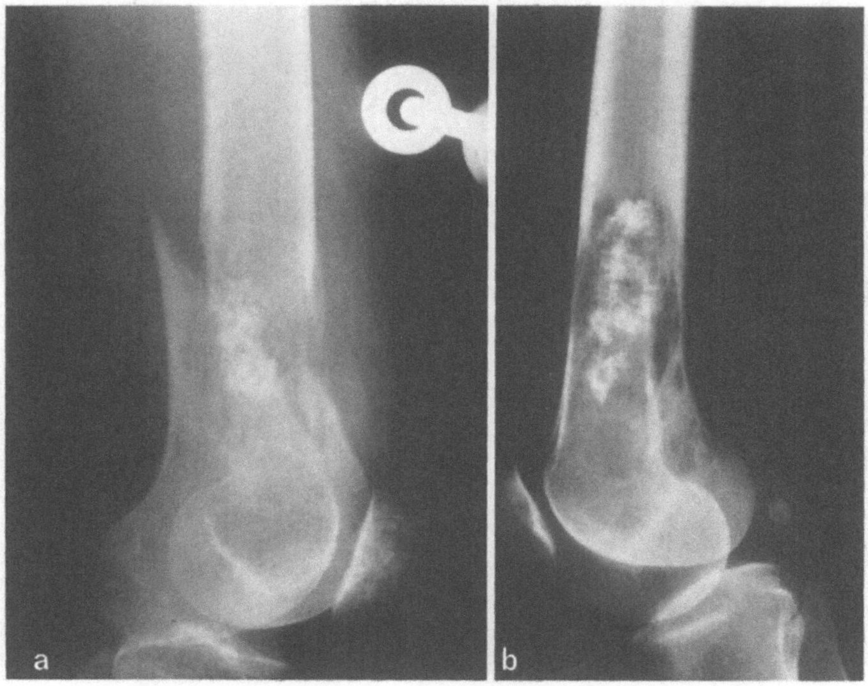

Fig. 2. a Pathologic fracture through a distal femoral dedifferenciated chondrosarcoma in a 75-year-old female. **b** Low-grade chondrosarcoma of distal femur with surrounding radiolucency in a 44-year-old female. Histologically a malignant fibrosarcoma pattern with marked anaplasia corresponded to the more lytic areas

Microscopically, the well-differentiated chondroid-matrix-producing component of this tumor may be so benign in appearance that some authors have suggested that these sarcomas may develop in the reactive tissue adjacent to an enchondroma as well as in the vicinity of a low-grade chondrosarcoma.

The possibility of dedifferentiation of a low-grade cartilage tumor requires that all such tumors be thoroughly sampled and examined histologically to determine if this change is present. Pathologists should also question whether a lesion identified as a malignant fibrous histiocytoma or a fibrosarcoma of bone in an elderly patient could in fact be the anaplastic component of a dedifferentiated cartilage tumor [3, 4, 8, 13, 18].

Mesenchymal chondrosarcoma is a variant with certain radiographic features often characteristic enough to suggest the diagnosis in younger patients. It is much rarer than dedifferentiated sarcoma. It is characterized by islands of hyaline-cartilage-producing cells of relatively well-differentiated appearance surrounded by a second component made up of undifferentiated, closely packed, round cells resembling Ewing's sarcoma. Very often these highly malignant areas are arranged in cords or nests bordering endothelium-lined vascular channels, giving a vascular or hemangiopericytoma pattern (Fig. 3). The chondroid areas may show extensive calcification, giving these tumors a characteristic stippled radiodense appearance. The facts that they tend to develop eccentrically in bone and that about one-third actually arise in soft tissue adjacent to bone are useful in radiographic diagnosis (Fig. 4). The most common sites are the ribs, vertebrae, pelvis, jaws, long bones, and scapula. They also occur in the skull, and meningeal involvement has been reported.

Mesenchymal chondrosarcomas are radioresistant, and they tend to recur and metastasize, sometimes 5–10 years after initial surgery [1, 6, 7, 11, 12, 19].

A third variant is *clear cell chondrosarcoma*, which is often radiographically indistinguishable from a chondroblastoma (Fig. 5) since they occur most often in the epiphyseal ends of long bones. They are well-defined intraosseous radiolucencies without associated cortical destruction or periosteal reaction in their early phases of growth. Some, but not all, contain central areas of radiodensity. They differ from chondroblastomas in that their clinical course is progressive, with a slow growth rate. The best treatment is wide en bloc resection, since local recurrence is the rule with lesser forms of therapy and metastasis to the lungs does occur. In five of 22 reported cases, the patients died of distant spread. These lesions also differ from chondroblastomas clinically in that they occur in older patients (range 19–68 years), with a peak incidence in the 3rd and 4th decades. The femur and humerus are the most common sites of involvement.

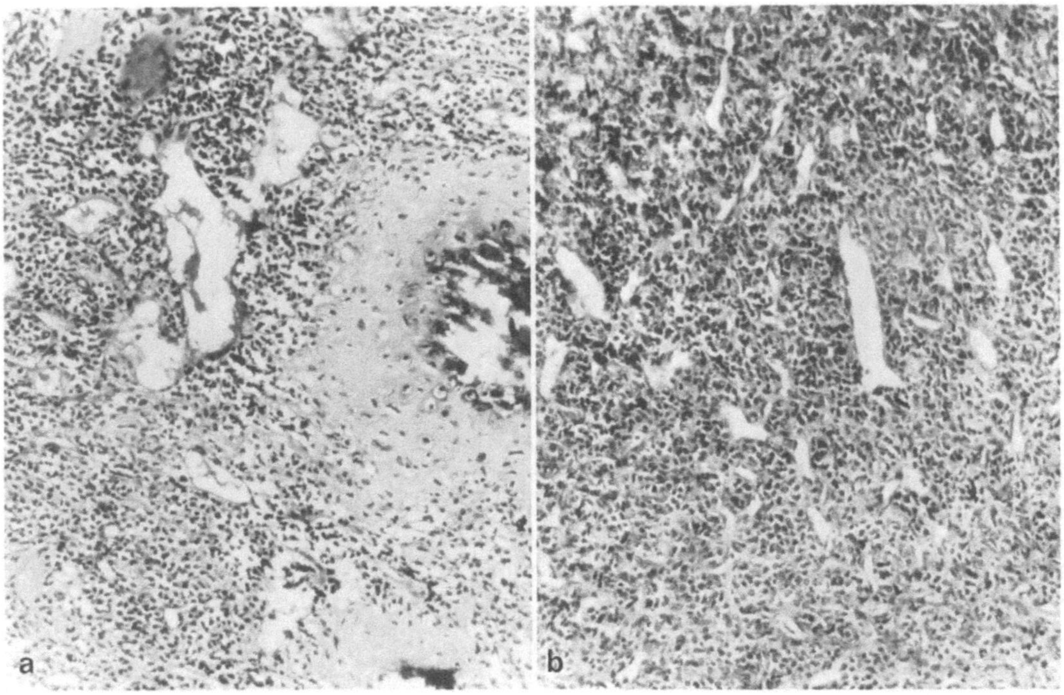

Fig. 3. a Mesenchymal chondrosarcoma in rib of a 10-year-old male. Low-grade chondrosarcoma area with calcification and undifferentiated round cell sarcoma areas. × 180. **b** Hemangiopericytoma-like pattern in a mesenchymal chondrosarcoma. × 180

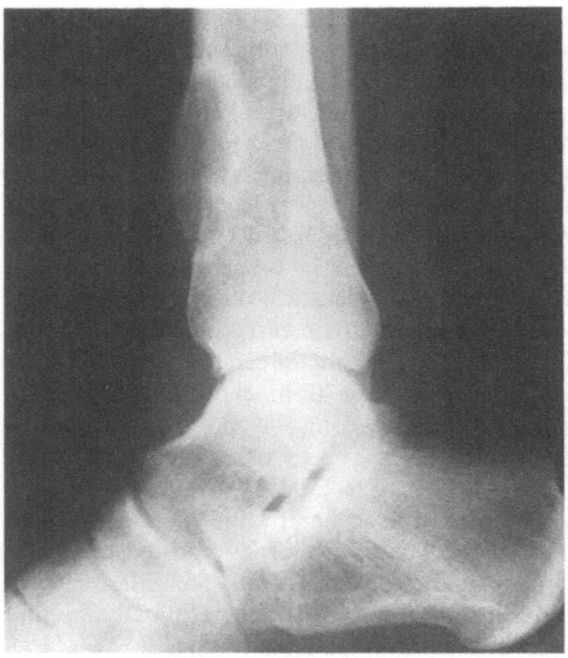

Fig. 4. Mesenchymal chondrosarcoma in distal tibia of a 24-year-old male

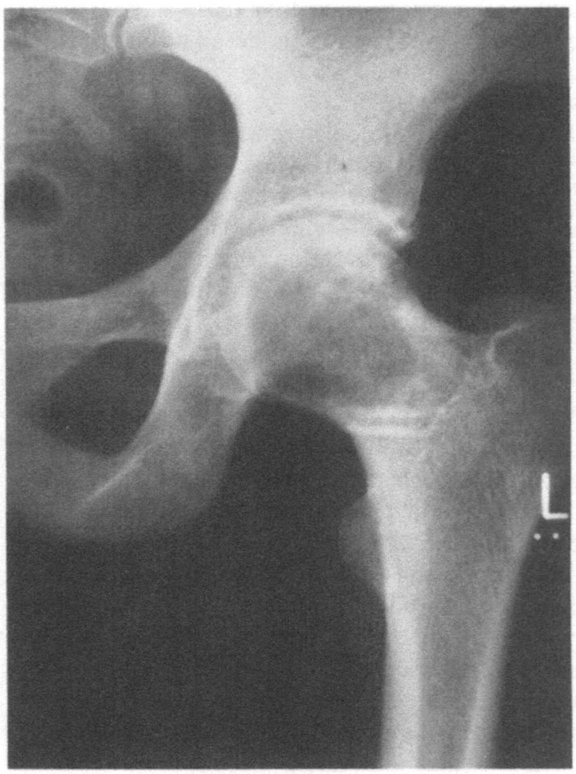

Fig. 5. Clear cell chondrosarcoma in proximal femur of a 36-year-old female. Note similarity to chondroblastoma

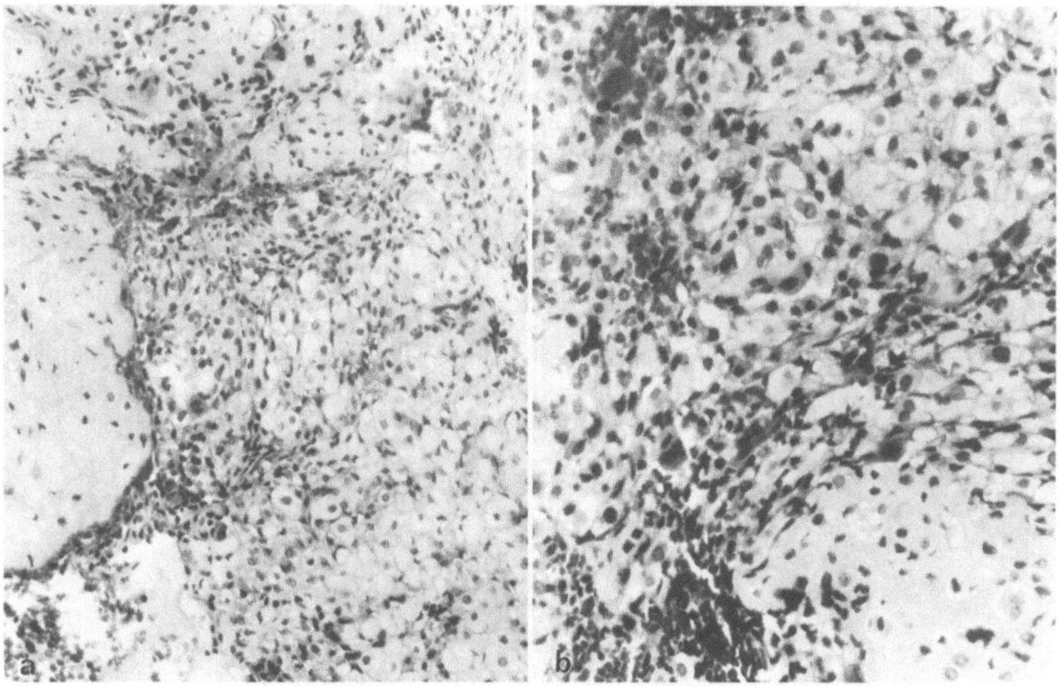

Fig. 6. **a** Clear cell chondrosarcoma of proximal femur. Note chondroid matrix island and sheets of clear cells. × 120. **b** Clear tumor cells have abundant cytoplasmic glycogen. × 200

Microscopically, these lobular lesions contain some areas of more conventional chondroid-producing tumor, but much of the neoplasm is composed of sheets of large cells with abundant clear cytoplasm, rich in glycogen (Fig. 6). The nuclei show little atypia. Multinucleated giant cells of the benign, osteoclastic type are a prominent feature of some tumors. The chondroid areas may show calcification between tumor cells, and trabeculae of osteoid and bone may be present, causing confusion with osteoblastoma microscopically. Some have been associated with areas resembling aneurysmal bone cysts.

References

1. Dahlin DC (1976) Chondrosarcoma and its "variants" in bones and joints. In: Ackerman LV, Spjut HJ, Abell MR (eds) IAP monograph. Williams & Wilkins, Baltimore, pp 300–311
2. Dahlin DC, Beabout JW (1971) Dedifferentiation of low grade chondrosarcomas. Cancer 28:461–466
3. Dahlin DC, Henderson ED (1962) Mesenchymal chondrosarcoma: further observations on a new entity. Cancer 15:410–417
4. Dowling EA (1964) Mesenchymal chondrosarcoma. J Bone Joint Surg [Am] 46:747–754
5. Evans HL, Ayala, AG, Romsdahl MM (1976) Prognostic factors in chondrosarcoma of bone: a clinicopathologic analysis with emphasis on histologic grading. Cancer 40:818–831
6. Faraggiana T, Sender B, Glicksman P (1981) Light and electron-microscopic study of clear cell chondrosarcoma. Am J Clin Pathol 75:117–121
7. Forest M, LeCharpentier Y, Postel M, Tomeno B, Roux JP, Mayabraud A, Dandaouh B, Abelanet R (1978) Une nouvelle varieté de chondrosarcome: les sarcomes dits "chondroblastiques" ou "chondrosarcomes à cellules claires." Etude anatomoclinique et ultrastructurale de 5 observations. Arch Anat Cytol Pathol 26:5–11
8. Goldman RL (1967) "Mesenchymal" chondrosarcoma, a rare malignant chondroid tumor usually primary in bone: report of a case arising in extraskeletal soft tissue. Cancer 20:1494–1498
9. Heffelfinger MJ, Dahlin DC, MacCarty CS, Beabout JW (1973) Chordomas and cartilaginous tumors of the skull base. Cancer 32:410–420
10. Kahn LB (1976) Chondrosarcoma with dedifferentiated foci. A comparative and ultrastructural study. Cancer 37:1365–1375
11. Kahn LB, Wood FM, Ackerman LV (1969) Malignant chondroblastoma. Report of two cases and review of the literature. Arch Pathol 88:541–551
12. LeCharpentier Y, Forest M, Postel M, Tomeno B, Abelanet R (1979) Clear cell chondrosarcoma. A report of five cases including ultrastructural study. Cancer 44:622–629

13. Lichtenstein L, Bernstein D (1959) Unusual benign and malignant chondroid tumors of bone. A survey of some mesenchymal cartilage tumors and malignant chondroblastic tumors, including a few multicentric ones, as well as many atypical benign chondroblastomas and chondromyxoid fibromas. Cancer 12:1142–1157
14. McCarthy EF, Dorfman HD (1982) Chondrosarcoma of bone with dedifferentiation: a study of eighteen cases. Hum Pathol 13:36–40
15. Mirra, JM, Marcove RC (1974) Fibrosarcomatous dedifferentiation of primary and secondary chondrosarcoma. J Bone Joint Surg [Am] 56:285–296
16. Salvador AH, Beabout JW, Dahlin DC (1971) Mesenchymal chondrosarcoma; observations on 30 new cases. Cancer 28:605–615
17. Sanerkin NG, Woods CG (1979) Fibrosarcomata and malignant fibrous histiocytoma arising in relation to enchondromata. J Bone Joint Surg [Br] 61:366–372
18. Steiner GC, Mirra JM, Bullough PG (1973) Mesenchymal chondrosarcoma. A study of ultrastructure. Cancer 32:926–939
19. Unni KK, Dahlin DC, Beabout JW, Sim FH (1976) Chondrosarcoma: clear cell variant. A report of sixteen cases. J Bone Joint Surg [Am] 58:676–683

Radiology and Some of the Mechanical Principles of Orthopedic Surgery

M. T. Freedman

Sinai Hospital of Baltimore, Department of Radiology, Belvedere and Greenspring Avenues, Baltimore, MD 21215, USA

An understanding of the radiology of orthopedic procedures depends on an understanding of some of the mechanical features of these procedures, of the appliances, and of the biomechanics of bone. The greater one's understanding of these principles, the greater one's potential understanding of orthopedic radiology. This chapter will deal with some of the mechanical features of orthopedic procedures and with the mechanical structures of particular appliances and these appliances' biomechanical effects on bone.

The Effects of the Techniques of Orthopedic Surgery on the Postoperative Radiographic Appearance

Two of the common techniques of orthopedic surgery, overdrilling and periosteal stripping, can have dramatic effects on the postoperative radiographic appearance.

Overdrilling. It is common to overdrill when a screw is to be used to pull two pieces of bone together. In this technique, the hole drilled in the bone fragment closest to the side plate of the appliance or to the head of the screw is made larger than the screw so that the screw can slide freely within it. This large hole results in radiolucency around a portion of the appliance, simulating the appearance of loosening or infection (Fig. 1). Since overdrilling is often used, only radiolucency around the tip of a screw device can be considered as abnormal, unless serial films can show that the radiolucency has developed, after operation.

Periosteal Stripping. When a plate is attached to bone, the surgeon has the option of stripping the periosteum from the bone. When this is done, the formation of callus may be quite limited, simulating disease.

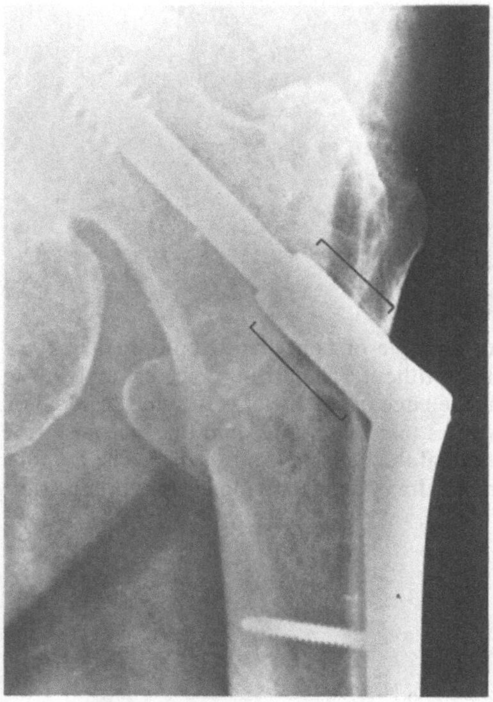

Fig. 1. An example of the effect of overdrilling. Well-defined radiolucency is present around the barrel of this compression screw (*brackets*), resulting from the drilling of an oversized hole at the time of surgery

Orthopedic Appliances and Their Effect on Adjacent Bone

Shifting of Fragments

Appliances designed to transfix fracture fragments are of two types: some permit controlled fragment shift, others are designed to prevent all fragment shift. This difference in design reflects two different philosophies of the fixation of fracture fragments. It is important for the radiologist to understand the difference between these two types of fixation, because should fragment shift

Radiology Today 2. Ed. by F. H. W. Heuck and M. W. Donner

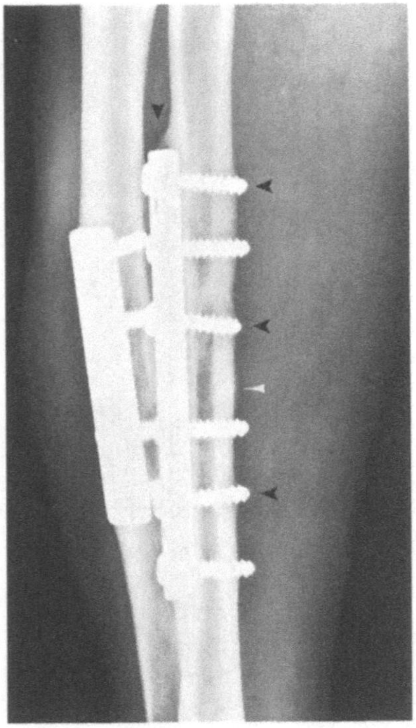

Fig. 2. An example of bone hypertrophy and of fracture healing without visible callus. Increased bone is present at the edge of the metal plates and at some of the screw holes (*black arrows*). Almost no callus is present at the radial fracture site (*white arrow*). The fracture has healed by direct bone formation across the fracture line

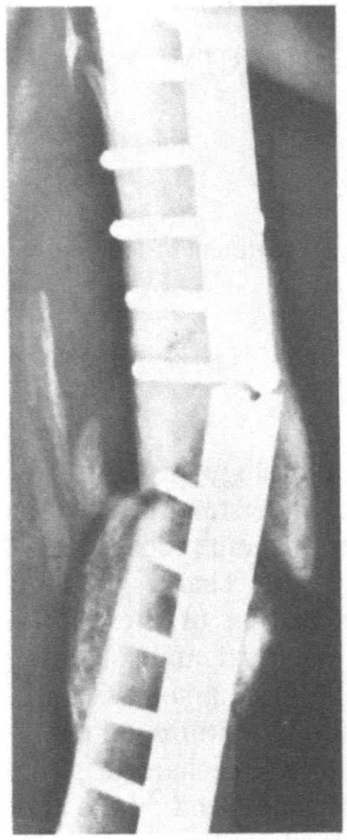

Fig. 3. An example of breakage of a plate on a femur at a screw hole with nonunion. This multihole femoral plate has broken at the screw hole just proximal to the fracture. Bone ends are smooth with no active callus formation, indicating atrophic nonunion

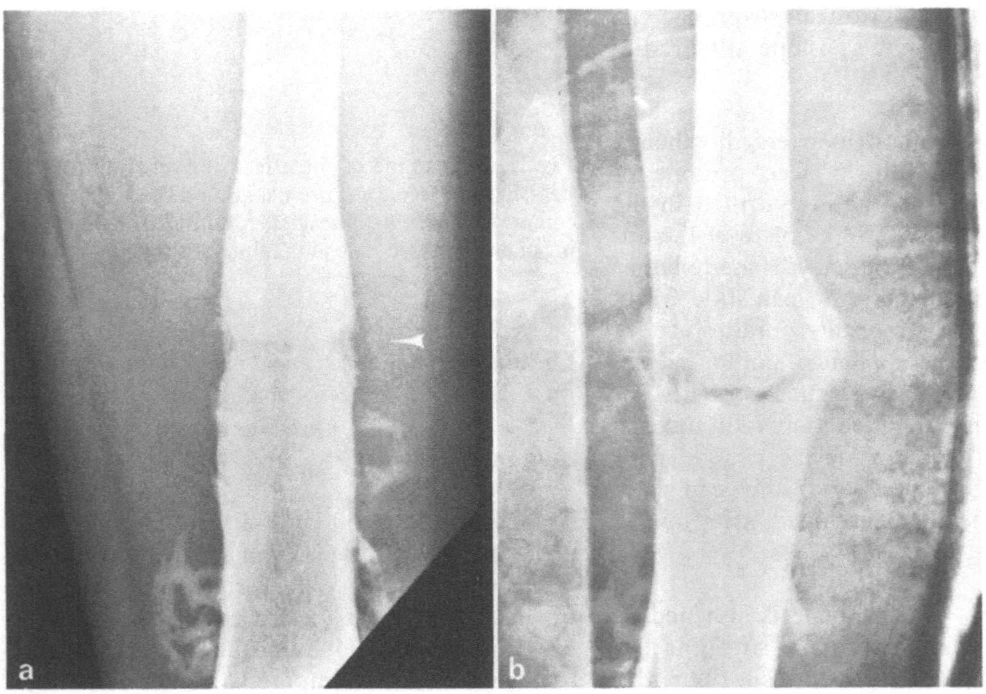

Fig. 4a, b. An example of late breakage through an infected pin tract. **a** An infected Hoffmann pin tract (*arrow*) 5 months after the removal of the pin is a continuing site of weakness in the bone. **b** Fracture through the infected pin tract occurred 2 months later (viewed in plaster)

occur with a device designed to prevent it, it is likely that further shift will occur with loss of reduction. Conversely, should rigid fixation accidentally occur with a device designed to permit controlled movement of bone fragments, delayed union or nonunion may result.

Response of Bone

All appliances change the mechanical properties of the adjacent bone. They can increase or decrease the local strength and can affect the amount of callus formed.

Increase in Strength

Many appliances that are firmly attached to bone increase the strength and rigidity of the bone at the site of fixation. This often results in slow atrophy of the bone within the fixed segment. Because of the increased strength, new fractures are more likely to occur at the edge of the appliance than within the area covered by the appliance. In general, if a new fracture is seen through the bone at the site of the appliance it implies that the appliance was loose or infected.

Hypertrophy is frequently seen around bone screw holes and at the edge of a firmly fixed appliance (Fig. 2). This increased bone formation is indicative of the rigidity of fixation.

Atrophy of bone between the screw holes and in regions protected from stress does occur and in some instances can simulate the appearance of infection.

Callus Formation

While there is a great amount of individual variability, rigid appliances tend to result in little or no callus formation while flexible appliances result in more callus. A rigidly held fracture may demonstrate no visible callus (Fig. 2), the fracture healing by direct repair with callus involved in little or none of the healing. Not seeing callus in a rigidly fixed fracture does not mean that the fracture will not heal, only that the sign of healing is the obliteration of the fracture line, not the formation of callus.

Stress-Raising Effect

Deformable substances such as bone and metal show a predictable decrease in strength at sites of holes. Both metal appliances and bone are most likely to break at the site of screw holes (Fig. 3). Holes in bone continue to serve as sites of raised stress for several months, after which time the strength of bone returns to normal. Late fracture through a screw hole implies that the bone has not reformed and strongly suggests the presence of infection (Fig. 4a, b).

Summary

Radiolucency around an appliance can result from the techniques of overdrilling or from the complications of loosening or infection. The extent of the radiolucency is the key for differentiating them; with overdrilling only that portion closest to the screw head or side plate of the appliance will be radiolucent.

Periosteal stripping may result in limited callus along one portion of a fracture.

Appliances that hold bone rigid may have limited callus or none at all. Any fragment shift with these appliances is a sign of impending failure of fixation. Appliances designed to provide nonrigid fixation and controlled fragment shift tend to have more callus. If these appliances are placed so that the bone is held rigid, delayed union or nonunion may occur.

Bone protected by a rigid appliance may atrophy, simulating infection. Hypertrophy occurs at sites of screw fixation and at the edge of a rigid appliance and indicates the firmness of fixation that is present. Failure of this atrophy and hypertrophy to occur may indicate the lack of firm fixation. Fracture through the bone encompassed by a rigid fixation type of appliance usually indicates that the appliance is loose or that infection is present.

Appliances and bone tend to break at the sites of holes. Holes in bone decrease strength for several months after they are made. Prolonged weakness with late fracture can indicate the presence of infection.

References

1. Burstein AH, et al. (1972) Bone strength: the effect of screw holes. J Bone Joint Surg [Am] 54:1143
2. Frankel VH, Burstein AH (1970) Orthopedic biomechanic. Lea & Febiger, Philadelphia
3. Frankel VH, Nordin M (1980) Basic biomechanics of the skeletal system. Lea & Febiger, Philadelphia, pp 47–55
4. Freedman MT (1979) The radiology of the postoperative hip. Wiley & Sons, New York

Paraneoplastic Osteopathy

F. H. W. Heuck

Katharinenhospital, Radiologisches Institut, Zentrum für Radiologie, Kriegsbergstrasse 60, 7000 Stuttgart, FRG

Recent advances in the knowledge of *paraneoplastic syndromes and diseases* (divided into endocrine, hematologic, cutaneous, and neuromuscular paraneoplasias and metabolic changes caused by tumors) have explained many relationships between the tumors of different organs and skeletal disorders. Metabolic changes in paraneoplastic endocrinopathies are caused by malignant tumors of tissues that normally have no endocrine function [15, 44]. Different kinds of *paraneoplastic endocrinopathies* have been observed from which secondary skeletal diseases can arise:

1. Paraneoplastic hypercalcemic syndrome (parathormone, pseudohyperparathyroidism)
2. Ectopic adrenocorticotropic hormone syndrome
3. Ectopic gonadotropin syndrome
4. Rare endocrinopathies (thyroid-stimulating hormone and somatotropic hormone syndrome, multiple paraneoplastic endocrinopathies)

By tracing protein molecules which can be produced by tumor cells and have an effect similar to that of hormones, the pathogenesis of different kinds of paraneoplastic osteopathies could be identified as the origin of known paraneoplastic hypercalcemia. The following list shows some hormones and hormone-like proteins which are important for bone metabolism and transformation and which have been found in patients with paraneoplastic endocrinopathies [30, 32]:

Parathormone
Bronchogenic carcinoma, Renal carcinoma, Ear/nose/throat carcinoma, Genital carcinoma, Acute leukopathies

Calcitonin
Bronchogenic carcinoma, Thyroid carcinoma, Mammary carcinoma

Adrenocorticotropic Hormone
Bronchogenic carcinoma, Thymoma, Pancreatic carcinoma

Androgens/Estrogens
Ovarian carcinoma, Testicular carcinoma, Bronchogenic carcinoma, Adrenal carcinoma

Somatotropic Hormone
Pulmonary carcinoma, Bronchogenic carcinoma

Anti-Vitamin D Factor
Bone tumors, Tumors of blood vessels

Prostaglandins
Pheochromocytoma, Melanoma, Thyroid carcinoma, Renal carcinoma

In some tumors, especially in undifferentiated lung carcinoma, oat cell bronchial carcinoma, and renal carcinoma, a synthesis of different endocrinologically effective substances and hormones has been discovered.
Ectopic production of *parathormone* or parathormone-like substances by tumors results in *hypercalcemia* and hypophosphatemia, known as *pseudohyperparathyroidism* [5, 20, 21]. It seems possible that a variety of tumors can produce parathormone and that this is a mechanism of hypercalcemia in those patients. In some patients with tumors it is not easy to differentiate between primary hyperparathyroidism and pseudohyperparathyroidism (Table 1). Measurements of parathormones in patients with primary hyperparathyroidism reveal a level of parathormone biological activity much higher than that of the hormone produced by the tumor, but if the tumor is of adequate size, a generalized osteopathy or a fibrous ostitis may result. Another possibility is that tumors can metabolize vitamin D to one of its active forms.
Plasma values of *human growth hormone* were measured in 12 patients by Steiner et al. [42]. In this series four patients had lung cancer and fin-

Radiology Today 2. Ed. by F. H. W. Heuck and M. W. Donner

Table 1. Criteria for differentiation of pseudohyperparathyroidism and primary hyperparathyroidism (from Wahl and Röher 1973 [45])

Pseudohyperparathyroidism	Primary hyperparathyroidism
Parathyroid glands normal	Hyperplasia and adenoma of parathyroids
Production of parathyroid-like substance by malignant tumor	Production of parathormone
Improvement of disease after removal of malignant tumor	Improvement of disease after removal of parathyroid glands
Mostly male patients	Mostly female patients
Short duration of illness (2–6 months)	Long duration of illness (1–10 years)
Nearly no renal calculi	Frequently renal calculi
Great loss of weight	Nearly no loss of weight
Rarely fibrous cystic ostitis	Frequently fibrous cystic ostitis
Often serum calcium higher than 14 mg/100 ml	Rarely serum calcium higher than 14 mg/100 ml
Varying calcium values	Constant calcium values
Alkaline phosphatase increased only for skeletal and liver metastases	Alkaline phosphatase mostly increased
Mostly normal serum chloride	Serum chloride mostly increased
Serum phosphate decreased	Serum phosphate decreased
Frequently hyperuricemia	Frequently hyperuricemia
Reduced tubular reabsorption	Reduced tubular reabsorption

ger clubbing, and one had *osteoarthropathy* and a *very high plasma level* of human growth hormone. After resection of the adenocarcinoma in the left upper lung lobe, the plasma range decreased and knee and ankle pain disappeared. The pathogenesis of hypertrophic osteoarthropathy is not yet well known, but the behavior of the plasma level of growth hormone and the postoperative disappearance of joint pain in this case may explain ectopic growth hormone production by the pulmonary tumor.

With reference to *paraneoplastic hypercalcemia*, the *prostaglandins* are of special importance for bone resorption by tumorous tissue. It has been demonstrated that prostaglandins E and F are synthesized in tumorous tissue, [19, 27, 31, 41]. Prostaglandins stimulate bone cells, especially osteoclasts, and therefore play an important role in the growth of bone metastases. Prostaglandin E2 is produced by bone tissue and probably promotes bone resorption, but the metabolic activities and functions of prostaglandins are still not fully understood. Acetylsalicylic acid and Indomethacin have been found to be inhibitors of prostaglandins.

The main question in the biology and pathology of tumors is: Which biological mechanisms are necessary for a differentiated cell to produce metabolically active proteins without humoral or nervous regulation?

Generalized Skeletal Changes

Paraneoplastic osteopathy is a *secondary* disease of the skeleton, accompanying the tumorous disease and *independent of skeletal metastases. Generalized diffuse skeletal changes* may result, resembling a *diffuse osteoporosis,* or following accompanying vitamin D changes the bone may have an osteomalacic appearance [3, 10, 16, 35, 37]. In the literature we find very few cases *of generalized osteoporosis or osteomalacia* being the first stage of a paraneoplastic bone disease [25]. Figure 1 shows pronounced diffuse osteoporosis in the skeleton of a 65-year-old man with oat cell carcinoma.

If the disease includes a *malacic component,* then pathological fractures or Looser's transformation zones and collapsed vertebral bodies should occur, as seen in the X-ray of a 70-year-old women suffering from carcinoma of the breast (Fig. 2). Autopsy excluded metastases in the osteomalacic bones. Similar observations have been published by Fornasier and Czitrom [14].

Hypertrophic Osteoarthropathy: A Special Kind of Paraneoplastic Osteopathy

Roentgen appearance of a *special kind of paraneoplastic osteopathy* called "hypertrophic os-

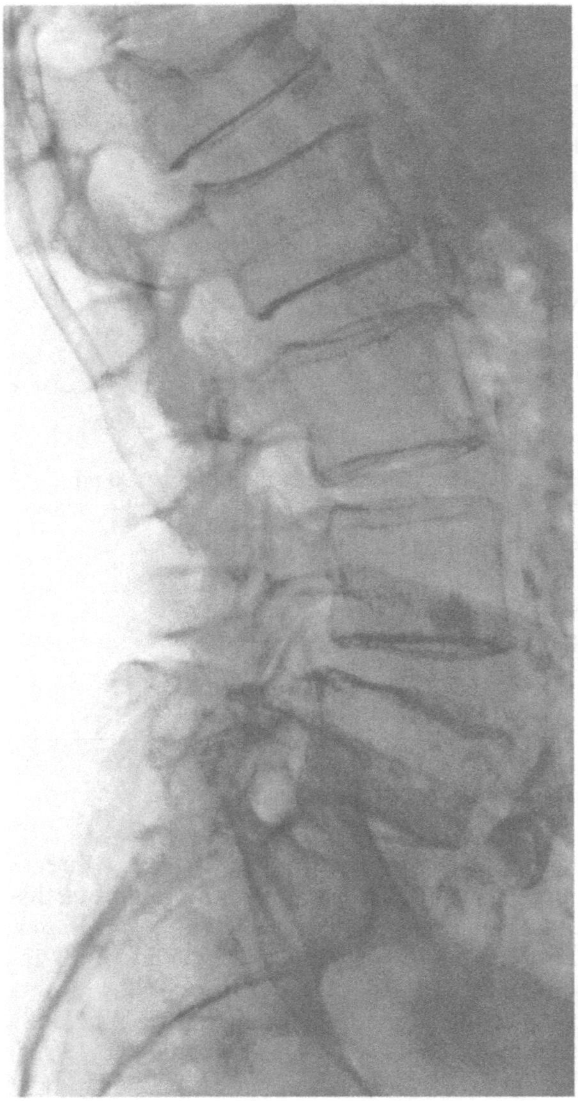

Fig. 1. Severe osteoporosis in the spine of a 65-year-old man with oat cell carcinoma of the lung

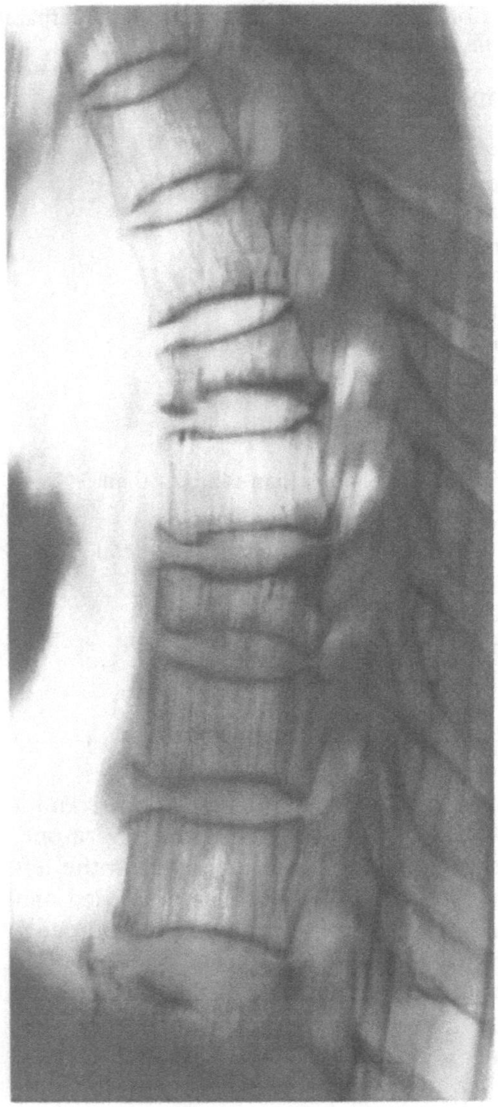

Fig. 2. Paraneoplastic osteopathy with a malacic component in a 70-year-old man with carcinoma of the lung. Collapsed vertebral bodies demonstrated by tomography

teoarthropathy" is reflected by a high rate of transformation of bone tissue and apposition of new periosteal bone around the diaphysis of tubular bones. In the future follow-up studies will help to determine if *generalized skeletal disorders* are the first stage of well-known hypertrophic osteoarthropathy.

In 1889 Bamberger [6] and in 1890 Marie [29] first observed and published their findings on hypertrophic osteoarthropathy in patients suffering from inflammatory lung disease and lung or bronchial tumors. Conditions such as bronchiectases, lung abscess, congenital heart disease, bacterial endocarditis, and inflammatory bowel disease were also associated with hypertrophic osteoarthropathy.

Later the same disorders were found in patients with tumors in organs other than the lungs. At present, *primary lung cancer* is the entity most frequently associated with the condition. In some series 0.7%–12.0% of patients with bronchogenic carcinoma have osteoarthropathy.

The frequency of appearance of hypertrophic osteoarthropathy in patients with other malignant tumors varies in the literature from 0.4% to 1.2%. It is proposed that the more or less circular new periosteal bone formations are observed in combination [9, 18, 34] with *inflammatory signs in the joints.* The clinical appearance of hypertrophic osteoarthropathy is characterized by the following triad:

1. Periosteal new bone formation
2. Clubbing of fingers and occasionally toes
3. Synovitis

The first report of clubbed fingers in a patient with emphysema was made by Hippocrates. The combination of clubbed fingers with hypertrophic osteoarthropathy was first reported in 1915 by Locke [28]. The disorders were interpreted as generalized diseases of the skeleton with structural and morphological bone changes. Morphological investigation revealed layers of *periostal appositions* around the diaphysis and the metaphysis, with a preference for peripheral regions of the skeleton (Fig. 3a). Huge periosteal new bone formations also have been found (Fig. 3b). Later, general disorders of bone metabolism and transformation of bone tissue were realized to be the reason for the growth of these appositions. The pathological structure of bones can be demonstrated by X-ray if the skeletal changes are distinct and strongly marked [1, 17, 18].

The painful *synovitis* accompanied by swelling is caused by changes in the microvessels, which can be recognized in histological sections. Schumacher 1976 [40] found small dense particles in the synovial vessels and an increased number of leukocytes in the synovial fluid. In patients with digital *clubbing* the X-rays of the hands show spur-like overgrowth of bone in the cortex of some terminal phalanges. Fischer [11] published X-rays of hands for which he had used the *soft tissue technique* to demonstrate *thickening of the tendon sheaths.* Furthermore, the hand skeleton showed discrete *periosteal reactions* and trans-

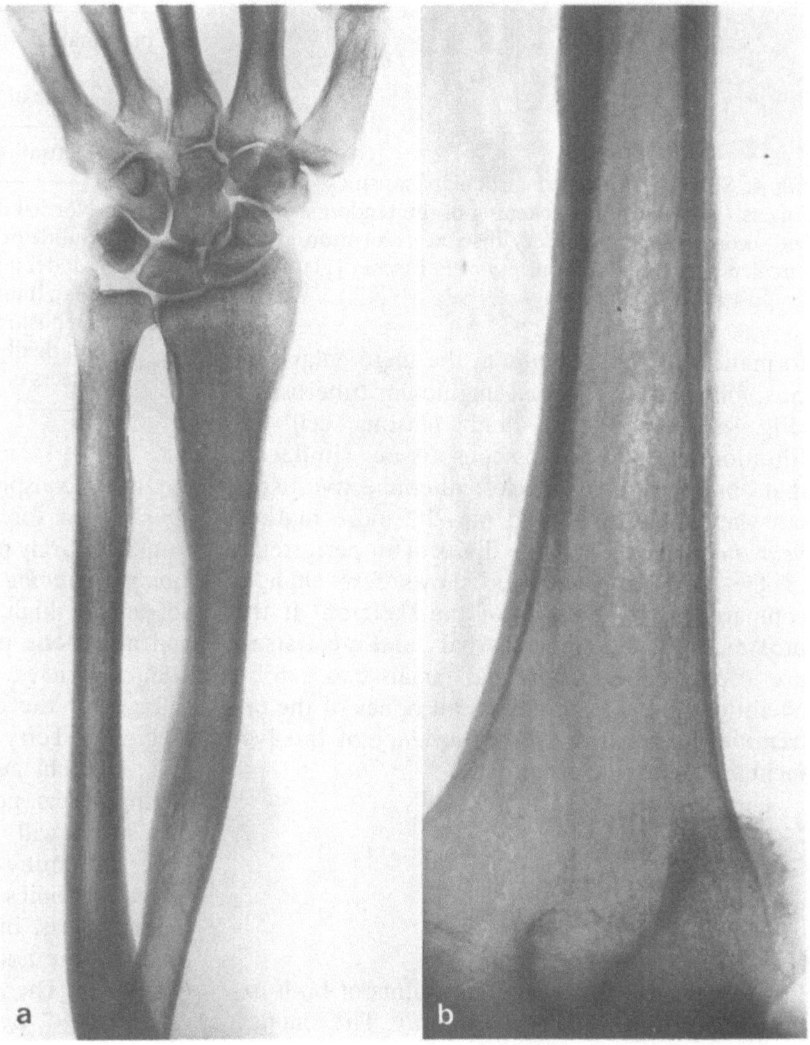

Fig. 3. a Periosteal appositions on the diaphysis and meta-physis of ulna and radius in a 57-year-old man with lung cancer. **b** Unusual periosteal new bone formations on the femoral diaphysis in a 56-year-old man with lung cancer. X ray of the right femur taken by magnification technique

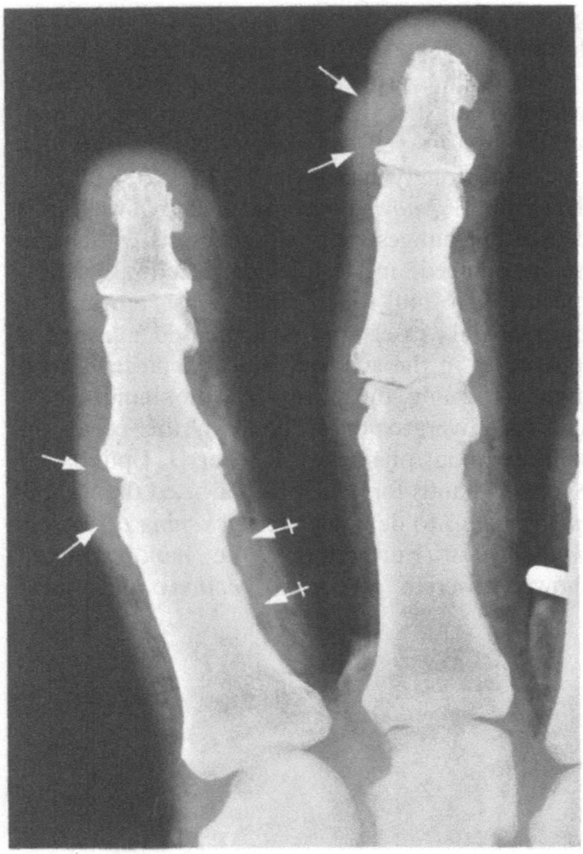

Fig. 4. Slightly thickened articular capsules of two fingers (→) as well as thickening of the tendon sheat of the second finger (→). Very discrete resorption at the unguicular processes. (Courtesy of E. Fischer [11])

Table 2. Regional involvement of skeleton by hypertrophic pulmonary osteoarthropathy (from Ali et al. [2])

Region	No. regions in grades[a] 0	1	2	3	4	Total positive	% positive
Skull	28	10	8	1	1	20	42
Clavicle	32	1	10	2	3	16	33
Scapula	15	8	20	2	3	32	67
Humerus, P	41	3	3	0	1	7	15
Humerus, D	18	11	13	3	3	30	63
Radius-ulna, P	8	5	21	6	8	40	83
Radius-ulna, D	7	6	20	10	5	41	85
Hands and carpus	6	8	29	3	2	42	88
Femur, P	13	2	16	10	7	35	73
Femur, D	6	4	16	13	9	42	88
Patella	24	7	10	7	0	24	50
Tibia-fibula, P	2	3	17	16	10	46	96
Tibia-fibula, D	3	5	12	13	15	45	94
Feet	9	11	16	7	5	39	81
Ribs	47	0	1	0	0	1	2
Pelvis	47	...	...	...	1	1	2

P = proximal; D = distal

[a] Grading scale of radionuclide deposition in bones

Grade	Definition
0 . . .	Normal deposition of radiopharmaceutical
1 . . .	Subtle but definitely increased deposition
2 . . .	Moderately increased deposition, but less than lumbar spine
3 . . .	Deposition equal to lumbar spine
4 . . .	Markedly increased deposition: clearly in excess of lumbar spine

formations with *resorption* at the unguicular process, followed by rounded unguicular tuberosities (Fig. 4). Lymphocytic and plasma cell infiltrations in the extraosseous tissue, similar to that observed in extraperiosteal connective tissue elsewhere, is present, and may be more marked *near the distal ends* of the digits. The periosteum of the terminal phalanges shows few changes compared to other parts of the skeleton. If the proximal phalanges, metacarpals, and metatarsals are affected, the carpals and tarsals can exhibit alterations later. In *rare cases* all bones of the extremities are involved. The *frequency* of involvement, in decreasing order, is:

1. Radius and ulna
2. Tibia and fibula
3. Humerus and femur
4. Metacarpals and metatarsals
5. Phalanges

It is remarkable that bones and joints of both extremities are involved *symmetrically*. The changes are most conspicuous on the *concavity of long bones* of the forearms and legs. The bones of the trunk are rarely morphologically involved.

Isotope scanning of the skeleton reveals early involvement, high turnover in the affected bones, and also bone transformation in the skull, sternum, clavicles, and vertebral bodies before changes in the extremities are perceptible radiologically. Terry et al. [43], Rosenthall and Kirsh [39], Albrecht and Ellegast [1], and Ali et al. [2], among others, pointed out that increased nuclide deposition will be found in the torso and the lower extremities, mostly in trabecular bone, e.g., vertebral bodies, ribs, and epiphyseal and metaphyseal parts, but in the bones of the upper extremities the nuclide concentration will be lower (Table 2). The generalized metabolic bone disease caused by paraneoplastic hormone pro-

Table 3. Radionuclide deposition in bones by hypertrophic osteoarthropathy in 48 patients (Ali et al. [2])

Region	Negative	Positive
Proximal tibia and fibula	2	46
Distal tibia and fibula	3	45
Distal femur	6	42
Hands + carpals	6	42
Distal radius and ulna	7	41
Proximal radius and ulna	8	40
Feet	9	39
Proximal femur	13	35
Scapula	15	33
Distal humerus	18	30
Patella	24	24
Skull	28	20
Clavicle	32	16
Proximal humerus	41	7
Ribs	47	1
Pelvis	47	1

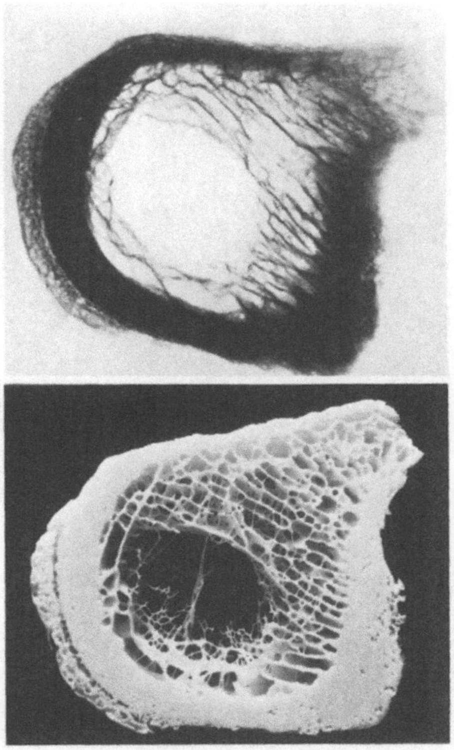

Fig. 5. Sharply demarcated layer of new bone during the early stage of periosteal proliferation in a 47-year-old man suffering from lung cancer. Cross-section of the femur

duction and activity of hormonal metabolism, which is of importance for bone transformation, is verified by the distribution of nuclide activity. Ali et al. [2] have listed 48 cases of various tumors, especially lung carcinomas, followed by hypertrophic osteoarthropathies and the resulting increased deposition of radionuclide in skeletal regions (Table 3). *Scintigraphy* is a sensitive indicator of the early stage of a generalized paraneoplastic osteopathy, which can be followed by a more pronounced localized hypertrophic osteoarthropathy characterized by periosteal appositions.

The first *morphological changes* to be seen on X-ray are periosteal proliferations of *new bone*, which become progressively greater, in some parts irregular, rough, and undulated. At the beginning the layer of new bone is sharply demarcated from the old cortical bone (Fig. 5), but later the new bone becomes thicker and more compact and *merges* with the cortex. Various types of periosteal elevation can be noted:

1. *Single-layer* elevation, caused by lifting of the periosteum with a narrow area of connective tissue between old and new bone
2. *Onion-skin-like* or spur-like appearance of elevated periosteum
3. *Irregular* periosteal deposition
4. *Solid bone formation* with undulated or uneven surface
5. *Thickening of the cortex* without sharp demarcation between old and new bone tissue

Studies of the layers of new bone indicate different *stages* of the process, enabling one to reconstruct the *history* of the disease. Thus it is established that the new periosteum is formed layer by layer (Fig. 6a). The result is a *lamellar appearance* of the newly formed structure; usually the new periosteum envelops the old cortex like the bark enveloping a tree, where the surface has an irregular porous or wart-like appearance (Fig. 6b).

It is significant that *osteoporosis* is also present in bones with or without periosteal apposition. The secondary paraneoplastic bone disease originates not primarily from the periosteum, but from the cortex. If this is true, the process is similar to that of hyperparathyroidism with porotic osteoperiostitis. The designation "pseudohyperparathyroidism" is therefore exactly correct. Considerably thickened and *disfigured but not elongated bones* result.

Figure 7 illustrates a case of hypertrophic osteoarthropathy in a 46-year-old man with a pulmonary neoplasm, demonstrating the radiological and anatomical picture of periosteal apposition

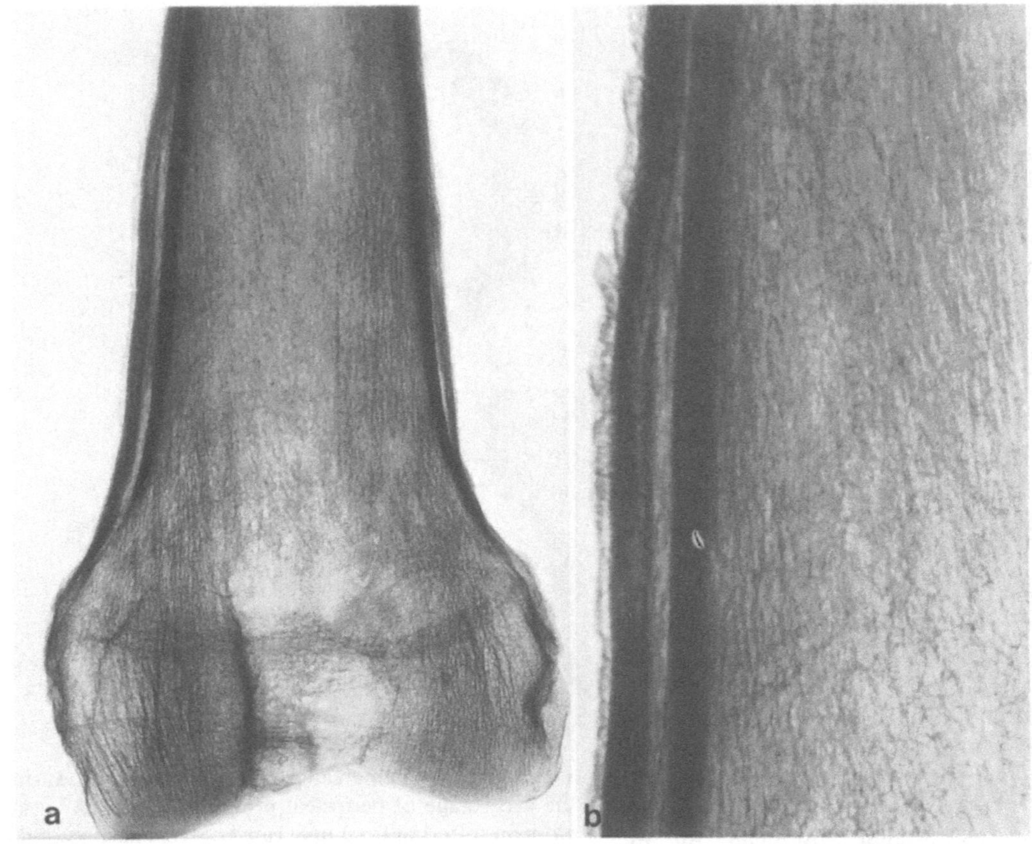

Fig. 6 a, b. Different stages of new bone formation in the distal femur of a 61-year-old man with pleural sarcoma. **a** New periosteum forming layer by layer. **b** The new surface is irregular

on both forearms and both hands. Analysis of the structure of the new periosteal bone by X-ray reveals in cross section the onion-skin-like layers of apposition.

At the beginning of the disease, *histology* shows periosteal thickening and inflammation with perivascular infiltrations of lymphocytes, plasma cells, and occasionally leukocytes, which can also be found in the surrounding connective tissue. Differentiation of the internal periosteal cambium and the external layer, with inflammatory infiltrations, is possible. The fibrillary tissue is then replaced by osteoid, from which palisades of new bone develop perpendicular to the old cortex. Between these palisades, formation of edematous and fully vascularized *connective tissue* is observed (Fig. 8). After transformation of the new bone tissue, lamellar trabecular bone develops and the fibrous marrow is replaced by *fatty* marrow. In addition to osteoid seams with osteoblasts, osteoclasts are to be found. The newly formed periosteal bone seems to merge with the old cortex, but histology and microradiography show the borderline still represented very clearly by cement lines. The endosteal region of the cortex shows bone resorption and structural changes.

Comparative microradiographic and histological studies have revealed differences in the mineral density up to the cellular level in bone tissue. Juster and Crespo [26] were the first to apply the microradiographic technique in studies of the new bone formation in hypertrophic osteoarthropathy, in which the distinction between the old original cortey and the new bone is obscured. Continuation of this resorptive trend ultimately results in similar cancellous structures in both new periosteal and old cortical bone. The shaft is therefore markedly thickened but of more cancellous character. The *mineralization* of bone in the different new layers varies greatly. *Microdensitometry* demonstrates the differences in mineral concentration in the periosteal bone.

The number of osteocytes is nearly normal. Osteocyte lacunae are larger than in normal bone tissue

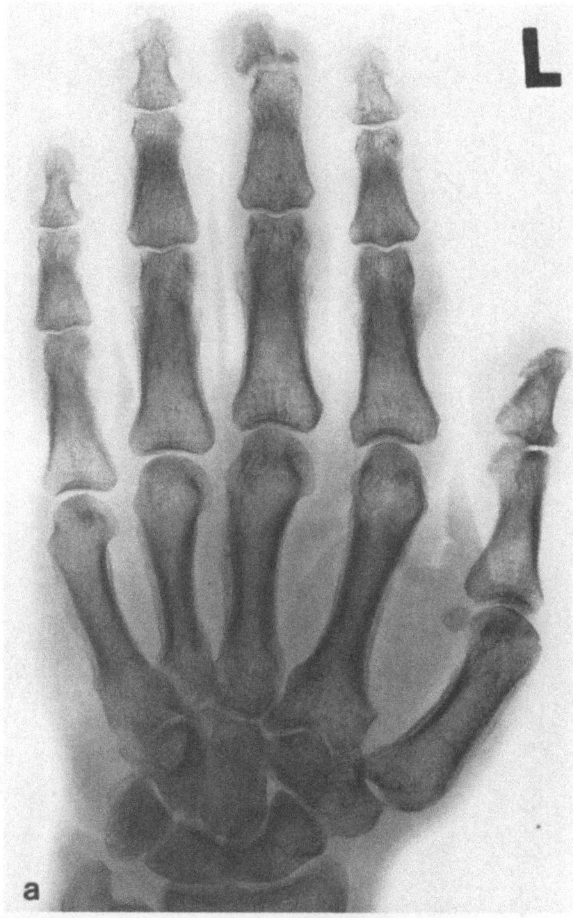

Fig. 7a–c. Hypertrophic osteoarthropathy in a 46-year-old man suffering from a pulmonary neoplasm. **a** Periosteal appositions on the phalanges and metacarpals. **b, c** Slight periosteal bone formation on the forearms

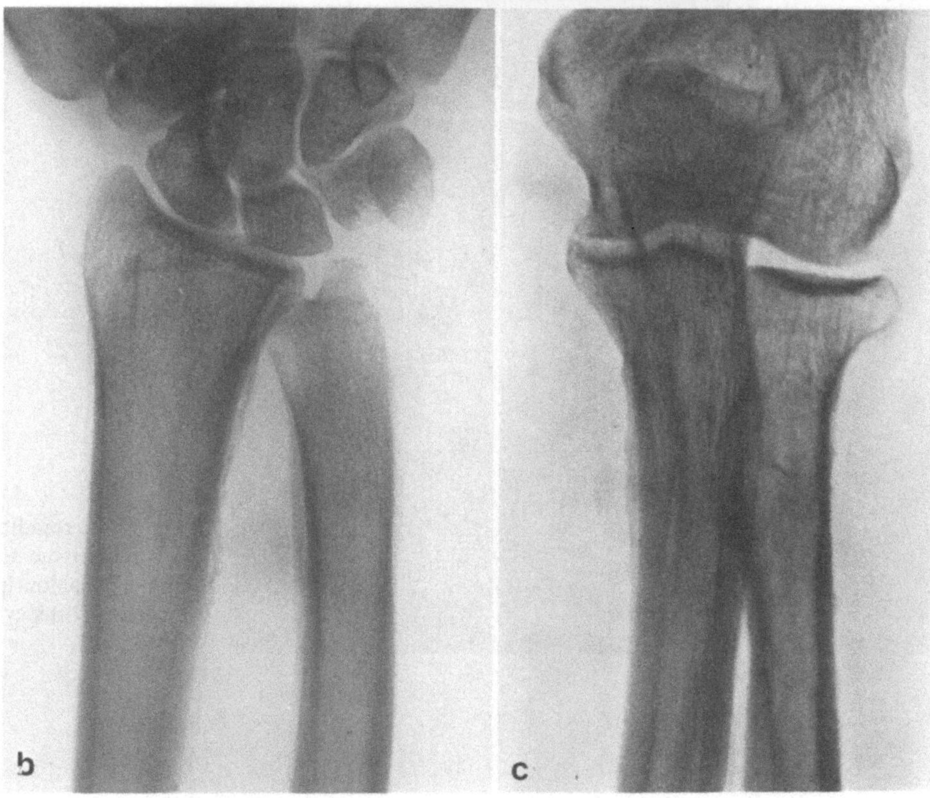

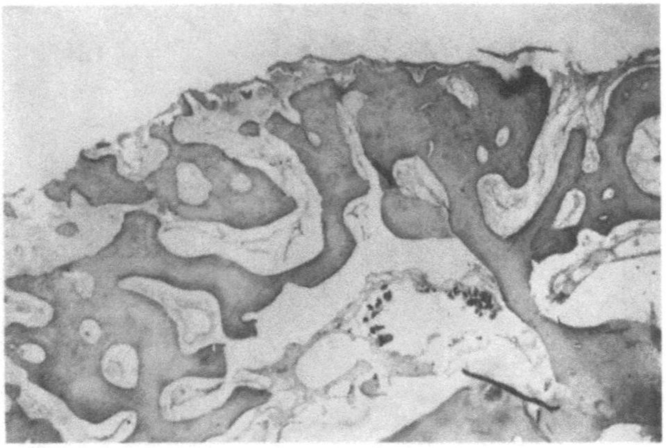

Fig. 8. Connective tissue between the palisades of new bone formation in the ulna of a 57-year-old man with lung cancer. Histology of decalcified bone tissue

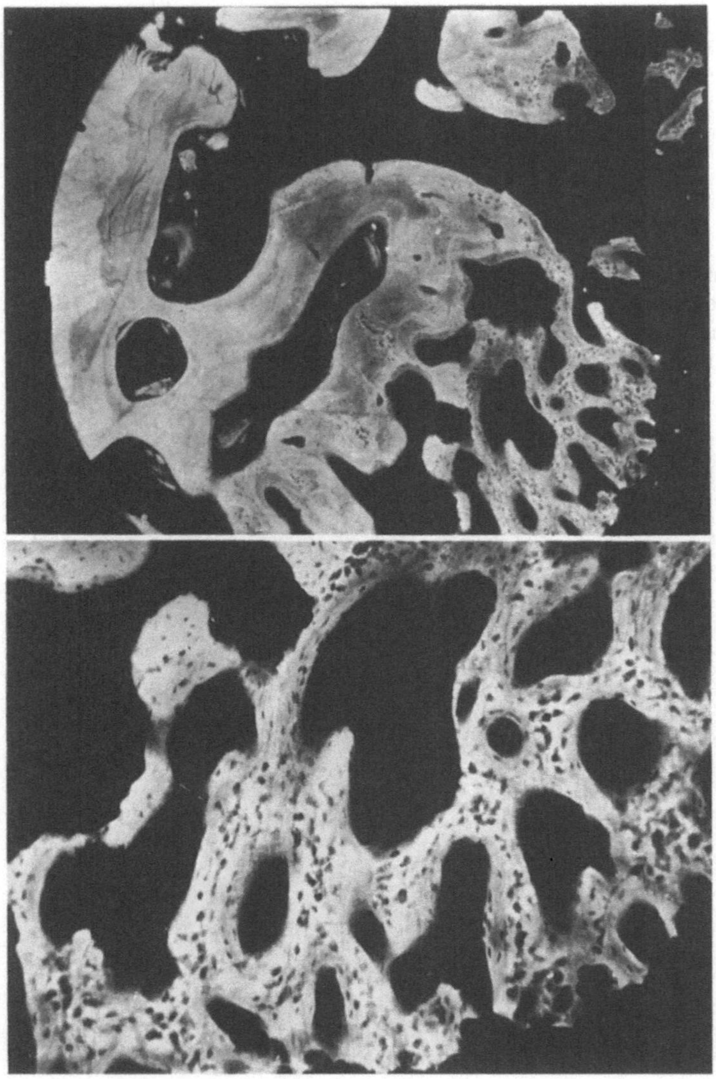

Fig. 9. Microradiography of periosteal new bone tissue demonstrates differences and regional low mineralization, large lacunae of osteocytes, and partly osteocytic osteolysis

and surrounded by low-density halos. In some places osteocytic osteolysis [7, 8, 22, 23] appears side by side with new bone formation (Fig. 9).

After *tumor removal* the new bone appositions disappear rapidly by transformation over a period of weeks or months. If not much new bone has been formed, *total resorption* is possible; if the proliferation has been greater, it *remains as a portion of the diaphysis.* The symptoms of this entity frequently resolve with amazing speed after treatment of the primary lesion, but *reappearance* of symptomatology has been seen after recurrence of the tumor or spreading of metastases [33, 46].

Some patients had neither signs nor symptoms of hypertrophic osteoarthropathy at the time of initial diagnosis. The hypertrophic osteoarthropathy was diagnosed by bone scintigraphy when the metastatic disease became clinically apparent.

The pathogenesis of hypertrophic osteoarthropathy is still unknown. Besides humoral factors such as hormonal influences, paraneoplastic endocrinopathy and circulatory disorders have been discussed. Follow-up studies of the development at macroscopic level, histological and microradiographic investigations, and isotope studies of the turnover of new periosteal bone tissue demonstrate the *dynamics* of the disease. *Osteogenesis* and partial or total bone resorption are probably induced by *more than one factor.* Systematic analysis of the different types and manifestations of paraneoplastic osteopathy is necessary to discover their pathogenesis.

References

1. Albrecht HJ, Ellegast HH (1979) Osteoarthropathie hypertrophicans Pierre Marie-Bamberger. In: Schinz, Baensch, Frommhold, Glauner, Uehlinger, Wellauser (eds) Lehrbuch der Röntgendiagnostik, vol II/2 (6th edn). Thieme, Stuttgart
2. Ali A, Tetalman MR, Fordham EW, Turner DA, Chiles JT, Patel SL, Schmidt KD (1980) Distribution of hypertrophic pulmonary osteoarthropathy. Am J Roentgenol 134:771–780
3. Azzopardi JG, Whittaker RS (1969) Bronchial carcinoma and hypercalcemia. J Clin Pathol 22:718–724
4. Azzopardi JG, Williams ED (1968) Pathology of "nonendocrine" tumors associated with Cushing's syndrome. Cancer 22:274–286
5. Azzopardi JG, Freeman E, Poole G (1970) Endocrine and metabolic disorders in bronchial carcinoma. Br Med J 4:528–530
6. Bamberger E (1889) Vorstellung von 2 Fällen mit hypertrophischer Osteoarthropathie. Wien Klin Wochenschr 2:226–227
7. Bélanger LF (1969) Osteocytic osteolysis. Calcif Tissue Res 4:1–12
8. Bélanger LF (1971) Osteocytic resorption. In: Bourne GH (ed) The biochemistry and physiology of bone, vol 3. Academic, New York
9. Denck H, Titscher R (1973) Pseudohyperparathyreoidismus. In: Mlczoch, Seidel (eds) Aktuelle Fragen in der Lungenpathologie. Thieme, Stuttgart
10. Drezner MK, Feinglos MN (1977) Osteomalacia due to 1-25-dihydroxychole-calciferol deficiency. Association with a giant cell tumor of the bone. J Clin Invest 60:1046–1053
11. Fischer E (1979) Die Weichteilveränderungen der Finger bei der rheumatischen Polyarthritis. Ergebnisse nach Weichstrahlaufnahmen in drei Ebenen. Radiologe 19:119–137
12. Fischer E (1981) Low kilovolt radiography. In: Resnick, Niwayama (eds) Diagnosis of bone and joint disorders. Saunders, Philadelphia
13. Fischer E, Manolakis P (1967) Das röntgenologische Frühzeichen der rheumatischen Polyarthritis nach Noorgard bei der Osteopathia hypertrophicans toxica. Fortschr Geb Röntgenstr Nuklearmed Ergänzungsband 106:844–847
14. Fornasier VL, Czitrom AA (1978) Collapsed vertebrae: a review of 659 autopsies. Clin Orthop 131:261–265
15. Gordan GS (1967) Hormonal effects on nonendocrine tumors with special reference to the hypercalcemia of breast cancer. In: Segaloff, Meyer, DeBakey (eds) Current concepts in breast cancer. Williams and Wilkins, Baltimore
16. Gordan GS (1974) Hyper- and hypocalcemia: pathogenesis and treatments. Ann NY Acad Sci 230:181–186
17. Greenfield GB, Escamilla CH, Schorsch HA (1967a) Hand as an indicator for generalized disease. Am J Roentgenol 99:736–745
18. Greenfields GB, Schorsch HA, Shkolnik A (1967b) The various roentgen appearances of pulmonary hypertrophic osteoarthropathy. Am J Roentgenol 101:927–931
19. Hamberg M, Samuelsson B (1972) On the metabolism of prostaglandin E_1 and E_2 in man. J Biol Chem 247:3495–3502
20. Hayduk K, Kaufmann W (1973) Ektope paraneoplastische Endokrinopathien mit Störungen des Wasser- und Elektrolythaushaltes. Klin Wochenschr 51:361–376
21. Heath H, Weller RE, Mundy GR (1980) Canine lymphosarcoma: a model for study of the hypercalcemia of cancer. Calcif Tissue Res 30:127–133
22. Heuck F (1966) The osteolytic action of the osteocytes in disorders of bone metabolism. 4th Europ Symp Calc Tiss, Leiden, 1966. Excerpta Medica Congress Ser no 120
23. Heuck F (1968) Investigations of the mineral content of the osteocyte halos. Calcif Tissue Res 2 [Suppl] 81–81A

24. Heuck F (1972) Die Struktur des Knochens bei Osteoarthropathie hypertrophicans (Pierre Marie-Bamberger Syndrom). 53. Tagung der Deutschen Röntgen-Gesellschaft, Stuttgart, 1972. Thieme, Stuttgart
25. Heuck F (1982) Paraneoplastische Osteopathie. In: Diethelm L, Heuck F (eds) Osteopathien. (Handbuch der medizinischen Radiologie, vol 5/5) Springer, Berlin Heidelberg New York
26. Juster M, Crespo I (1979) Estudio microradiografico en la Osteoartropatia hipertrofiante neumica o enfermedad de Pierre Marie-Bamberger. Rev Interam Radiol 4:44–58
27. Karim SMM, Rao B (1976) Prostaglandins and tumors. In: Karim SMM (ed) Prostaglandin: physiological, pharmacological, and pathological aspects. MTP Press, Lancaster
28. Locke E (1915) Secondary hypertrophic osteoarthropathy and its relation to simple clubfingers. Arch Intern Med 15:659–713
29. Marie P (1890) De l'ostéoarthropathie hypertrophiante pneumonique. Rev. Med Interne 10: 1–36
30. Munson PL, Tashjian AH, Levine L (1965) Evidence for parathyroid hormone in nonparathyroid tumors associated with hypercalcemia. Cancer Res 25:1062–1067
31. Oelz O, Knapp HR, Roberts LJ, Oelz R, Sweetman, BJ, Oates JA, Reed PW (1978) Calcium-dependent stimulation of thromboxane and prostaglandin biosynthesis by ionophorese. Adv Prostaglandin Thromboxane Res 3:147–158
32. O'Grady AS, Morse LJ, Lee JB (1965) Parathyroid hormone-secreting renal carcinoma associated with hypercalcemia and metabolic alkalosis. Ann Intern Med 63:858–868
33. Perkins PJ (1978) Delayed onset of secondary hypertrophic osteoarthropathy. Am J Roentgenol 130:561–562
34. Ponchon Y, Chelloul N, Roujeau J (1969) Contribution a l'étude anatomo-pathologique de l'hippocratisme digital. Sem Hop Paris 45:2604–2611
35. Powell D, Singer FR, Murray TM, Minkin C, Potts JT (1973) Nonparathyroid humoral hypercalcemia in patients with neoplastic diseases. New Engl J Med 289:176–181
36. Raisz LG, Koolemans-Beynen AR (1974) Inhibition of bone collagen synthesis by prostaglandin E_2 in organ culture. Prostaglandin 8:374
37. Raisz LG, Mundy GR, Luben RA (1974a) Skeletal reactions to neoplasms. Ann NY Acad Sci 230:473–475
38. Raisz LG, Sandberg AL, Goodson JM, Simmons HA, Mergenhagen SE (1974b) Complement-dependent stimulation of prostaglandin synthesis and bone resorption. Science 185:789–791
39. Rosenthall L, Kirsh J (1976) Observation of radionuclide imaging in hypertrophic pulmonary osteoarthropathy. Radiology 120:359–362
40. Schumacher, R (1976) Articular manifestations of hypertrophic pulmonary osteoarthropathy in bronchogenic carcinoma. Arthrit Rheum 19: 629–636
41. Seyberth HW (1978) Prostaglandin-mediated hypercalcemia: a paraneoplastic syndrome. Klin Wochenschr 56:373–387
42. Steiner H, Dahlbäck O, Waldenström J (1968) Ectopic growth hormone production and osteoarthropathy in carcinoma of the bronchus. Lancet I:783–785
43. Terry DW, Isitman AT, Holmes RA (1975) Radionuclide bone images in hypertrophic pulmonary osteoarthropathy. Am J Roentgenol 124:571–576
44. Thomas C, Windt T, Grom E (1974) Hämatologische und endokrine Formen des paraneoplastischen Syndroms. Schattauer, Stuttgart
45. Wahl AR, Röher, H-D (1973) Pseudohyperparathyreoidismus als paraneoplastisches Syndrom bei einem Fall von Magenkarzinom. Dtsch Med Wschr 98:565–568
46. Wierman WH, Clagett DT, McDonald JR (1954) Articular manifestations in pulmonary diseases. J Am Med Wom Assoc 155:1459–1463

Bone Scanning for the Early-Detection of Metastases

W. Bessler

Radiologisches Institut, Kantonsspital Winterthur, 8401 Winterthur, Switzerland

Skeletal scintigraphy is one of the most frequently performed examinations in nuclear medicine. There are no longer any important differences over technique and procedure. ^{99m}Tc-labeled phosphorus complexes have been used as tracer substances for 11 years and there is general agreement on the indications for bone scanning and on its results. New developments cannot be expected in the near future.

This chapter will give a general view of the practical use of bone scanning, which is still the most important diagnostic tool for the evaluation of the skeleton in cancer patients.

The major *advantages* of skeletal scintigraphy are:

1. The entire skeleton can be examined in one procedure.
2. Bone lesions are visualized with a high degree of sensitivity.
3. Osteogenetic reactions of the skeleton to pathologic processes can be evaluated.

There are also *limits* to the information obtained by bone scanning:

1. It has a low degree of specificity. Bone pathology is documented simply by an increase or a decrease of tracer uptake.
2. There is no visualization of the pathologic process itself.
3. Additional diagnostic examinations are necessary for the interpretation of a bone scan, e.g., radiography, conventional tomography, computed tomography, or bone biopsy.

The *mechanism of the tracer uptake* seems to be determined by the amount of the mineral surface available for interaction with a bone imaging agent, by the blood flow, which influences the supply of the tracer substance, and by the rate of modeling and remodeling of bone. Extraosseous tracer uptake can occasionally be seen in liver metastases of intestinal tumors, in large necrotic breast tumors, in neuroblastomas with calcifications, in fibrothorax after pneumonectomy, in lung calcifications due to primary or secondary hyperparathyroidism, and in lung metastases of osteosarcomas.

The *technique* of bone scanning is standardized. The patient receives 15 mCi[^{99m}Tc]methylenediphosphonate intravenously, and if desired scintigrams can be obtained immediately after injection to study the blood supply of the body and the skeleton. The scans of different parts of the skeleton are performed 4 h after injection, the patient lying supine for one series and prone for another.

To obtain quantitative information, counts per minute can be measured at regions of interest and bone/bone or bone/soft tissue ratios calculated.

Practically every skeletal disease can be an *indication* for bone scanning. It is the method of choice for the detection of bone metastases. At the time of diagnosis of a primary tumor the osseous metastases can still be small and asymptomatic. The high sensitivity of bone scanning enables *early diagnosis.* Malignant tumors can spread to every part of the skeleton, which should therefore be examined in its entirety.

Figure 1 shows the scintigrams and roentgenogram of the left leg of a 74-year-old patient with a lung carcinoma. Prior to the planned pneumonectomy, skeletal scintigraphy demonstrates a local increase of radioactivity in the distal portion of the left femoral shaft. The scintigraphic diagnosis of a metastasis is confirmed by the X-ray examination, which shows a solitary osteolytic lesion. This case is an example of a clinically occult metastasis found by bone scanning and confirmed by roentgenogram. As curative treatment is no longer possible, pneumonectomy is abandoned and radiotherapy of the lung carcinoma and the metastasis initiated.

Figure 2 shows the roentgenograms of the thoracic spine and the skeletal scintigrams of a 82-year-old patient with a 10-month history of pain in the region of the ribs and spine. The alka-

Radiology Today 2. Ed. by F. H. W. Heuck and M. W. Donner

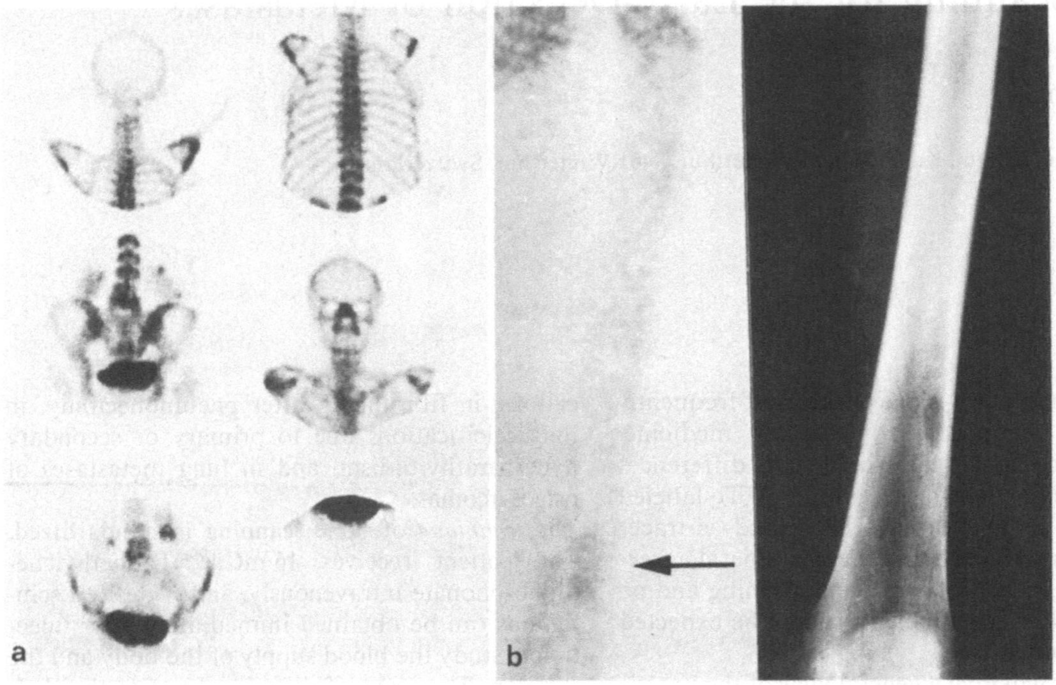

Fig. 1 a, b. A 74-year-old patient with a lung carcinoma and a solitary osteolytic metastasis in the distal portion of the left femoral shaft, detected by bone scanning. **a** Scintigram; **b** roentgenogram

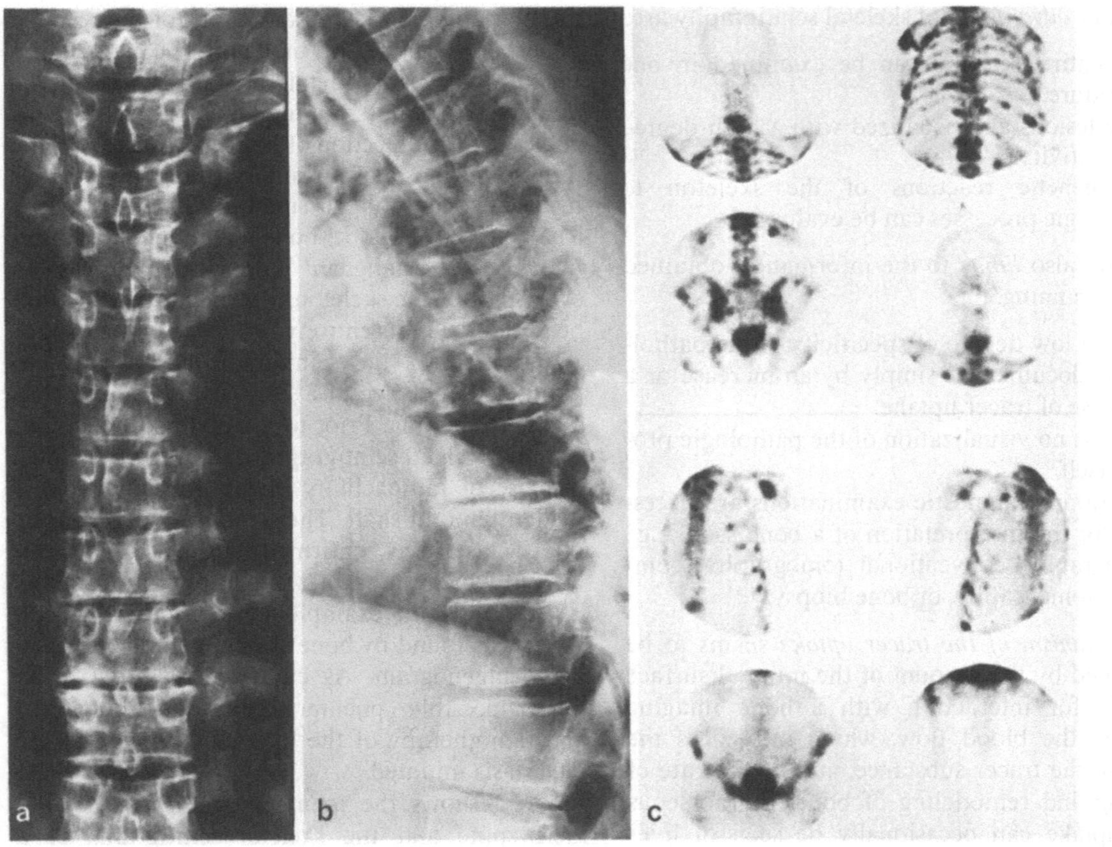

Fig. 2 a–c. An 82-year-old patient with multiple metastases of a prostatic carcinoma. The metastases are only visible on the bone scans (**c**). The roentgenographic examinations of the thoracic spine and of the other parts of the skeleton (**a, b**) are negative

line, acid, and prostate phosphatase activities are elevated. On rectal palpation the prostate is large and indurated. On the roentgenogram of the spine and pelvis only minor degenerative changes can be noted. The bone scan findings are surprising – typical for metastatic involvement of the entire skeleton. The further course of the disease proves the presence of a prostatic carcinoma with multiple osseous metastases. In this case the clinically suspected metastases were proven by bone scanning, having been occult on the roentgenograms.

Skeletal scintigraphy is the best method to check the *effect of treatment* of bone metastases. The amount of osteogenetic reaction around the tumor is in most cases proportional to tumor activity. If tracer uptake decreases to normal values, the metastases have become inactive and a good result has been obtained. Such effects can be noted after radiotherapy as well as after systemic treatment of bone metastases.

Figure 3a shows the bone scans of a 69-year-old patient with multiple metastases of a prostatic carcinoma, located especially in the ribs and the spine. After 7 months of hormonal treatment (Fig. 3b) the bone metastases have partially regressed. The uptake of radioactivity has decreased at the sites of the lesions.

Since the introduction of the computer, there have been attempts to quantify nuclear medical diagnostic results. Ritsema [7] has recently proved that the sensitivity of bone scanning for the detection of metastases cannot be increased by measurements of the whole body retention of nuclide or by the determination of bone to soft tissue count ratios. This seems logical if one considers that the tracer uptake in the skeleton is not specific for tumor involvement and that the scintigraphic diagnosis of bone metastases depends on the type of localization and distribution of focal radioactive deposits.

In the rare cases of diffuse tumorous infiltration of large parts of the skeleton there can be a general increase in tracer uptake. Measurement of counts per minute in regions of interest and the calculation of bone to bone or bone to soft tissue ratios can be the only way of reaching the right diagnosis in such cases.

The roentgenologic and scintigraphic findings in 183 patients with bone metastases proven by biopsy, autopsy, or further clinical course were compared. Ten skeletal regions were examined separately in every patient, and it was found that 405 of the total 1830 regions included metastases. Seventy-one percent of the metastases were found on the roentgenograms, 90% on the scintigrams.

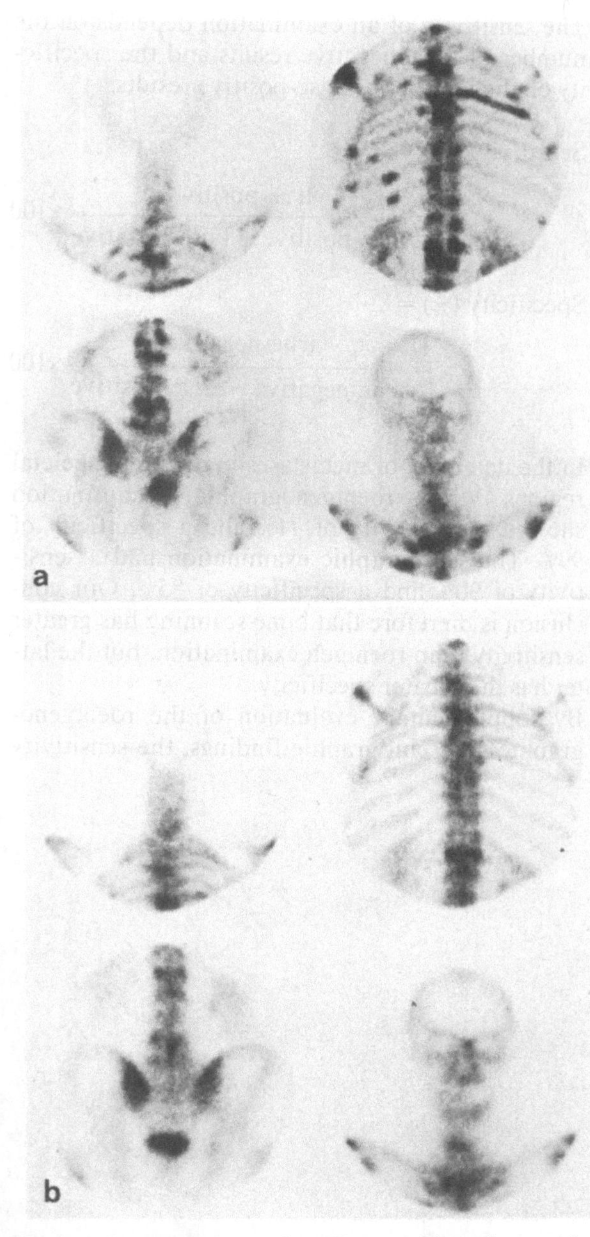

Fig. 3 a, b. Bone scans of a 69-year-old patient with multiple metastases of a prostatic carcinoma before (**a**) and after (**b**) 7 months hormonal treatment. Regression of the metastases under treatment

Of the diseased skeletal regions, 6% of the roentgenographic and 6% of the scintigraphic examinations were equivocal. On roentgenography 23% and on scintigraphy 4% of the metastases were not recognized. At 15 vertebral sites fractures were recognizable; neither by roentgenographic nor by scintigraphic examination was it possible to decide whether these fractures were due to metastases or to osteoporosis. At 195 sites positive scintigraphic findings were caused by degenerative disease.

The sensitivity of an examination depends on the number of false-negative results and the specificity on the number of false-positive results:

$$\text{Sensitivity (\%)} = \frac{\text{true-positive}}{\text{true-positive} + \text{false-negative}} \times 100$$

$$\text{Specificity (\%)} = \frac{\text{true-negative}}{\text{true-negative} + \text{false-positive}} \times 100$$

In the detection of metastases in different skeletal regions the roentgenographic examination showed a sensitivity of 71% and a specificity of 99%. The scintigraphic examination had a sensitivity of 90% and a specificity of 85%. Our conclusion is therefore that bone scanning has greater sensitivity than roentgen examination, but the latter has the greater specificity.

By supplementary evaluation of the roentgenographic and scintigraphic findings, the sensitivity and specificity of the combined examination can be increased to almost 100%.

There is often no or only low osteogenetic reaction in cases of multiple myeloma, reticular cell sarcoma, or leukemia, as well as in some cases of metastasis of thyroid carcinoma, lymphoma, or renal cell carcinoma. Such tumorous processes often cannot be visualized by bone scanning, which thus gives false-negative results.

For multiple myeloma, Waxman et al. [8] found on a patient basis a sensitivity for roentgenograms of 94% and for bone scans of 78%. On a site basis the sensitivity for roentgenograms was 82% and for bone scans only 46%. In spite of these poor results, we think that bone scanning has a role to play in the evaluation of multiple myeloma and should routinely be used.

Figure 4a shows the scintigrams of a 50-year-old patient with multiple myeloma. Myelomatous lesions can be seen in the skull, spine, pelvis, and femoral shafts. The roentgenogram of the pelvis taken at the same time (Fig. 4b) is negative. Only 5 months later (Fig. 4c) can multiple osteolytic myelomatous lesions be seen in the pelvic bones.

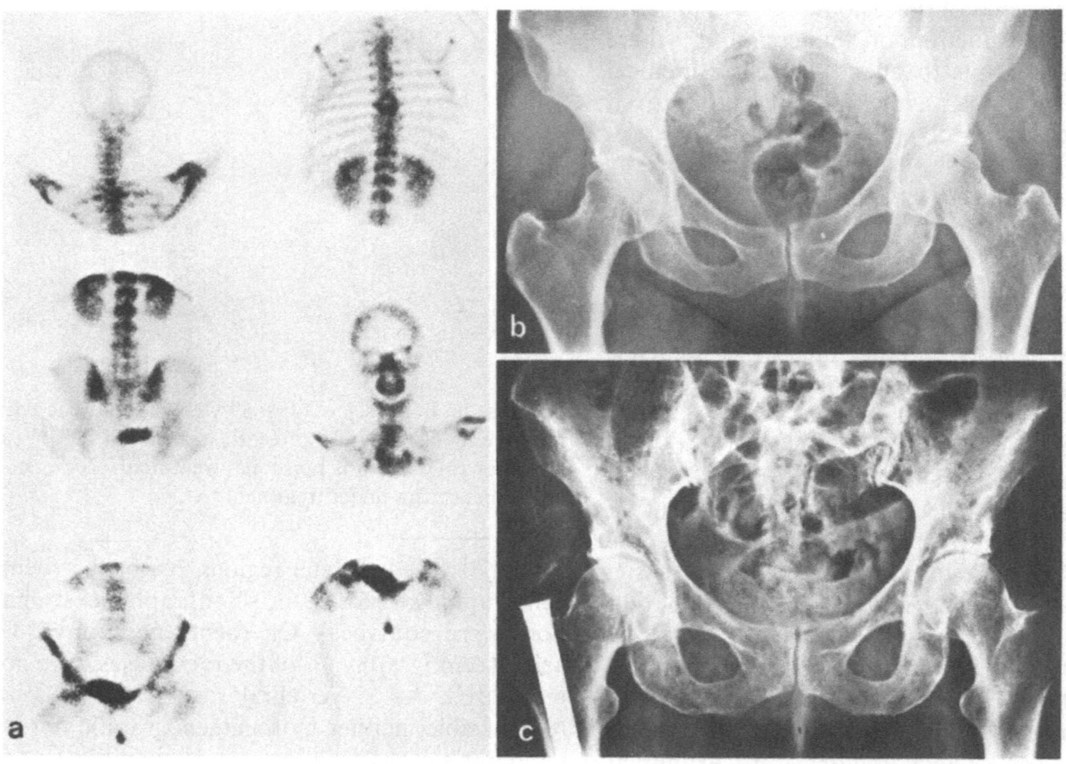

Fig. 4. A 50-year-old patient with multiple myeloma. The bone scan (**a**) reveals multiple lesions in the skull, spine, pelvis, proximal ends of both femora, and right femoral shaft. The roentgenogram of the pelvis at the time of the bone scan (**b**) is negative; the myelomatous involvement of the pelvis and the femoral bones can only be seen on the roentgenograms 5 months later (**c**)

Table 1. Procedure for roentgenographic and scintigraphic evaluation of patients with known or possible bone metastases

Clinical situation	Sequence of examinations	Information
Known → *metastases*	Rg → Sc	Possible additional metastases
Possible metastases		
With local symptoms	Rg+ → Sc...	Possible additional metastases
	RG– → Sc...	Roentgenographically occult metastases
Without local symptoms	Sc–.........	Probably no metastases
	Sc+ → Rg+..	Clinically occult metastases
	Rg– ..	Clinically and roentgenographically occult metastases

Another lesion in the midportion of the right femoral shaft has led to a pathologic fracture, treated with intramedullary nailing.

The indications for bone scanning in the detection of metastases can be summarized as follows:

1. If skeletal metastases are known, bone scanning has to be performed to determine the extent of the metastatic involvement of the skeleton.
2. The effect of local treatment by radiotherapy or systemic treatment can be controlled by scintigraphy.
3. If clinical examination arouses suspicion of metastases, bone scanning should be performed to prove or exclude osseous involvement.
4. For the staging of malignant tumors skeletal scintigraphy is indispensable.

Table 1 outlines the procedure for roentgenographic and scintigraphic evaluation of patients with suspected or proven bone metastases. Known metastases must have their exact location, local appearance, and extent demonstrated by roentgenogram. Skeletal scintigraphy has to be routinely performed to detect possible additional metastases. If metastases are suspected and local symptoms are present, at first a roentgenogram has to be taken. Bone scanning is indicated after a positive roentgenogram to look for additional metastases and after a negative roentgenogram to find possible roentgenographically occult metastases.

In patients without local symptoms skeletal scintigraphy should be performed first. If the result is negative, metastases are probably not present. If the result is positive, roentgenograms must be taken, and if they are also positive it has to be ascertained whether a clinically occult metastasis or another bone disease is the cause of the increased tracer uptake. If the roentgenogram is negative, a clinically and roentgenographically occult metastasis is probably present. This should be checked if possible by local biopsy or bone puncture.

References

1. Bessler W (1977) Bone scanning in breast cancer staging. In: Progress in clinical and biological research. Vol. 12, ed. Montague ACW, Stonesifer GL, Lewison EF, Bessler WT, Handley RS, Siegenthaler P, Witkin E. Liss, New York, pp 303–312
2. Bessler W (1978) Skelettszintigraphie. In: Lehrbuch der Röntgendiagnostik, vol. 2/1, Skelett, ed. Schinz HR, Baensch WE, Frommhold W, Glauner R, Uehlinger E, Wellauer J. Thieme, Stuttgart, pp 279–306
3. Bessler W (1980) Szintigraphie bei Knochentumoren. In: Klinisch-radiologisches Seminar, vol. 10, Knochentumoren, ed. Frommhold W, Gerhardt P. Thieme, Stuttgart, pp 68–78
4. Brady LW, Croll MN (1979) The role of bone scanning in the cancer patient. Skeletal Radiol 3:217–222
5. Genant HK, Bautovich J, Singh M, Lathrop KA, Harper PV (1974) Bone-seeking radionuclides: an in vivo study of factors affecting skeletal uptake. Radiology 113:373–382
6. Khandekar JD (1979) Role of routine bone scans in operable breast cancer: an opposing viewpoint. Cancer Treat Rep 63:1241–1244
7. Ritsema GH (1982) Quantifications and sensitivity in bone scanning in the detection of metastases. Diagn Imaging 51:99–106
8. Waxman AD, Siemsen JK, Levine AM, Holdorf D, Suzuki R, Singer FR, Bateman J (1981) Radiographic and radionuclide imaging in multiple myeloma. The role of gallium scintigraphy: concise communication. J Nucl Med 22:232–236

Quantitative Computed Tomography for Assessment of Metabolic Bone Diseases

H. K. Genant

Department of Radiology, Medicine and Orthopedic Surgery, University of California, San Francisco, CA 94143, USA

The principal application of computed tomography (CT) in metabolic bone disorders is the quantitative assessment of bone mineral content in osteoporosis. Osteoporosis, or atrophy of bone, affects tens of millions of people in the United States, especially postmenopausal women; its complications result in considerable morbidity, mortality, and public health expenditure [35]. Several methods have been employed for quantitative assessment of the skeleton in osteoporosis. The most widely used techniques are radiogrammetry [12] and photon absorptiometry [3] of the peripheral appendicular skeleton. Techniques developed as research tools include dual-photon absorptiometry [21, 28] partial-body [17] and whole-body [10] neutron activation analysis, and Compton scattering [33]. To date, no single method has proved entirely satisfactory in the evaluation of metabolic bone disease.

Due to its ability to provide a quantitative image, CT has been widely investigated in recent years as a means for noninvasive quantitative bone mineral determination [1, 2, 4–9, 11, 13–16, 18, 19, 22–24, 26, 27, 29–32, 24]. Potential advantages of this technique over photon absorptiometry or neutron activation analysis are precise regional localization and spatial separation of cortical and cancellous bone [13]. Approximately 80% by weight of skeletal mineral content is cortical or compact bone, with trabecular or cancellous bone making up the remainder [32]. Trabecular bone, however, has a turnover rate approximately eight times that of compact bone, due to its high surface to volume ratio and to other physiologic factors. This high turnover rate makes trabecular bone more sensitive to metabolic stimuli than compact bone, leading to the observed clinical situation of osteoporotic fractures occurring first in the spine and distal radius, areas of predominantly trabecular bone.

Quantitative computed tomography (QCT) has been shown to measure changes in trabecular mineral content in the radius [11, 18, 22, 29, 30, 31] and the spine [1, 4–6, 9, 14, 15] with great sensitivity and precision. The extraction of this quantitative information from the CT image currently requires sophisticated calibration and positioning techniques [5, 14]. However, rapid technological advances in CT, especially in external localization capabilities, may mean that many of the 5000 advanced CT scanners in the United States may be modified for QCT measurements at relatively little cost [14]. Reductions in patient time, radiation exposure and cost make this an attractive technique for widespread application of noninvasive bone mass measurements.

Scanning Procedures

At the University of California, San Francisco, vertebral mineral content ise measured on a rotary fan-beam scanner (General Electric modified CT/T 7800 or standard CT/T 9800). The standard measuring sites are the midportions of the upper lumbar vertebrae, chosen for several reasons: (a) close correlation between cancellous mineral content in adjacent vertebrae, eliminating the need for a large number of measurement sites; (b) availability of a large measuring volume for cancellous bone to reduce variation from intravertebral inhomogeneities; and (c) avoidance of such sites as the lower lumbar vertebrae where degenerative disease may affect the measurement. During scanning, the patient lies on a crescent-shaped phantom that contains solutions of K_2HPO_4 (mineral equivalent) ethanol (fat), glycerol, and water (soft tissue) for calibration. Two different scanning procedures can be used. In the first, our standard technique (Fig. 1), the patient is positioned using a CT localization system so that the first axial slice is taken at the bottom of T12 and the last at the top of L3. Approximately 18 contiguous, 5-mm-thick slices are obtained

Radiology Today 2. Ed. by F. H. W. Heuck and M. W. Donner

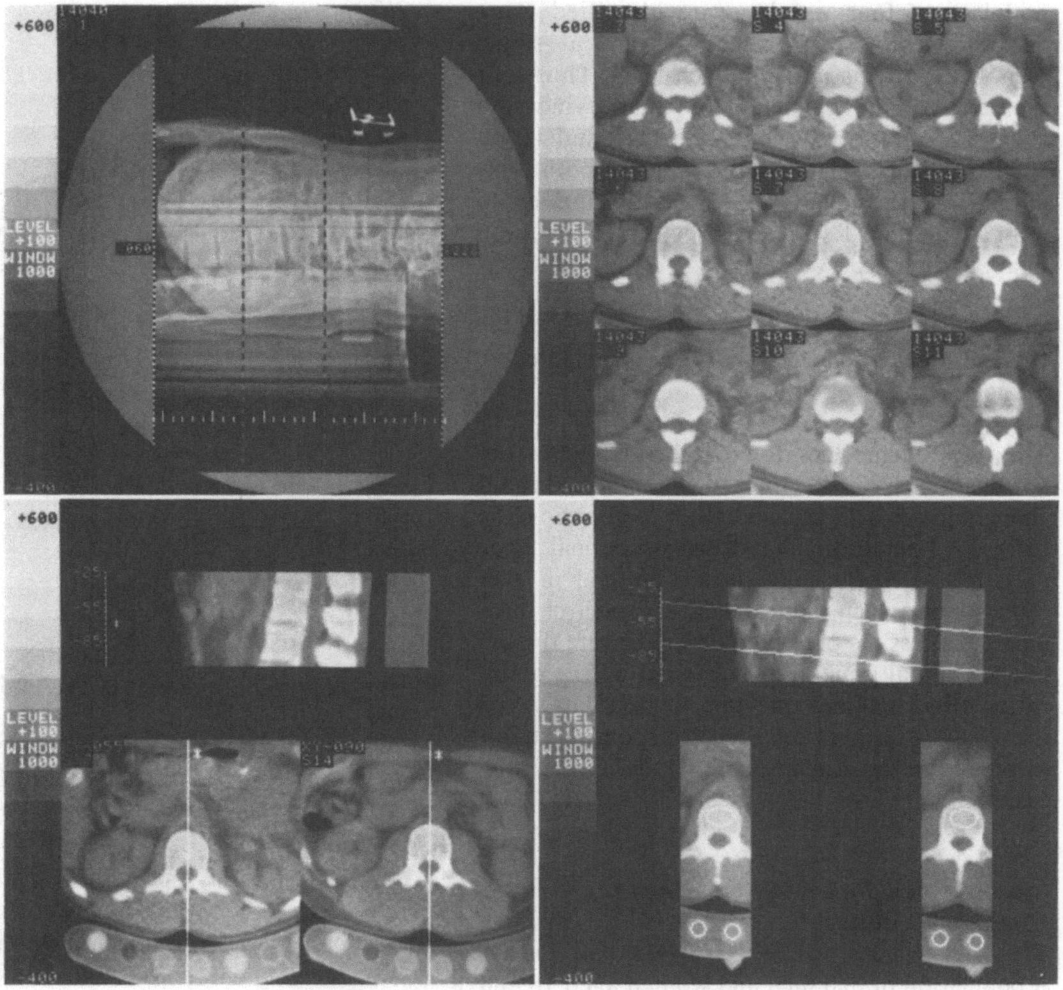

Fig. 1. A lateral computed radiograph (scout view) (*upper left*) provides gross localization to upper lumbar spine. A series of contiguous 5-mm-thick axial sections (*upper right*) are obtained. Using advanced computer software, a sagittal reformatted image (*lower left*) is generated. From the sagittal view, the midplanes of L1 and L2 are defined (*lower right*) and a new, 1-cm-thick synthesized image is generated in the axial plane, centered at the midplane and corrected for angulation. An oval region of interest in the synthesized images is used to determine vertebral mineral content and a circular region of interest is used to quantify the calibration solutions

providing complete coverage of the region of L1 and L2 at 80 kVp. Patient time on the scanner table is 10–15 min, and radiation dose to the region of L1 and L2 is 100–200 mrem [5, 31].

Analysis for mineral content is done by means of a specially programmed off-line computer. Precise positioning to the midplane of L1 and L2 is obtained with advanced image analysis software. The mean CT number in a 4-cm³ volume within each vertebral body is determined using an oval region of interest (Fig. 1) and the CT numbers from the calibration phantom scanned with the patient are used to calculate the mineral equivalent in each vertebra. Mineral content C_b is expressed as milligrams of K_2HPO_4 per cubic centimeter, using the relationship

$$C_b = \frac{H_b - H_w}{H_k - H_w} \times C_k,$$

where H is the CT number and b, k, and w refer to bone, K_2HPO_4, and water. The K_2HPO_4 calibration curve obtained from the phantom is linear in the region used for vertebral mineral determinations. The precision using these techniques is 1.6% (coefficient of variation) for in vivo vertebral mineral determination in human subjects [9].

A second simpler scanning approach also utilizes the computed radiographic system to obtain a lateral scout view of the lumbar spine [14]. The midplane of four vertebrae are identified using cursor-determined coordinates, and a single 1-cm-thick slice is made at each level. Thus four separate volume elements for quantifying and averaging are rapidly obtained. Normalization and expression of data are the same for both techniques, but the latter can be readily applied to most advanced CT scanners, providing a precision of approximately 3%–4%.

Clinical Applications of Quantitative Computed Tomography

The QCT techniques for vertebral mineral determination have been used to study skeletal changes in osteoporosis and other metabolic bone diseases. Longitudinal and cross-sectional bone mass measurements have been obtained in over 1500 patients seen clinically or on research protocols. The results presented here illustrate the use of QCT spinal mineral measurement in the delineation of normal and osteoporotic populations, in the serial assessment of skeletal response to treatment, and in the diagnosis of metabolic bone diseases.

Cross-sectional Studies of Normal and Osteoporotic Subjects

A population of 320 men and women aged 18–80 years was used to define the normal mean and range of vertebral cancellous mineral content for males and females as a function of age. All subjects were ambulatory and had neither a history of chronic debilitating illness or recognized calcium metabolic disorders nor vertebral fractures as assessed by lateral spinal radiographs. This normal population included normal volunteer subjects and Caucasian or Asian patients referred for CT scans of the abdomen or spine in whom the diagnosis was normal [6].

The normal male and female values for vertebral cancellous mineral are shown in Fig. 2 plotted as functions of age by decade. The normal mean value for control males is approximately 175 mg/cm³ over the age range of 20–45 years. The biological variability is 20–30 mg/cm³ or approximately 15% coefficient variation. There is normally a gradual loss of mineral with increasing age, so that by the age of 75 the mineral content is reduced by about 40% or approximately 2–3 standard deviations (SD) below the value in young adult males. The normal premenopausal

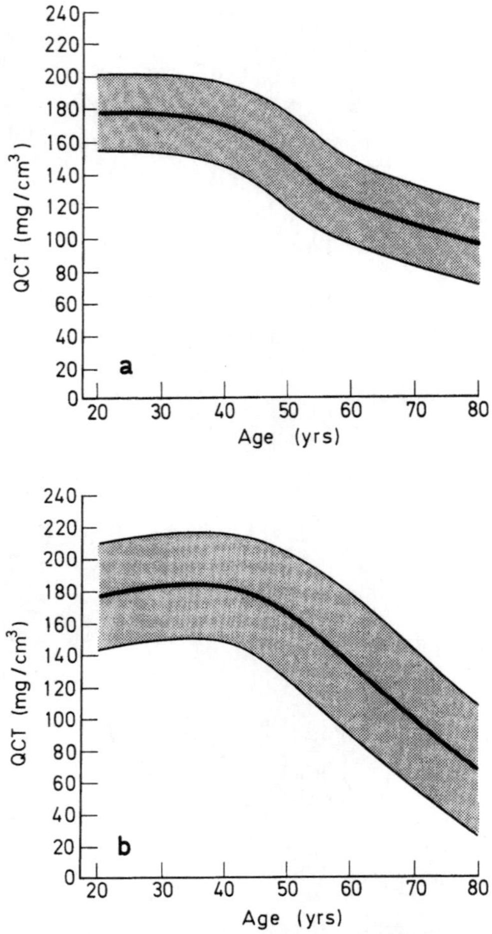

Fig. 2. Normal male (**a**) and female (**b**) values for vertebral cancellous mineral content by QCT (mean ± SD grouped by decade)

female mean for mineral content is also about 175 mg/cm³ over the age range of 20–45 years, with a biological variation of 35–40 mg/cm³, or about 20%. After age 45 or from about the time of menopause the vertebral mineral content decreases, initially rapidly, so that by the age of 75, normal mineral content is reduced by about 55% or approximately 3 SD below the premenopausal mean value.

Fifty-six women with clinically suspected osteopenia or proven osteoporosis were referred for evaluation of vertebral mineral content by QCT [6]. Twenty-two of them had vertebral crush fractures and so fit the clinical defintion of osteoporosis. Patients with osteopenia related to specific metabolic disorders such as Cushing's syndrome, renal osteodystrophy, or osteomalacia were excluded from this grouping. The majority of women referred for osteopenia or osteoporosis had vertebral mineral values by QCT below the age-matched normal mean (Fig. 3). The women with clinical osteoporosis had cancellous mineral values of 28–112 mg/cm³, while only five of 34 patients without fractures fell below 100 mg/cm³, and none below 77 mg/cm³. It appears that a vertebral mineral content of about 100 mg/cm³, or 2 SD below the premenopausal mean, is a significant risk factor for vertebral fracture in osteoporosis. Thus the QCT measurement of spinal cancellous mineral content may be a good predictor of fracture risk for patients with osteopenia in whom osteoporosis is not yet clinically evident.

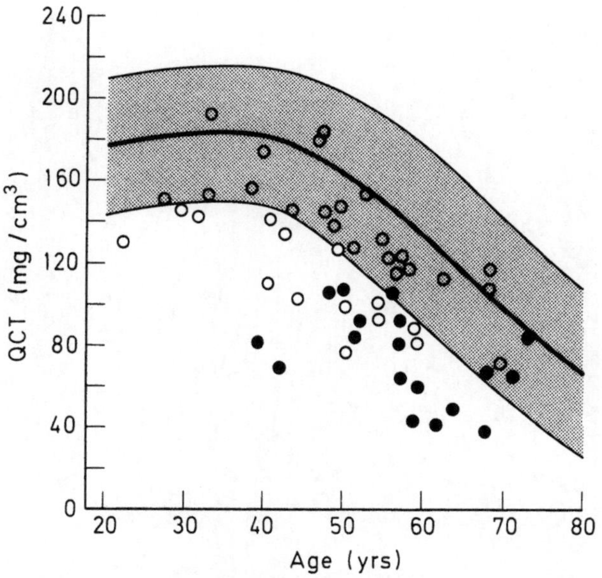

Fig. 3. Vertebral cancellous mineral content (mean ± SD) for women referred for osteopenia or osteoporosis. *Open circles* are osteopenic patients with at least one atraumatic vertebral crush fracture

Longitudinal Studies of Postoophorectomy Bone Loss

A small group of premenopausal women who have recently undergone total hysterectomy and oophorectomy are being studied in a serial fashion to determine bone mineral changes in the axial and peripheral skeleton after loss of ovarian function [1, 9, 14–16]. They have received either a placebo or conjugated estrogens (Premarin) in doses ranging from 0.15 to 0.60 mg/day to determine the minimum osteotrophic dose of estrogen, previous work by Lindsay et al. [20] and Recker et al. [25] having shown that specific higher doses of other estrogen compounds reduce or prevent postmenopausal bone loss.

Bone mineral measurements are made before the commencement of treatment and after 6, 12, 24, and 36 months. In addition to spinal QCT, three separate measures of peripheral cortical bone are made: combined cortical thickness (CCT) of the second metacarpal midshafts [2] and Norland-

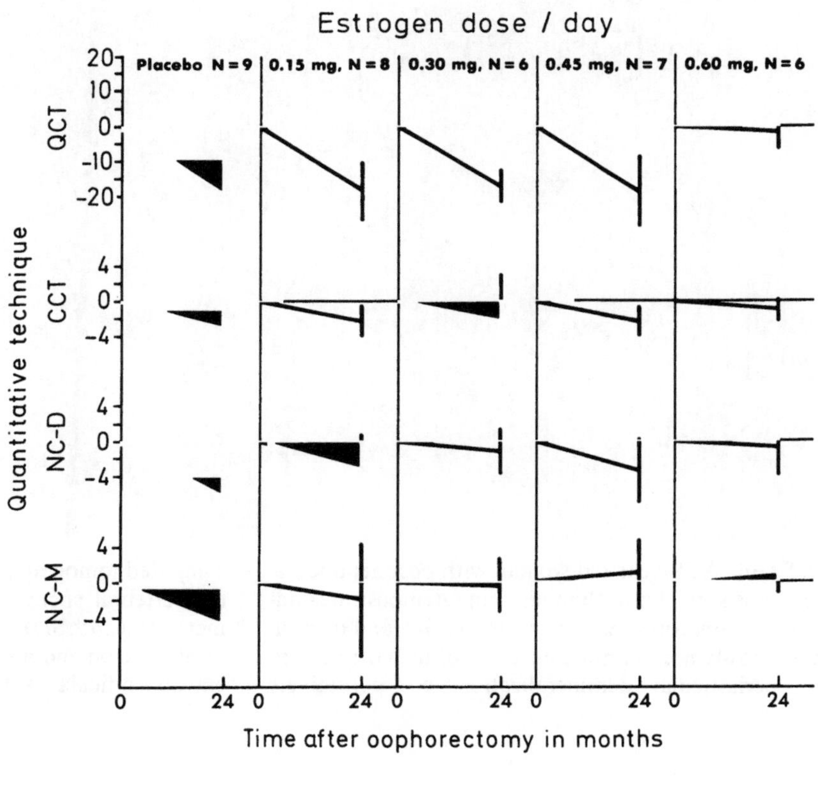

Fig. 4. The mean percentage mineral loss 24 months after oophorectomy in a group of 36 premenopausal women as a function of quantitative technique and estrogen therapy

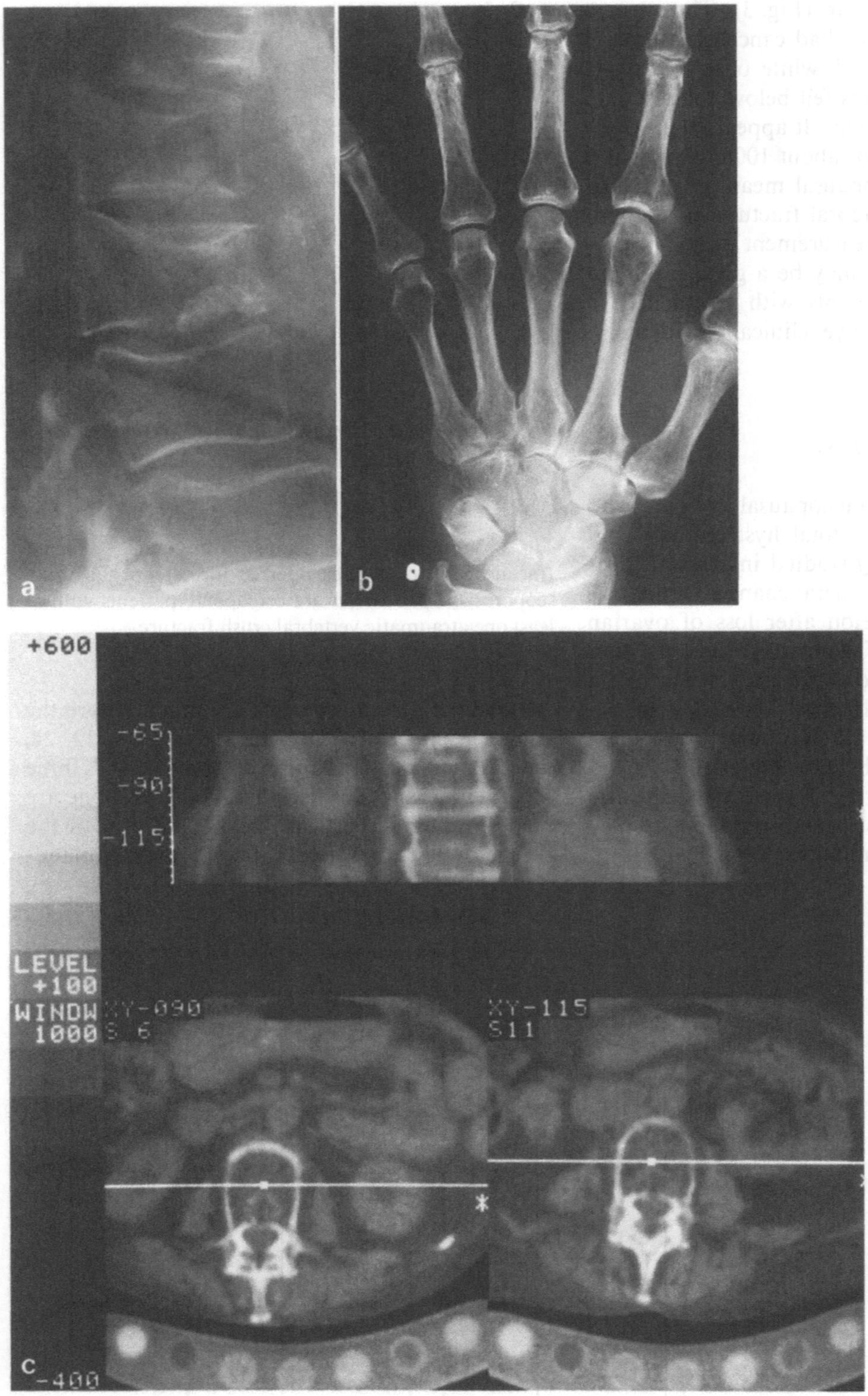

Fig. 5a–d. A 59-year-old woman with postmenopausal osteoporosis. **a** Thoracolumbar spine demonstrates advanced osteoporotic vertebral fractures. **b** Hand demonstrates grossly normal mineralization of the cortices and mild periarticular demineralization. **c** Qualitatively computed tomography demonstrates marked lucency of the vertebral spongiosum. **d** By quantitative measurements (mean ± SD), there is severe osteopenia of the axial skeleton and normal mineralization of the peripheral appendicular skeleton for age and sex

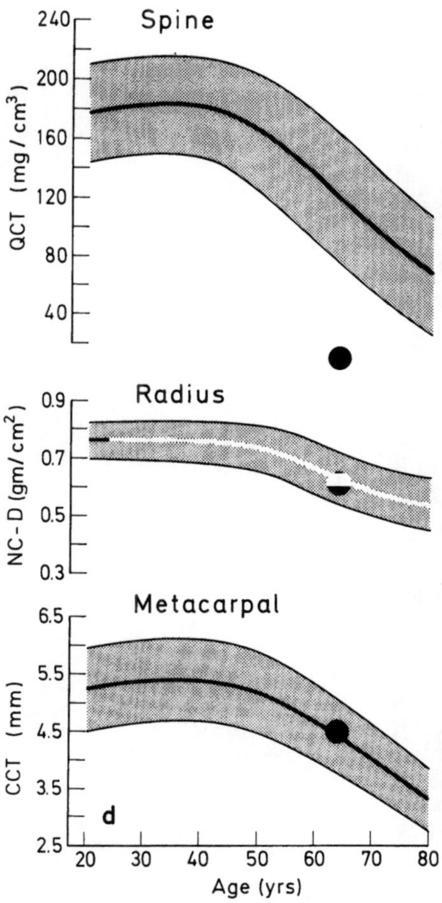

Fig. 5d (Legend see p. 194)

Cameron photon absorptiometry of the radial diaphyses (NC-D) and metaphyses (NC-M). Precision for these measurements at our center is 3% for both CCT and NC-D and 5% for NC-M. Thirty-six subjects have completed at least 2 years of the study protocol, and seven have completed 3 years.

The results at 24 months by the four quantitative techniques are illustrated in Fig. 4. The mean (±SD) cumulative bone mineral losses observed in the 30 subjects receiving *less than* 0.6 mg of conjugated estrogen daily were as follows: QCT, -17.40 ± 9.86 ($P < 0.001$); CCT, -2.44 ± 2.80 ($P < 0.001$); NC-D, -3.86 ± 3.82 ($P < 0.001$); and NC-M, -1.44 ± 5.02 (ns). The magnitude of bone mineral loss observed in the placebo and low-dosage treatment groups were greater by QCT than by any of the standard peripheral appendicular measurements.

The correlation between mean peripheral cortical bone loss and vertebral cancellous bone loss was significant ($r = 0.471$, $P \pm 0.05$) for the group as a whole, but considerable dispersion about the regression line precludes an accurate prediction of spinal loss from peripheral measurements for individual subjects. Furthermore, the slope of the regression line indicates a more than fivefold greater bone mineral loss from the spinal spongiosa than from the appendicular cortex.

The vertebral mineral losses at 24 and 36 months for seven placebo-treated women completing 3 years of study were analyzed. Three of the seven had their treatment changed to 0.6 mg conjugated estrogen daily at 24 months, and not only was further bone loss averted but two of these regained a substantial amount of mineral (± 9.89 and + 9.33%) during the ensuing 12 months. The four subjects remaining on placebo continued to lose vertebral mineral. These results, although preliminary, suggest the ability of QCT to monitor the course of disease and therapeutic response in the individual patient.

Diagnostic Studies in Selected Metabolic Bone Disorders

The clinical results of radiographic and quantitative analyses of the axial and peripheral skeleton in a number of common metabolic bone disorders are illustrated in Figs. 5–7. Examples are given of postmenopausal osteoporosis, Cushing's syndrome, and renal osteodystrophy. The necessity of measuring at several skeletal sites to detect or monitor disease is underscored by the poor correlation between spinal trabecular and peripheral cortical bone mass in some patients. For example, in the relatively common disorder of postmenopausal osteoporosis (Fig. 5), it is not uncommon to observe marked demineralization of the axial skeleton while the peripheral skeleton remains normal for age and sex. Similarly, disproportionate loss of cancellous compared to cortical bone in response to an excess of corticosteroids (Fig. 6) is reflected by the large reduction in vertebral mineral compared to appendicular cortical mineral. Conversely, marked demineralization of the peripheral cortex in renal osteodystrophy (Fig. 7) may be accompanied by sclerosis of the vertebral cancellous bone, producing a rugger-jersey spine. It may be concluded that measurements of peripheral *and* axial as well as compact *and* cancellous bone provide the best overall assessment of skeletal status in many metabolic bone disorders.

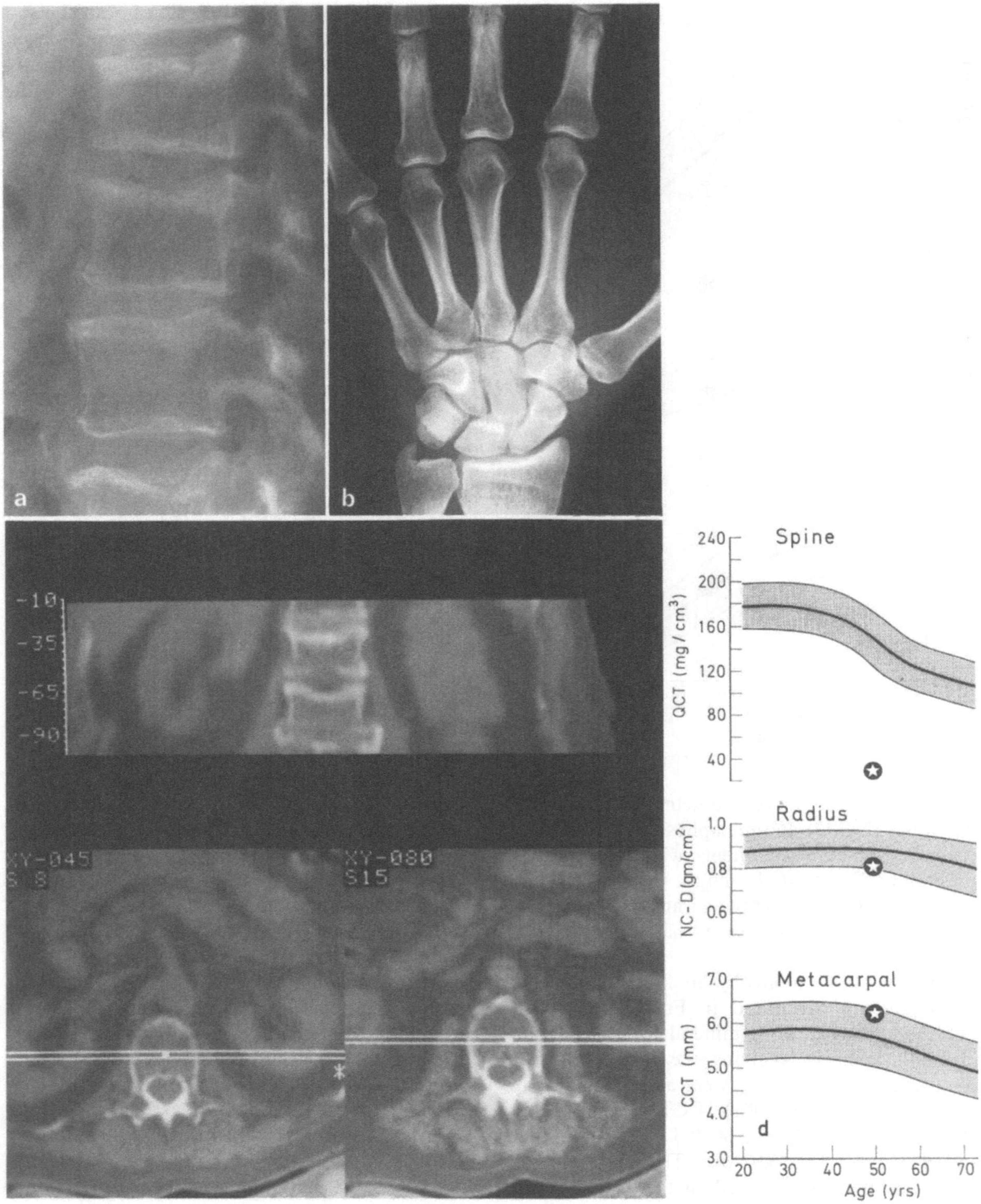

Fig. 6a–d. A 50-year-old man with Cushing's disease. **a** Lateral lumbar spine demonstrates marked osteoporosis with vertebral collapse and marginal condensation of the endplates. **a** Hand demonstrates normal mineralization of the cortices. **c** (*lower left*) Computed tomography qualitatively demonstrates lucency of the spongiosum and increased intra- and retroperitoneal fat. **d** By quantitative measurements (mean ± SD), there is severe osteopenia of the axial skeleton and normal mineralization of the peripheral appendicular skeleton

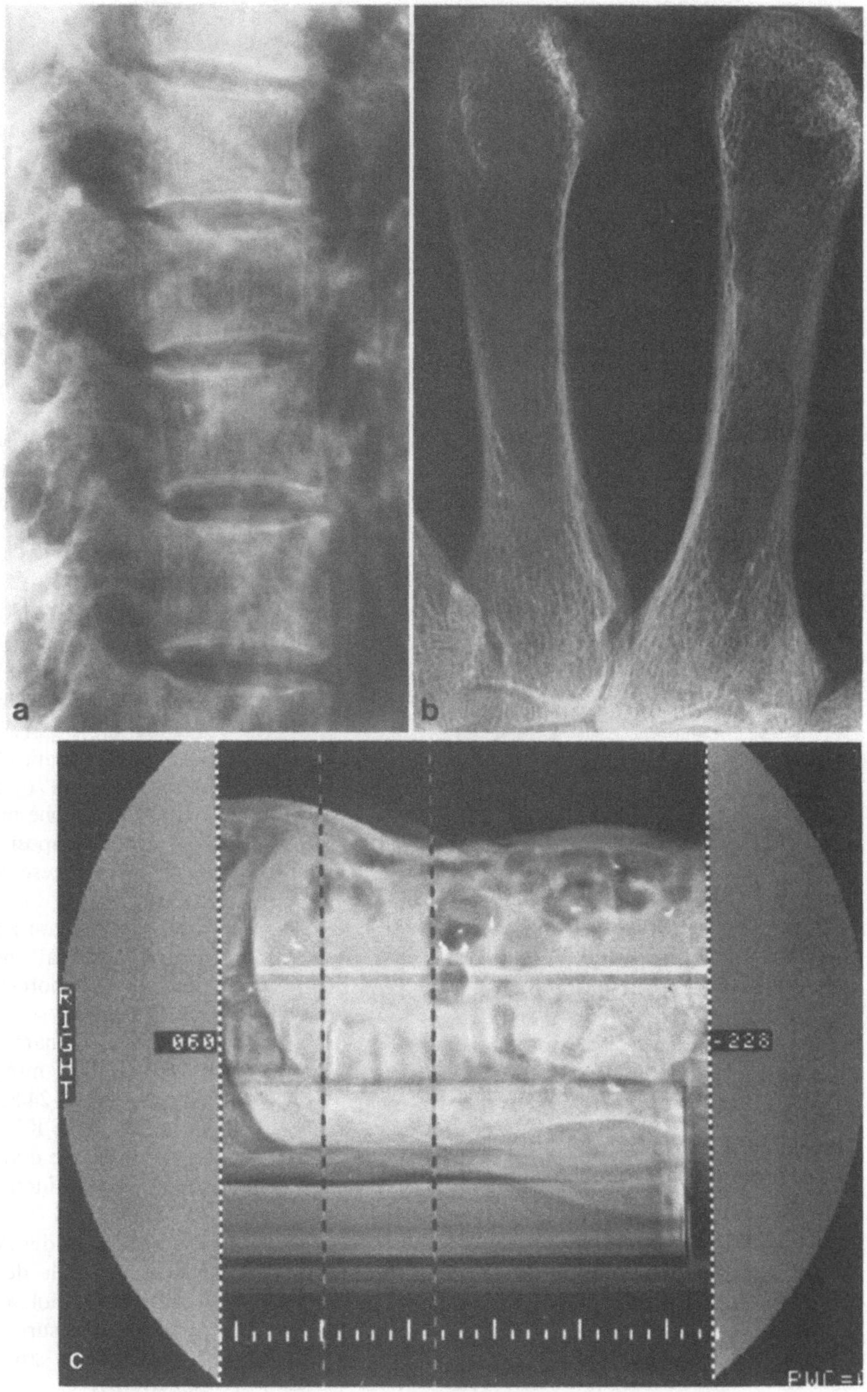

Fig. 7a–d. A 69-year-old woman with renal osteodystrophy. **a** Magnification radiograph demonstrates severe demineralization of the metacarpals accompanied by increased intracortical bone resorption. **b** Thoracic spine demonstrates mild osteosclerosis of the spongiosum. **c** Lateral scout view demonstrates irregular bands of sclerosis in the thoracolumbar spine (rugger-jersey spine). **d** (see p. 198)

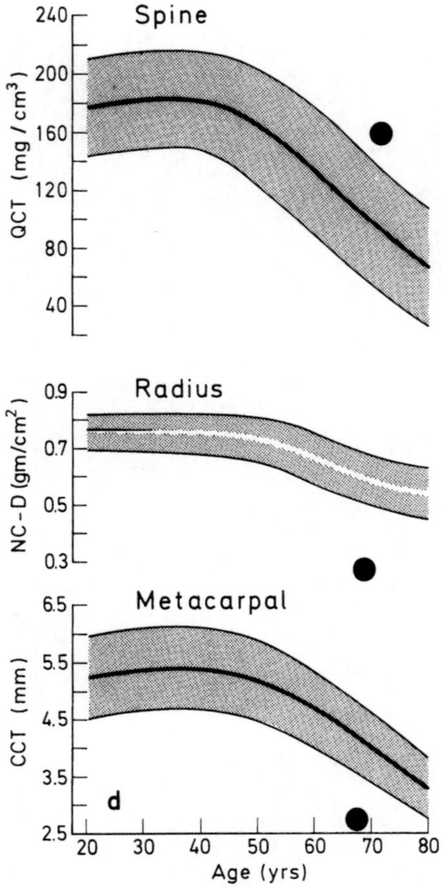

Fig. 7. d By quantitative measurements (mean ± SD), there is increased mineralization of the axial skeleton and severe demineralization of the peripheral appendicular skeleton

Conclusion

The greatest advantage of spinal QCT for noninvasive bone mineral measurement lies in the high precision of the technique and the high sensitivity of the vertebral spongiosa measurement site. The clinical results presented here suggest that QCT provides the clinician with a powerful tool for evaluating and monitoring the many forms of osteoporosis and its various treatments.

Acknowledgments. Partial support for this work was provided by NIH grant AM27926, NASA Contract NAS9-15887, and by Ayerst Laboratories. Assistance in preparation of the manuscript was provided by Mrs. Denice Nakano.

References

1. Abols Y, Genant HK, Rosenfeld D, Boyd DP, Ettinger B, Gordan GS (1980) Spinal bone mineral determination using computerized tomography in patients, controls and phantoms. In: Mazess RB (ed) Proceedings of the 4th international conference on bone measurement. US Government Printing Office, Washington (NIH Publication 80–1938, pp 297–308
2. Bradley JG, Huang HK, Ledley RS (1978) Evaluation of calcium concentration in bones from CT scans. Radiology 128:103–107
3. Cameron JR, Mazess RB, Sorenson JA (1968) Precision and accuracy of bone mineral determination by the direct photon absorptiometric method. Invest Radiol 3:141–150
4. Cann CE (1981) Low-dose CT scanning for quantitative spinal mineral analysis. Radiology 140:813–815
5. Cann CE, Genant HK (1980) Precise measurement of vertebral mineral content using computed tomography. J Comput Assist Tomogr 4:493–500
6. Cann CE, Genant HK (1982) Cross-sectional studies in vertebral mineral content. J Comput Assist Tomogr 6:216–217
7. Cann CE, Genant HK (to be published) Models of immobilization osteoporosis and applications of quantitative bone mass measurements. In: Proceedings of the symposium of models and techniques in radiological research, Tucson/Arizona, March 29–30, 1980
8. Cann CE, Genant HK, Young DR (1980) Comparison of vertebral and peripheral mineral losses in disuse osteoporosis in monkeys. Radiology 134:524–529
9. Cann CE, Genant HK, Ettinger B, Gordan GS (1980) Spinal mineral loss in oophorectomized women. JAMA 244:2056–2059
10. Cohn SH, Ellis KJ, Wallach S, et al. (1974) Absolute and relative deficit in total skeletal calcium and radial bone mineral in osteoporosis. J Nucl Med 15:428–435
11. Exner GH, Prader A, Elsasser U, Anliker M (1980) Effects of high dose oestrogen and testosterone treatment in adolescents upon trabecular and compact bone measured by ^{125}I computed tomography. A preliminary study. Acta Endocrinol (Copenh) 94:126–131
12. Garn SM (1970) The earlier gain and later loss of cortical bone. In: Nutritional perspective. Thomas, Springfield, p 146
13. Genant HK, Boyd DP (1977) Quantitative bone mineral analysis using dual-energy computed tomography. Invest Radiol 12:545–551

14. Genant HK, Cann CE (1981) Vertebral mineral determination using quantitative computed tomography. In: DeLuca HF, Frost HM, Jee WSS, Johnston CC, Parfitt AM (eds) Osteoporosis: Recent advances in pathogenesis and treatment. University Park Press, Baltimore, pp 37–47
15. Genant HK, Cann CE, Ettinger B, Gorden GS (1982) Determination of bone mineral loss in the axial and appendicular skeleton of oophorectomized women (Abstr). J Comput Assist Tomogr 6:217–218
16. Genant HK, Cann CE, Ettinger B, Gordan GS (to be published) Quantitative computed tomography of vertebral spongiosa: a sensitive method for detecting early bone loss after oophorectomy. Lancet
17. Harrison JE, McNeill KG, Meema S, et al. (1974) Partial body calcium measurement by *in vivo* neutron activation analysis. J Nucl Med 15:929–934
18. Jensen PS, Orphanoudakis SC, Baron R, Lang R, Rauschkolb EN, Rasmussen H (1979) Determination of bone mass by CT and correlation with quantitative histomorphometric analysis. J Comput Assist Tomogr3:847
19. Laval-Jeantet M, Laval-Jeantet AM, Lamerque JL, Demoulin B (1979) Evaluation de la minéralisation osseuse vertebrale par tomographie computerisée. J Radiol 60:87–93
20. Lindsay R, Hart DM, Aitkin JM, et al. (1976) Long-term prevention of postmenopausal osteoporosis by oestrogen. Lancet 1:1038–1041
21. Madsen M, Peppler W, Mazess RB (1975) Vertebral and total body bone mineral content by dual photon absorptiometry. Proceedings of XI European Symposium on Calcified Tissues, 1975
22. Orphanoudakis SC, Jensen PS, Rauschkolb EN, Lang R, Rasmussen H (1979) Bone mineral analysis using single energy computed tomography. Invest Radiol 14:122–130
23. Posner I, Griffiths HJ (1977) Comparison of CT scanning with photon absorptiometric measurement of bone mineral content in the appendicular skeleton. Invest Radiol 12:524–544
24. Pullan BR, Roberts TE (1978) Bone mineral measurement using an EMI scanner and standard methods: a comparative study. Br J Radiol 51:24–28
25. Recker RR, Saville PD, Heaney RP (1977) Effect of estrogens and calcium carbonate on bone loss in postmenopausal women. Ann Intern Med 87:649–755
26. Reich NE, Seidelmann FE, Tubbs RR, MacIntyre WJ, Meaney TF, Alfidi RJ, RG: Determination of bone mineral content using CT scanning. AJR 127:593–594
27. Revak CS (1980) Mineral content of cortical bone measured by computed tomography. J Comput Assist Tomogr 4:342–351
28. Roos B, Rosengren B, Skoldborn H (1979) Determination of bone mineral content in lumbar vertebrae by a double gamma-ray technique. In: Cameron JR (ed) Proceedings of bone measurement conference. USAEC Conf. 700515, pp 243–254
29. Ruegsegger P, Elsasser U, Anliker M, et al. (1976) Quantification of bone mineralization using computed tomography. Radiology 121:93–97
30. Ruegsegger P, Anliker M, Dambacker M (1981) Quantification of trabecular bone with low dose computed tomography. J Comput Assist Tomogr 5:384–390
31. Schneider VS, Hinderling T, Vogel JM, Rambaut R (1979) CT ^{125}I gamma-ray densitometry (CT scanner): noninvasive measurement of trabecular bone mineral. J Comput Assist Tomogr 3:847–848
32. Synder W (1975) Report of the task group on reference man. ICRP23, Pergamon, Oxford
33. Webber CE, Kennett KJ (1976) Bone density measured by Compton photon scattering. I. A system for clinical use. Phys Med Biol 21:760–769
34. Weissberger MA, Zamenhof RG, Aronow S, Neer RM (1978) Computed tomography for the measurement of bone mineral in the human spine. J Comput Assist Tomogr 2:253–262
35. Whedon GD (1981) Osteoporosis. N Engl J Med 305:397–399

Value of Different Imaging Modalities in Peripheral Soft Tissue Tumors

P. E. Peters and G. Friedmann

Institut für Klinische Radiologie, Westfälische Wilhelms-Universität, Albert-Schweitzer-Strasse 33, 4400 Münster, FRG

The somatic soft tissues are defined as the mesodermal tissues excluding skeleton, viscera, and skin [13]. According to a WHO proposal, they can be further divided into *internal* (mediastinum, mesentery, retroperitoneum, orbitas) and *peripheral* soft tissues [2]. This chapter will discuss only tumors of the peripheral soft tissue, including the abdominal and thoracic wall, with special emphasis on malignant neoplastic lesions.

Soft tissue tumors and tumor-like lesions can arise from fibrous, adipose, or tendosynovial tissue, from muscle, vessels, or peripheral nerves. In addition, there are rare extraskeletal bone tumors and miscellaneous soft tissue tumors (see classification of soft tissue tumors according to Hajdu [11], Table 1).

The exact incidence of soft tissue tumors is unknown. While benign neoplastic lesions such as lipoma and fibroma are very common, malignant soft tissue tumors are estimated to represent only 1% of all malignancies [14]. The responsibility of the diagnostic radiologist in patients with soft tissue tumors is the definition of the *location*, *nature*, and *extent* of the disease. The applicable imaging modalities include conventional radiography and xeroradiography, ultrasonography (US), computed tomography (CT), and arteriography.

Our own experience is based upon comparative studies of different imaging modalities in 67 patients with malignant peripheral soft tissue tumors. In addition, three patients with soft tissue metastases and 20 patients with various benign tumors and tumor-like lesions were included in the study (see Table 2).

* We wish to acknowledge the valuable contributions made by Prof. Dr. R. Fischer (Dept. of Pathology), PD Dr. F. Ghussen (Dept. of Surgery), and PD Dr. D. Beyer (Dept. of Radiology). We are particularly indebted to Mrs. M. Bischofsberger, R. T., for her skillfull work in the CT laboratory and to Mrs. G. Schade who prepared the illustrations

Radiology Today 2. Ed. by F. H. W. Heuck and M. W. Donner

Conventional Radiography and Xeroradiography

Conventional radiography using the low-kVp technique will detect soft tissue masses only if there are marked attenuation differences or if the lesion is large enough to deform adjacent fascial fat planes. Such attenuation differences are present in tumors containing fat and/or calcifications (Fig. 1).

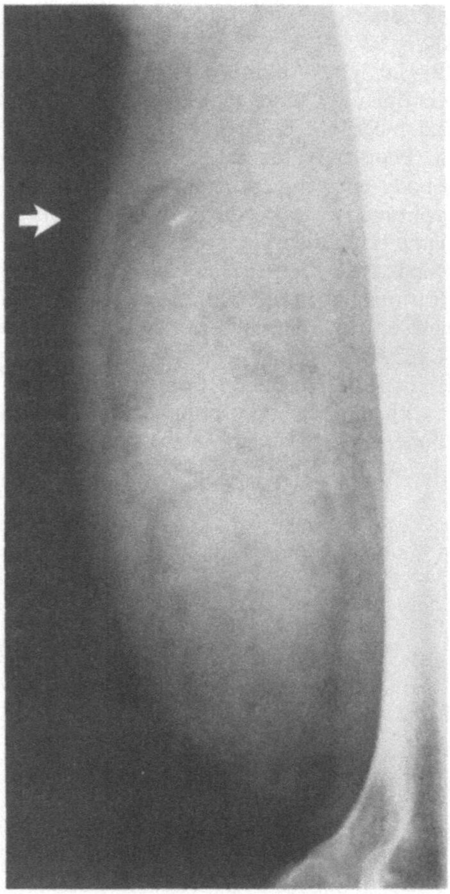

Fig. 1. *Liposarcoma* of the dorsal thigh with small calcifications of the upper pole (→). Conventional radiogram with low-kVp technique

Table 1. Classification of soft tissue tumors and tumor-like lesions (abridged from Hajdu [11])

Site	Non-neoplastic lesions	Benign neoplastic lesions	Malignant neoplastic lesions
Fibrous tissue	Fasciitis Keloid Fibromatosis	Benign fibrous histiocytoma (fibroblastic, histiocytic, pleomorphic) Fibroma	Malignant fibrous histiocytoma (fibroblastic, histiocytic, pleomorphic) Desmoid tumor (agressive fibromatosis) Fibrosarcoma
Tendosynovial tissue	Tendosynovial cyst Tendosynovitis Synovial chondromatosis	Fibroma Lipoma Villonodular synovitis	Tendosynovial sarcoma Clear cell sarcoma Malignant giant cell tumor
Adipose tissue	Lipogranuloma Adiposis dolorosa Steatopygia	Lipoma Angiolipoma Angiomyolipoma	Liposarcoma (well-differentiated, myxoid, lipoblastic, fibroblastic, pleomorphic)
Muscle	Atrophy Dystrophy Myositis ossificans	Leiomyoma Angiomyolipoma Rhabdomyoma	Leiomyosarcoma Leiomyoblastoma Rhabdomyosarcoma (embryonal, pleomorphic) Rhabdomyoblastoma
Vessels	Arteriovenous fistula Hereditary hemorrhagic teleangiectasia	Hemangioma Glomus tumor Lymphangioma Lymphangiomyoma	Hemangiopericytoma Hemangiosarcoma Kaposi's sarcoma Lymphangiosarcoma
Peripheral nerve	Traumatic neuroma Degeneration Hypertrophy	Neurofibroma Neurofibromatosis Benign schwannoma	Malignant schwannoma (neurogenic sarcoma)
Extraskeletal bone tumors	Chondroid metaplasia Osteoid metaplasia	Chondroma Osteochondroma Osteoma	Osteogenic sarcoma Chondrosarcoma Ewing's sarcoma
Miscellaneous soft tissue tumors		Benign mesenchymoma Benign granular cell tumor	Malignant mesenchymoma Malignant granular cell tumor Alveolar soft tissue sarcoma Undifferentiated soft tissue sarcoma Postirradiation sarcoma

Nonspecific calcifications have been observed in synovial sarcoma (30%), liposarcoma (15%), and malignant fibrous histiocytoma (10–15%) [20]. Ring-like or "popcorn" calcifications within the soft tissues may suggest extraskeletal chondrosarcoma, while amorphous calcifications seem to be more common in extraskeletal osteosarcoma [7]. Metaplastic bone and cartilage formation has recently been reported as a new radiological sign in malignant fibrous histiocytoma of soft tissue [5].

The single most important feature of conventional radiography is its ability to demonstrate *bone involvement* in a suspected soft tissue mass. It may be very difficult to differentiate primary soft tissue tumors with osseous invasion from bone tumors extending into the soft tissues. Certain soft tissue tumors, e.g., rhabdomyosarcoma and malignant fibrous histiocytoma, are known to metastasize frequently to the skeleton [22]. However, cortical thickening might also reflect benign hyperostosis reactive to the overlying soft tissue tumor [24].

Since it is more important to visualize the bones adequately, we use the *bone technique* for conventional radiography when peripheral soft tissue tumors are suspected.

Our own experience with *xeroradiography* in soft tissue tumors is limited. Campani et al. (Radio-

Table 2. Soft tissue tumors and tumor-like lesions: own material

Site	Non-neoplastic lesions	Benign neoplastic lesions	Malignant neoplastic lesions
Fibrous tissue	–	–	18
Tendosynovial tissue	2	–	3
Adipose tissue	–	4	9
Muscle	–	1	10
Vessels	1	3	8
Peripheral nerve	–	3	5
Extraskeletal bone tumors	–	–	5
Miscellaneous soft tissue tumors	6	–	9
Soft tissue metastases	–	–	3
Total	9	11	70

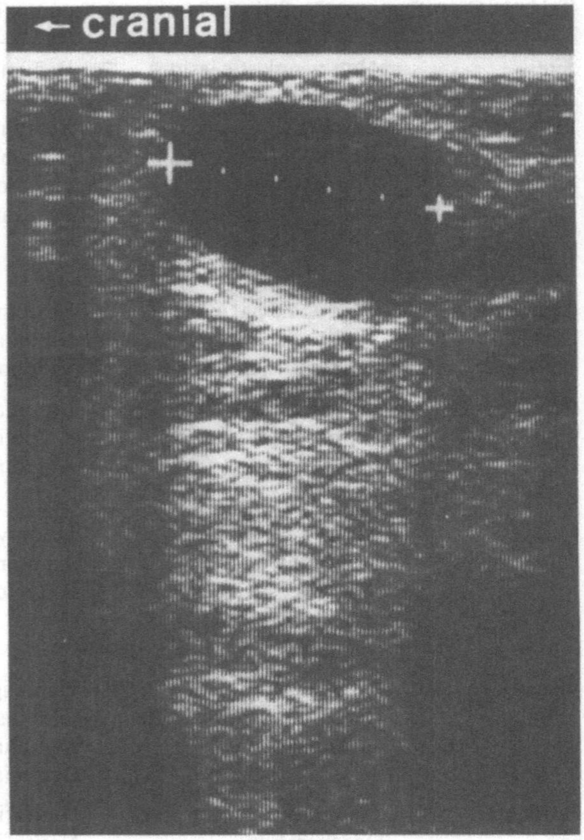

Fig. 2. *Malignant fibrous histiocytoma* of the right dorsal thigh. Real-time US (3-MHz probe). Echo-poor lesion with increased through transmission

logical Approach to Soft Tissue Masses, this volume p. 213) discuss its potential in more detail. The edge enhancement of this radiographic modality allows better analysis of the fascial planes and the boundaries of the tumor. These data, however, can also be obtained by US and CT, so there is no obvious reason to invest in special xeroradiographic equipment if these widely applicable imaging modalities are available. In a recent comparative study, Bernardino et al. [1] came to the same conclusion.

Ultrasonography

Ultrasonography can detect soft tissue lesions either by differences in acoustic impedance between the mass and the surrounding normal tissue or by gross anatomical distortion (displacement of normal fat planes). Depending upon the internal consistency of the lesion, the image may be *cystic* (echo-free with increased through transmission), *solid* (echogenic), or show a *complex* or *mixed* echo pattern. Most soft tissue tumors are less echogenic than the surrounding muscle and connective tissue, exception of fatty tumors, which are highly echogenic (Figs. 2, 3).

US may be performed as a *static* (compound technique) or *dynamic* (real-time) investigation. Each has its advantages and drawbacks. With new computerized real-time devices featuring exchangeable probes ranging from 3.5 to 10.0 MHz, the spatial resolution is as good as in the best compound machines. The relationship of a soft tissue mass lesion to the vascular bundle can better be studied by real-time US, while compound images offer the advantage of large-scale cross-sectional images which are better reproducible.

At our institution preference is given to dynamic real-time US. Every patient with a soft tissue mass which cannot be diagnosed by palpation and clinical findings is taken to the sonographic laboratory for a rapid study, possibly including US-guided puncture. The latter applies mainly to cystic lesions such as hematomas, seromas, or lymphoceles presenting as soft tissue masses.

Fine-needle biopsy of solid soft tissue tumors is only performed when surgical removal is difficult or impossible. The tremendous problems of histological calssification of soft tissue tumors mean

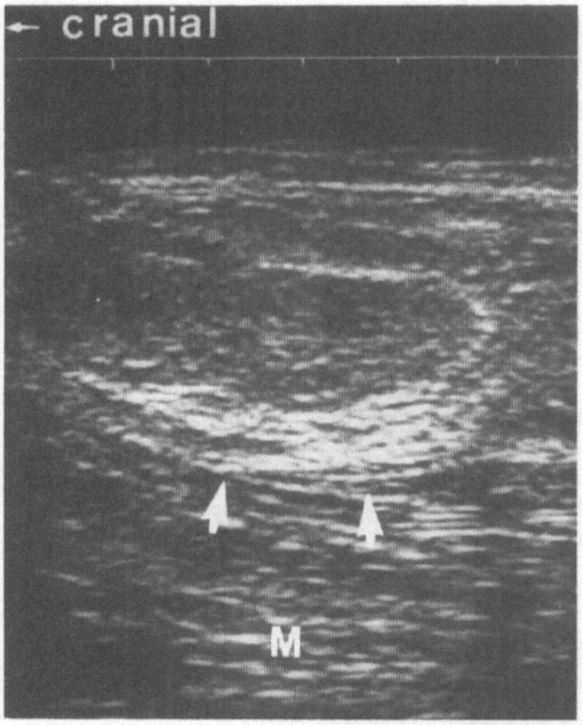

Fig. 3. *Lipoma* of the thigh. Real-time US (5-MHz probe). Highly echogenic mass with capsule formation (→). *M*, underlying muscle

that it is extremely difficult to secure a reliable diagnosis from minute needle biopsy sample.

Real-time US has the advantage of imaging the soft tissue tumor in the most appropriate direction and perpendicular to it. Since there is no geometric distortion, *size*, *shape*, and *location* of the mass can be determined exactly.

We cannot confirm that the absence of an acoustic interface indicates invasion of the adjacent fascial planes [20]. In our experience, US findings are entirely *nonspecific*. Even a malignant soft tissue tumor may present as an echo-poor lesion with increased through transmission, resembling a hematoma with clotted material [9].

However, once the nature of the lesion is known, US is the best, easiest, and certainly the most economical imaging modality for follow-up studies after chemotherapy or radiation therapy [1, 20].

Computed Tomography

Detection of soft tissue tumors with CT is by density differences between the lesion and the surrounding normal tissues and by gross anatomical distortion. In most cases valuable additional information may be obtained after contrast enhancement.

In accordance with most reports from the literature, *location* and *extent* of benign and malignant soft tissue neoplasms could be determined exactly in all our cases [12, 17, 27]. Egund et al. [6] missed one tumor, which turned out to be a 12-mm fibrosarcoma, in 36 investigated mass lesions. Grabbe et al. [10], using a translate-rotate scanner, failed to detect two of 50 malignant soft tissue tumors. Bernardino et al. [1] found determination of lesion length to be less accurate by CT than by US.

In general, however, most authors agree that CT is well suited for determining the extent of a peripheral soft tissue tumor as well as the involvement of adjacent structures, including bone. The tumor margins and the presence of calcifications or low-density necrotic areas could be outlined better by CT than by any other imaging modality [18, 19, 25, 30].

On the other hand, the contribution of CT to clarifying the *nature* of a given soft tissue mass remains very small. Levine et al. [19] found CT useful in establishing the primary diagnosis of soft tissue tumor in two of 15 cases (13%). Even in liposarcoma, which offers rather impressive CT findings, a specific CT diagnosis was only possible in four of 17 cases (22%) [26].

There are three major radiological signs in CT which can help in assessing the nature of a lesion:

1. Density difference
2. Signs of invasive growth
3. Contrast enhancement

The importance of these signs will now be discussed using tumors of the adipose tissue as an example.

Density Difference

The most striking density differences are undoubtedly present in tumors of adipose tissue. *Lipomas* are among the most common benign soft tissue neoplasms. They are usually solitary but occasional cases of multiple lipomas are encountered. Located deep within the limb, they may grow within muscles (*intramuscular* type) or between muscles (*intermuscular* type) [15]. On CT the simple lipoma presents as a homogenous, sharply demarcated, low-density mass with attenuation values in the range of −100 HU (Fig. 4). The *infiltrating-type lipoma* reveals projections of fatty tissue into adjacent structures.

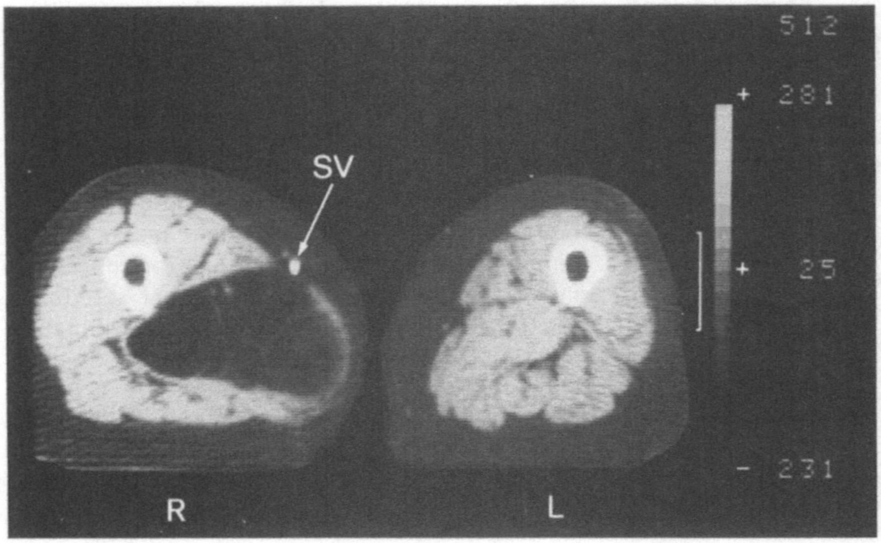

Fig. 4. *Intramuscular lipoma* of the right thigh. CT after injection of contrast medium at the dorsum of the right foot. Hypodense, well-defined lesion within the great adductor muscle. →, enhanced saphenous vein (*SV*)

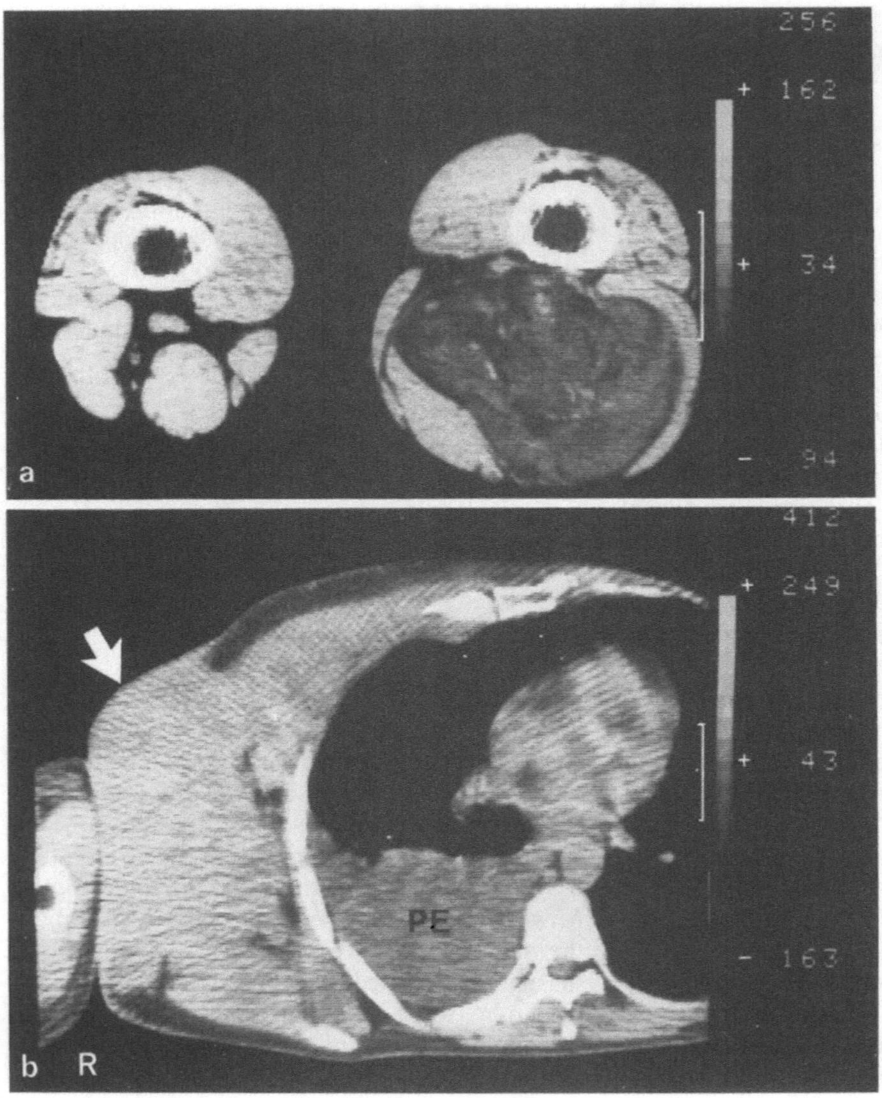

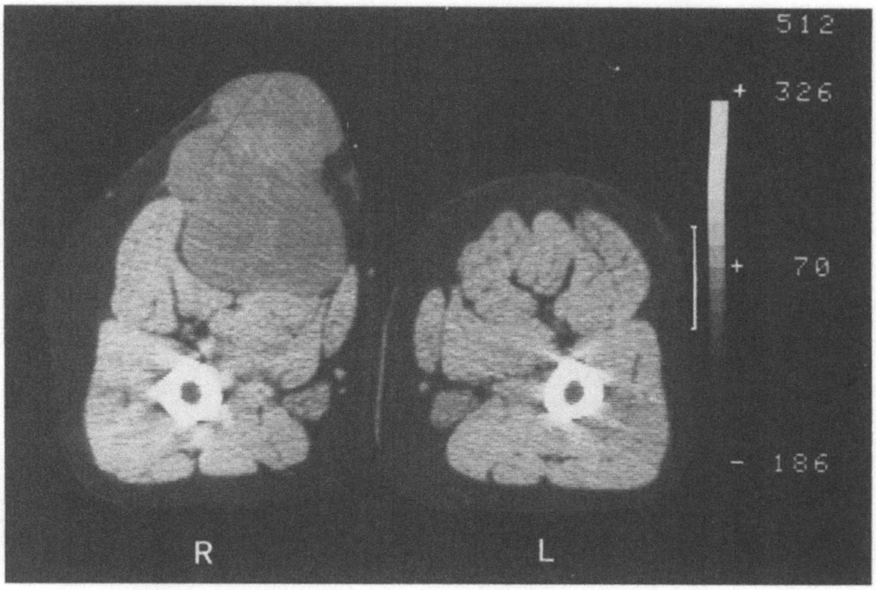

Fig. 6. *Liposarcoma* of the right dorsal thigh. Postcontrast CT in prone position. Well-defined tumor with attenuation values of + 16 HU. No enhancement after bolus injection of contrast medium

There is no contrast enhancement in either type. Definitive diagnosis can be made on the basis of CT findings [13].

Liposarcomas occur at the rate of about one for every 120 lipomas [28]. Depending upon their internal consistency, i.e., the amount of fatty tissue present, they show rather different attenuation values, ranging from − 10 to + 20 HU. They often contain fibrous septa and calcifications (Fig. 5a). Correct diagnosis can be made on the basis of typical CT findings in well-differentiated and lipoblastic forms, but fibroblastic and myxoid liposarcomas may contain very little fatty tissue, rendering them indistinguishable from other soft tissue tumors (Fig. 5b).

In general, attenuation values in malignant soft tissue tumors tend to be lower than those of the surrounding muscles. According to Grabbe et al. [10] the majority of cases were in the range + 15 to + 40 HU. However, the same applies to abscesses, focal myositis, and intramuscular hematomas, which may perfectly mimic CT findings of soft tissue malignancies [16, 21]. Even an accessory soleus muscle must be taken into differential diagnostic considerations [4].

Signs of Invasive Growth

The benign lesions studied in this series were well demarcated without any signs of invasive growth (Fig. 4). The only exceptions to this rule were recurrences of benign soft tissue tumors after incomplete resection. In these cases, due to postoperative scar formation the contours were obscured and the separating fat planes distorted.

More important, though, is the observation that well-differentiated malignant soft tissue tumors may present as well-defined masses without any evidence of invasive growth (Fig. 5a). Therefore in our experience, CT signs of invasive growth are of very limited value, since they may be present in recurrent *benign* lesions and are absent in many well-differentiated *malignant* soft tissue tumors.

Contrast Enhancement

In most malignant soft tissue tumors there seems to be a close correlation between vascularity and malignancy: higher vascularity tends to occur in the more malignant neoplasms [13, 15]. Again, in

Fig. 5. a *Liposarcoma* of the left distal thigh. Precontrast CT. Well-defined, inhomogeneous tumor with attenuation values between − 10 HU and + 20 HU. Scattered fibrous septa. Displacement of muscles without signs of invasive growth. **b** *Fibroplastic liposarcoma* of the right axilla. Precontrast CT. Large malignant soft tissue tumor with attenuation values similar to muscle tissue (ca. 40 HU) invading the axilla and the anterior chest wall and infiltrating the skin (→). Separating fat planes and fascias are distorted. Large right pleural effusion (*PE*)

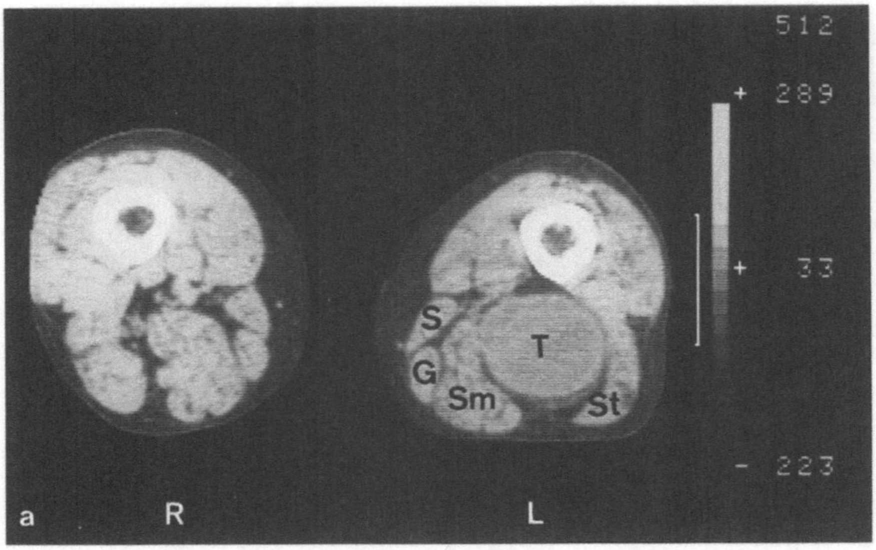

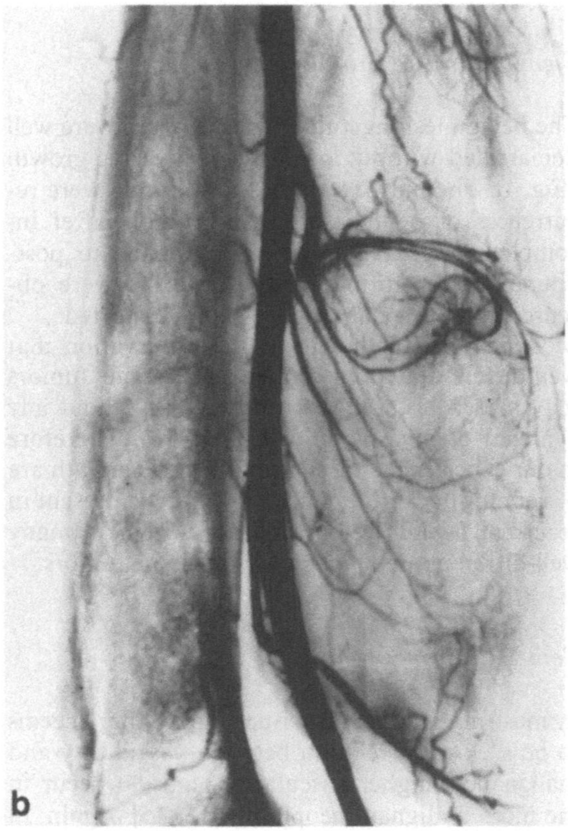

Fig. 7 a, b. *Neurogenic sarcoma.* **a** Precontrast CT. Well-defined mass (*T*) in the left lower thigh displacing the muscles. *S*, m. sartorius; *G*, m. gracilis; *Sm*, m. semimembranosus; *St*, m. semitendinosus. **b** Angiography, lateral view. Displacement of muscular branches of distal femoral artery. Corkscrew vessels at the upper pole of the lesion

CT studies these findings are best demonstrated in malignant tumors of adipose tissue: the well-differentiated types are easily recognized by virtue of their low-density fatty content (Fig. 6). After bolus injection of contrast medium there is very little enhancement within the tumor.

The less-differentiated types of liposarcoma look different even in precontrast scans (Fig. 5 b) and enhance in much the same way as other malignant soft tissue tumors.

Contrast enhancement is of particular interest in desmoid tumors (synonym: aggressive fibromatosis). To confuse matters even more, benign vascular lesions such as angiolipoma may perfectly simulate CT findings of liposarcoma [3] and benign tumors of vascular origin such as hemangiomas cannot be distinguished from malignant soft tissue tumors by CT.

Thus contrast enhancement in CT, while often indicating a vascularized malignant soft tissue tumor, might also be misleading. In order to clarify those situations we continue to perform angiography.

Angiography

Angiography was previously the radiographic method of choice in evaluating peripheral soft tissue tumors, but currently it is reserved for the problems left unresolved by the less invasive procedures. The main indications are:

- Closer diagnostic approach to the *nature* of a given neoplasm by analysis of tumor vascularity.

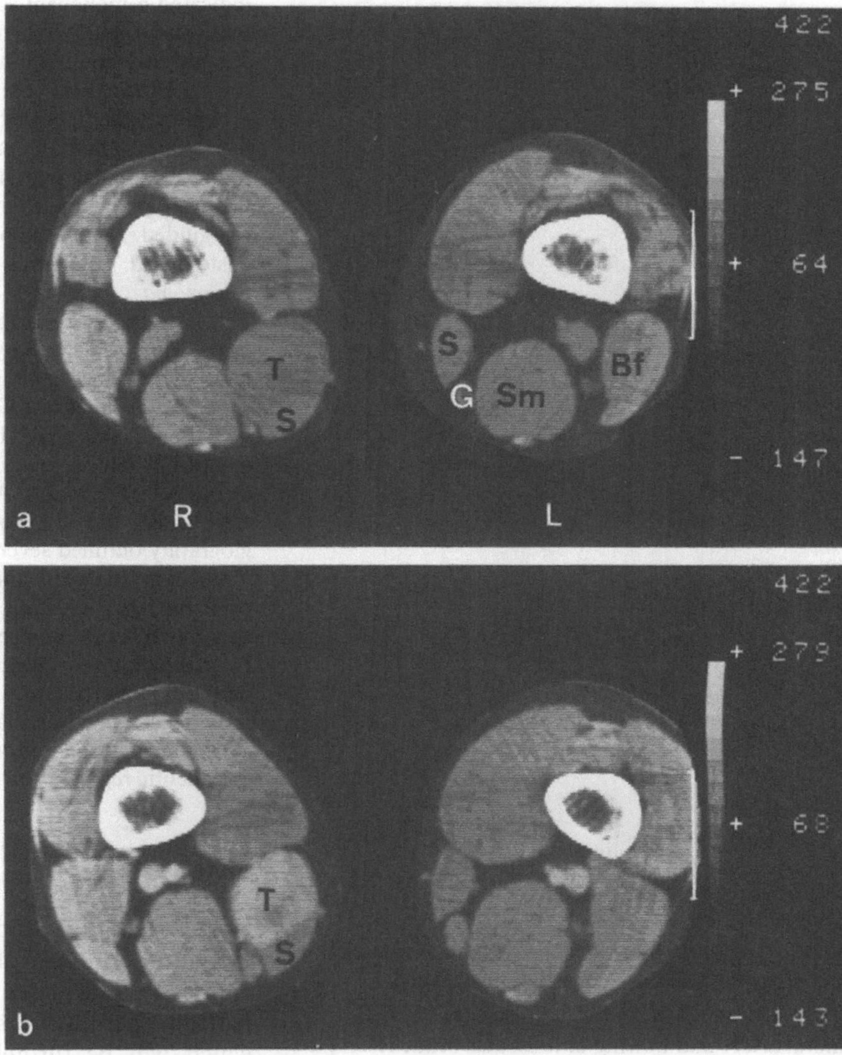

Fig. 8a–c. *Malignant fibrous histiocytoma* of the right sartorius muscle. **a** Precontrast CT showing a hypodense soft tissue tumor (*T*) developing within the fascia of the right sartorius muscle (*S*). *G*, m. gracilis; *Sm*, m. semimembranosus; *Bf*, m. biceps femoris. **b** After i.v. bolus injection of contrast medium, marked enhancement of the tumor, which is now hyperdense as compared to the surrounding muscle tissue. **c** see p. 208

- Study of the *vascular supply* in peripheral soft tissue tumors planned for isolated hyerthermic perfusion with cytostatic drugs [8].
- *Transcatheter therapy*, e.g., preoperative or palliative tumor embolization [20].

Unfortunately, there are no absolute angiographic criteria of malignancy [23, 29]. So-called tumor vessels or malignant neovascularity can also be seen in benign soft tissue tumors as well as in inflammatory lesions. Hemangiomas, benign schwannomas, myositis, and abscesses have been confused angiographically with malignant neoplasms. However, in conjunction with CT cross sections and density measurements before and after bolus injection of contrast medium, angiographic pitfalls of that kind are less likely. Our comparative study indicates that CT and angiography are truly *complementary* imaging modalities in soft tissue neoplasms, as the following case reports will show.

Figure 7 shows CT and angiography of a 41-year-old male patient who complained of dull pain and a mass in the left lower thigh region with a slow-growing tendency. CT revealed a well-defined space-occupying lesion in the left lower thigh, located dorsally to the vascular bundle with attenuation values of + 20 HU. Angiography demonstrated displacement of the distal

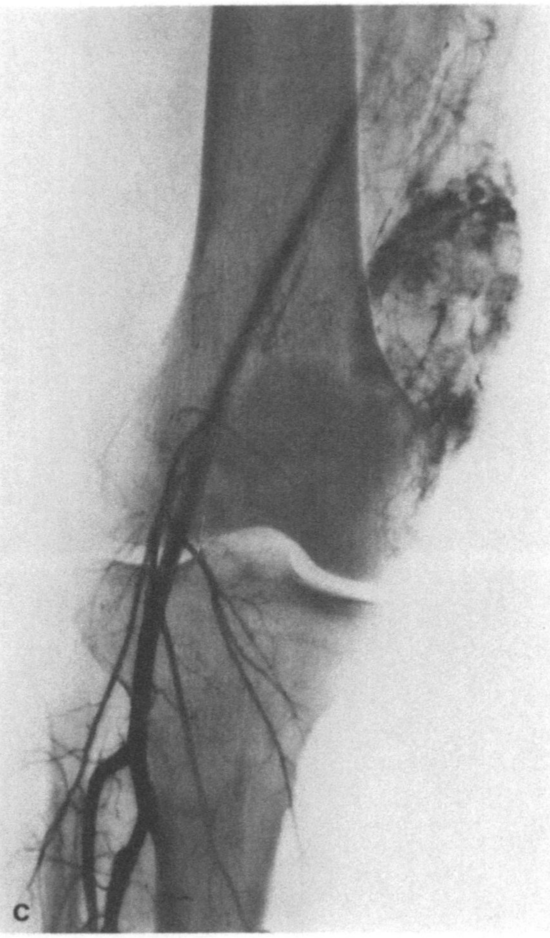

Fig. 8. **c** Angiography reveals neovascularity and pooling of contrast medium, suggesting malignancy

femoral artery and bowing of muscular branches. At the upper pole a few corkscrew vessels were seen, prompting us to suspect malignancy. The tumor was removed in toto. Histological diagnosis was *neurogenic sarcoma.*

A 37-year-old male patient observed a slowly growing mass at the inner surface of the right distal thigh (Fig. 8). On CT, the volume of the right sartorius muscle was greater than that of the left one. A hypodense soft tissue mass displaced the muscle itself dorsally but did not penetrate the fascia. After bolus injection of contrast medium the lesion proved to be highly vascular with a central necrotic or less vascularized core. Angiographically bizarre neovascularity and pooling of contrast medium was seen, again suggesting malignancy in spite of the smooth contours of the lesion on CT. Histological examination disclosed *malignant fibrous histiocytoma.*

Soft tissue tumors arising from vessels such as hemangiosarcomas and hemangiopericytomas are particularly well suited for angiographic study. Figure 9 illustrates the case of a 24-year-old female patient admitted to the hospital because of a rapidly growing soft tissue mass of the right thigh. Lymphography had been performed at an outside hospital, and clinical findings indicated a malignant soft tissue tumor. CT revealed a bulky soft tissue tumor with an highly invasive growth pattern and multiple hypodense areas. Angiography was performed in preparation for possible hyperthermic isolated perfusion therapy. It demonstrated intense staining and a lobulated structure, resembling the radiated vascular pattern reported by Yaghmai [32] in hemangiopericytoma. The patient refused surgery, so a CT-guided needle biopsy was carried out (Fig. 9c). Histological diagnosis was *malignant hemangiopericytoma.*

The last case emphasizes the value of angiography in *desmoid tumors.* The 35-year-old female patient noticed a slowly growing tender mass in the right gluteal region (Fig. 10). Postcontrast CT demonstrated an ill-defined hyperdense mass which had replaced part of her gluteal muscles. There were several hypodense areas scattered throughout the lesion. A previous biopsy had already established the diagnosis of desmoid tumor. Angiography outlined several areas of neovascularity. The tumor was removed and the diagnosis of the biopsy confirmed. In less than a year the patient presented again with recurrent disease. Desmoid tumors are rated by pathologists as low-grade fibrosarcomas [11]. It has been our experience and that of others that angiographic evidence of neovascularity indicates an higher degree of malignancy and should be taken into account in therapeutic regimen and prognostic considerations [31].

Conclusion

Our comparative study of the different imaging modalities in peripheral soft tissue tumors, although so far based upon a limited number of patients, permits some preliminary conclusions which will be further evaluated in an ongoing prospective protocol:

1. Conventional radiography using the low-kVp technique contributes very little to the diagnosis and management of soft tissue tumors. It has thus been replaced by conventional radiography using the *bone technique* in order to detect calcifications and/or osseous involvement.
2. Xeroradiography has been replaced by *real-time US* because of the latter's better delineation of location and extent of soft tissue masses. However, in spite of tremendous research effort put into tissue characterization by US, we currently consider US findings entirely nonspecific as far as the nature of disease is concerned. In selected cases, US-guided puncture or fine– needle biopsy may be the diagnostic procedure of choice. We consider real-time US the best, easiest, and certainly most economical imaging modality for follow-

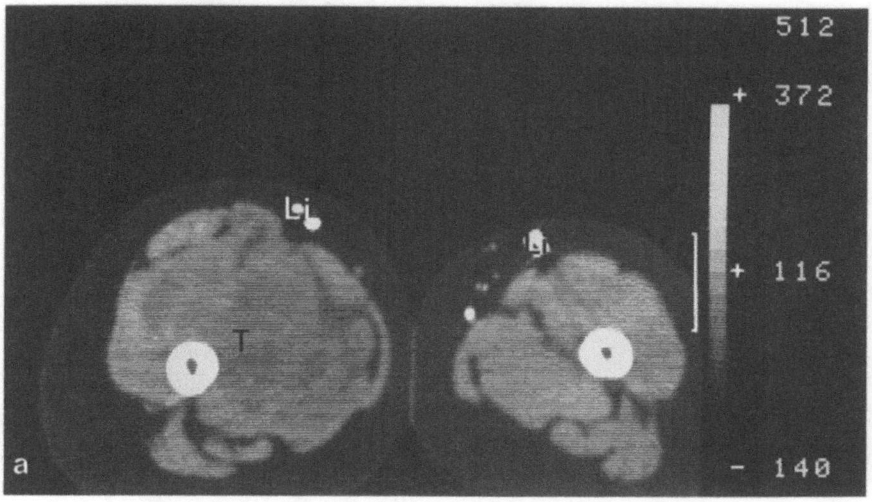

up studies after chemotherapy or radiation therapy.

3. The ability of CT to define anatomy in cross-sectional scans and its superior spatial resolution as compared to US have proved clearly advantageous to both the radiologist and the referring physician. The location and extent of the soft tissue mass, as well as the involvement of adjacent structures, including bone, can be determined exactly. By virtue of density measurements, certain benign and malignant tumors of adipose tissue can be identified with a sufficiently high degree of accuracy. The assessment of the vascularization of the lesion by means of bolus injection of contrast medium permits further differential-diagnostic considerations concerning the nature of soft tissue tumors. Consequently, CT is considered to be the most valuable imaging modality in soft tissue neoplasms.
4. *Angiography* has been an important diagnostic tool in soft tissue tumors. In definition of the location and extent of a given mass, it is *inferior* to CT, but it may identify soft tissue tumors arising from vessels, such as hemangiomas, and may provide useful additional information concerning the nature of a soft tissue tumor, e.g., desmoid tumor. Angiography can help in selecting the most appropriate biopsy site in large masses and must be performed in cases where isolated hyperthermic extremity perfusion with cytostatic drugs is planned.

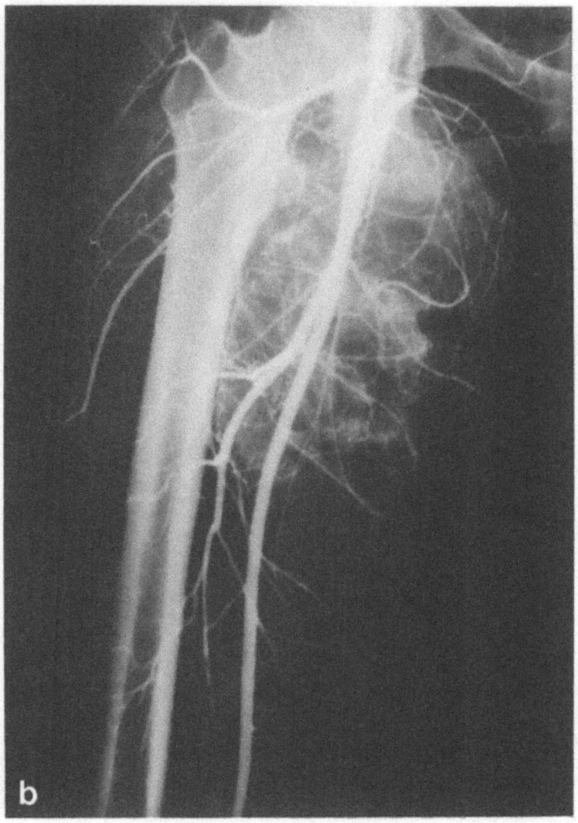

Fig. 9a, b. *Malignant hemangiopericytoma* of the right thigh. **a** Precontrast CT. Large soft tissue tumor (*T*) invading the muscles of proximal thigh. *Li*, oily contrast medium (Lipiodol) in superficial inguinal lymph nodes. **b** Angiography. Soft tissue tumor with hypervascularity, lobulated appearance, and radiated arterial vascular pattern compatible with hemangiopericytoma

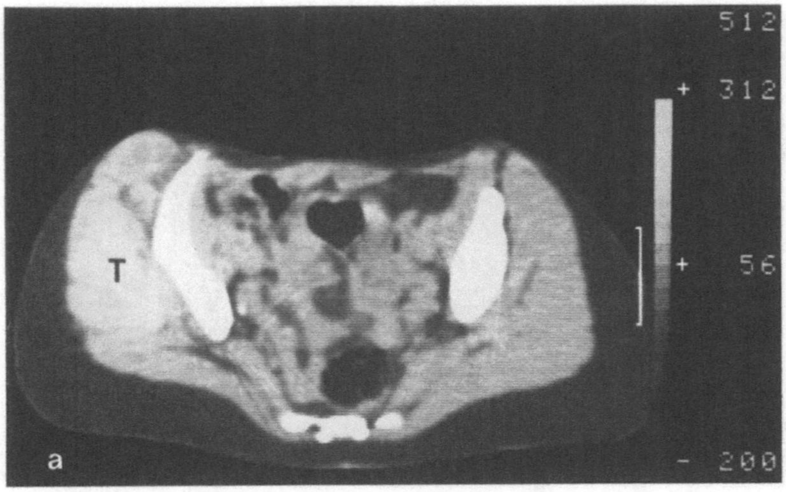

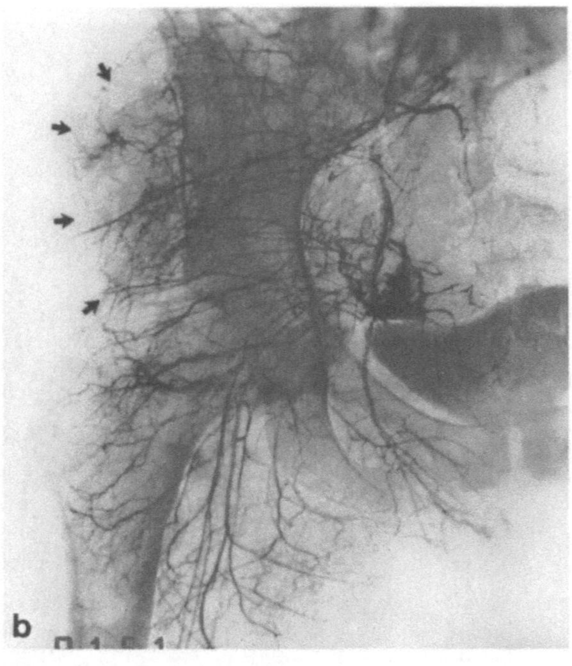

Fig. 10a, b. *Desmoid tumor* of the right gluteal muscle. **a** CT after drip infusion of 100 ml 65% contrast medium reveals a hyperdense mass lesion (*T*) infiltrating the musculature. **b** Angiography shows several areas of neovascularity (→) compatible with malignancy (low-grade fibrosarcoma)

References

1. Bernardino ME, Jing BS, Thomas JL, Lindell MM, Zornoza J (1981) The extremity soft-tissue lesion: a comparative study of ultrasound, computed tomography, and xeroradiography. Radiology 139:157–163
2. Bünte H, Einhoff E, Klaus A, Jost JO (1977) Benigne periphere Weichteiltumoren. Dtsch Aerztebl 74:71–78
3. Chew FS, Hudson TM, Hawkins IF (1980) Radiology of infiltrating angiolipoma. AJR 135:781–787
4. Dokter G, Linclau LA (1981) Case report *β*. The accessory soleus muscle: symptomatic soft tissue tumor or accidental finding. Neth J Surg 33:146–149
5. Dorfman HD, Bhagavan BS (1982) Malignant fibrous histiocytoma of soft tissue with metaplastic bone and cartilage formation: a new radiologic sign. Skeletal Radiol 8:145–150
6. Egund N, Ekelund L, Sako M, Persson B (1981) CT of soft-tissue tumors. AJR 137:725–729
7. Forrester DM, Becker TS (1977) The radiology of bone and soft tissue sarcomas. Orthop Clin North Am 8:973–978
8. Ghussen F, Stock W (1980) Aktueller Stand der Therapie maligner Weichteiltumoren. Dtsch Med Wochenschr 105:166–169
9. Goldberg BB (1975) Ultrasonic evaluation of superficial masses. J Clin Ultrasound 3:91–94
10. Grabbe E, Heller M, Böcker W (1979) Computertomographie bei Weichteilsarkomen. RoFo 131:372–378
11. Hajdu SI (1979) Pathology of soft tissue tumors. Lea & Febiger, Philadelphia
12. Heelan RT, Watson RC, Smith J (1979) Computed tomography of lower extremity tumors. AJR 132:933–937
13. Hunter JC, Johnston WH, Genant HK (1979) Computed tomography evaluation of fatty tumors of the somatic soft tissues: clinical utility and radiologic-pathologic correlation. Skeletal Radiol 4:79–91
14. Jost JO, Bünte H, Senftleben E, Clemens M, Schwering H (1980) Periphere Weichteiltumoren. Dtsch Med Wochenschr 105:341–346
15. Kindblom LG, Angervall L, Stener B, Wickbom I (1974) Intermuscular and intramuscular lipomas

and hibernomas, a clinical, roentgenologic, histologic, and prognostic study of 46 cases. Cancer 33:754
16. Lackner K, Hofmann P, Grauthoff H, Brecht G, Thurn P (1978) Computertomographischer Nachweis von Muskelhämatomen bei Haemophilie. RoFo 129:298–302
17. Laursen K, Reiter S (1980) Computed tomography in soft tissue disorders of the lower extremity. Acta Orthop Scand 51:881–885
18. Levine E (1981) Computed tomography of musculoskeletal tumors. CRC Crit Rev Diagn Imaging 16:279–309
19. Levine E, Lee KR, Neff JR, Maklad NF, Robinson RG, Preston DF (1979) Comparison of computed tomography and other imaging modalities in the evaluation of musculoskeletal tumors. Radiology 131:431–437
20. Levinsohn EM, Bryan PJ (1979) Computed tomography in unilateral extremity swelling of unusual cause. J Comput Assist Tomogr 3:67–70
21. Lindell MM, Wallace S, de Santos LA, Bernardino ME (1981) Diagnostic technique for the evaluation of the soft tissue sarcoma. Semin Oncol 8:160–171
22. Martel W, Abell MR (1973) Radiologic evaluation of soft tissue tumors Cancer 32:352–366
23. Ney FG, Feist JH, Altemus LR, Ordinario VR (1972) The characteristic angiographic criteria of malignancy. Radiology 104:567–570
24. Rich PJ, King W (1982) Benign cortical hyperostosis underlying soft-tissue tumors of thigh. AJR 138:419–422
25. Santos LA de, Goldstein HM, Murray JA, Wallace S (1978) Computed tomography in the evaluation of musculoskeletal neoplasms. Radiology 128:89–94
26. Santos LA de, Ginaldi S, Wallace S (1981) Computed tomography in liposarcoma. Cancer 47:46–54
27. Stephenson TF (1980) Computerized tomography of soft tissue abnormalities. Comput Tomogr 4:181–188
28. Viamonte M, Viamonte M (1981) Radiology and pathology of fat. CRC Crit Rev Diagn Imaging 16:93–123
29. Viamonte M, Roen S, LePage J (1973) Nonspecificity of abnormal vascularity in the angiographic diagnosis of malignant neoplasms. Radiology 106:59–63
30. Weinberger G, Levinsohn EM (1978) Computed tomography in the evaluation of sarcomatous tumors of the thigh. AJR 130:115–118
31. Yaghmai I (1977) Angiographic features of fibromas and fibrosarcomas. Radiology 124:57–64
32. Yaghmai I (1978) Angiographic manifestations of soft-tissue and osseous hemangiopericytomas. Radiology 126:653–659

Radiological Approach to Soft Tissue Masses

R. Campani, M. Lombardi, M. Alerci, G. Di Giulio,
F. Alessi Grassi, A. Vacchino, and D. De Nile

Istituto di Radiologia, Università di Pavia, Policlinico S. Matteo, Piazzale Golgi, 27100 Pavia PV, Italy

Diagnosis of soft tissue masses has always been difficult and is often inconclusive. An accurate preoperative diagnosis is unusual, except in some well-defined pathological conditions such as the classical subcutaneous lipomas [1, 8]. Angiography has sometimes been used to determine vascular changes [8, 9]. Great improvement has been achieved through xeroradiography (XR) [2, 3, 5, 11–14, 16, 17]. Nevertheless, even XR is of little or no help in many cases. Ultrasonography (US) has been proposed by many authors, including Braunstein et al. [1], Golding [6], and Gooding [7], but its proper role and efficacy in the evaluation of soft tissue masses have not yet been determined. It has been shown to be useful in many cases, even those where angiography is not possible, such as in anticoagulated patients [1].

The role and efficacy of computed tomography (CT) have been stressed but this method cannot be employed as a first-step examination [4, 8].

In this study some new imaging techniques were combined, the aim being to determine the logical sequence of these methods and the results which may be expected.

Material and Methods

Since 1976, a total of 964 patients with soft tissue masses have been studied at the Institute of Radiology, University of Pavia, Italy. Among these, a group of 84 patients underwent XR and US in 1981 and 1982. CT was performed in 28 patients; in five cases angiography was added.

This study focuses mainly on benign lesions, which represented the majority of the pathological conditions examined. A future publication will deal with the subject of malignant soft tissue masses.

Xeroradiography was performed by means of the Xerox Medical 125 System, set at maximum electrostatic voltage (conditioner "D" setting) and maximum powder quantity (processor "D" setting). Nearly all examinations were developed in the negative mode.

Ultrasonography was performed with a digital compound gray scale equipment Sonia (Compagnie Generale de Radiologie), using a 7.0-MHz transducer with 7-mm diameter focused at 15 mm. Both longitudinal and transverse scans were performed with respect to the axes of the mass to be examined.

Computed tomography was performed with the Siemens Somatom 2, sometimes with sagittal or coronal reconstruction of the image. In eight cases contrast medium was injected.

Results

To be of use in the diagnosis of soft tissue masses the procedures employed must yield sufficient data to evaluate the following parameters:

1. The demonstration of a clinically suspected lesion and its site
2. The depth of the mass with regard to the skin and the distance between the lesion and the adjacent bony structures

Fig. 1 a–d. Superficial lipomas. **a** Xeroradiography of a small lipoma. **b** Ultrasonography of the same case in a longitudinal plane. **c** Xeroradiography of a larger lipoma. **d** Ultrasonography of the same case

Fig. 2. **a** Xeroradiography. The clinically existing lipoma is not visible. **b** Ultrasonsography clearly showing the lipoma not visible in **a**

Radiology Today 2. Ed. by F. H. W. Heuck and M. W. Donner

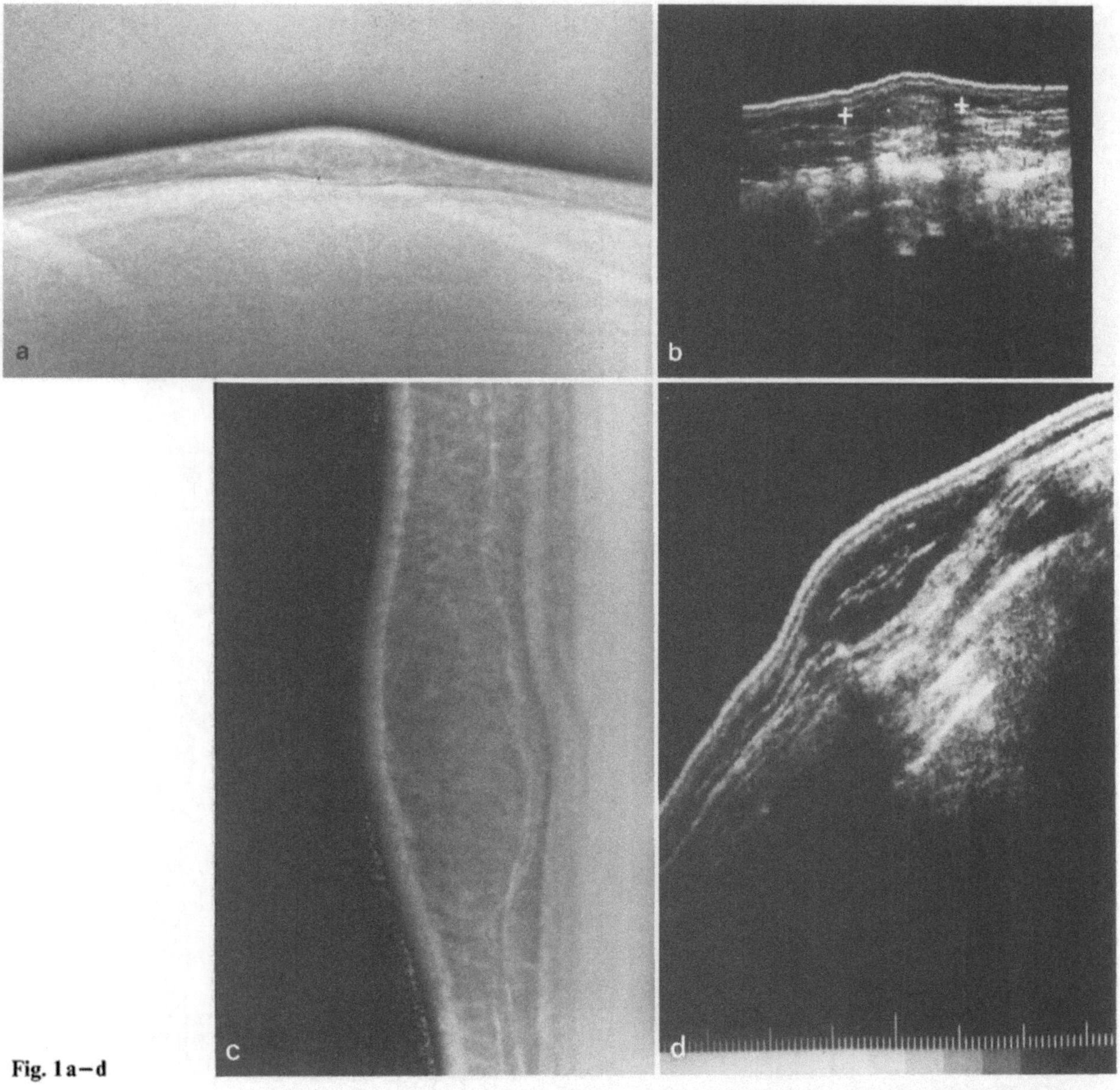

Fig. 1 a–d

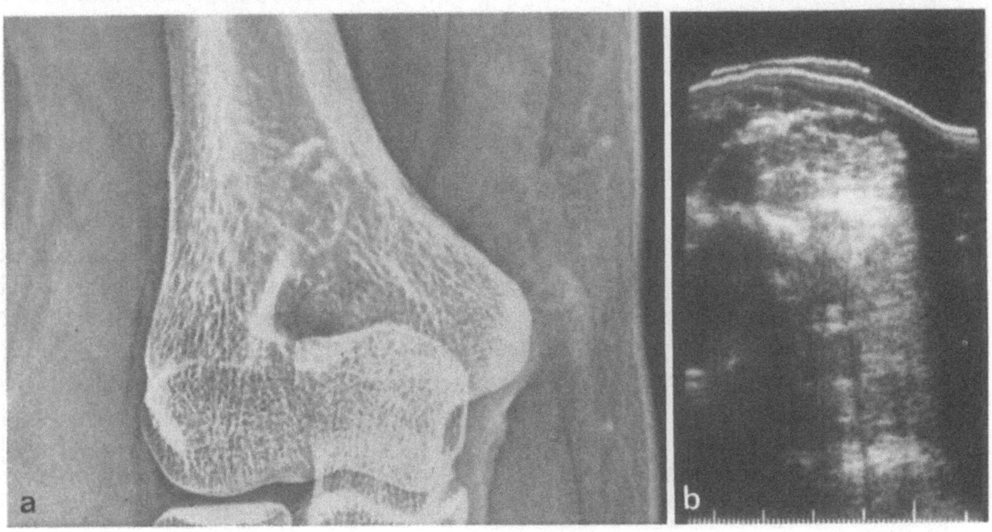

Fig. 2 a, b

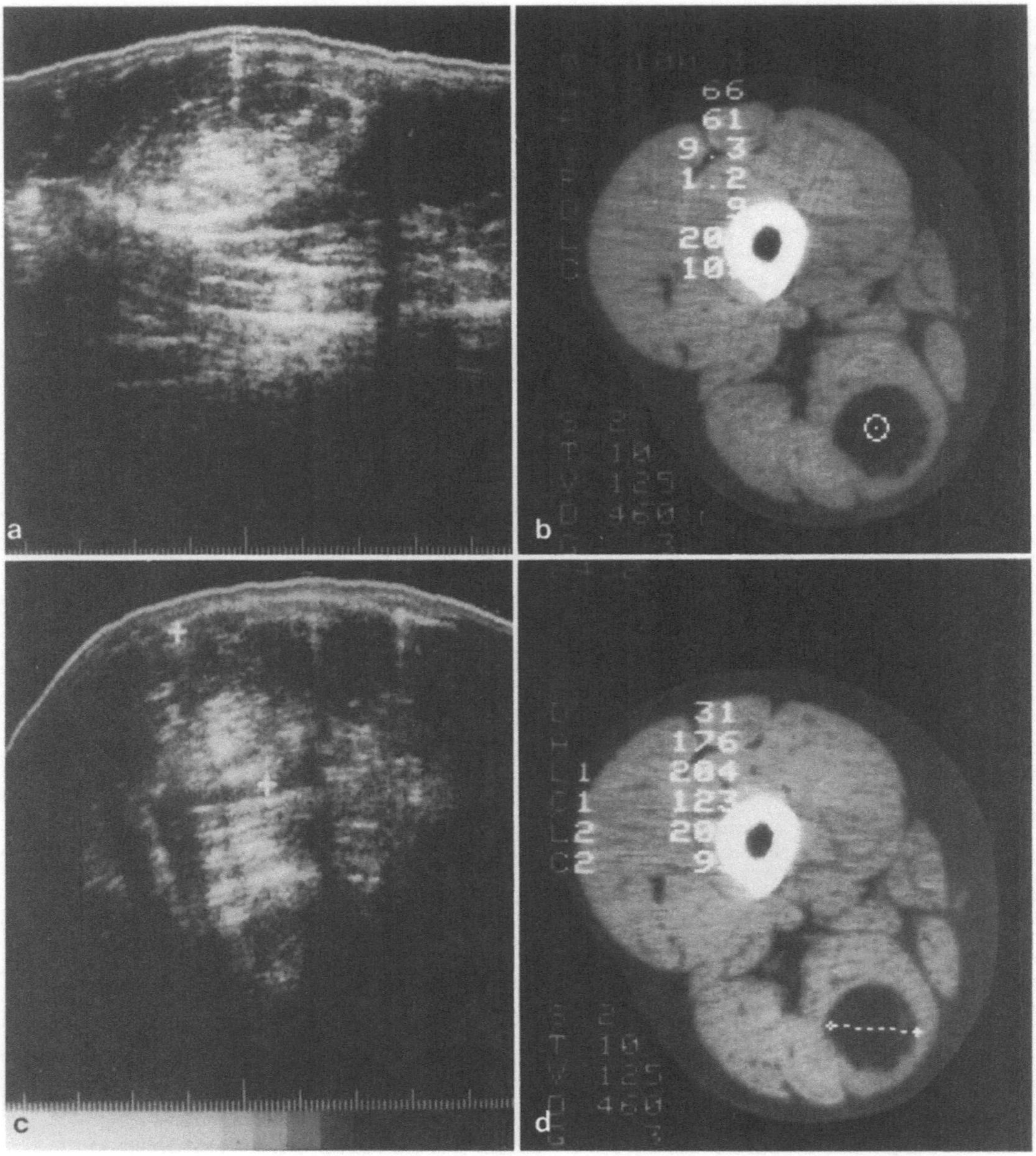

Fig. 3. **a** Typical aspect of a lipoma with US. **b** The same with CT. **c** Accurate measurement obtained through US. **d** The same with CT

3. The presence of surgical planes
4. The dimensions, shape and contours of the lesion and the possible presence of a capsule
5. The density and homogeneity of the lesion
6. Gross benign or malignant signs, even in respect of vascularization
7. The extension to adjacent structures and the relationships with anatomical structures
8. Anatomopathological correlations

These parameters are all of great importance in making the correct diagnosis and in establishing a subsequent prognosis. Their primary importance, however, lies in the determination of the correct therapeutic approach (radiological, surgical). Many different soft tissue masses were examined; the majority of cases turned out to be adipose tissue tumors. The results obtained can be summarized as follows.

Lipomas

Usually solitary, in some cases lipomas may be dispersed over the entire body (one of our patients had 27). They are found more frequently in the limbs and their dimensions may vary greatly.

XR findings have been well described in the literature [3, 8, 9, 13]. A simple lipoma is shown as a radiolucent area, round or oval in shape with smooth well-defined contours, often capsulated. When superficial, the lipomas usually compress the adjacent soft tissues and the muscular layers without infiltrating them (Fig. 1). Intramuscular lipomas are usually deeply situated with their longer axis parallel to that of the muscles. They are usually oval but can change shape during muscle contraction.

In both cases XR showed a translucent area with well-defined contours, sometimes capsulated and sometimes partially or completely lobulated. In five of our cases lipomas were not demonstrable by means of XR (Fig. 2). US features were characteristic, showing a solid echo structure with medium echogenicity, rarely homogeneous due to the presence of highly echogenic areas (usually in the center) and poorly echogenic areas (in the peripheral zone).

Sometimes an echogenic border and posterior wall enhancement were visible. When present, calcifications were easily identified by their typical appearance.

CT scans provided precise transverse anatomical pictures. Lipomas appeared as homogeneous masses with regular contours. The absorption coefficient was approximately − 50 HU, similar to subcutaneous fat. Sometimes strands of solid tissue were visible (Fig. 3). No enhancement followed the injection of contrast medium. Only the structures peripheral to the tumor were regularly enhanced, due to compression of surrounding tissues.

If calcifications were present, CT showed them quite easily.

Liposarcomas

On XR liposarcomas usually appeared as radiopaque asymmetrical or round areas with irregular contours. Their density was high and heterogeneous; often strands of solid tissue were visible and the masses were lobulated. There was lack of pseudocapsule and often the surrounding soft tissues appeared infiltrated. Two of nine liposarcomas appeared as translucent areas with irregular contours.

US showed an ill-defined mass with irregular contours and high echogenicity. The echoes were ir-

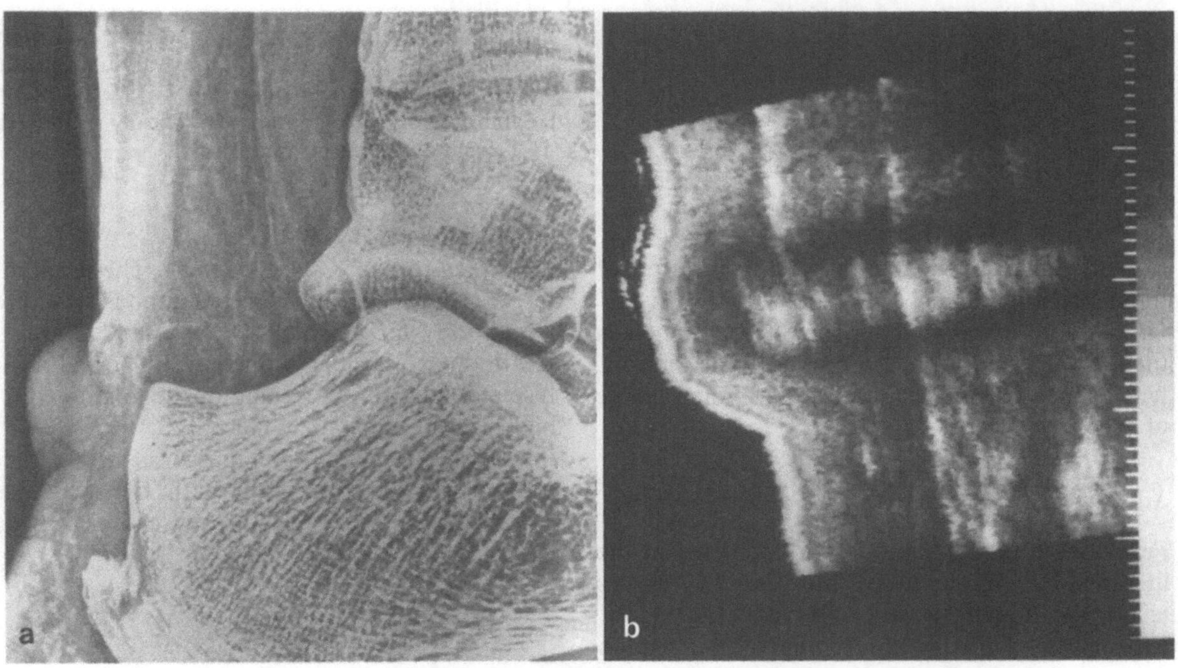

Fig. 4 a, b. Achilles tendon xanthomatosis. **a** Xeroradiographic findings. **b** Ultrasonographic findings

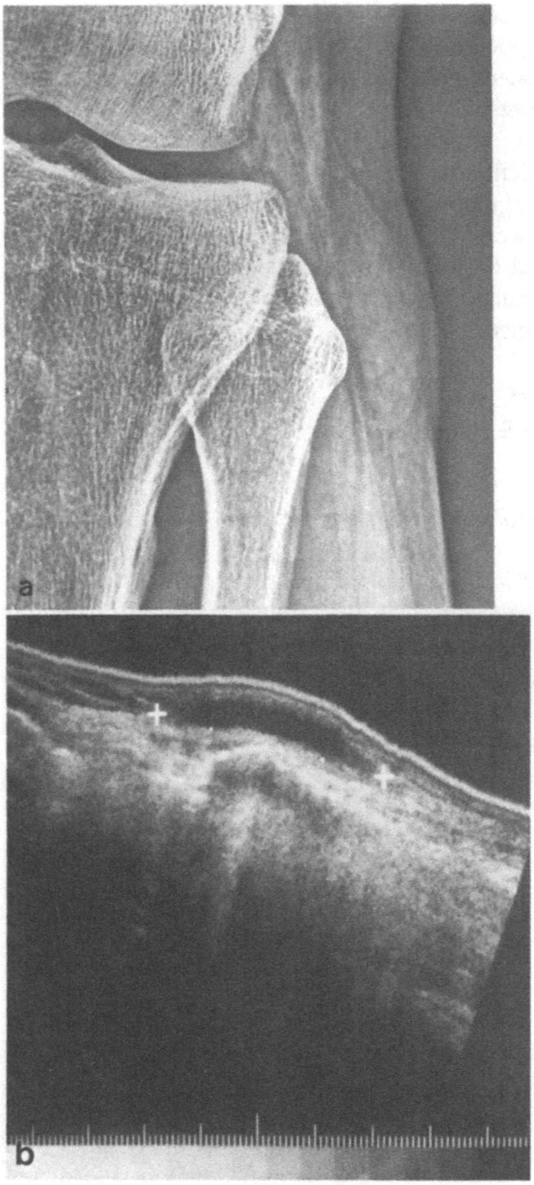

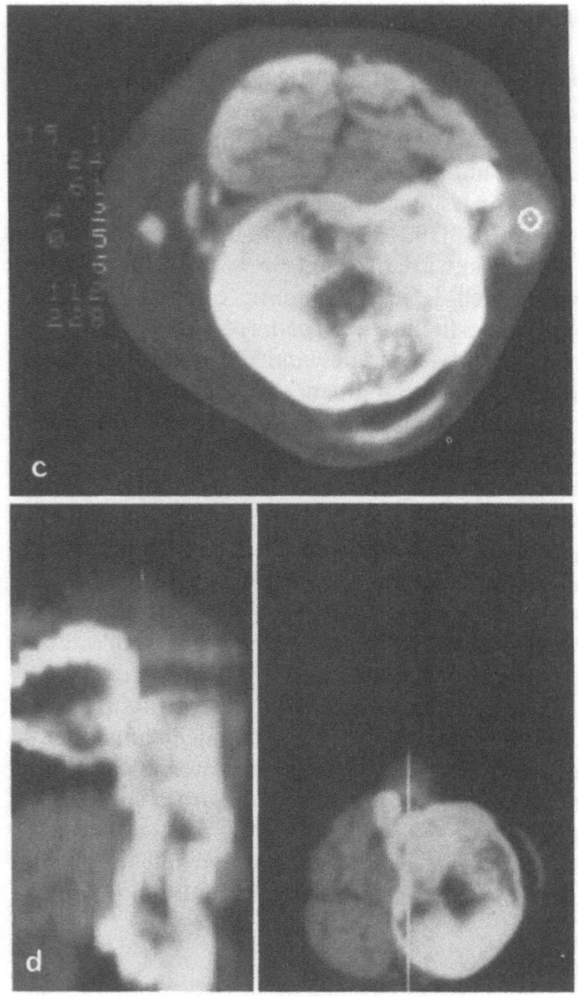

Fig. 5a–d. Tendinous cyst of the external collateral ligament. **a** Xeroradiography. The oval subcutaneous cyst is easily seen. **b** Echotomography. Perfect superimposability with **a.** **c** CT. The mean density is 15.1 HU. **d** CT. Sagittal reconstruction

regularly distributed and showed infiltration of the surrounding tissues.

On CT, a mass was visible with a density between that of water and fat. According to some authors, heterogeneity of the lesion means a higher degree of malignancy.

Xanthomatosis

Few cases of xanthomatosis are described in the literature [15]. In our study, four cases of Achilles tendon xanthomatosis were observed.

XR showed a diffuse thickening of the tendon throughout its entire length with a reduction of the dimensions of Kager's triangle. The usual differences between muscle and tendinous structures were poorly appreciable.

US findings in a longitudinal scan showed a diffuse and uniform thickening of the tendon with a higher echogenicity than normal.

In two cases a small, round mass was visible, radiopaque with XR, echo-free with US, with posterior wall enhancement. In each case it was determined to be a cyst (Fig. 4).

Tendinous and Synovial Cysts

Thirty-six patients had round bulges located mainly in the knee along the medial or lateral collateral ligaments.

The XR findings have been well described in the literature and our results agree precisely: a radiopaque image, usually oval with well-defined superficial contours, easily distinguishable from superficial soft tissues, but rarely differentiated from the deep tissues (Fig. 5).

They generally compress and dislocate the surrounding structures. In our cases there were no signs of infiltration. Sometimes small calcifications were visible.

US quite easily determined the presence of an echo-free area which exactly reproduced the XR image and showed no signs of infiltration of the surrounding tissues (Fig. 6). The deeper muscular planes could not always be differentiated from the surrounding tissues.

Oleogranulomas

In some patients bulges localized in the glutei were observed.

On XR they usually appeared as round radiopaque masses with smooth well-defined contours. Peripheral calcifications were often present. US showed echo-free areas with posterior wall enhancement. When present, peripheral calcifications were seen with their typical shadow.

CT showed a homogeneous mass with smooth and regular contours. The approximate mean density was 21 HU, indicating a liquid content. CT clearly indicated the exact delimitation of the mass, the presence of peripheral calcifications, and the absence of infiltration of the surrounding muscular planes.

In one case a fibrotic strand was shown in the anterior wall of the mass; this was subsequently also seen on XR and US (Fig. 7).

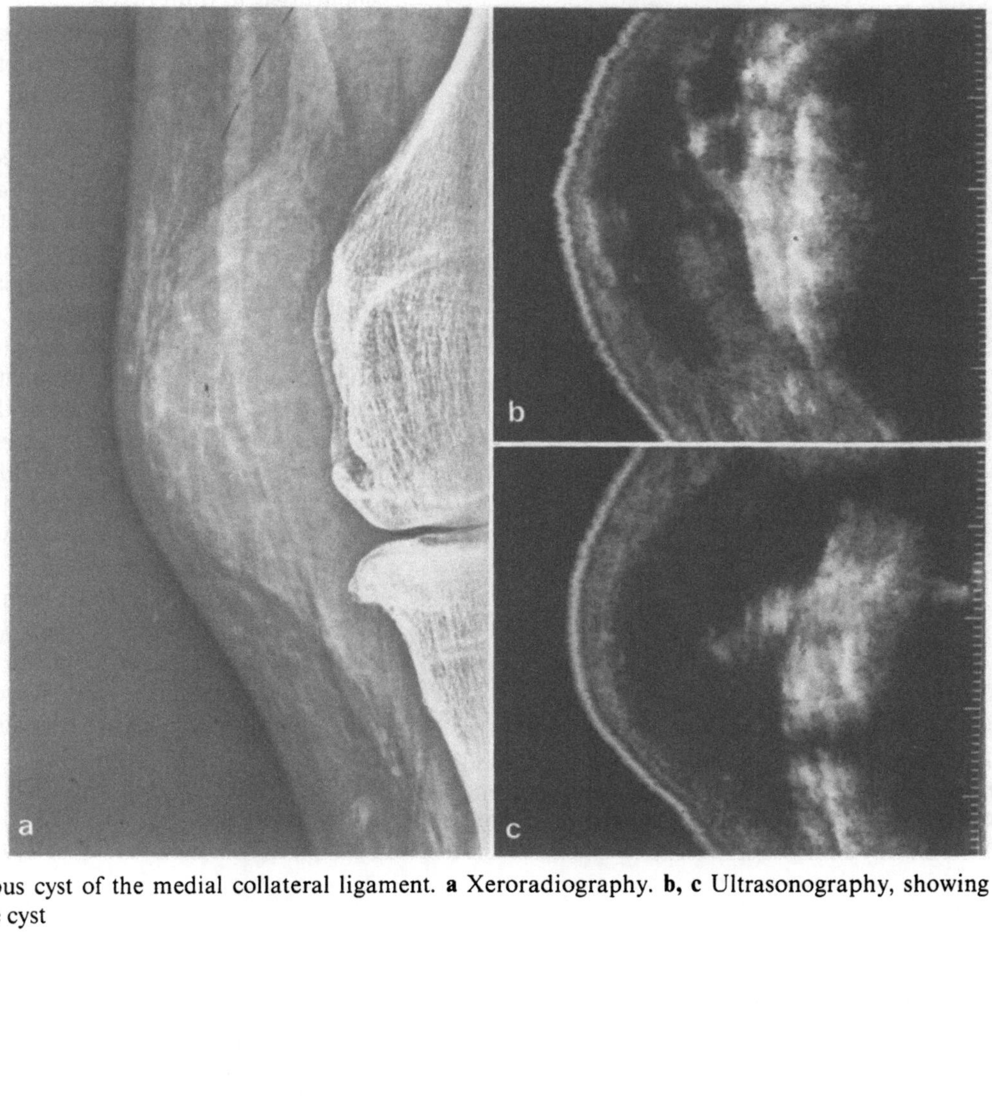

Fig. 6a–c. Tendinous cyst of the medial collateral ligament. **a** Xeroradiography. **b, c** Ultrasonography, showing the lobulation of the cyst

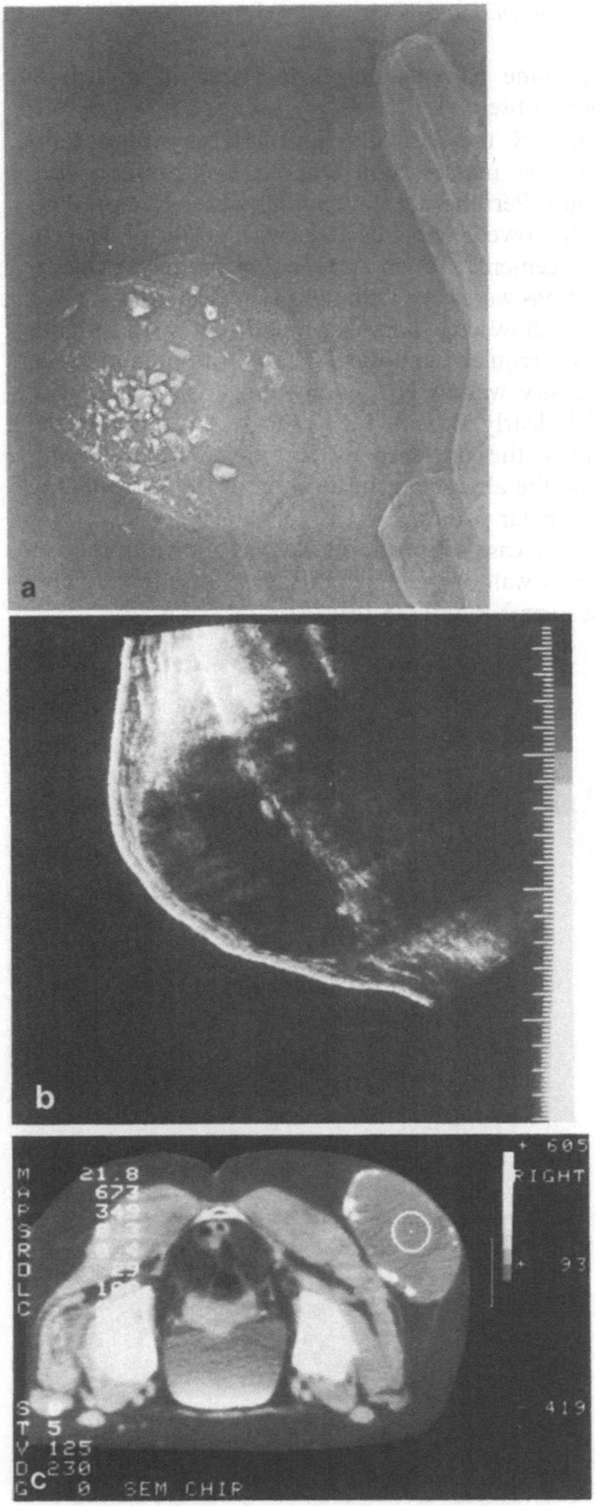

Fig. 7a–c. Cicatricial oleogranuloma. **a** Xeroradiography. **b** Ultrasonography, showing the same findings. **c** CT adds at great amount of information about the anatomical structures surrounding the mass

Parotid Gland Tumors

Some cases of parotid gland tumors studied with CT are reported in the literature [6, 7]. In recent months we have examined 13 patients with soft tissue bulges localized in the parotid or submandibular glands.

Due to the proximity of the ascending or the horizontal branches of the mandible, XR yielded poor results. It showed a radiopaque image with superficial smooth or irregular contours. XR never showed the deep contours of the mass, nor was it able to provide data concerning homogeneity. The thickness of the skin and the subcutaneous tissues was normal or slightly reduced.

US added more information on the anatomopathological correlations, showing a solid heterogeneous structure with some peripheral poor or echo-free areas. It also showed a thinning of superficial tissue layers (Fig. 8). At surgery these lesions were found to be pleiomorphic adenomas; a striking correspondence was found between US and surgical findings, the echo-free areas corresponding to necrotic tissue and the highly echogenic areas to solid tissue.

Similar pictures were seen in patients diagnosed as having benign parotid oncocytomas (Fig. 9). In these cases XR data was poor, but US allowed differentiation from the pleiomorphic adenomas, showing a higher number of echoes inside the mass with more homogeneous and regular echo distribution. The contours of the oncocytomas were better defined that those of the pleiomorphic adenomas; the US appearance of the soft superficial tissues was the same.

Similar findings to those in pleiomorphic adenomas and oncocytomas were made in some patients with bulges located along the lateral margin of the sternocleidomastoid muscle. In none of these cases did XR add much information to that obtained from clinical examination. In addition, XR often showed only one or two masses, while with other methods there appeared to be more. US either yielded a poor number of echos or showed echo-free areas with well-defined contours, usually not infiltrating the surrounding soft tissues. At surgery they were diagnosed as tubercular lymph nodes in caseous necrosis.

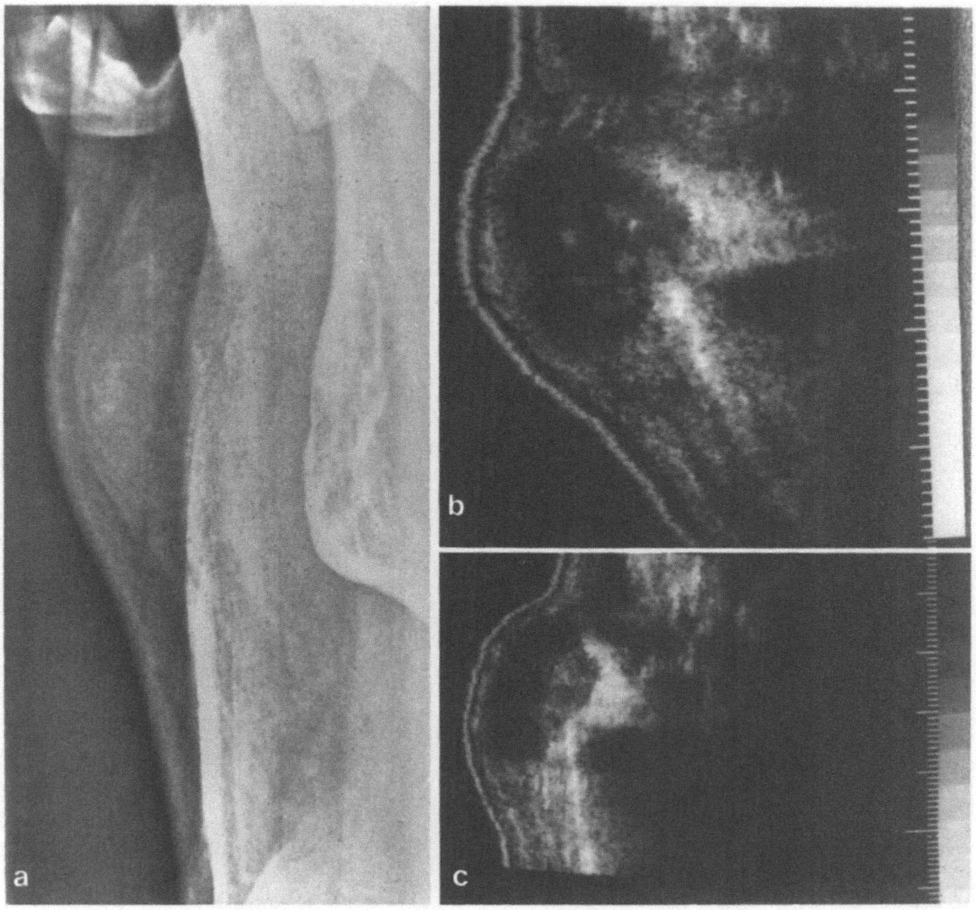

Fig. 8a–c. Pleiomorphic adenoma of the parotid gland. **a** Xeroradiography. **b, c** Ultrasonography. Heterogeneous distribution of the echoes

Discussion and Conclusions

Although the findings of this study varied widely, some positive conclusions can still be drawn in light of the techniques employed. The first parameter, existence of the lesion, was demonstrated accurately by all methods except XR, which failed to show five of 38 lipomas (19%) and two of 36 tendinous cysts (7%).

With the exceptions previously described, all methods were able to verify the site of the mass and its depth from the skin, and all were able to demonstrate the distance of the lesion from the upper and lower skeletal planes, with the greatest degree of accuracy obtained from CT. XR often failed to detect surgical planes, especially if deeply situated.

The dimensions of the masses were accurately demonstrated by all methods. In fact, the images obtained from the various techniques were perfectly superimposable.

Regarding the morphology of the lesions and their encapsulation, the greatest accuracy was with CT. XR demonstrated only the radiopacity or translucency of the mass examined, but no data was supplied on its average density. US offered intermediate results.

The diagnosis of benignity of malignancy was again most accurate with CT, followed by XR and US. However, US was sometimes more precise than XR in distinguishing extension to surrounding tissues and structures.

Pathological typing of the tumor was limited to CT, but in many cases US supplied important information. XR allowed a pathological diagnosis only in those cases in which the morphological aspect was pathognomonic.

Only CT with the injection of contrast medium provided information concerning vascularization of the lesion.

CT clearly emerges as the most complete and accurate method in the diagnosis of soft tissue mas-

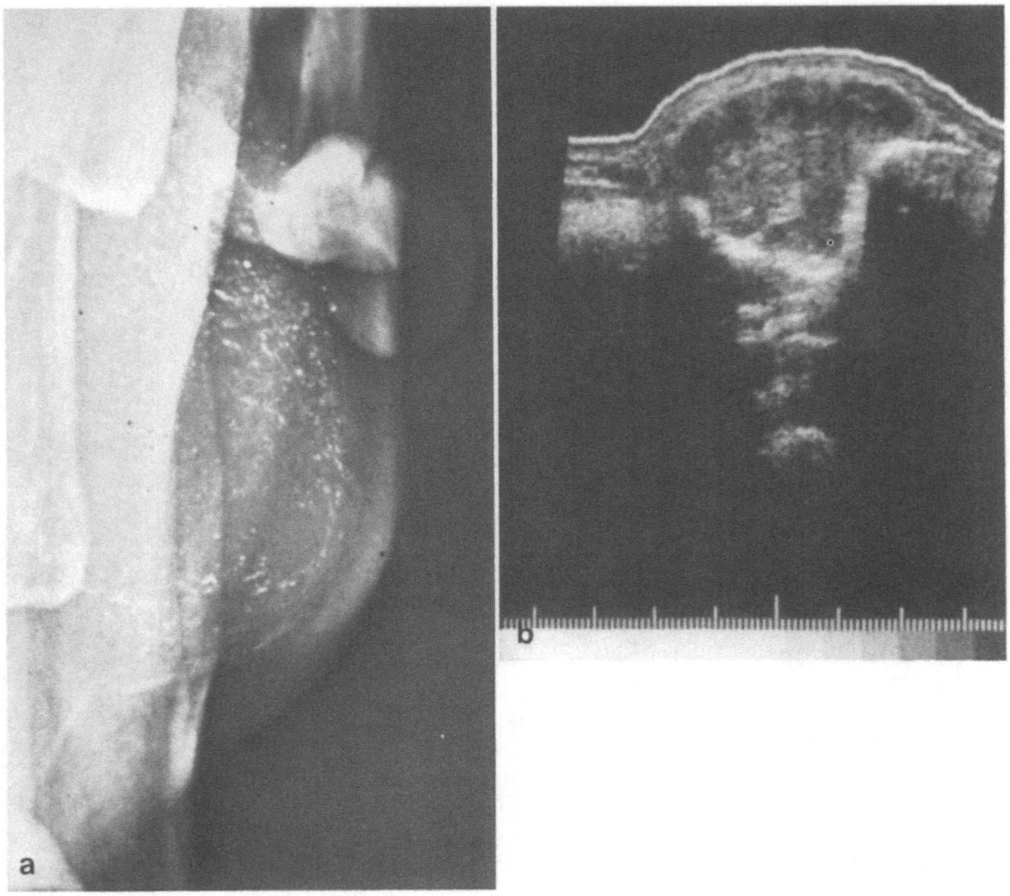

Fig. 9a, b. Benign oncocytoma of the parotid gland. **a** Xeroradiography. Presence of contrast medium used in a previous scialography. **b** Ultrasonography. The echo structure is quite homogeneous

ses. However, in choosing the method to be employed, certain problems (clinical, logistical, economic, etc.) must be taken into account. On the basis of these problems and our personal experience, our preliminary conclusion is to consider XR as the first approach; in fact in about 28% of our cases this method resolved diagnostic, prognostic, and therapeutic problems. US, which correctly diagnosed another 37% of cases, may be added as a second examination. CT had to be used in the remaining 35% of cases.

References

1. Braunstein EM, Silver TM, Martel W, Jaffe M (1981) Ultrasonographic diagnosis of the extremity masses. Skeletal Radiol 6:157–163
2. Campani R, Alerci M, Pricca P, Rota L (1980) La xeroradiografia nello studio della patologia dei tessuti molli. Radiol Med [Suppl] (Torino) 1:275–282
3. Campani R, Ferrari Ciboldi F, Benazzi M, Meissner M, Rota L (1981) Xeroradiographie zur Diagnostik pathologischer Befunde an den Weichteilen des Kniegelenkes. Roentgenberichte 10:274–284
4. De Santos LA, Goldstein H, Murray J, Wallace S (1978) Computed tomography of musculoskeletal neoplasms. Radiology 128:89–94
5. Di Guglielmo L, Campani R, Garbagna P, Mira E (1977) Xeroradiography in otorhinolaryngology. Excerpta Medica, Amsterdam
6. Golding S (1982) Computed tomography in the diagnosis of parotid gland tumours. Br J Radiol 55:182–188

7. Gooding GAW (1980) Gray scale ultrasound of the parotid gland. AJR 134:469–472
8. Hunter JC, Johnston WH, Genant HK (1979) Computed tomography evaluation of fatty tumours of the somatic soft tissue: clinical utility and radiologic-pathologic correlations. Skeletal Radiol. 4:79–91
9. Kindblom LG, Angervall L, Steiner B, Wickbom I (1974) Intermuscular and intramuscular lipomas and hibernomas. Cancer 33:754–762
10. Kramer FL, Kurtz AB, Rubin C, Goldberg BB (1979) Ultrasound appearance of myositis ossificans. Skeletal Radiol 4:19–20
11. Nessi R (1977) La xeroradiografia nello studio delle parti molli. Radiol Med (Torino) 63:1083–1092
12. Nessi R, Freri F, Coopmans De Yoldi G (1979) Xeroradiography of bone and soft tissue tumours. Tumori 65:255–263
13. Nessi R, Gattoni F, Mazzoni R, Coopmans De Yoldi G (1980) Lipoblastic tumours of somatic soft tissues: a xerographic evaluation of 67 cases. Skeletal Radiol 5:137–143
14. Otto RC, Pouliadis GP, Kumpe DA (1976) The evaluation of pathologic alterations of iuxtaosseous soft tissues by xeroradiography. Radiology 120:297–302
15. Piasco D (1981) L'aspetto ecografico della xantomatosi del tendine di Achille. Ultrasuonodiagnostica 2:59–61
16. Reichmann S, Astrand K, Deichgraber E, Olsson B (1976) Soft tissue xeroradiography of the shoulder joint. Acta Radiol (Stockh) 46:572–576
17. Reinhard B, Evers R, Fischedick O (1974) Skelett und Weichteildarstellung in der Xeroradiographie. RoFo 120:209–215

Neuroradiology

Neuroradiology: Overview

A. E. Rosenbaum, H. S. Ahn, and S. B. Rosenbloom *

Department of Radiology and Neurosurgery, The Johns Hopkins Hospital, 600 N. Wolfe Street, Baltimore, MD 21205, USA

In the past 2 years there have been many revolutionary advances in neuroradiologic imaging. Their importance may be ranked as follows:

- Digital techniques: computed tomography (CT) digital angiography, emission tomography, and, most excitingly, nuclear magnetic resonance (NMR)
- High-resolution CT studies, particularly of the pituitary gland and sella and the middle ear
- Diagnosis of diseases of the spine and its neural contents on plain CT
- New nonionic contrast media for CT myelography – iopamidol(Squibb), iohexol(Nygaard/Winthrop), and iotrol(Schering) and cerebral angiography – metrizamide, iohexol
- Head and neck diseases reassessed in the CT era
- Dynamic scanning of cerebral and spinal compartments
- The effects of high technology in reducing or obviating plain films and geometric tomography
- The supplanting of many plain roentgenographic examinations by computed radiography – Scoutview (General Electric), Topogram (Siemens), DeltaView (TechnicAre), etc.
- Digital arterial angiography (with the need for higher matrix and higher line rate television chains if this technique is to supplant "conventional" angiography to any significant degree
- Large-field image intensifiers for routine, indirect cerebral angiography and interventional radiology
- Intraoperative ultrasonography in the localization of surgical planes and lesions
- Routine stereoradiography via a single tube (Siemens Stereolix)
- The advent of biplane large-field fluoroscopy and imaging systems for cerebral angiography (Siemens Angioskop-N, Philips biplane Polydiagnost-I)
- Acceptance of CT-guided stereotaxis with the development of improved frames (e.g., Lexsell's, Brown, Roberts, Wells) and even a therapeutic scanner

The advances have been particularly significant in two fields.

Digital Angiography. Intravenous injection was originally promoted as the great advantage of this method, but arterial injections using only fractions (e.g., 10%–20%) of the standard amounts of iodinated 60% contrast material diluted to 1/10–1/5 (6%–12%) strength have been shown to provide excellent images with truly minimal or even undetectable morbidity (Figs. 1–3).

Magnetic Resonance. Imaging of the brain by this technique is essentially unaffected by motion and dense bone. "Hounsfield artifacts," which characteristically degraded the imaging of the posterior fossa to a great extent, no longer pose problems (Fig. 4).

Shielding is projected to be the major problem area for NMR installations in the near future. As larger magnets are used, separate buildings will be needed to provide adequate shielding, because of the effect of external influences on the homogeneity of the magnetic field. This may therefore significantly reduce the number of NMR scanners per installation and militate for the continued use of several CT scanners. The use of NMR will depend on whether imaging analysis or spectrometric analysis, is considered more desirable.

* The authors wish to thank Dr. Manfred Pfeiler and Mr. K. von Bünnau of Siemens A.G. and Mr. John S. Carey, Jr. of Siemens Corporation for their assistance in obtaining the NMR images

Radiology Today 2. Ed. by F. H. W. Heuck and M. W. Donner

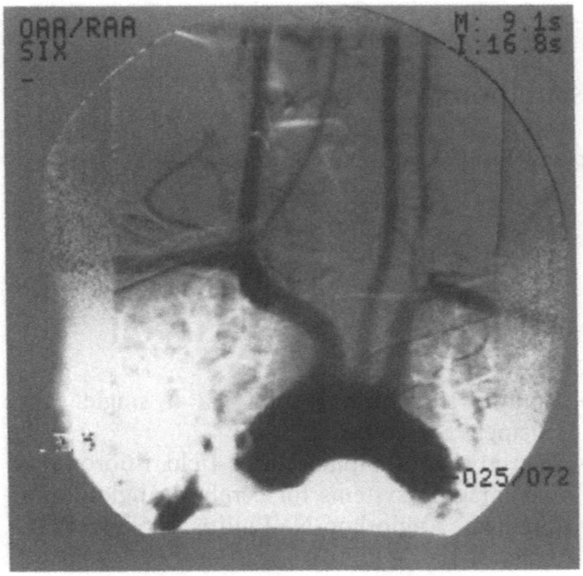

Fig. 1. Intravenous digital angiography. Normal aortic arch study, reversed gray scale, 6F pintail catheter positioned in inferior vena cava. Injection rate: 15 ml/s for 30 cc total volume Hypaque (meglumine) 75%

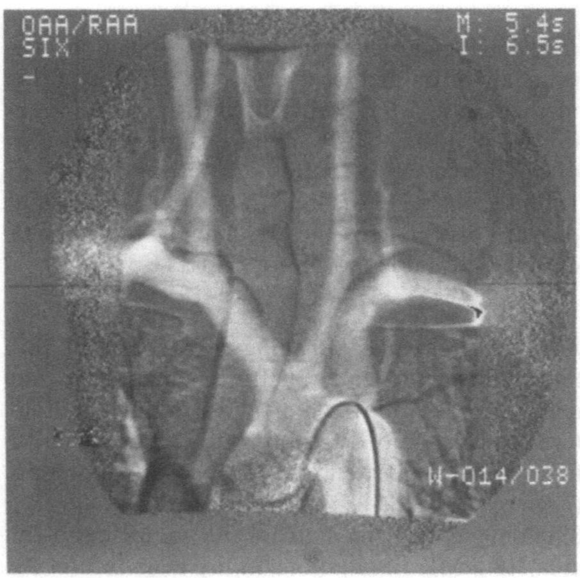

Fig. 2. Intravenous digital angiography. Normal aortic arch study, common anatomic variant. The left common carotid artery arises from the innominate artery

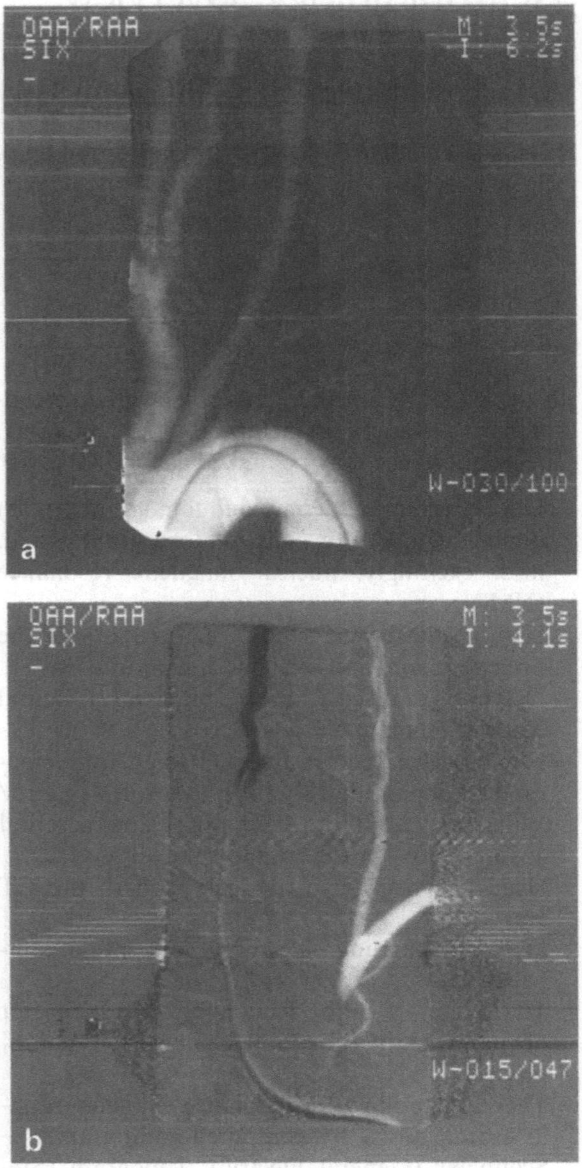

Fig. 3 a, b. Left subclavian artery occlusion. **a** Intravenous digital angiography. Transfemoral inferior vena cava injection results in opacification of the aortic arch, showing occlusion of the subclavian artery just distal to its origin. Injection volume: 30 cc delivered in 2 s. **b** Intra-arterial digital angiography. Transfemoral catheterization of the right vertebral artery (*black vessel*) shows reflux down the left vertebral artery and demonstrates the superior aspect of the occluded left subclavian artery and its more distal portion

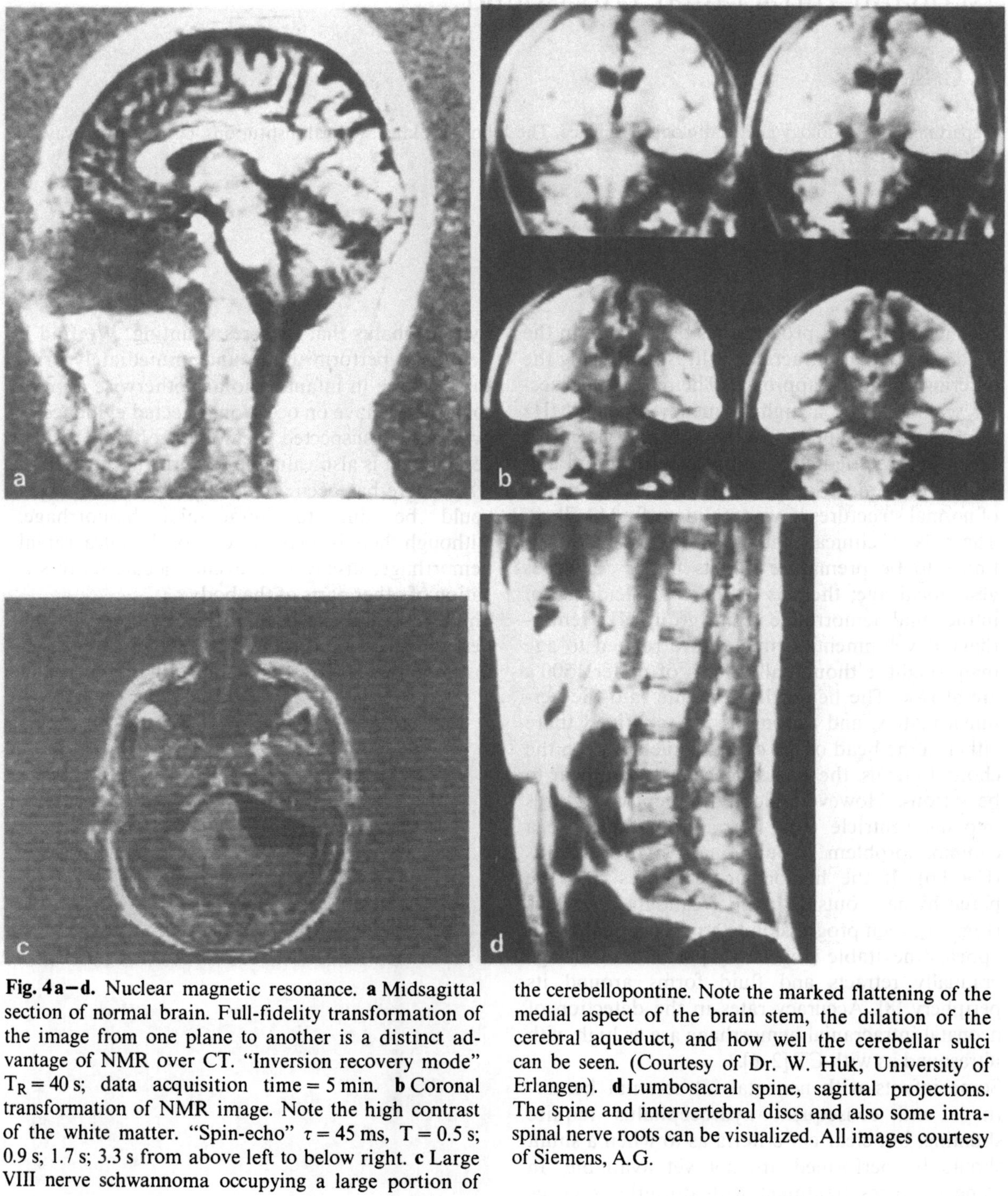

Fig. 4a–d. Nuclear magnetic resonance. **a** Midsagittal section of normal brain. Full-fidelity transformation of the image from one plane to another is a distinct advantage of NMR over CT. "Inversion recovery mode" $T_R = 40$ s; data acquisition time = 5 min. **b** Coronal transformation of NMR image. Note the high contrast of the white matter. "Spin-echo" $\tau = 45$ ms, T = 0.5 s; 0.9 s; 1.7 s; 3.3 s from above left to below right. **c** Large VIII nerve schwannoma occupying a large portion of the cerebellopontine. Note the marked flattening of the medial aspect of the brain stem, the dilation of the cerebral aqueduct, and how well the cerebellar sulci can be seen. (Courtesy of Dr. W. Huk, University of Erlangen). **d** Lumbosacral spine, sagittal projections. The spine and intervertebral discs and also some intraspinal nerve roots can be visualized. All images courtesy of Siemens, A.G.

Neonatal Intracranial Ultrasound

R. C. Sanders

Department of Radiology and Radiological Science, The Johns Hopkins Medical Institutions, 601 N. Broadway, Baltimore, MD 21205, USA

Further significant progress has been made in the field of neonatal intracranial ultrasound using the anterior fontanelle approach. The mechanical sector scanner using a high-frequency 5- or 7-MHz transducer continues to be the optimal system for this area. Detailed correlations of ultrasound and pathological material have been made. A number of normal structures have been identified [3, 7].

The bulk of clinical material in the neonate continues to be premature infants under 32 weeks gestational age; there is about 40% incidence of intracranial hemorrhage in this group [4]. Hemorrhage development is much more related to age than weight, although all infants of under 1500 g are at risk. The hemorrhage occurs into the germinal matrix, and as long as it is confined there either in the head of the caudate nucleus or in the choroid plexus, the consequence do not appear to be serious. However, blood frequently ruptures into the ventricle (Fig. 1a), and in that case a common problem is subsequent hydrocephalus (Fig. 1b). If the hemorrhage ruptures into the parenchyma outside the caudate nucleus (Fig. 2a), then progression to a porencephalic cyst appears inevitable (Fig. 2b) [5]. The hemorrhage gradually retracts and fluid forms around its periphery [8]. Accuracy rates in the detection of neonatal intracranial hemorrhage are as high with ultrasound as with CT [2, 6].

Some infants with neonatal intracranial hemorrhage and consequent hydrocephalus require shunting, but clear-cut criteria as to when a shunt should be performed are not yet available. In some instances treatment with diuretics such as Diamox or with "benign neglect" is sufficient. It is not clear how frequently ultrasound needs to be performed.

Hemorrhage usually develop within the first 72 hours of life so the initial ultrasound examination should be performed after this date. If a hemorrhage is discovered, it would appear that examinations at weekly intervals are sufficient to detect hydrocephalus that requires shunting. We find it helpful to perform ultrasound immediately prior to discharge in infants who are otherwise asymptomatic; we have on occasion detected evidence of previous unsuspected hemorrhage and hydrocephalus. It is also valuable to perform ultrasound when there has been a clinical catastrophe which could be due to intracranial hemorrhage. Although there is no treatment for the intracranial hemorrhage, discovery prevents needless investigation of other parts of the body.

Shunt insertion can be significantly aided by the performance of ultrasound [9]. Operative shunt insertion under ultrasound control has shown that

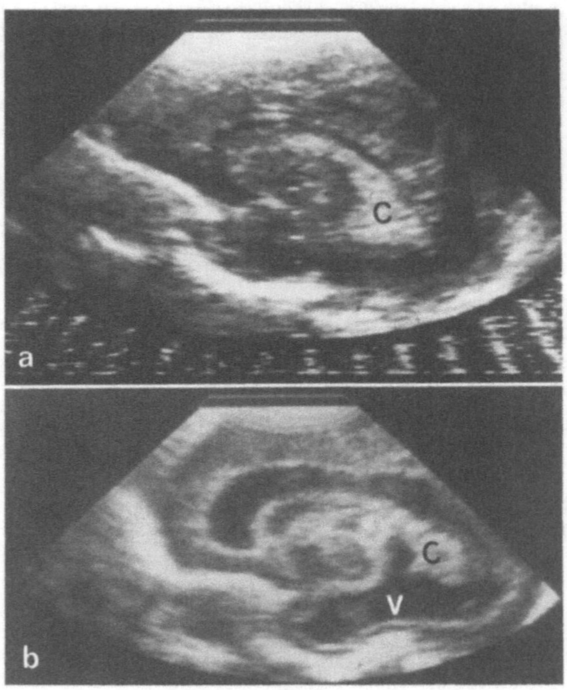

Fig. 1. a Sagittal section of the left ventricle, showing the ventricle entirely filled with echogenic clot (*C*). **b** The clot (*C*) has contracted and the ventricle (*V*) has expanded after a weeks delay

Radiology Today 2. Ed. by F. H. W. Heuck and M. W. Donner

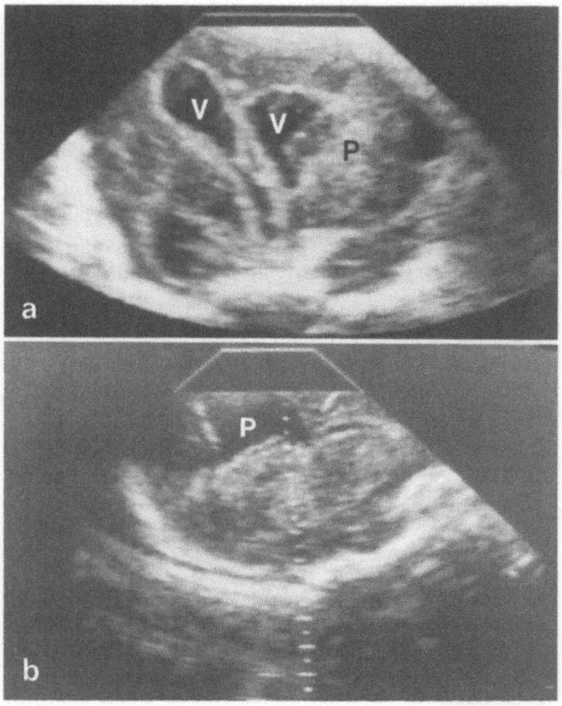

Fig. 2. **a** Coronal section showing ventricular enlargement (*V*). An echogenic parenchymal hemorrhage (*P*) is present. There is midline shift. **b** A porencephalic cyst (*P*) developed at the site of the hemorrhage over the course of the next month. Sagittal section through the left ventricle

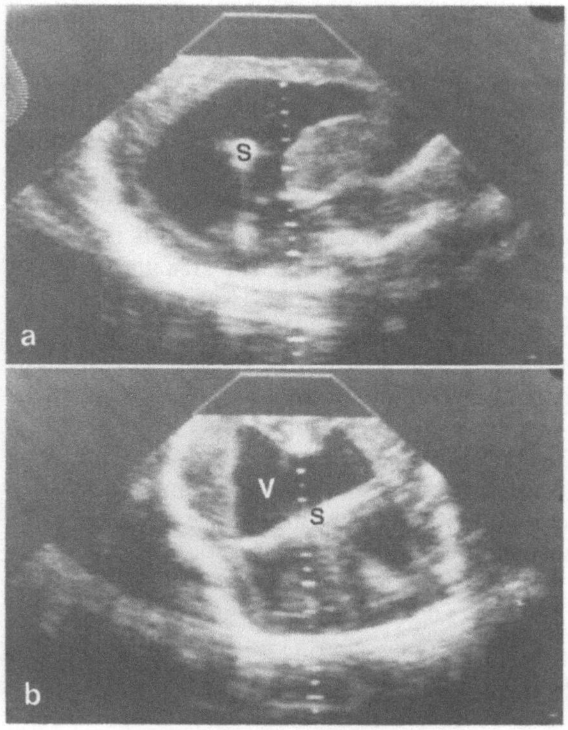

Fig. 3. **a** Sagittal section through a hydrocephalic ventricle with a shunt (*S*). **b** Coronal section at the arterial level, showing the shunt (*S*) crossing the dilated ventricle (*V*)

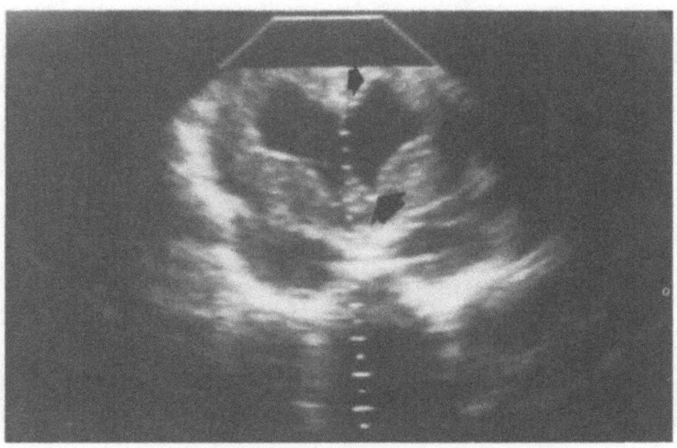

Fig. 4. Child with Arnold-Chiari malformation. Note the superior and inferior tenting of the ventricles (*arrows*)

shunts are frequently placed within the choroid plexus or in the parenchyma. The ideal site for a shunt is thought to be in the anterior horn. Guidance into this horn can be performed with ultrasound control. It is not uncommon to see shunts placed without ultrasound control which drain only one ventricle or are embedded in brain parenchyma (Fig. 3). Such complications can easily be detected with ultrasound.

A number of congenital anomalies have been detected and reported with neonatal intracranial ultrasound [1]. Many examples have been seen of the Arnold-Chiari malformation (Fig. 4), in which several typical ultrasound features have been described. These include partial absence of the septum pellucidum, tenting of the superior and inferior aspects of the lateral ventricles, a large massa intermedia, and decreases in cerebellar size and in the area below the tentorium. There is often asymmetry of the lateral ventricles.

Another cause of hydrocephalus, which can be difficult to identify, is the Dandy-Walker syndrome. In this syndrome a large posteriorly located cystic area is seen in the region where the cerebellum should be and is thought to represent enlargement of the fourth ventricle. There is usually secondary lateral ventricular hydrocephalus, and the third ventricle is enlarged.

A condition which can be mistaken for the Dandy-Walker syndrome is vein of Galen aneurysm. The vein enlarges and is located in the midline immediately posterior to the lateral ventricles, which usually show some secondary hydrocephalus, and superior to the tentorium. The condition is associated with heart failure because a large AV shunt occurs.

Holoprosencephaly is another condition which has been recognized several times on ultrasound. There is a common central ventricle replacing the lateral ventricles. Considerable distortion of the brain parenchyma, takes place but this is not recognizable with ultrasound. The size and shape of the area of holoprosencephaly varies.

Porencephalic cysts have been seen in the absence of intracranial hemorrhage in the neonate. It is thought that they probably represent a consequence of in utero hemorrhage.

Tumors in this age-group are very rare, but have been seen, notably in the cerebellum, and have an acoustic texture quite different from that of the surrounding brain parenchyma.

References

1. Babcock DS (1981) Cranial ultrasonography of infants. Williams & Wilkins, Baltimore
2. Babcock DS, Han BK (1981) The accuracy of high resolution, real-time ultrasonography of the head in infancy. Radiology 139:665–676
3. Fiske CE, Filly RA, Callen PW (1981) The normal choroid plexus: ultrasonographic appearance of the neonatal head. Radiology 141:467–471
4. Grant EG, Borts FT, Schellinger D, McCullough DC, Sivasubramanian KN, Smith Y (1981) Real-time ultrasonography of neonatal intraventricular hemorrhage and comparison with computed tomography. Radiology 139:687–691
5. Grant EG, Kerner M, Schellinger D, et al. (1982) Evolution of porencephalic cysts from intraparenchymal hemorrhage in neonates: sonographic evidence. AJNR 3:47–50
6. Johnson ML, Rumack CM, Mannes EJ, Appareti KE (1981) Detection of neonatal intracranial hemorrhage utilizing real-time and static ultrasound. J Clin Ultrasound 9:427–433
7. Pigadas A, Thompson JR, Grube GL (1981) Normal infant brain anatomy: correlated real-time sonograms and brain specimens. AJR 137:815–820
8. Slovis T (1982) Neonatal intracranial ultrasound. In: Roger C. Sanders (ed) Ultrasound annual. Raven, New York
9. Skolnick A, McLone DG (1982) Intra-operative real-time ultrasonic guidance of intracranial shunt tube placement in infants. Radiology 144:573–576

Computed Tomography in Spinal Disease: Overview

K. Sartor

Washington University School of Medicine, Mallinckrodt Institute of Radiology, 510 South Kingshighway, St. Louis, MO 63110, USA

Development

Historically, computed tomography (CT) of the juxtaspinal structures, vertebral column, and intraspinal soft tissues (spinal CT) has evolved from CT of the cranium. The first pertinent paper – on CT in syringomyelia – was published by Di Chiro et al. [14] as early as January 1975. The equipment used, the ACTA scanner, had a wide aperture and a tiltable gantry and permitted the examination of virtually every part of the body, as interposition of absorption-equilibrating water was unnecessary. Shortly thereafter, further clinical results were communicated from the same group [23]. Because of the poor resolution of the early whole-body machines, however, spinal CT remained limited to the visualization of rather gross lesions. Scanning times were also unduly long, and level localization presented a problem. Only with the advent of third- and fourth-generation CT scanners were these initial difficulties overcome. Nevertheless, spinal CT is still far from being as established a procedure as cranial CT, though the end of its development has not yet been reached.

Methodology

Like any other neuroradiological procedure, spinal CT has to be tailored to the individual diagnostic problem. However, the absence of "routine" procedures should not impede the standardization of examination techniques where this is feasible and useful.

Scanning and Imaging

At present, most diagnoses are carried out with section thicknesses of between 4 and 8 mm. In special situations and when reformatting of the image data is required in coronal, sagittal, oblique, or "subaxial" planes, scanning with thinner sections may be advisible. The time involved with the latter methods has led several authors to successfully try direct coronal CT of the spine in children [24] as well as adults [48]. The selection of scanning levels and optimal gantry angulation for standard axial transverse CT studies no longer presents a problem since it is done by means of digital radiographs produced with the scanner and displayed on the monitor. Major hard- and software developments have made measurements of all kinds easier and more reliable. Following the introduction of high-resolution CT of the cervical spine and spinal cord by Ethier et al. [17], significant further progress has also been made in noninvasive imaging of lower parts of the spine and its contents [20, 32, 46]. Careful adjustment to allow for variations in physical factors among individual patients and regions to be studied are of utmost importance when high-quality scans are to be obtained. Short scanning times have eliminated most of the artifacts caused by biologic motion. Sedation or general anesthesia are only rarely necessary, and this also holds true for suppression of intestinal peristalsis by glucagon or similarly acting pharmacologic substances. Patient positioning is important also: The necessity to change constantly the gantry angulation in order to produce correct transverse cuts is reduced by straightening of the spinal region of interest prior to scanning. Straightening of the thoracic spine is unfortunately rather limited. Displacement of the examination table should be in one direction only and with precise increments. To keep the radiation dose of the patient to a minimum, excess overlapping of tomographic slices has to be avoided.

Contrast Enhancement

There are two major modes of creating diagnostically favorable changes in relative tissue density.

Radiology Today 2. Ed. by F. H. W. Heuck and M. W. Donner

Intrathecal enhancement, developed by Di Chiro and Schellinger [13], leads to better delineation of cord, nerve roots, and other normal or pathologic intraspinal structures surrounded/bordered by CSF. Usually, the necessary application of a suitable watersoluble contrast medium (Metrizamide, Iopamidol) is done by the lumbar route. The dose needed for adequately increasing the density of the subarachnoid space rarely exceeds half of the amount that would be used for conventional myelography. In most situations, solutions at or close to isotonicity (170 mg I/ml), known to cause least morbidity, are sufficient. The distribution of the contrast medium in the spinal canal can be promoted by placing the patient in the head-down position for a short period of time [42], or may be left entirely to CSF dynamics [13]. Spinal scanning performed after opacification of the subarachnoid space in this way is called "primary CT myelography," whereas "secondary CT myelography" denotes scanning after the completion of conventional filming (supplementary study, [42]. Therefore, secondary CT myelography, albeit very informative when used selectively (third plane), is associated with the higher morbidity of conventional myelography.

Intravenous enhancement, on the other hand, again developed by Di Chiro et al. [15], improves the visualization of vascular tissue in general. The higher the blood iodine level in the region of interest, the better the structures (normal or abnormal) with prominent vascularity can be differentiated from structures with less vascularity. This is the reason why bolus injections of contrast medium immediately prior to scans may give the best results. Extravasation of contrast material secondary to local breakdown of the blood-neural-tissue barrier may be of diagnostic importance in certain tumors of the spinal cord and possibly in other (e.g., inflammatory) lesions as well [41].

Xenon enhancement, by inhalation [34] or contact with the spinal cord [9], has not yet obtained importance in clinical practice. Other modes of contrast enhancement have not left the experimental stage.

Clinical Results

Since the very first clinical examinations were carried out using spinal CT, it has been employed increasingly by a growing number of physicians. Meanwhile, the list of publications dealing with all aspects of the new method has reached an impressive length and is still expanding. The references given in the following passages should, therefore, be regarded as representative only.

Normal Anatomy

With regard to visualization of the *paravertebral soft tissues*, CT is superior to conventional radiography, (intravenous) contrast medium rarely being necessary. The *bony spinal canal* is also optimally shown, provided sectioning planes are precisely transverse. Noninvasive CT demonstration (i.e., by scanning without intrathecal contrast application) of the intraspinal soft tissues is still somewhat limited, however. According to Haughton and associates [20, 46], the following can presently be stated: The *dural sac*, most easily differentiated where it is surrounded by fat and connective tissue (below C2), is normally seen as a smooth, almost round structure appearing slightly more dense than CSF. The *spinal cord* also has a more or less round shape and attenuation values higher than the subarachnoid space. In the cervical region, it is seen quite well, whereas in the thoracic region – provided the technical standard is high – it is seen well in about one-third of cases, it is discernible in another third, and is not distinguishable from the other intraspinal structures in the rest. From this it follows that in a considerable number of clinical situations, intrathecal contrast enhancement is still unavoidable. Differentiation of gray and white matter, which is now always possible on high quality brain scans, has yet to be achieved. Intrathecal enhancement is also necessary when the *nerve roots* are to be demonstrated. The *root sleeves* can be readily distinguished from the surrounding epidural fat on plain scans, particularly in the lumbar region. The *ganglion of the spinal nerve* is also visible as an enlargement in the lateral root sheath (just outside the neural foramen). Of the larger *intraspinal vessels*, only the vertebral arteries (in the uppermost cervical canal) can be regularly seen, especially on intravenously enhanced scans. The *spinal ligaments* can be best recognized as separate structures where they have considerable thickness (like the ligamenta flava in the lumbar region) or where they are surrounded by fatty tissue (like the inter- and supraspinous ligaments). The *intervertebral disk* is well demonstrated as long as partial volume averaging with the adjacent bony endplates is avoided by a proper selection of scanning angle and section thickness. The posterior margin of the normal disk is slightly concave. Important papers on the (CT myelographic) morphology of the normal spinal cord in infants, children, and adults including linear measurements have been published by Thijssen et al. [47] and Resjö et al. [37]. Recently, Raskin [35] has shown that in selected cases, the lumbar nerve roots can be demonstrated by unenhanced CT on axial as well as reformatted oblique images.

Developmental Disorders

One of the earliest publications on the use of CT in spinal disease dealt with diastematomyelia. Weinstein et al. [50] were able to show all the vertebral anomalies associated with this dysrhaphic disease. They found that the cross-sectional (nonenhanced) images obtained were much more informative than conventional radiographs, particularly in demonstrating the – bony or fibrous – midline septum, which is a pathognomonic symptom of the disease. Since then, numerous articles on CT in developmental disorders have appeared in the literature. In large centers, CT has become the major examination modality in the roentgendiagnostic workup of children with spinal dysrhaphism of any kind, including the low medullary conus syndrome as well as congenital intra- and paraspinal masses, such as neurenteric cysts, dermoid cysts, teratomas, and lipomas [36, 38]. Primary CT myelography with very little contrast medium may be the method that still gives the best results on a routine basis, but if high-quality scanning equipment is available noninvasive CT should be tried first. Not infrequently, proceeding in this way yields enough information and spares the young patient the lumbar puncture. Arredondo et al. [2] were able to define subtle but characteristic differences in the hemicords in diastematomyelia and diplomyelia without the use of intrathecal enhancement. Developmental stenosis of the spinal canal has become another important diagnostic field for CT, particularly since measurements of the various diameters have gained more reliability. The interest has focused more or less on the lumbar region [49].

Traumatic Disorders

Since initial reports on its use in the diagnosis of atlas fractures [25] and traumatic narrowing of the dorsolumbar spinal canal secondary to fragment displacement [12], CT has gained wide acceptance as a valuable diagnostic tool in trauma to the spinal column. More recently, injuries to the intraspinal soft tissues including epidural hematomas have also been shown [11, 16, 39]. Of the bony structures that can be far better evaluated by CT than by conventional radiography, the neural arch has to be mentioned first [11, 39]. This is of particular importance in the cervical region where the arch is the most frequently fractured vertebral element of all (Fig. 1). Fractures possibly involving the articular processes or compression injuries with multiple vertical fracture lines in the vertebral bodies are also good indications for CT [31, 45]. Any narrowing of the spinal canal is easily detected, and small fragments not seen on conventional films may be found [11, 39]. Dural tears may be demonstrated by CT myelography [7]. Rupture of ligaments is usually better recognized on conventional (functional) studies. To demonstrate fracture lines running more or less horizontally (transversely), lateral, coronal, or other image reformation can be indispensable. Paravertebral hematomas of sufficient size are usually not very difficult to diagnose, which is also true of injuries of other structures adjacent to the spine.

Neoplastic Disorders

When an intraspinal tumor is suspected, the signs to look for on nonenhanced CT scans are deformation/displacement of the cord/nerve roots,

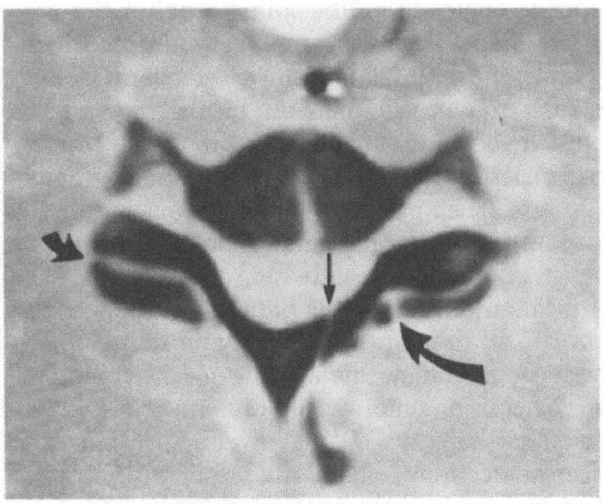

Fig. 1. Fracture of C6 with involvement of vertebral body and neural arch (*straight arrow*). *Large curved arrow* points to bony fragment probably originating from lower articular process of C5. *Small curved arrow* points to intact zygoapophyseal joint on opposite side. Density posterior to arch represents lowermost portion of spinous process of C5 (no fragment!) (Courtesy of Dr. Rath, Munich)

locally abnormal densities, and changes in width/shape of the vertebral canal. Intravenous enhancement may be of value because many lesions are quite vascular. Of the intramedullary masses, the ones in the cervical region pose the least problems, as narrowing of the subarachnoid "ring" can be far better discerned here than in the thoracic region. If the question "tumor vs. syringo(hydro)myelia" arises, the differentiation can usually be made. For the demonstration of thoracic and thoracolumbar cord masses, intrathecal enhancement is still the better choice in most instances [38]. The recognition of regressive changes within the neoplastic tissue, e.g., calcification or cyst formation, is largely possible at all levels. The same applies to fat as a component of certain congenital masses [40]. Extramedullary-intradural masses, mostly neurinomas and meningiomas, fortunately often have features that make them recognizable, for instance, meningiomas may be of the psammomatous type, therefore containing considerable amounts of calcium (Fig. 2). Other tumors are vascular and become readily visible on intravenous enhancement. Frequently, the masses are well circumscribed, and their topographic relationship to the spinal cord is obvious. When this is not the case, intrathecal enhancement may clarify the point [4, 33, 38, 40, 42, 44]. Among the extradural spinal tumors, the ones originating from the vertebral column and featuring primarily bony changes are not difficult to diagnose. CT may be very important in lesions that are prone to encroach on the spinal canal or the neural foramina, such as giant cell tumors, aneurysmal bone cysts, chondromas, osteochondromas, osteoblastomas, osteomas. In masses with a combined involvement of bone and intra- and/or extraspinal soft tissue, CT may also be extremely valuable. This applies to benign lesions with bony erosion, e.g., hourglass neurinomas, as well as malignant processes with bony destruction. The delineation of the borders between neoplastic and normal soft tissue can frequently be improved by intravenous enhancement. The paravertebral tumor extension is most easily discerned in the thoracic region [3, 29, 33]. CT myelography may be necessary to show reliably the presence or absence of intraspinal extension in tumors of paravertebral origin (Resjö et al. 1979). In patients with lumbosacral radiculopathy and a normal or atypically pathologic myelogram, CT should be the next diagnostic step: Not infrequently, neoplastic processes (often malignant) are found unsuspectedly, or neoplastic masses that have already been recognized can be better judged with regard to their involvement with the spine, the sacrum, and the paravertebral/presacral soft tissue [18, 22, 53]. CT may also be used to guide biopsy of the spine in tumors and various other diseases [1].

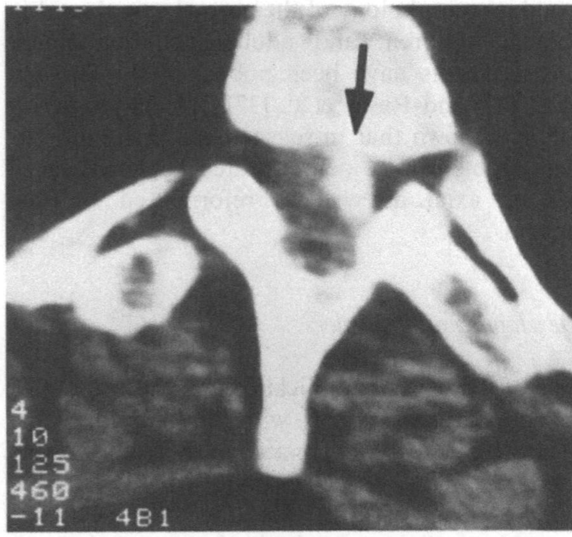

Fig. 2. Psammomatous thoracic meningioma. *Arrow* points to massive calcification within spinal canal. Plain scan (Courtesy of Prof. Kühne, Essen)

Inflammatory Disorders

Experience with CT in myelitis of any kind is still very limited, there being only a few cases – with questionable findings – documented in the literature [10, 41]. Much better established is the role of CT as a useful diagnostic method in infections involving the meninges, the epidural space, the vertebral column, and the paravertebral soft tissues [23, 28, 41]. Of particular importance is the possibility of early recognition of primary or postoperative disk-space infection. Paravertebral abscess formation may, however, mimic neoplastic processes with central necrosis (and vice versa), and therefore should be diagnosed by clinical correlation only. CT has also been used effectively in selected cases of spinal disease of rheumatic origin [26, 41].

Degenerative Disorders

Atrophic changes of the spinal cord are associated with corresponding (localized or generalized) widening of the subarachnoid space. In the cervical region, the diagnosis can usually be made without any contrast application. In the clinically less important thoracic region, the demonstration of a thin cord may be possible only after intrathecal enhancement. Calcification of the posterior longitudinal ligament with its inherent danger of compressive myelopathy is another disease in which CT can be of great diagnostic importance; it is still relatively rarely seen in whites [30] (Fig. 3). The greatest field of application of CT, however, is in disorders associated with degenerative changes of the vertebrae (including apophyseal joints) and intervertebral disks. The aim is either to supplement conventional radiography (third plane), or reduce the number of invasive procedures, particularly myelography. For instance, CT may be used to evaluate the exact topography of cervical spondylophytes dangerously narrowing the spinal canal or neural foramina [41]. It may also be of assistance in the examination of the lateral (lumbar) recesses encroached upon by hypertrophic intervertebral joints or other degenerative changes [27]. Since promising early reports [52], CT has been increasingly successful in the noninvasive diagnosis of herniated lumbar disks and may, provided expert examination techniques and image interpretation are employed, replace myelography in many, if not the majority, of cases [8, 21] (Fig. 4). Herniations recurring after operation still pose serious diagnostic difficulties as the extruded disk material can be indistinguishable from scar tissue.

Miscellaneous Disorders

Apart from the above-mentioned disease groups, CT has been employed in a considerable number of other disorders, but only a few can be considered here. Since the first pertinent report by Di

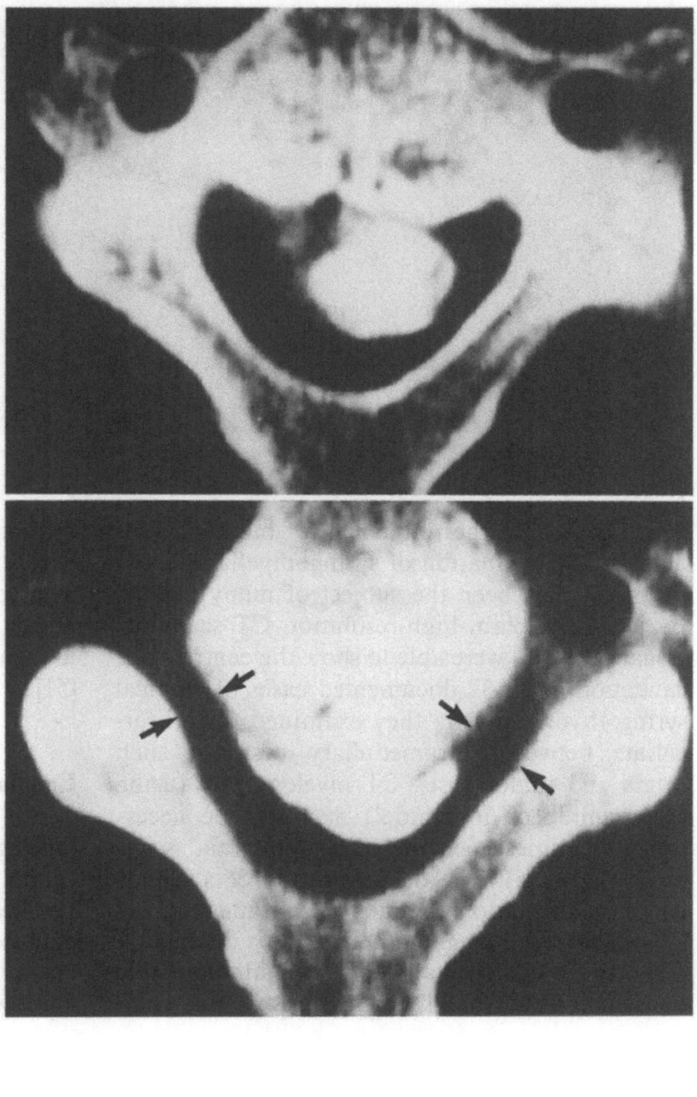

Fig. 3. Osteoma-like spondylophyte with calcification of posterior longitudinal ligament at level of C3/C4. Marked narrowing of spinal canal without significant encroachment on intervertebral canals (*bottom, arrows*)

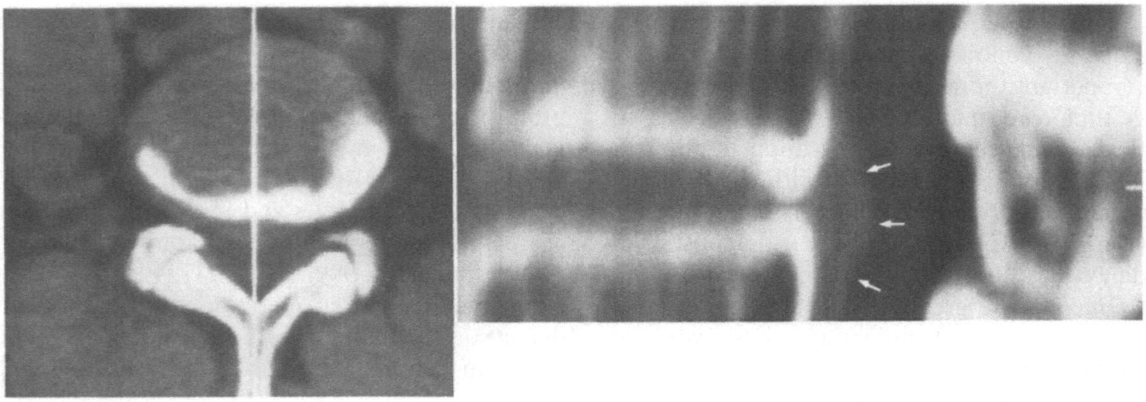

Fig. 4. Medial herniation of L3/L4 intervertebral disk. Axial view (*top*) showing focal dorsal displacement of disk margin, reformatted midplane image (*bottom*) showing herniated disk material (*arrows*) at level of interspace. Plain scan (Courtesy of Prof. Kühne, Essen)

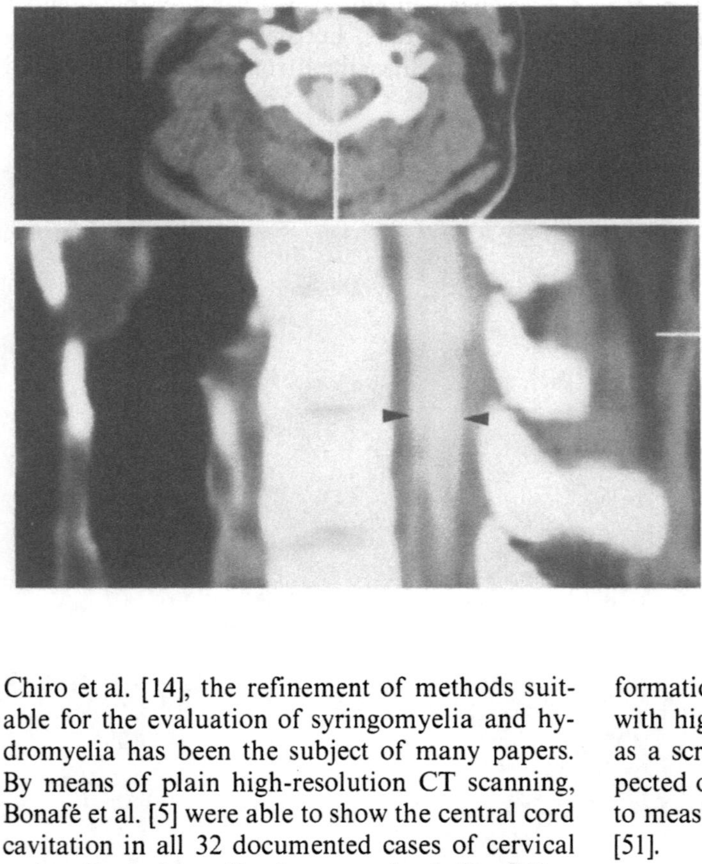

Fig. 5. Cervical hydromyelia with contrast (metrizamide)-filled cavity. Axial view (*top*) showing somewhat excentrically located "cyst;" reformatted midplane image (*bottom*) showing longitudinal extent of "cyst" (*arrowheads*) (Courtesy of Prof. Kühne, Essen)

Chiro et al. [14], the refinement of methods suitable for the evaluation of syringomyelia and hydromyelia has been the subject of many papers. By means of plain high-resolution CT scanning, Bonafé et al. [5] were able to show the central cord cavitation in all 32 documented cases of cervical syringo(hydro)-myelia they examined. To differentiate between intramedullary cysts of such origin and tumor cysts, CT myelography (using Metrizamide or Iopamidol) may still be necessary, sometimes even including sequential scanning [6] (Fig. 5). The demonstration of a Chiari type I malformation on scans at or somewhat below the foramen magnum helps in this distinction [19]. As Di Chiro et al. [15] were already able to demonstrate spinal cord arteriovenous malformations prior to the advent of fast scanners with high-resolution, CT may today be regarded as a screening procedure if such a lesion is suspected on clinical grounds. CT has also been used to measure the bone mineral content of the spine [51].

Conclusion and Outlook

During the 7 years since its first clinical application, spinal CT has gained acceptance slowly but steadily. The main attraction of this roentgendiagnostic method lies in its capacity to visualize noninvasively the intraspinal soft tissues as well as the low-density structures closely adjacent to the vertebral column. This capacity, however, depends largely on the resolution of the scanner used in the examination, and is still limited in many respects, even with the best machines. Nevertheless, spinal CT can definitely be helpful in many diagnostic situations, either as a primary or a secondary (supplementary) procedure. Fortunately, the numerically predominant degenerative disorders, particularly the ones involving the vertebral column, are accessible to plain, nonenhanced CT. The same is true of most developmental and traumatic lesions. Numerous extramedullary neoplasms, benign or malignant, are richly vascularized and, therefore, often demonstrated after intravenous enhancement. Even when CT myelography becomes necessary, the examination still remains relatively innocuous as the amount of contrast medium can be kept very low. A severe problem remains, though: As an examination of the entire spine is unrealistic in routine spinal CT, the clinician has to provide exact information regarding the level of the suspected pathology. Because this is frequently not the case (or often impossible), the radiologist is forced to examine long portions of the spine. Under such circumstances, myelography, which can be done very fast, would be preferable. For this reason, careful case selection is of the utmost importance; patients with nonspecific neurologic symptomatology and patients with multilevel lesions are usually not suitable candidates for spinal CT. What might the future development of spinal CT bring? Some improvement in intraspinal contrast resolution can be awaited from the new scanners, that are being developed and the capacity to distinguish gray and white matter of the cord might be achieved in the not too distant future. A major breakthrough comparable to the introduction of fast-rotate-only scanners with high spatial and contrast resolution, is not very likely. Rather more likely, however, is competition with nuclear magnetic resonance.

References

1. Adapon BD, Legada BD, Lim EVA, Silao JV, Dalmacio-Cruz A (1981) CT-guided closed biopsy of the spine. J Comput Assist Tomogr 5:73–78
2. Arredondo F, Haughton VM, Hemmy DC, Zelaya B, Williams AL (1980) The computed tomographic appearance of the spinal cord in diastematomyelia. Radiology 136:685–688
3. Balériaux-Waha D, Terwinghe G, Jeanmart L (1977) The value of computed tomography for the diagnosis of hourglass tumors of the spine. Neuroradiology 14:31–32
4. Böker DK, Sartor K (1981) Computed tomography in tumors of the spinal region. Adv Neurosurg 9:467–473
5. Bonafé A, Ethier R, Melançon D, Bélanger G, Peters T (1980) High resolution computed tomography in cervical syringomyelia. J Comput Assist Tomogr 4:42–47
6. Bonafé A, Manelfe C, Espagno J, Guiraud B, Rascol A (1980) Evaluation of syringomyelia with metrizamide computed tomographic myelography. J Comput Assist Tomogr 4:797–802
7. Brant-Zawadzki M, Jeffrey RB, Minagi H, Pitts LH (1982) High resolution CT of thoracolumbar fractures. AJNR 3:69–74
8. Claussen C, Grumme T, Treisch J, Lochner B, Kazner E (1982) Die Diagnostik des lumbalen Bandscheibenvorfalls. Computertomographische und myelographische Ergebnisse. RöFo 136:1–8
9. Coin CG, Coin JT (1980) Contact enhancement by xenon gas in computed tomography of the spinal cord and brain: Preliminary observations. J Comput Assist Tomogr 4:217–221
10. Coin CG, Hucks-Folliss A (1979) Cervical computed tomography in multiple sclerosis with spinal cord involvement. J Comput Assist Tomogr 3:421–422
11. Coin CG, Pennink M, Ahmad WD, Keranen VJ (1979) Diving-type injury of the cervical spine: Contribution of computed tomography to management. J Comput Assist Tomogr 3:362–372
12. Colley DP, Dunsker SB (1978) Traumatic narrowing of the dorsolumbar spinal canal demonstrated by computed tomography. Radiology 129:95–98
13. Di Chiro G, Schellinger D (1976) Computed tomography of spinal cord after lumbar intrathecal introduction of metrizamide (computer assisted myelography) Radiology 120:101–104
14. Di Chiro G, Axelbaum SP, Schellinger D, Twigg HL, Ledley RS (1975) Computerized axial tomography in syringomyelia. N Engl J Med 292:13–16
15. Di Chiro G, Doppman JL, Wener L (1977) Computed tomography of spinal cord arteriovenous malformations. Radiology 123:351–354
16. Donovan Post J, Seminer DS, Quencer RM (1982) CT diagnosis of spinal epidural hematoma. AJNR 3:190–192
17. Ethier R, King DG, Melançon D, Bélanger G, Taylor S, Thompson C (1979) Development of high resolution computed tomography of the spinal cord. J Comput Assist Tomogr 3:433–438
18. Federle MP, Moss AA, Margolin FR (1980) Role of computed tomography in patients with "sciatica". J Comput Assist Tomogr 4:335–341
19. Forbes WS, Isherwood I (1978) Computed tomography in syringomyelia and the associated Arnold-Chiari Type I malformation. Neuroradiology 15:73–78
20. Haughton VM, Svertsen A, Williams AL (1980) Soft tissue anatomy within the spinal canal as seen on computed tomography. Radiology 134:649–655

21. Haughton VM, Eldevik OP, Magnaes B, Amundsen P (1982) A prospective comparison of computed tomography and myelography in the diagnosis of herniated lumbar disks. Radiology 142:103–110
22. Heller M, Grabbe E, Hagemann J, Jend HH (1981) Computertomographische Befunde bei Kreuzbeindestruktionen. Computertomographie 1:74–79
23. Hübener KH, Schmitt WGH (1979) Die computertomographische Diagnostik von Abszeßbildungen. RoFo 130:53–57
24. Kaiser MC, Pettersson H, Harwood-Nash DC, Fitz CR, Armstrong E (1981) Direct coronal CT of the spine in infants and children. AJNR 2:465–466
25. Kershner MS, Goodman GA, Perlmutter GS (1977) Computed tomography in the diagnosis of an atlas fracture. AJR 128:688–689
26. Kramer LD, Krouth GJ (1978) Computerized tomography. An adjunct to early diagnosis in the cauda equina syndrome of ankylosing spondylitis. Arch Neurol 35:116–118
27. Lackner K, Schroeder S (1980) Computertomographie der Lendenwirbelsäule. RöFo 133:124–131
28. Lee BCP, Kazam E, Newman AD (1978) Computed tomography of the spine and spinal cord. Radiology 128:95–102
29. Miller EM, Norman D (1979) The role of computed tomography in the evaluation of neck masses. Radiology 133:145–149
30. Murakami J, Russell WJ, Hayabuchi N, Kimura S (1982) Computed tomography of posterior longitudinal ligament ossification: Its appearance and diagnostic value with special reference to thoracic lesions. J Comput Assist Tomogr 6:41–50
31. Naidich TP, Pudlowski RM, Moran CJ, Gilula LA, Murphy W, Naidich JB (1979) Computed tomography of spinal fractures. Adv Neurol 22:207–252
32. Naidich TP, King DG, Moran CJ, Sagel SS (1980) Computed tomography of the lumbar thecal sac. J Comput Assist Tomogr 4:37–41
33. Nakagawa H, Huang YP, Malis LI, Wolf BS (1977) Computed tomography of intraspinal and paraspinal neoplasms. J Comput Assist Tomogr 1:377–391
34. Pullicino P, du Boulay G, Kendall BE (1979) Xenon enhancement for computed tomography of the spinal cord. Neuroradiology 18:63–66
35. Raskin SP (1981) Demonstration of nerve roots on unenhanced computed tomographic scans. J Comput Assist Tomogr 5:281–284
36. Resjö IM, Harwood-Nash DC, Fitz CR, Chuang S (1978) Computed tomographic metrizamide myelography in spinal dysraphism in infants and children. J Comput Assist Tomogr 2:549–558
37. Resjö IM, Harwood-Nash DC, Fitz CR, Chuang S (1979) Normal cords in infants and children examined with computed tomographic metrizamide myelography. Radiology 130:691–696
38. Resjö IM, Harwood-Nash DC, Fitz CR, Chuang S (1979) CT metrizamide myelography for spinal and paraspinal neoplasms in infants and children. AJR 132:367–372
39. Sartor K (1980) Computertomographie bei Verletzungen der Halswirbelsäule und der oberen Brustwirbelsäule. RöFo 132:132–138
40. Sartor K (1980) Computertomographie bei spinalen Tumoren. RöFo 132:391–398
41. Sartor K (1980) Spinale Computertomographie. Neue Perspektiven in der Diagnostik der Wirbelsäule und des Rückenmarks. Radiologe 20:485–493
42. Sartor K, Richert S (1979) Computertomographie des zervikalen Spinalkanals nach intrathekalem Enhancement: Zervikale CT-Myelographie. RöFo 130:261–269
43. Schellinger D, Di Chiro G, Axelbaum SP, Twigg HL, Ledley RS (1975) Early clinical experience with the ACTA scanner. Radiology 114:257–261
44. Spallone A, Tanfani G, Vassilouthis J, Dazzi M (1980) Benign extramedullary foramen magnum tumors: Diagnosis by computed tomography. J Comput Assist Tomogr 4:225–229
45. Steppé R, Bellemans M, Boven F, de Smedt E, Potvliege R (1981) The value of computed tomography scanning in elusive fractures of the cervical spine. Skeletal Radiol 6:175–178
46. Taylor AJ, Haughton VM, Doust BD (1980) CT imaging of the thoracic spinal cord without intrathecal contrast medium. J Comput Assist Tomogr 4:223–224
47. Thijssen HOM, Keyser A, Horstink MWM, Meijer E (1979) Morphology of the cervical spinal cord on computed myelography. Neuroradiology 18:57–62
48. Van Waes PFGM, Zonneveld FW (1982) Direct coronal body computed tomography. J Comput Assist Tomogr 6:58–66
49. Verbiest H (1979) The significance and principles of computerized axial tomography in idiopathic developmental stenosis of the bony lumbar vertebral canal. Spine 4:369–378
50. Weinstein MA, Rothner D, Duchesneau P, Dohn DF (1975) Computed tomography in diastematomyelia. Radiology 118:609–611
51. Weissberger MA, Zamenhof RG, Aronow S, Neer RM (1978) Computed tomography scanning for the measurement of bone mineral in the human spine. J Comput Assist Tomogr 2:253–262
52. Williams AL, Haughton VM, Syvertsen A (1980) Computed tomography in the diagnosis of herniated nucleus pulposus. Radiology 135:95–99
53. Yang WC, Zappulla R, Malis L (1981) Neurolemmoma in lumbar intervertebral foramen. J Comput Assist Tomogr 5:904–905

Nosography of Constitutional Narrowness of the Lumbar Spinal Canal

A. Wackenheim

Institut de Radiologie, Faculté de Médecine, 11, rue Humann, 67085 Strasbourg Cedex, France

We still know very little about the etiopathogeny of narrowness of the lumbar spinal canal. To a certain extent, however, radiopediatric data can contribute to a better understanding of the mechanisms involved. According to Maroteaux's studies, we may distinguish two main groups of constitutional bone disease: (1) diseases without known pathogeny; (2) diseases in which the pathogenic processes are more or less known, e.g., metabolic diseases, chromosome aberrations. From a very general point of view, constitutional canalar stenoses occur in diseases of the first group; their occurrence in diseases of the second group only is coincidental.

The constitutional bone diseases without known pathology are divided into two groups – osteochondrodysplasia and dysostosis. Osteochondrodysplasia is a generalized disturbance of bone and cartilage growth, whereas dysostosis is a malformation of a single or of several bones. In the present study, we consider the canalar stenosis as the main anomaly and analyze its distribution in osteochondrodysplasia and dysostosis.

Osteochondrodysplasia

Achondroplasia and its related diseases comprise a more or less marked stenosis of the lumbar spinal canal. The presence of such a lumbar canalar stenosis may be expected in cases of osteochondrodysplasia associated with micromelia, i.e., achondroplasia, chondrodysplasia punctata, diastrophic dysplasia, metatropic dysplasia, mesomelic dwarfism, and diverse other forms of dysplasia, such as spondyloepiphyseal dysplasia, spondyloepiphysometaphyseal dysplasia, and acrodysostosis. For spondyloepiphyseal dysplasia, the reader is referred to Megret and Marsault's contribution [1]. With regard to a transitional form, we studied the correlations between acrodysostosis and cheirolumbar dysostosis [6]. The prototype of osteochondrodysplasia with lumbar canal stenosis is, however, achondroplasia (Figs. 1, 2). In patients suffering from achondroplasia, these are extreme shortness of the predicles, anomalies of the vertebral bodies consisting of the wedging of several vertebrae, scalloping, and, above all, the progressive reduction from L1 to L5 of the interpedicular distance. The diminution of the anterior width of the spinal canal is a radiologic sign indicating achondroplasia. As a matter of fact, the other above-mentioned forms

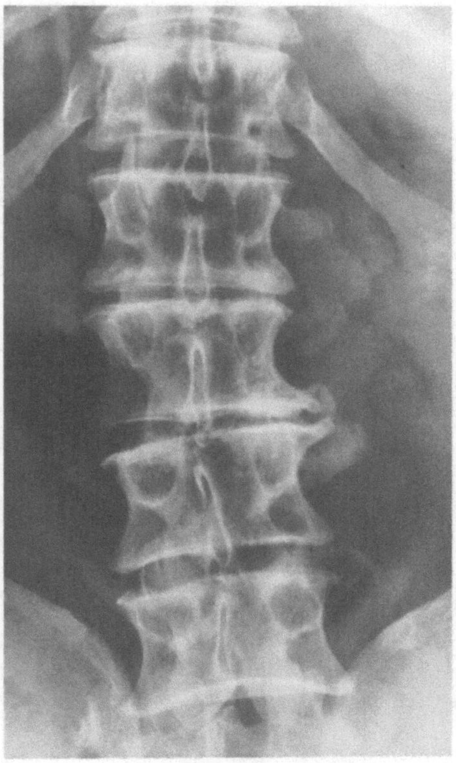

Fig. 1. Achondroplasia. Note the signs of canalar stenosis: Progressive narrowing – from T12 to L5 – of the interpedicular distance, hypertrophied pedicles, significant diminution of the posterior intervertebral spaces

Radiology Today 2. Ed. by F. H. W. Heuck and M. W. Donner

of osteochondrodysplasia may also determine canalar stenosis, but if so, this is never evident from the radiologic symptomatology and it is less often responsible for a neurologic deficit. This is true to such an extent that pseudoachondroplastic dysplasia (epiphysometaphyseal dysplasia) may be distinguished from achondroplasia by the fact that it has marked anomalies of the vertebral bodies but normal pedicles and canalar dimensions.

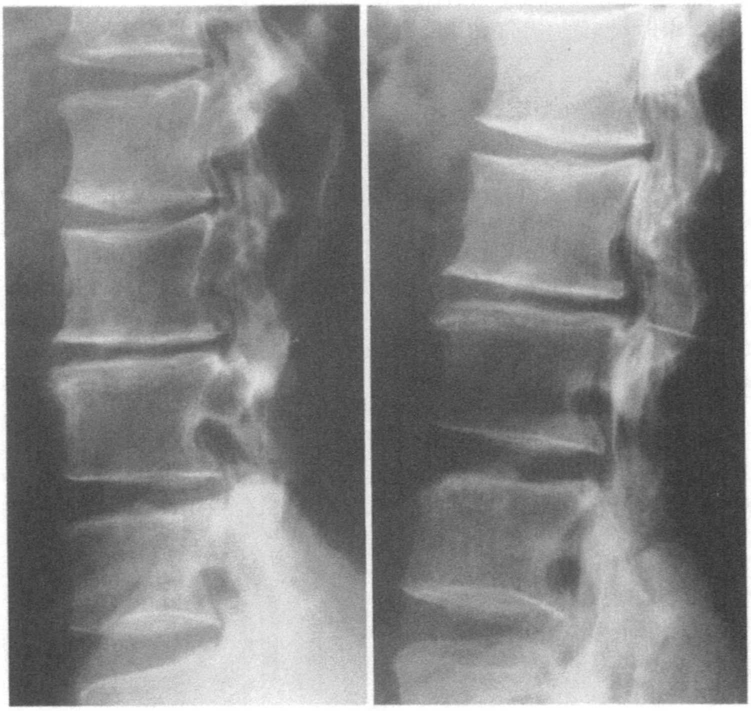

Fig. 2. Achondroplasia. Note the signs of canalar stenosis: markedly reduced AP diameter of the canal, poorly visible intervertebral foramina, radiculosaccography (*right*) very difficult to carry out, poor opacification due to the narrowness of the subarachnoidal spaces

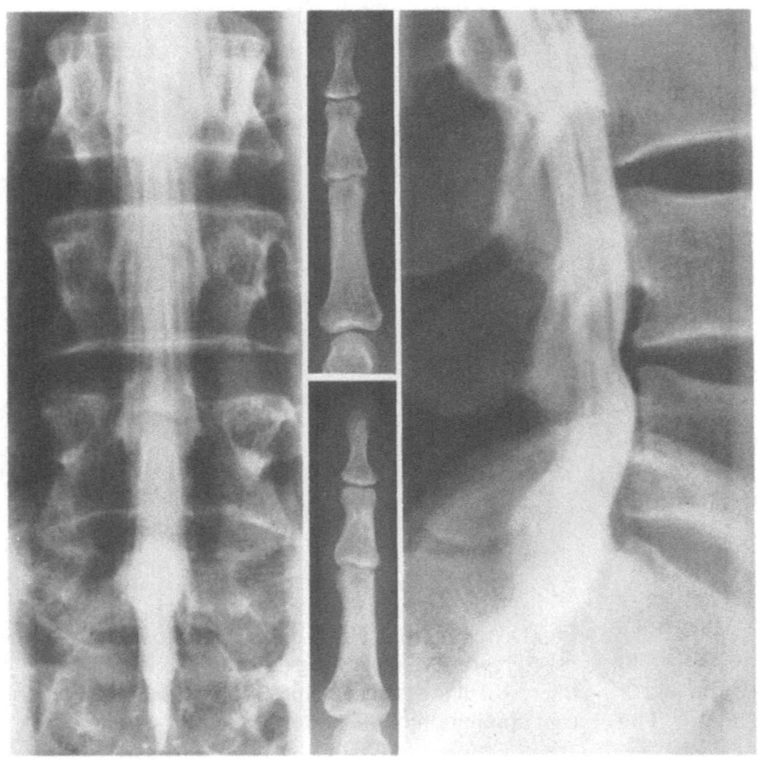

Fig. 3. Mild form of cheirolumbar dysostosis. Progressive narrowing of the lumbar spinal canal from L2 to L5; bilateral brachymesophalangia of the V

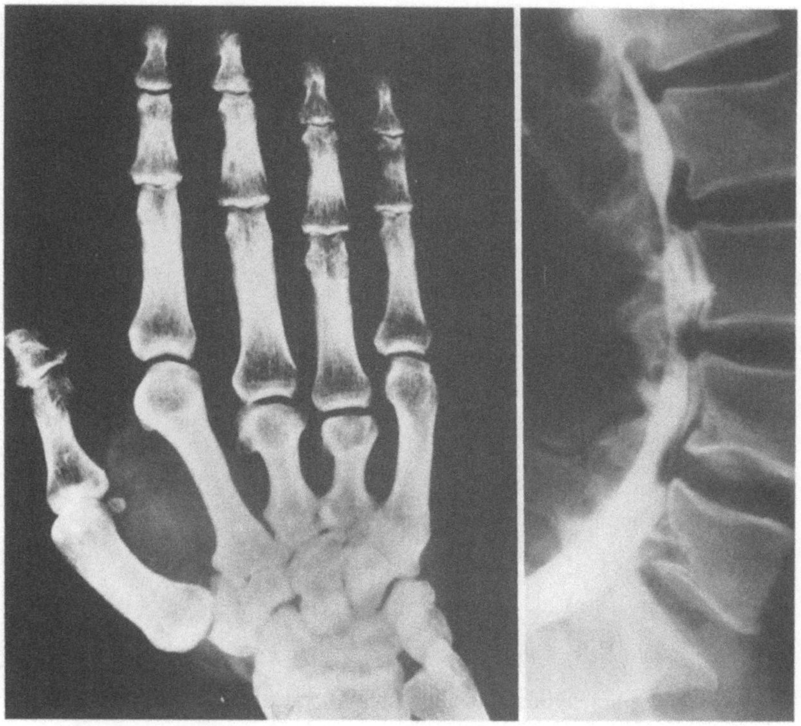

Fig. 4. Severe form of cheirolumbar dysostosis characterized by brachymetacarpia of digiti III and IV and brachytelephalangia of the thumb associated with significant narrowness of the lumbar canal

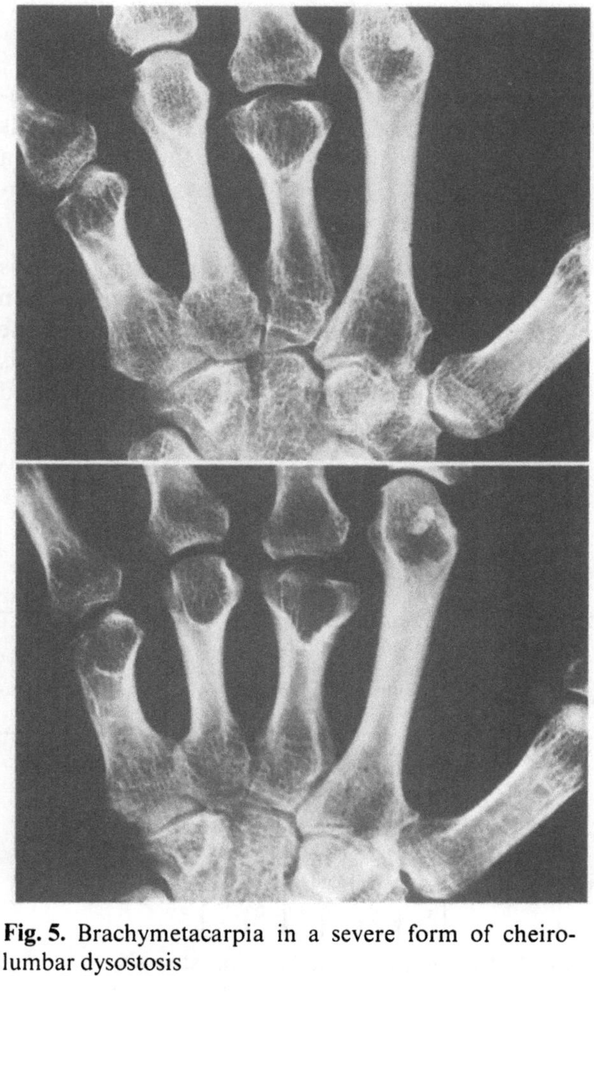

Fig. 5. Brachymetacarpia in a severe form of cheirolumbar dysostosis

Dysostosis

Two forms of dysostosis can be distinguished:

a) Isolated constitutional stenosis of the lumbar spinal canal was described by Verbiest in 1949 [2]. We do not insist on the roentgenologic symptomatology in this form of lumbar vertebral stenosis and refer the reader to Verbiest's studies and to the general review we published concerned with this question [3].
b) Constitutional stenosis associated with diverse forms of brachydactyly (brachyphalangia, brachymetacarpia) is a condition we term cheirolumbar dysostosis. Heredity factors are dominant as we were able to demonstrate in a family in which certain members had brachydactyly without lumbar canal stenosis, some members had lumbar canal stenosis without brachydactyly, and others had a cheirolumbar syndrome [4, 5]. In practice, the milder forms are common (Fig. 3), whereas severe forms are rare (Fig. 4). The involvement of the hands is marked to a greater or lesser extent according to the degree of shortening of the bones, but it is also dependent on the topographic distribution of the disturbance: involvement of one or several phalanges (Fig. 3), involvement of

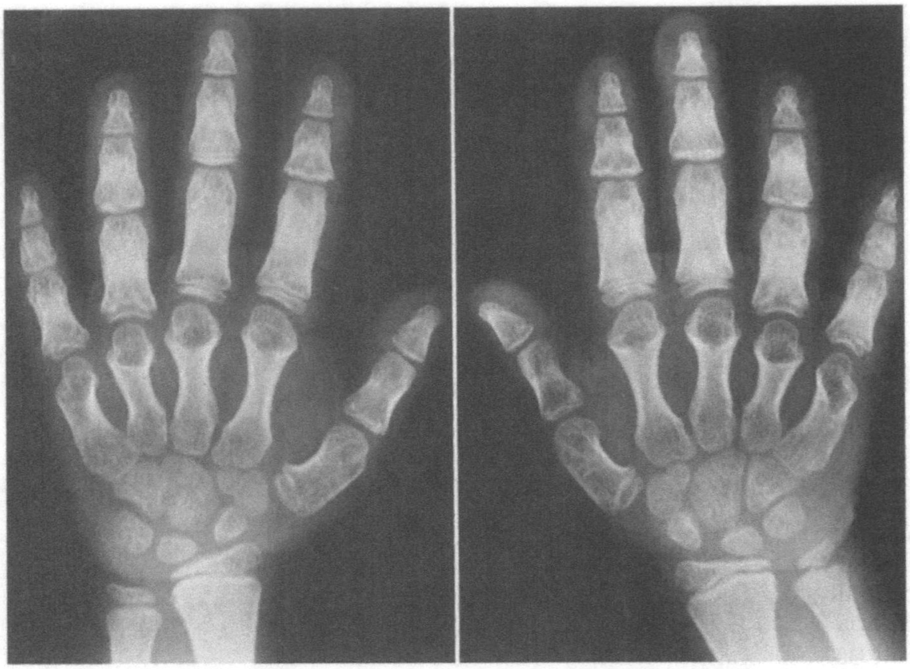

Fig. 6. Diffuse brachyphalagia and brachymetacarpia (peripheral dysostosis) in a case of cheirolumbar dysostosis

one or several metacarpals (Fig. 5), involvement of both phalanges and metacarpals (Fig. 4), or diffuse involvement producing a true peripheral dysostosis associated with lumbar canal stenosis (Fig. 6).

It should be noted that the lumbar canal stenosis is identical in Verbiest's isolated form and in cheirolumbar dysostosis. The same is true of the brachydactyly, which in cheirolumbar dysostosis has no particular form with regard to isolated brachydactyly.

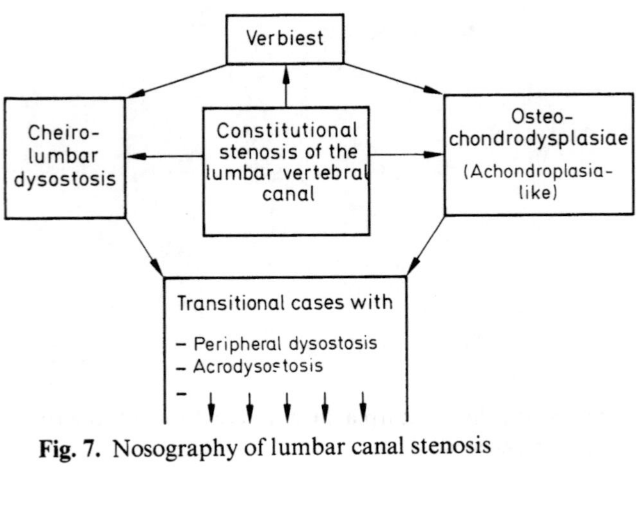

Fig. 7. Nosography of lumbar canal stenosis

Conclusion

The nosography of lumbar canal stenosis is relatively easily dealt with in light of the present state of knowledge. It may be viewed schematically as seen in Fig. 7.

References

1. Megret M, Marsault C (1980) Gas myelography in Verbiest's developmental spinal canal stenosis. In: Wackenheim A, Babin E (eds) The narrow lumbar canal. Springer, Berlin Heidelberg New York, pp 39–58
2. Verbiest H (1949) Sur certaines formes rares de compression de la queue de cheval. In: Hommage à Clovis Vincent. Maloine, Paris, 161–174
3. Verbiest H (1980) Stenosis of the bony lumbar vertebral canal. In: Wackenheim A, Babin E (eds) The narrow lumbar canal. Springer, Berlin Heidelberg New York, pp 115–146
4. Wackenheim A (1980) Cheirolumbar dysostosis. Springer, Berlin Heidelberg New York
5. Wackenheim A, Babin E (eds) 1980 The narrow lumbar canal. Springer, Berlin Heidelberg New York
6. Wackenheim A, Bourjat P, Marescaux C (1981) A transitional form of cheirolumbar dysostosis. J Belge Radiol 64:179–188

Four Malformations of the Cervico-Occipital Region

A. Wackenheim

Institut de Radiologie, Faculté de Médecine, 11, rue Humann, 67085 Strasbourg Cedex, France

This paper is a brief account of four malformations of the cervico-occipital region which we have identified and described.

Constitutional Fusion of the Anterior Arch of the Atlas with the Odontoid Process. This condition was first described in 1971 [1]. Later on we published further cases [2, 5–8, 10], including that of a child in whom it had been possible to follow up roentgenologically the progressive fusion of the anterior arch of the atlas with the odontoid process. This anomaly may exist as a simple malformation without any associated bone anomaly and without clinical symptoms, but may also be associated with other malformations. Figure 1 shows a very incomplete form of the anomaly, i.e., scalloping of the anterior aspect of the odontoid process produced by the anterior arch of the atlas. This condition corresponds to an intermediate ossification phase in the above-mentioned case [8].

Dens Tripartitus. We published the first case of dens tripartitus in 1974 [3]. We believe it to be the

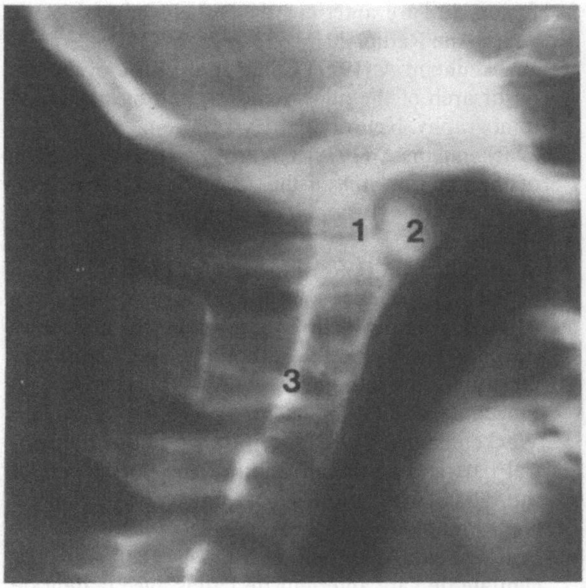

Fig. 1. Minor malformation of the cervico-occipital joint. *1,* Scalloping of the anterior aspect of the odontoid process, a minor form of C1-C2 block; *2,* Anterior arch of the atlas; *3,* C2-C3 block vertebra

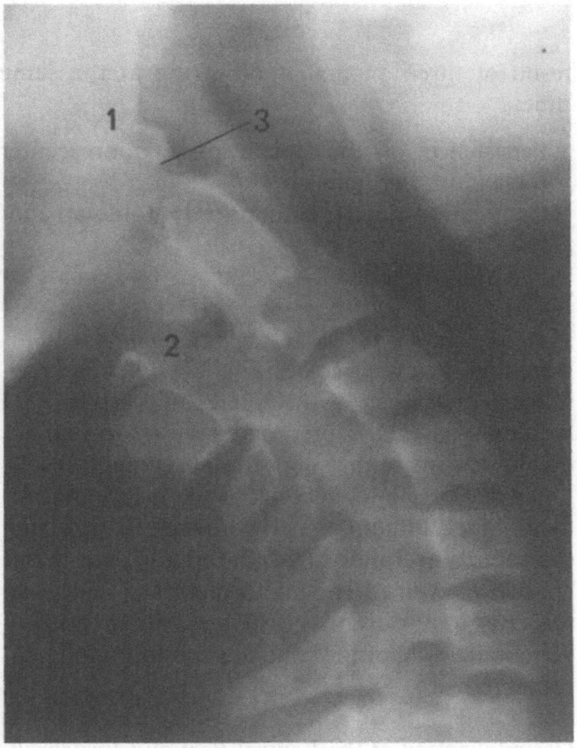

Fig. 2. Occipitalization and vertebralization of C1: retroflexed position of the head. *1,* Fusion of the anterior arch of the atlas with the occipital bone; *2,* Fusion of the posterior arches of C1 and C2; *3,* Normal space between the anterior arch of the atlas and the odontoid process

Radiology Today 2. Ed. by F.H.W. Heuck and M.W. Donner

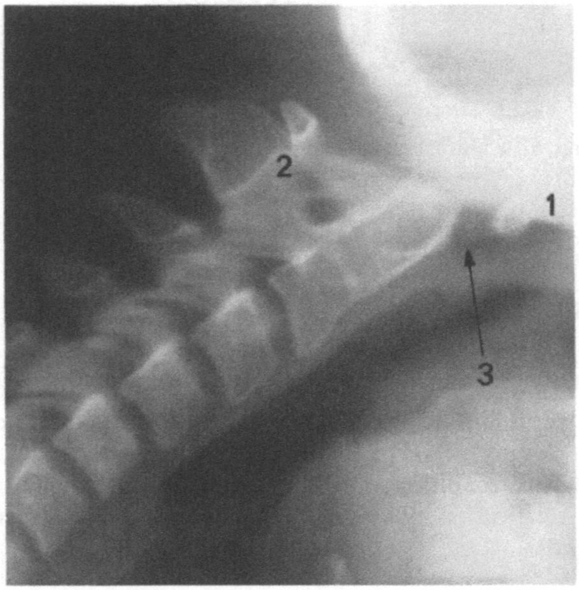

Fig. 3. Occipitalization and vertebralization of C1: flexed position of the head. *1,* Fusion of the anterior arch of the atlas with the occipital bone; *2,* Fusion of the posterior arches of C1 and C2; *3,* Widened space between the anterior arch of the atlas and the odontoid process

result of three anomalies occurring at the same time:

- Persistence of the apical ossification center (ossiculum Bergmann)
- Ossification defect, as in an odontoideum mobile
- Persistence of the C1-C2 disc

Vertebralization of the Occipital Condyles. This condition involves free occipital condyles and narrowness of the cervico-occipital canal [4]. In 1974 we observed a case of progressive quadriparesis due to stenosis of the suboccipital segment, resulting from free and very close-set occipital condyles. Since surgery, which consisted of widening the cervico-occipital canal, the quadriparesis has not become worse. The malformation is seldom so severe as in our original case, but milder forms of vertebralization of the condyles are commonly encountered.

Occipitalization of the Ventral Part and Vertebralization of the Dorsal Part of the Atlas with Insufficient Transverse Ligament. In contrast to simple total or partial occipitalization of the atlas, which is well known and well documented, occipitalization of the ventral part of the atlas and vertebralization of its dorsal part [9] is rare. In the extended (retroflexed) position of the head (Fig. 2) the space between the anterior arch of the atlas and the odontoid process is normal, but a film taken in the flexed position of the head (Fig. 3) shows it to be widened. This variation is characteristic for concomitant insufficiency of the transverse ligament.

References

1. Wackenheim A (1971) Densaplasia with atlanto-axial fusion. A special and stable form of dens-aplasia. Neuroradiology 2 [2]: 76–79
2. Wackenheim A (1974) Une forme d'odontoïde mobile stabilisé spontanément par la fusion de l'arc antérieur de l'atlas avec le corps de l'axis. Sem Hop Paris 50 [30]: 2087–2091
3. Wackenheim A (1974) Dens tripartitus Neuroradiology 8 [3]: 181
4. Wackenheim A (1974) Roentgen diagnosis of the craniovertebral region. Springer, Berlin Heidelberg New York
5. Wackenheim A (1977) Une malformation osseuse mal connue de la charnière cervicooccipitale: la fusion de l'arc antérieur de l'atlas et du corps de l'axis. Ann Radiol 20 [5]: 523–525
6. Wackenheim A (1977) Congenital fusion of the anterior arch of the atlas demonstrated by computed tomography. Neuroradiology 14: 41–42
7. Wackenheim A (1978) C1/2 block vertebra, fusion of the anterior arch of the atlas with the axis. Follow-up of the fusion in a child. Neuroradiology 16: 416–417
8. Wackenheim A (1978) Eine seltene Fehlbildung am Schädel-Hals-Uebergang: die Fusion des vorderen Atlas-Bogens mit dem Epistropheus bei Densaplasia oder Dysplasie. In: Pathologie und Klinik der Okzipito-Zervikalregion. Die Wirbelsäule in Forschung und Praxis 76: 49–51
9. Wackenheim A (1983) Occipitalization of the ventral part and vertebralization of the dorsal part of the atlas with insufficient transverse ligament. Neuroradiology
10. Wackenheim A, Dirheimer Y (1977) La fusion congénitale de l'arc antérieur de l'atlas avec la dent de l'axis. J Radiol Electrol 58 [8–9]: 525–526

New Contrast Medium for Myelography: Clinical Experience

S. Bockenheimer

Nordwest Krankenhaus, Neurologische Klinik, Steinbacher Hohl 2–26, 6000 Frankfurt 90, FRG

During the past 18 months we have performed 120 ascending thoracocervical myelographies and 135 radiculographies with the nonionic water-soluble contrast medium iopamidol at concentrations of 200 and 250 mg I/ml. We usually employed 10 ml iopamidol, i.e., the total iodine given never exceeded 2.5 g. The patients were aged 16–79 years (average 50.2 years).

In 30 patients, the EEG was recorded before, immediately after, and 6 and 24 h after myelography using 10 ml iopamidol at a concentration of 250 mg I/ml. No EEG changes due to the contrast medium could be detected in any of these patients. Other investigators [1–3], however, have reported such EEG changes, but they applied the contrast medium in higher concentrations of up to 370 mg I/ml and used up to 20 ml iopamidol, i.e., a total of over 6 g iodine. Carella et al. [2] reported general seizures in two patients examined using 20 ml iopamidol at a concentration of 300 mg I/ml. Doerstelmann (personal communication) reported one general seizure when 22 ml iopamidol at 300 mg I/ml was given via the C1/2 puncture route.

In our group of patients, adverse reactions were less severe. The side effects rarely exceeded complaints after simple lumbar puncture. In 25% of the patients, adverse reactions could be observed as shown in Table 1. Psychopathologic symptoms such as aphasia, hallucinations, psychic agitation, and euphoric or depressive states were not seen.

From the point of view of picture quality, there is no difference between iopamidol and other water-soluble contrast media of equal iodine concentration. The low viscosity gives excellent detailed information in radiculography (Fig. 1) as well as in myelography (Figs. 2, 3). Even functional diagnostic procedures are possible, as in chronic vertebrogenic myelopathy (Fig. 4). As a technical detail, it should be noted that we now tilt the patient in the opposite way to usual procedures to prevent the contrast medium from entering the

Table 1. The adverse reactions seen in 25% of the patients following the use of Iopamidol in myelography

Adverse reaction	Number of patients
Headache	51
Nausea	15
Vomiting	2
Dizziness	5
Radicular pain	9
Nuchal rigidity	3
Abnormal sleepiness	3
Hypotension	2

Number of patients suffering adverse reactions = 51

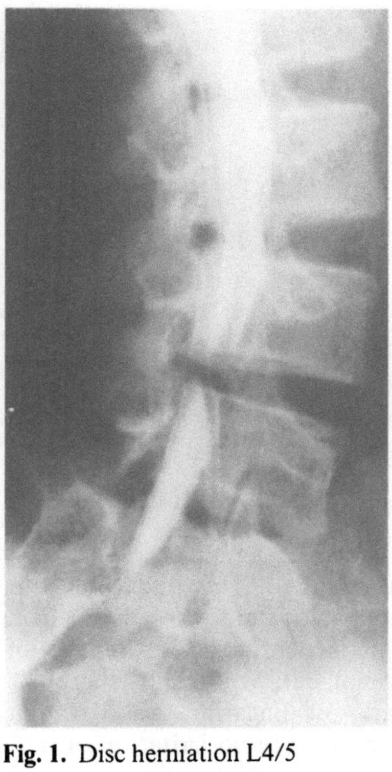

Fig. 1. Disc herniation L4/5

Radiology Today 2. Ed. by F. H. W. Heuck and M. W. Donner

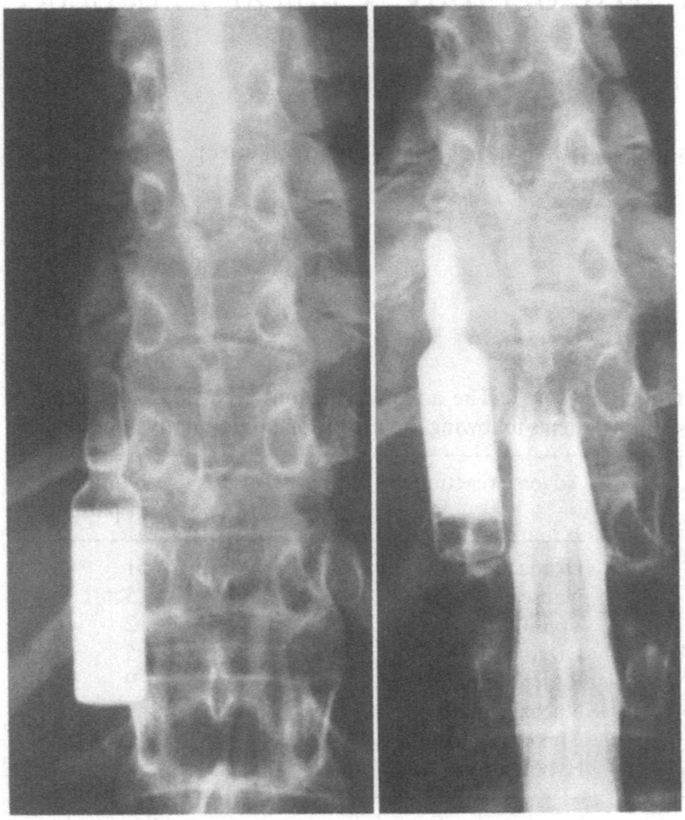

Fig. 2. Spinal neoplasm, after lumbar puncture block D11 (*right*); after suboccipital puncture upper block D10 (*left*)

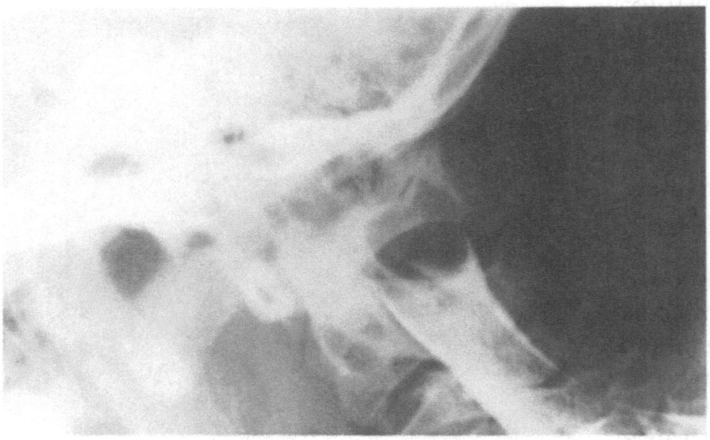

Fig. 3. Nuchal neurinoma C1/2

endocranium in excessive amounts when functional diagnosis is required. This underlines our opinion that although iopamidol is an excellent contrast material it is neurotoxic, as reports of general seizures point out. We cannot share the enthusiastic remarks of Bacarini et al. [1] that iopamidol seems to produce no irritation of nervous cells. Therefore, the concentration and total amount of iodine should be carefully chosen, especially as the lower concentration gives radiologically excellent detailed information.

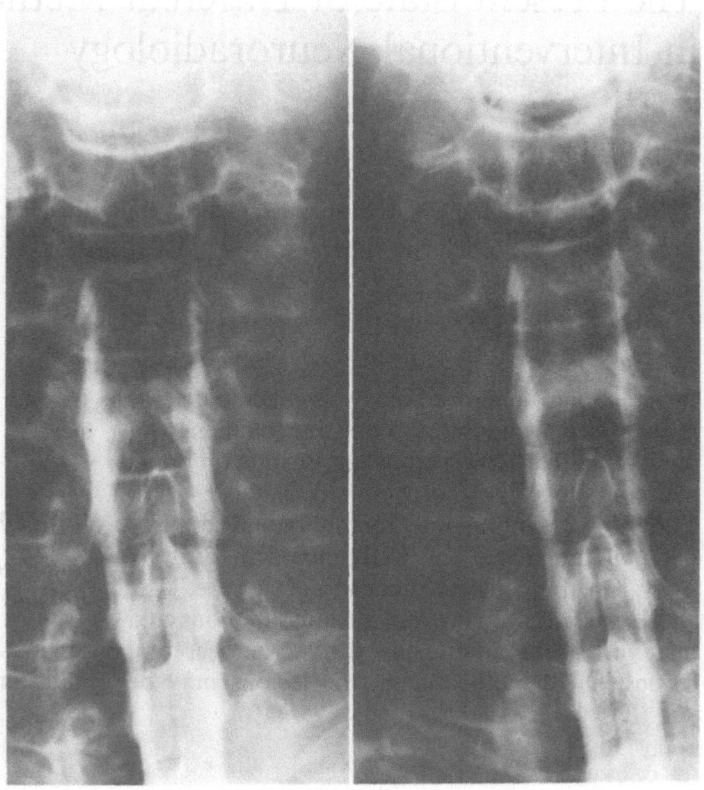

Fig. 4. Chronic vertebragenic myelopathy, in retroflection block C3/4 (*left*); in anteflection passage of the contrast medium (*right*)

References

1. Bacarini L, De Nicola T, Gasparini D, Orlando P, Vasallo A (1982) Iopamidol (B 15000), a nonionic water-soluble contrast medium for neuroradiology. Part I: Results of a clinical trial for myelography. Neuroradiology 23:81–84
2. Carella A, Federico F, Di Cuonzo F, Vinjau E, Lambert P (1982) Adverse side effects of metrizamide and iopamidolo in myelography. Neuroradiology 22:247–249
3. Liboni W, Benna P, Duca S, Fra L, Sicuro A (1982) Electrophysiological (EEG, BAEP, VEP, H-Reflex) patterns in myelography with nonionic water-soluble contrast media. Neuroradiology 22:227–278

The Present State of Different Methods and Techniques in Interventional Neuroradiology

K. Voigt

Abteilung für Neuroradiologie, Medizinisches Strahleninstitut der Universität, Osianderstrasse 22, 7400 Tübingen, FRG

Interventional neuroradiology is decidedly the most exciting and most promising challenge of our speciality. However, what is interventional neuroradiology?

Current interventional neuroradiology is certainly not a circumscribed and well-defined field of activity. On the contrary, depending on type, size, and localization, many and various methods and materials are available to attack craniocerebral lesions. On the other hand, the lesions may be treated in a more curative or only palliative manner.

Interventions in the External Carotid Territory

Superselective Angiography and Solid Embolization

High-standard superselective angiography is an indispensable prerequisite of solid embolization

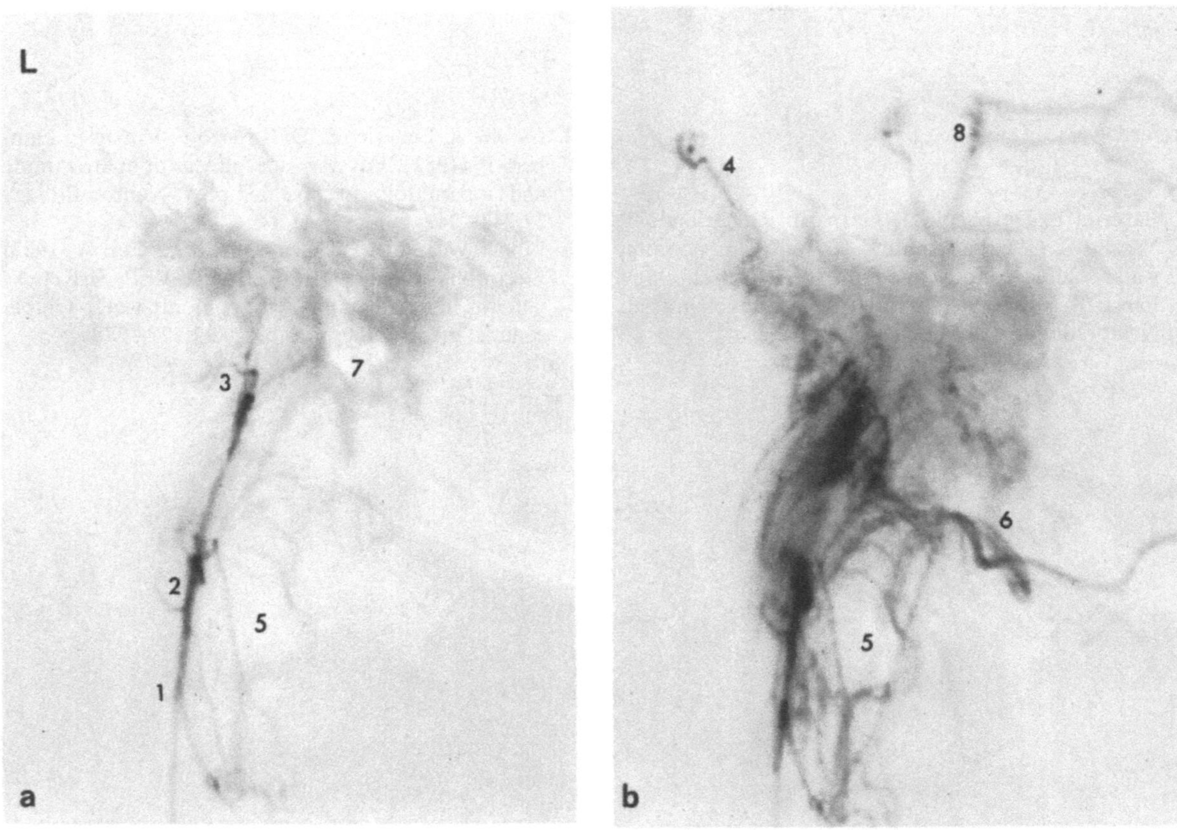

Fig. 1 a, b. Superselective angiography of normal left ascending pharyngeal artery. Arterial (**a**) and capillary (**b**) phases: *1*, main trunk; *2*, middle and caudal pharyngeal branches; *3*, cranial pharyngeal branch; *4* anastomotic branch to internal maxillary artery; *5*, muscular anastomotic branches to vertebral artery; *6*, atlantal loop of vertebral artery; *7*, dorsal branch of pharyngeal artery; *8*, collateral filling of basilar artery via anastomoses

Radiology Today 2. Ed. by F. H. W. Heuck and M. W. Donner

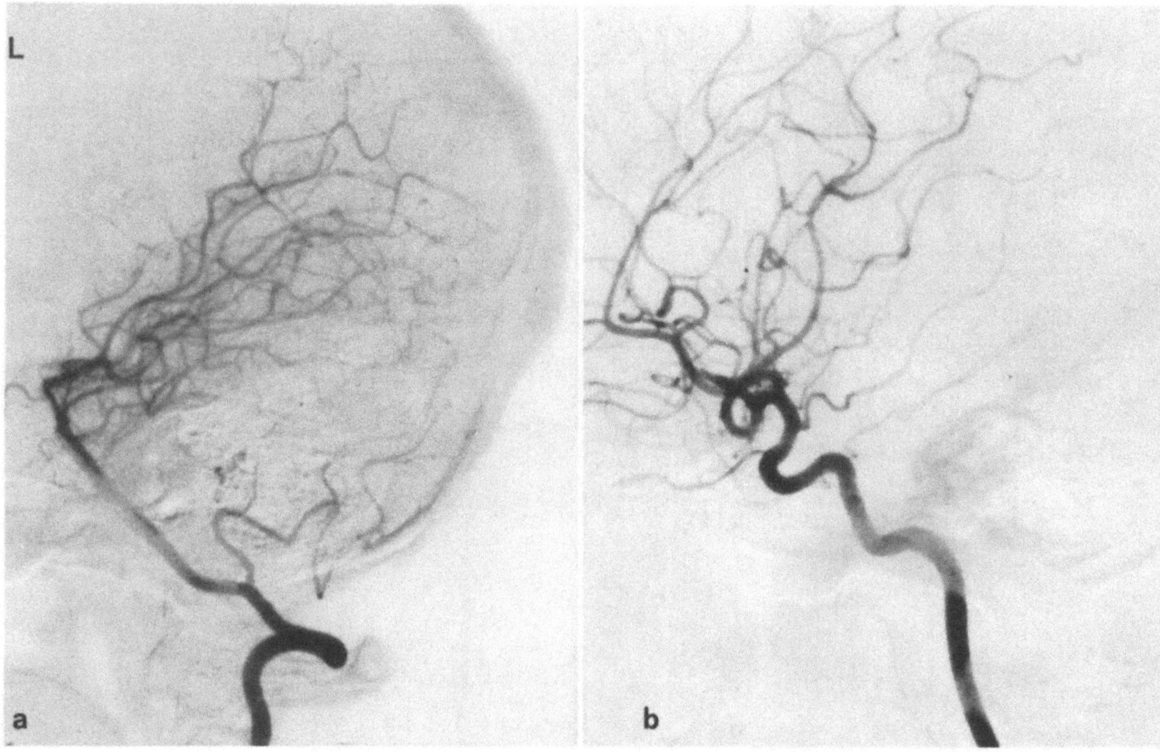

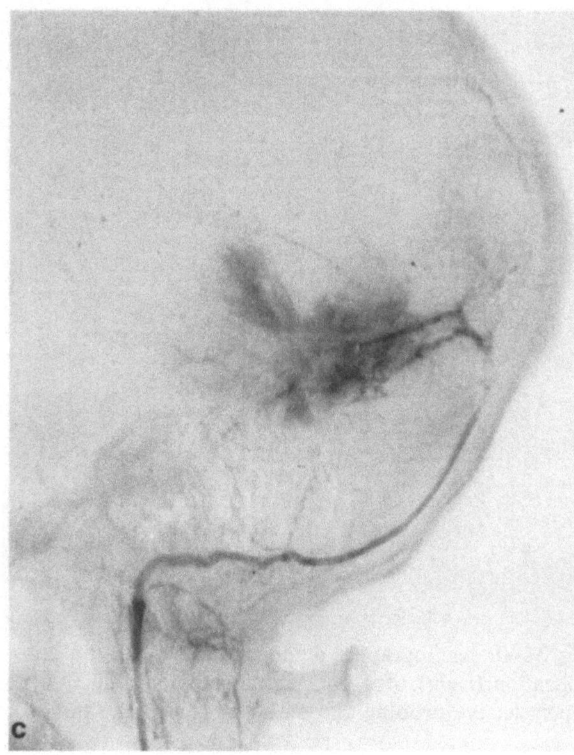

Fig. 2a–c. Selective and superselective angiography of a left-sided lateral tentorial meningioma. Left vertebral arteriography (**a**) shows no direct tumorous signs; left internal carotid arteriography (**b**) only demonstrates the tentorial artery; superselective arteriography of the left ascending pharyngeal artery (**c**) proves the diagnosis by opacification of the dorsal meningeal artery

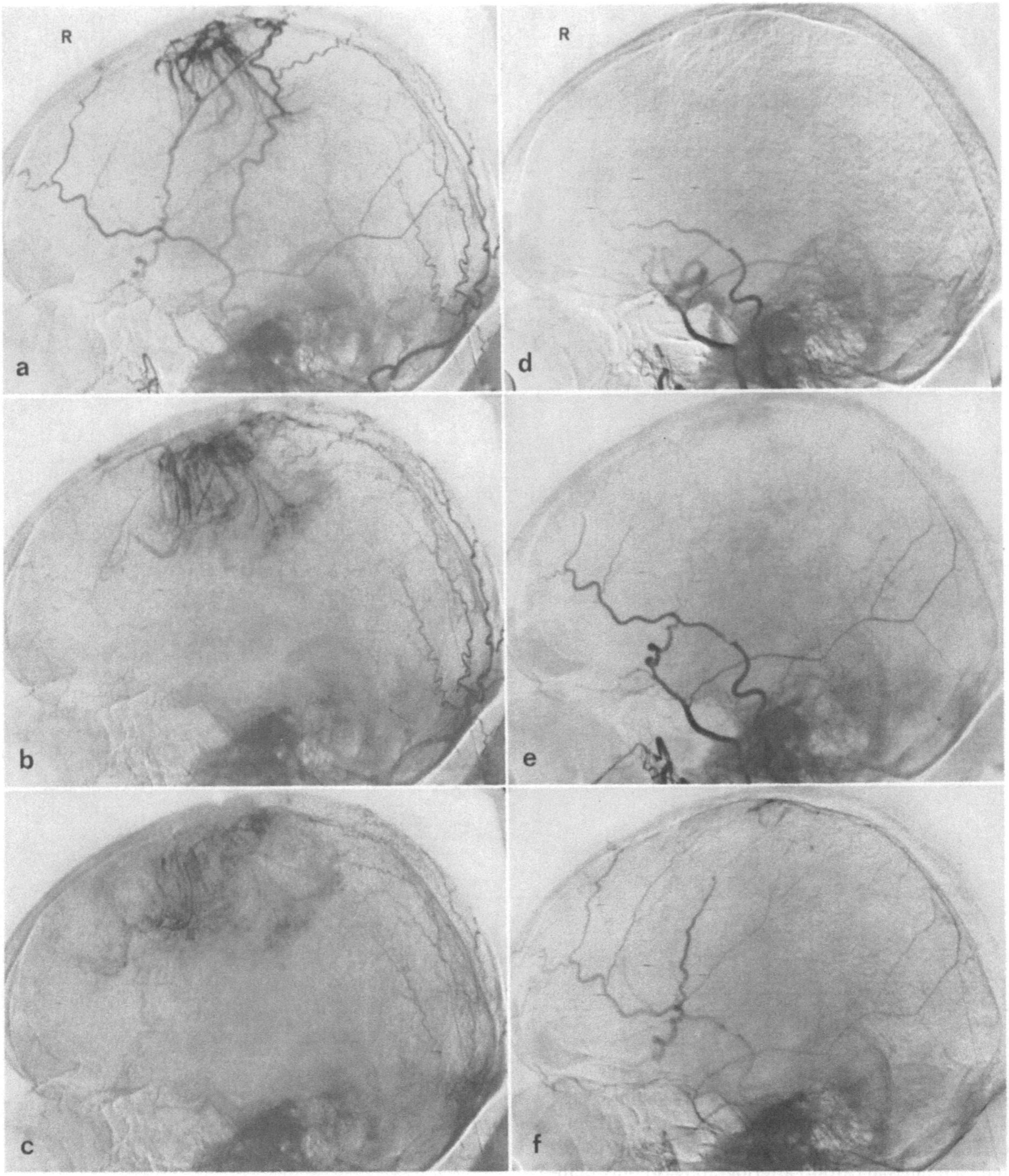

Fig. 3a–f. Angiographic demonstration (*left*) and embolization (*right*) of a parasagittal meningioma. After superselective probing and embolization of the tumor-feeding vessels (**a–c**), intratumorous placement of the emboli is proved by distal stasis of the tumor vessels (**d–f**) and lack of tumor stain

in the external carotid territory, first in order to avoid reflux emboli into the internal carotid artery and second to ensure embolization of only those vessels feeding the lesion. Superselective probing and opacification of every single branch of the external carotid artery is mandatory and should be routine for the examiner (Fig. 1).

In a number of cases the true nature of the pathological process to be diagnosed can only be discovered by means of superselective angiography, as shown in Fig. 2. In this case of lateral tentorial meningioma, vertebral angiography merely showed indirect signs of a space-occupying lesion (Fig. 2a) and internal carotid angiography just demonstrated a small tentorial artery (Fig. 2b); only when the ascending pharyngeal artery was superselectively filled could the typical blush and vasculature of the meningioma be shown by opacification of the dorsal meningeal artery (Fig. 2c).

After superselective angiography of tumor-feeding vessels these arteries may be occluded by embolization with particles of Gelfoam and/or lyophilized dura, as shown in the case of a large parasagittal meningioma (Fig. 3a–c). The intratumorous placement of the embolization particles (Fig. 3d–f) is of utmost importance, as only by this technique can collateral nutrition be avoided, resulting in central necrosis of the tumor. Besides the predominantly palliative treatment of meningiomas and/or tumorous and vascular malformations of the head, neck, and face, solid embolization is in our experience the curative therapeutic method of choice in external carotid–cavernous sinus fistulas [7].

Superselective Angiography and Liquid Embolization

The same technical and methodological conditions must be fulfilled for interventions with liquid embolization materials, which in some cases are more effective than solid particles because intratumorous placement may be obtained more easily and certainly. This is demonstrated in a left-sided glomus tumor which was fed by the left external occipital and ascending pharyngeal arteries (Fig. 4). Figure 5 shows the result of in-

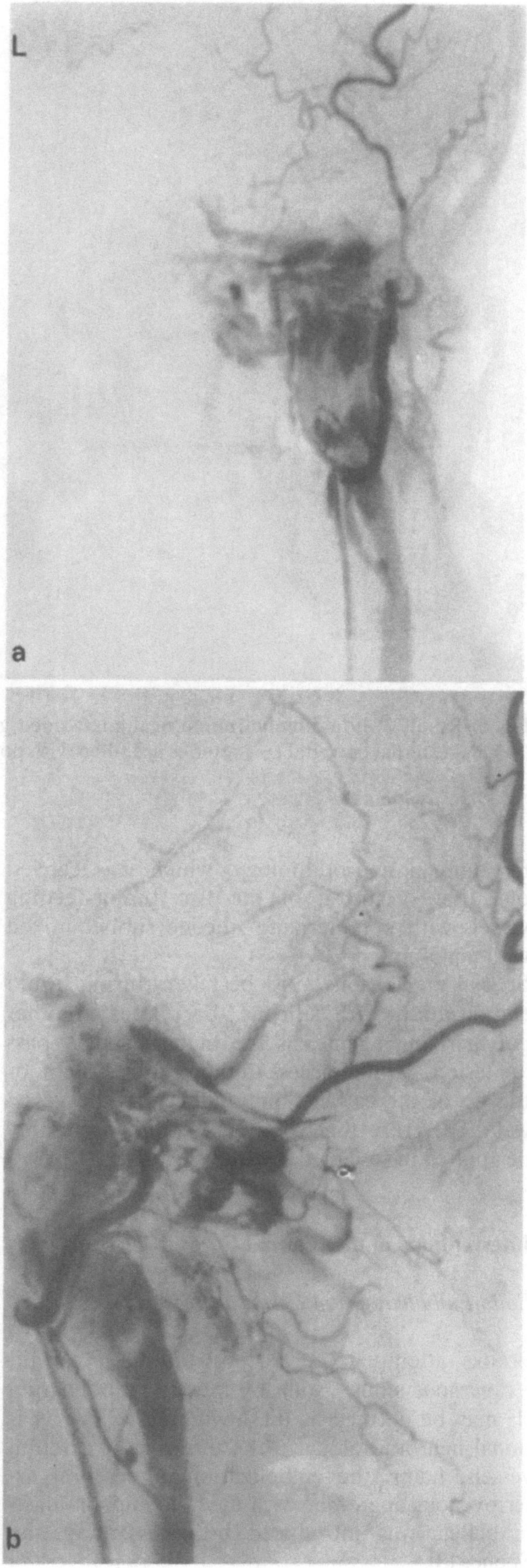

Fig. 4a, b. Superselective angiography of a left-sided glomus tumor. Anteroposterior (**a**) and lateral (**b**) views of the tumor stain fed by the left external occipital and ascending pharyngeal artery

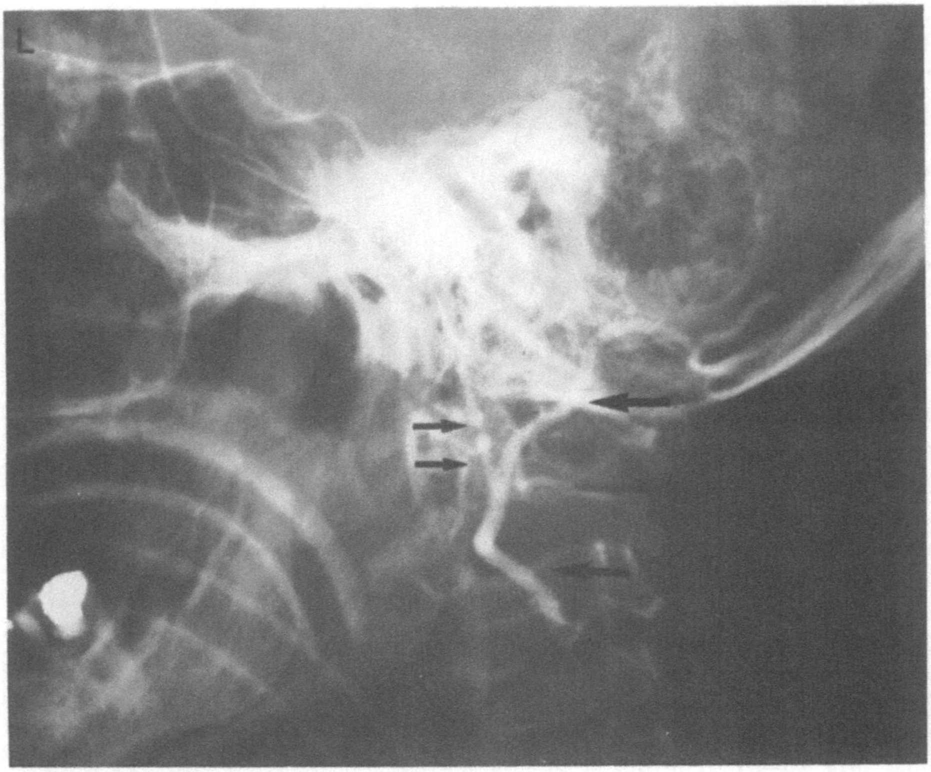

Fig. 5. Result of liquid embolization of the left-sided glomus tumor. The formerly feeding ascending pharyngeal (→) and external occipital (←) arteries are filled with polymerized silicone rubber mixed with tantalum

terventional neuroradiology, which was carried out after occlusion of the two tumor-feeding vessels with polymerizing silicone rubber mixed with tantalum.

Special precautions must be taken during liquid embolization with silicone, bucrylate, or other polymerizing agents, as the materials may pass the lesion, gaining access to the venous system, or the tip of the catheter may adhere to the vessel wall. Therefore the technique should preferably be applied in so-called low-flow lesions.

Interventions in the Internal Carotid Territory

Solid Embolization of Cerebral Vessels

Brooks' attempt to cure a post-traumatic carotid –cavernous sinus fistula by muscle embolization [1] may be defined as the beginning of interventional neuroradiology in the territory of cerebral vessels. Later, the embolization of cerebral arteriovenous angiomas with metallic and/or silastic pellets was introduced by Luessenhop and Spence [3]. Both of these techniques, however, involved noncontrollable injections of the embolization material after arteriotomy of the internal carotid artery in the neck. Moreover, it was shown by Luessenhop et al. [4, 5] that it may take up to 24 h for the pellets to reach their final, permanent position in the arteries. Because of the noncontrollable injection, some of the embolization particles may also pass the cerebral angioma or even reach other, nonfeeding cerebral vessels and by occluding them, lead to neurological deficits. This further, severe disadvantage of the technique, illustrated in Fig. 6, is one reason why solid embolization of cerebral vessels is still not generally accepted and should be restricted to some particular cases.

Catheter Techniques with Nondetachable Balloons

The nondetachable balloon technique was in the past used universally and is still used in some places for the elimination of internal carotid–cavernous sinus fistulas, the cure of which has long been a perplexing, unsolved problem in neuroradiology (Fig. 7a–c).

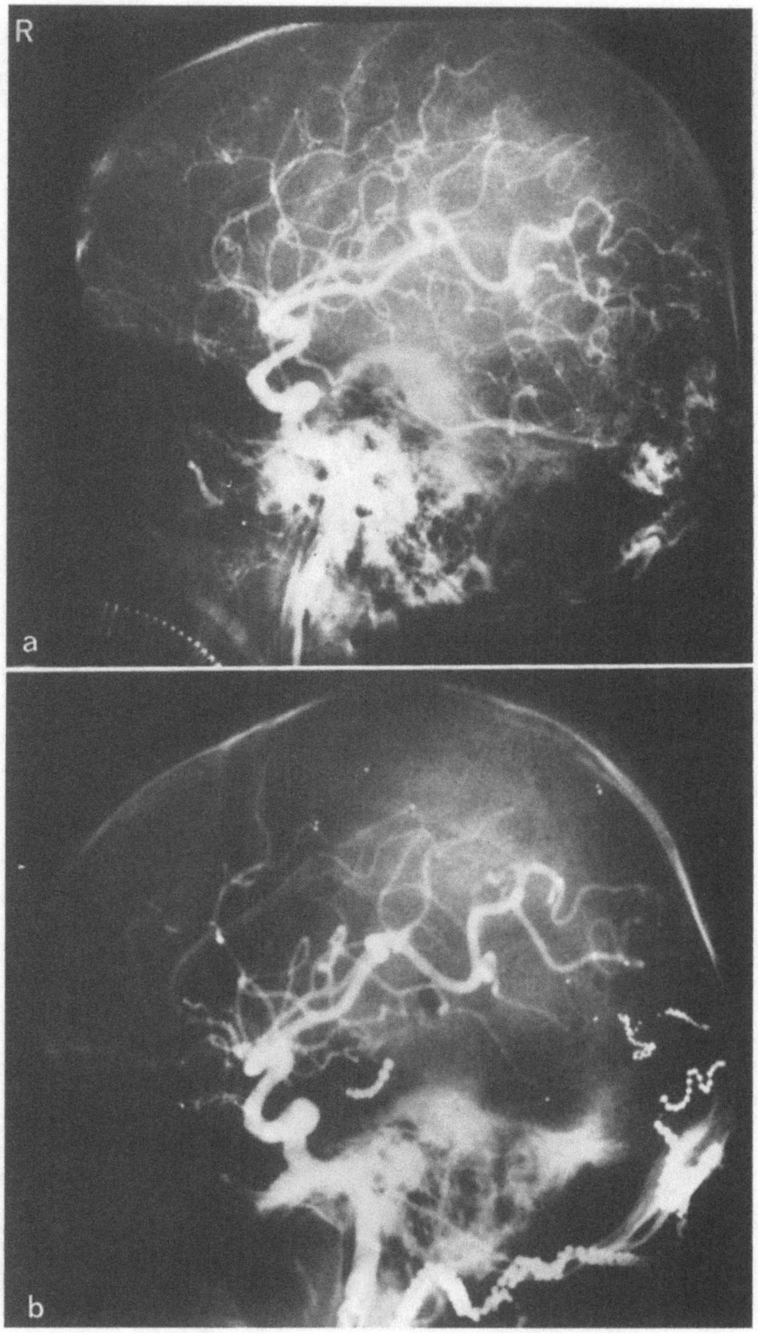

Fig. 6a, b. Angiographic demonstration (**a**) and pellet embolization (**b**) of a right-sided occipital arteriovenous angioma. After pellet embolization of the angioma (b), there is dissemination of pellets into nonfeeding cerebral vessels

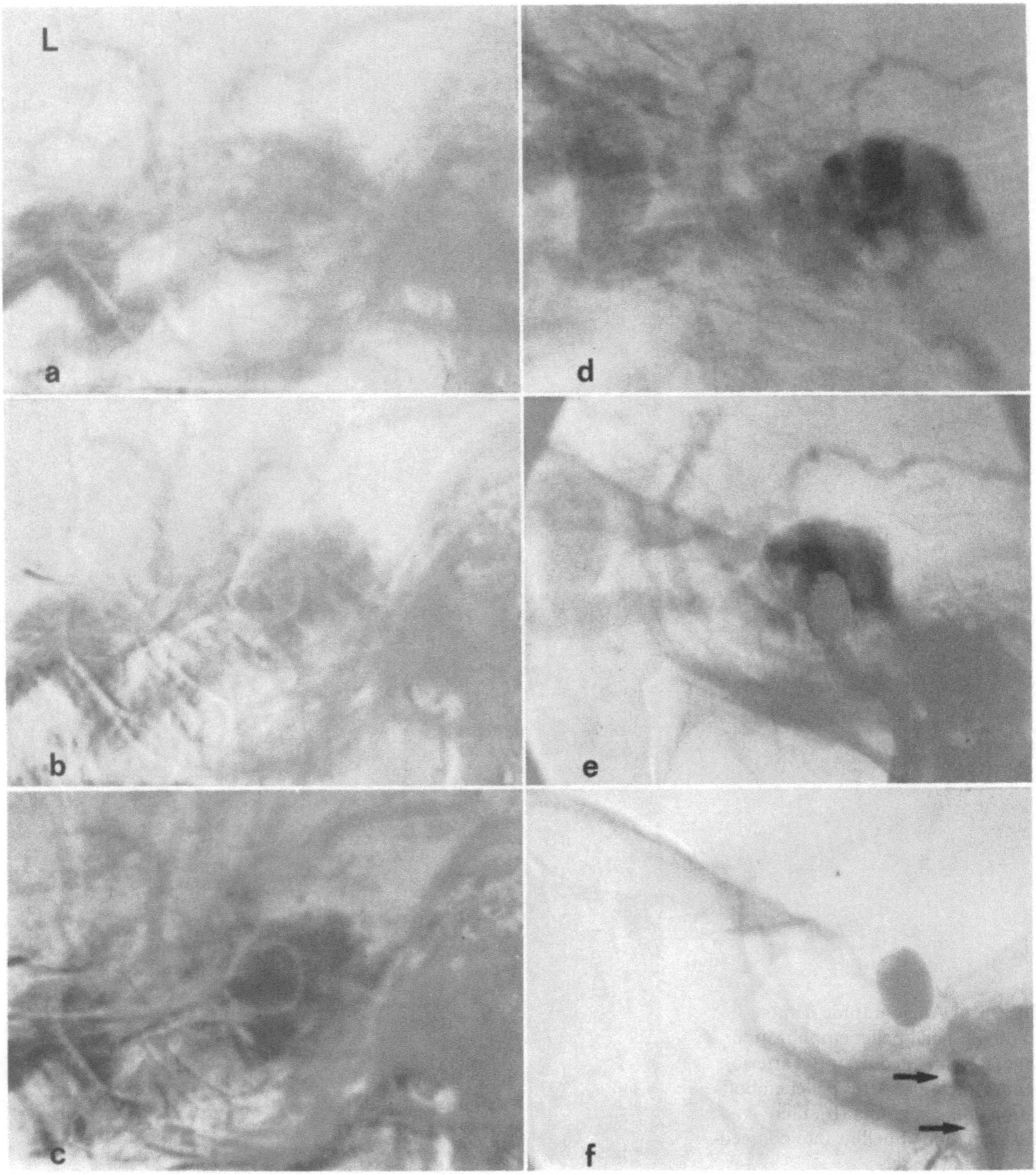

Fig. 7a–f. Angiographic demonstration (*left*) and balloon occlusion (*right*) of a traumatic internal carotid-cavernous sinus fistula. After different positioning and degree of insufflation (**d, e**) of the Fogarty balloon catheter, final occlusion of the fistula (**f**) and stasis of the formerly feeding internal carotid artery proximal to the inserted balloon (→)

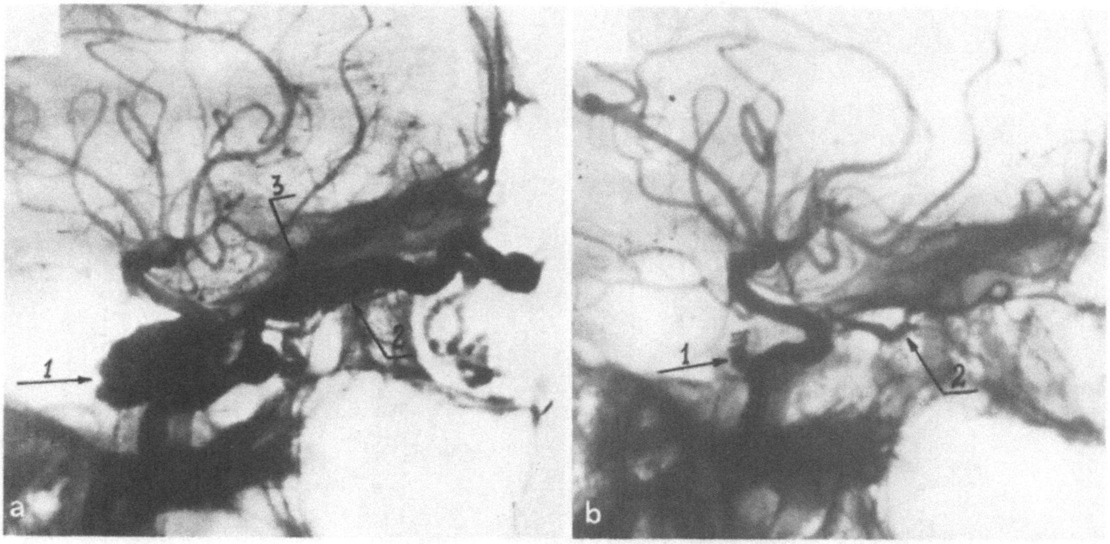

Fig. 8a, b. Angiographic demonstration (*left*) and reconstructive endovascular occlusion (*right*) of an internal carotid-cavernous sinus fistula. Carotid-cavernous fistula (**a**): *1*, fistula; *2*, ophthalmic artery; *3*, enlarged superior ophthalmic vein. Complete occlusion of the fistula with several detached balloons (**b**): *1*, markers of the detached balloons; *2*, ophthalmic artery. Note the patency of internal carotid artery after occlusion of the fistula

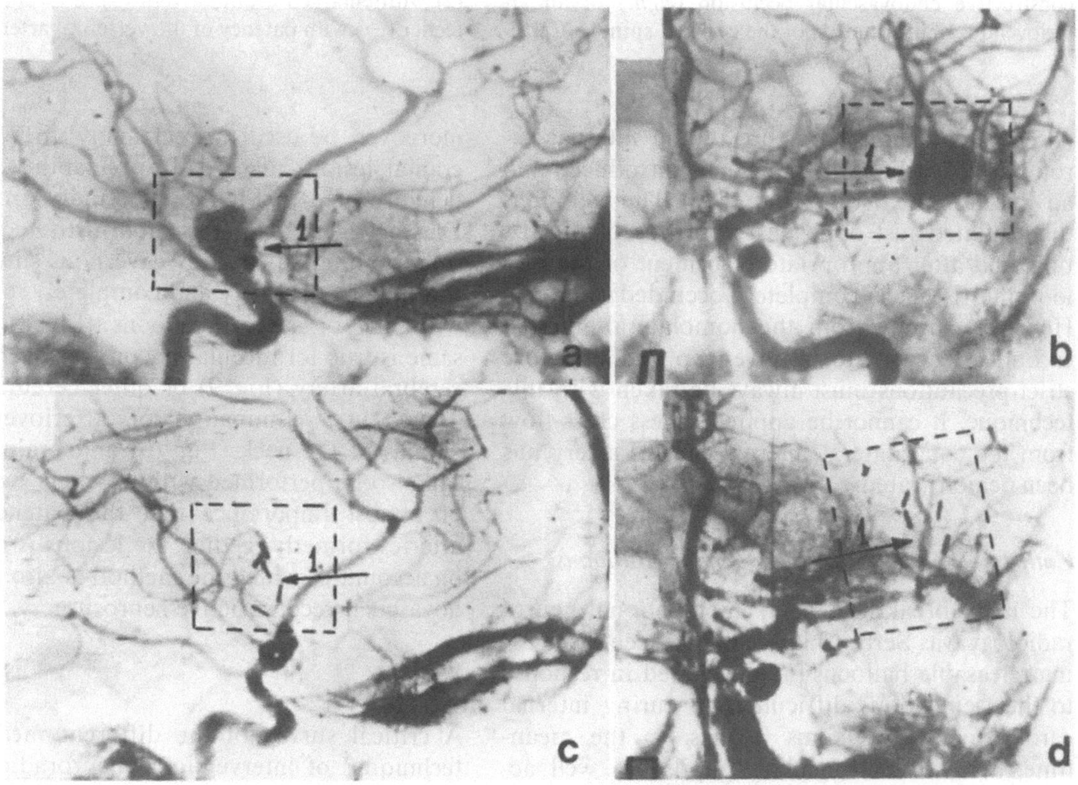

Fig. 9a–d. Angiographic demonstration (**a, b**) and reconstructive endovascular occlusion (**c, d**) of a saccular aneurysm (*1*) of the middle cerebral artery

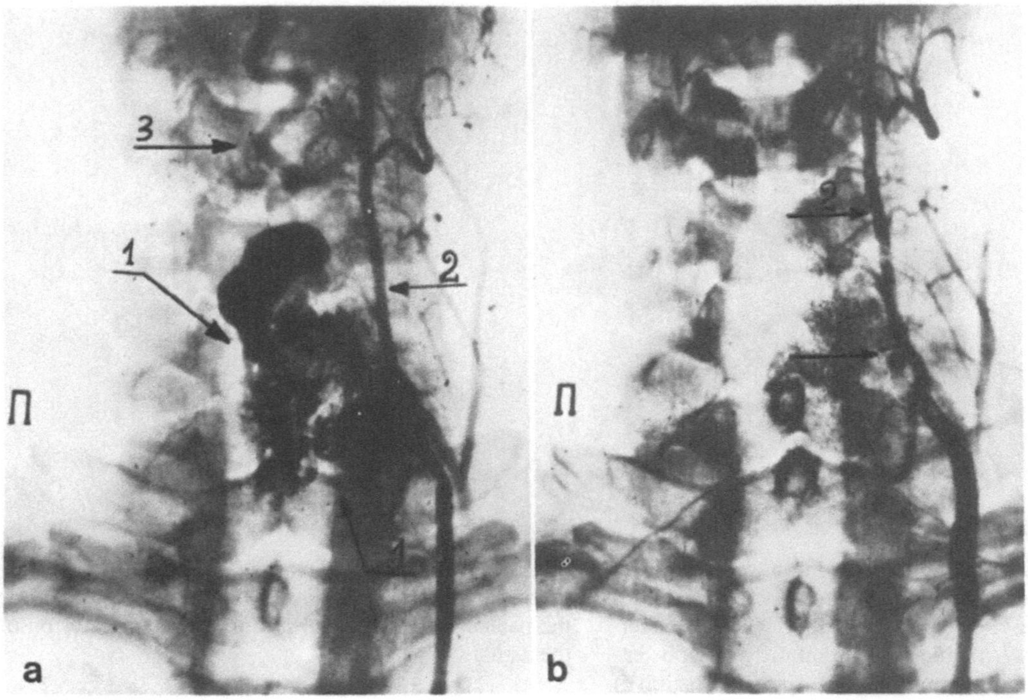

Fig. 10 a, b. Angiographic demonstration (*left*) and reconstructive endovascular occlusion (*right*) of an arteriovenous malformation of the cervical spine. **a** Cervical spinal angioma (*1*) fed by the left vertebral artery (*2*) with enlarged draining vein (*3*). **b** Occlusion of the feeder (→) with patency of the vertebral artery (**b**)

After percutaneous puncture of the internal carotid artery, a Fogarty catheter is introduced and advanced to the fistula (Fig. 7 d, e). The balloon is then inflated just opposite the orifice of the fistula, and after appropriate placement of the balloon the fistula is completely occluded (Fig. 7 f). However, supply from the homolateral internal carotid artery has to be given up and therefore strict precautions must always be taken with this technique. It cannot be applied unless cross-flow from the contralateral internal carotid artery has been demonstrated.

Catheter Techniques with Detachable Balloons

The latest breakthrough in interventional neuroradiology was Serbinenko's catheter technique using releasable balloons [6], developed in response to the tremendous difficulties in curing internal carotid–cavernous sinus fistulas. In the meantime, a lot of Serbinenko's pupils are well acquainted with, or have even modified, this endovascular interventional technique. In the West, most experience with these balloons has probably been gained by Debrun et al. [2].
Serbinenko's technique does not have any of the disadvantages of the Fogarty balloons and can, moreover, be used to treat many different intracranial lesions. Its broad applicability is briefly demonstrated in Figs. 8–11, kindly provided by Dr. Shcheglov, Kiev Research Institute of Neurosurgery. Internal carotid–cavernous sinus fistulas can now be routinely and completely, obliterated with one or several balloons (Fig. 8), and the same is true for saccular aneurysms of the middle cerebral artery (Fig. 9) or other cerebral vessels. Therapeutic elimination of arteriovenous angiomas of the neck (Fig. 10) and brain (Fig. 11) can also be performed with excellent results. It is of utmost importance that the patency of the arteries formerly feeding the lesions is preserved, on account of which the method is also called endovascular reconstructive neurosurgery.

Conclusion

A critical survey of the different methods and techniques of interventional neuroradiology employed to date reveals that superselective angiography and embolization with various materials has restricted indications in tumorous and vascular lesions of the external carotid artery territory. In arteriovenous fistulas of the external carotid artery, especially those of the cavernous

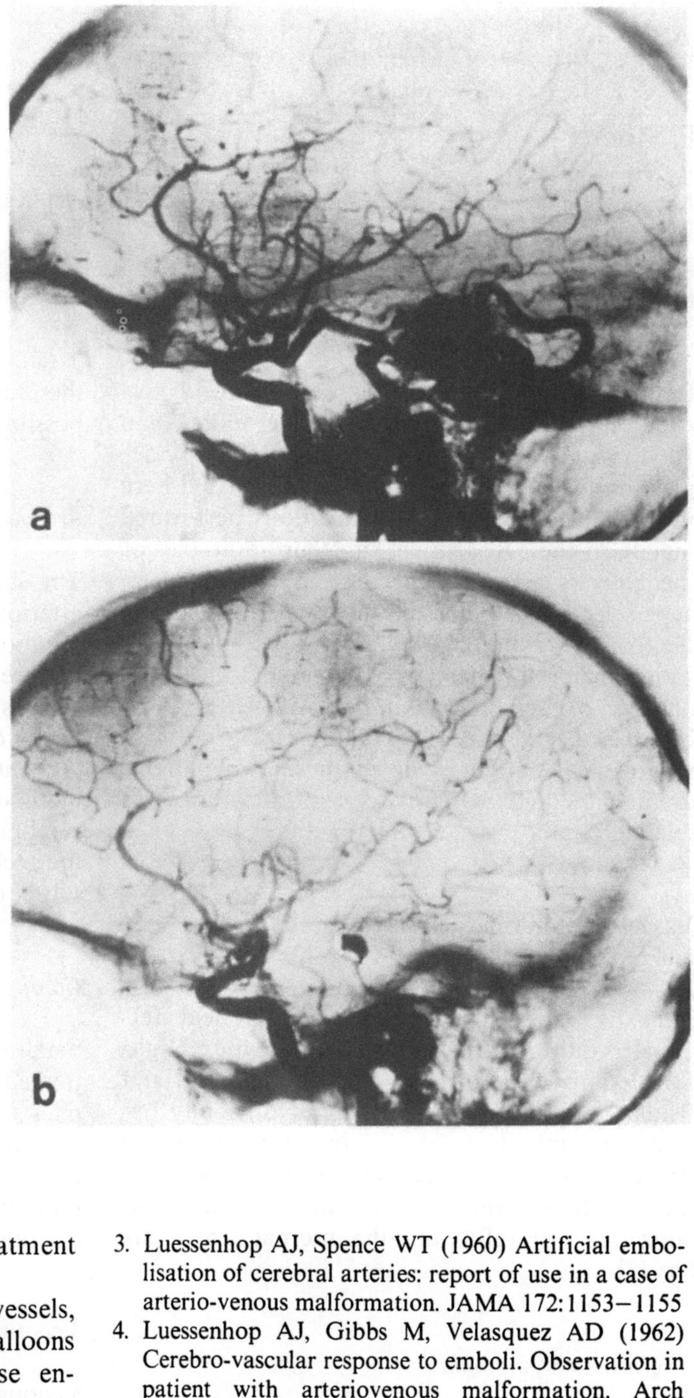

Fig. 11 a, b. Angiographic demonstration (**a**) and endovascular occlusion (**b**) of an occipital arteriovenous angioma. Distal occlusion of the formerly feeding posterior cerebral artery with a detached, contrast-filled balloon (**b**)

sinus, this technique is regarded as the treatment of choice.

In all kinds of vascular lesions of cerebral vessels, catheter techniques with detachable balloons yield the most promising results, because endovascular reconstructive intervention can be carried out with preservation of the arterial flow.

References

1. Brooks B (1930) The treatment of traumatic arteriovenous fistula. South Med J 23:100–106
2. Debrun G, Lacour P, Caron JP, Hurth M, Comoy J, Keravel Y (1978) Detachable balloon and calibrated leak balloon techniques in the treatment of cerebral vascular lesions. J Neurosurg 49:635–649
3. Luessenhop AJ, Spence WT (1960) Artificial embolisation of cerebral arteries: report of use in a case of arterio-venous malformation. JAMA 172:1153–1155
4. Luessenhop AJ, Gibbs M, Velasquez AD (1962) Cerebro-vascular response to emboli. Observation in patient with arteriovenous malformation. Arch Neurol Psychiat 7:264–274
5. Luessenhop AJ, Kachmann RJ, Sherling N (1965) Clinical evaluation of artificial embolisation in the management of large cerebral arterio-venous malformations. J Neurosurg 31:400–417
6. Serbinenko FA (1974) Balloon catheterization and occlusion of major cerebral vessels. J Neurosurg 41:125–145
7. Voigt K (1978) Neuroradiologische Diagnostik und Therapie von duralen Carotis-Cavernosus-Fisteln. Arch Psychiatr Nervenkr 225:359–377

Embolization Within the Territory of the External Carotid Artery

P. Stoeter

Abteilung für Neuroradiologie, Elisabethen-Krankenhaus, 7980 Ravensburg, FRG

Embolizations within the external carotid territory have been carried out since more than 10 years ago. The indications for this therapy depend on the type of lesion and are discussed here in the light of over 100 embolizations performed mainly in the Department of Neuroradiology of the University of Tübingen [4, 6]. In all cases, superselective catheterization was performed and Gelfoam or lyophilized dura was used as embolization material. There were three complications: one case of facial local skin necrosis, which could be excised, and two of incomplete restitution of neurological deficits. One of these two patients eventually died. Otherwise, embolization was tolerated well.

Vascular Malformations of the Neck, Face, and Skull

Neck, face, and skull malformations can be differentiated into high-flow and low-flow types. High-flow lesions, such as arteriovenous angiomas and fistulas, can be embolized without difficulty because the emboli are carried immediately to the shunt by the blood stream. In low-flow lesions, on the other hand, there is always the risk of overembolization with reflux into the internal carotid artery [5].

Arteriovenous Angiomas

In small angiomas with only one or two feeding vessels, embolization of the lesion can be complete and permanent cure is possible.

In these cases, unresorbable material such as bucrylate can also be used. However, the majority of angiomas are extensive with numerous afferent arteries, and not every single one can be embolized. If some shunts remain open, previously occluded or new feeding arteries will reopen, and therefore operation is advisible within 1 week if possible.

Arteriovenous Fistulas

The same rule applies to extra- and intracranial arteriovenous fistulas: If the afferent branches are not too numerous and if there is no participation by cerebral arteries, embolization can be curative. This is the case mainly in fistulas between external carotid branches and the cavernous sinus [3], but those into the sigmoid sinus are often more extensive with additional participation of cerebral arteries. These vessels may enlarge after the occlusion of the external carotid branches, and subsequent operation is necessary.

Capillary Angiomas and Epistaxis

Small telangiectases, as in Osler's disease, can be treated and cured by embolization. This also applies to cases of severe epistaxis, which is often due to small angiomas but sometimes has other causes, such as trauma, tumors, or hypertension. Embolization can be performed as a life-saving emergency procedure in these circumstances.

Venous Angiomas

Venous angiomas consist mainly of large venous caverns fed by a great number of capillary shunts [5]. Complete embolization of the malformation is usually impossible, but even if all shunts are occluded, the venous parts will not collapse because of retrograde filling through the efferent veins. The aims of embolization in venous angiomas are therefore the reduction of intraoperative bleeding and the prevention of recurrence by the elimination of the shunts.

Radiology Today 2. Ed. by F. H. W. Heuck and M. W. Donner

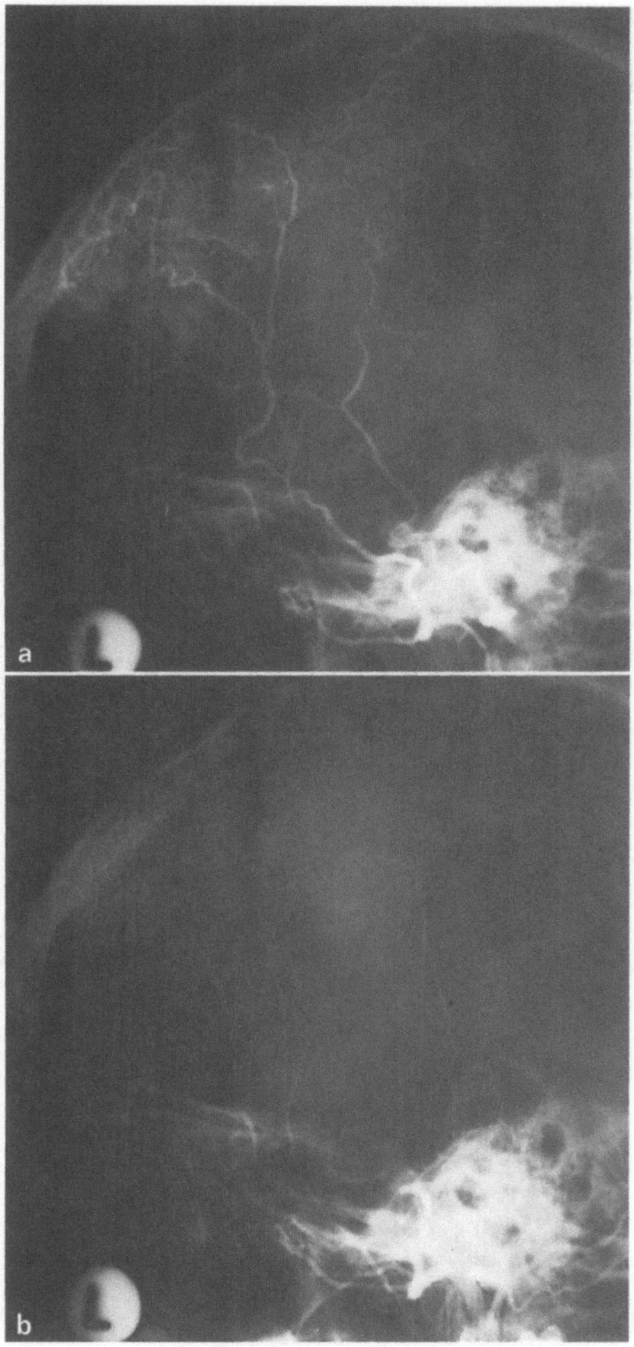

Fig. 1 a, b. Meningioma of the convexity. **a** Vascularization of the center by the middle meningeal artery. **b** After embolization

Highly Vascularized Tumors of the Face and Skull

In most of these growths, e.g., angiofibromas, glomus tumors, and malignancies, embolization plays a role as a preoperative or palliative measure, surgery following within 1 week if performed.

Juvenile Nasopharyngeal Fibromas

Juvenile nasopharyngeal fibromas have an extensive and on occasion bilateral blood supply from the maxillary and ascending pharyngeal arteries and sometimes also from the facial artery, and excision without preoperative embolization can be impossible. An intracranial extension of the fibroma is no contraindication to emboli-

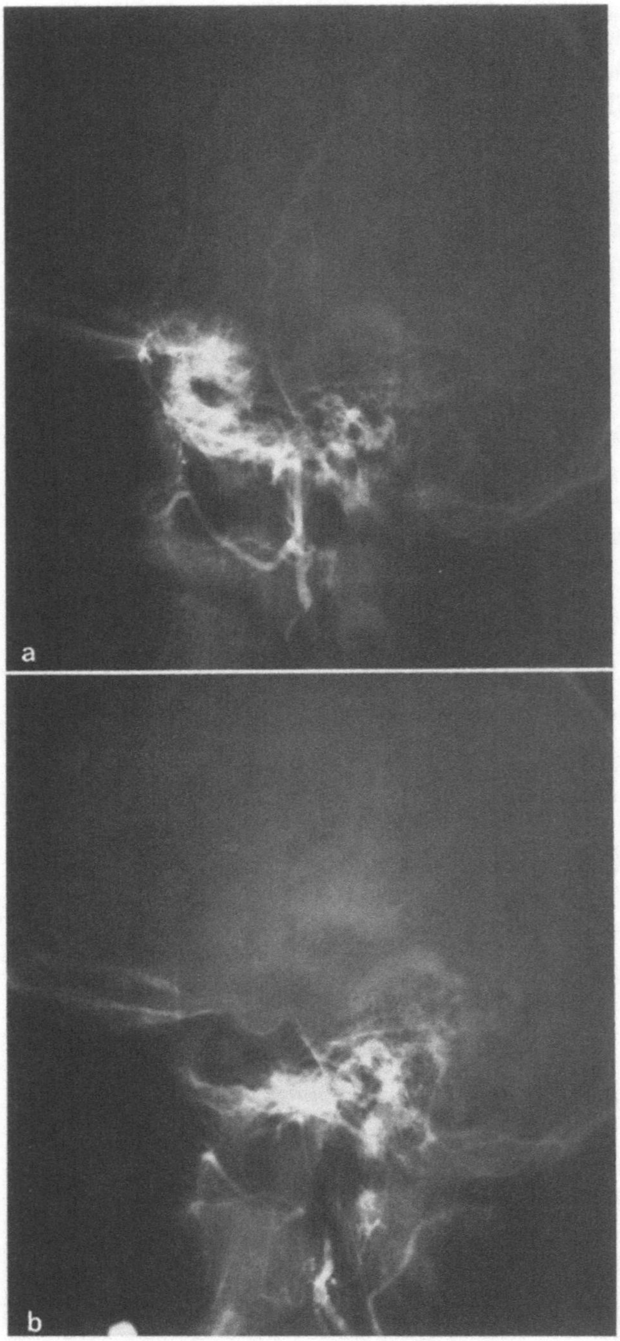

Fig. 2 a, b. Parasellar meningioma. **a** Heavy tumor stain via the middle meningeal artery and other small branches of the maxillary artery. **b** After embolization

zation, although success may be incomplete if the tumor also has tributaries from the internal carotid artery.

Glomus Tumors

The same applies to hypotympanic and jugular glomus tumors. In both types several external carotid branches may contribute to the blood supply as well as branches from the vertebral artery and, in large growths, intracranial vessels. Nevertheless, catheterization and embolization of the tributaries is carried out as superselectively and completely as possible and can be repeated in recurrences after subsequent operation. Even in an incompletely treated case the often troublesome bruit can be reduced.

Metastases

Malignancies cannot of course be cured by embolization, but reduction of their blood supply by facilitate operation or stop intractable bleeding. Embolization can also be combined with the injection of cytostatics.

Meningiomas

Meningiomas of the convexity and those of the middle cranial fossa and the sellar region are suitable for embolization if there is a demonstrable blood supply from the middle meningeal artery [1].

Meningiomas of the Convexity

In meningiomas of the convexity (Fig. 1), the centers are usually vascularized by the middle meningeal artery and can be embolized. Care has to be taken that small particles reach the tumor itself and do not merely occlude the afferent arteries. In some cases, mainly in elderly inoperable patients, a central necrosis has been observed by CT for several years [2], but in most cases, embolization is followed by operation because the periphery of the tumor is supplied by cerebral arteries which cannot be occluded.

Basal Meningiomas

Meningiomas of the sphenoid wings are often supplied by numerous branches of the middle meningeal and maxillary arteries, and excision of the tumors can be complicated by diffuse hemorrhage. Preoperative embolization can reduce the bleeding, but permant cure is not possible with embolization alone because of the great number of afferent arteries and additional branches from the internal carotid artery in parasellar meningiomas (Fig. 2).

Summary

As in other areas of the body, embolization within the external carotid territory is used mainly as a preoperative or palliative measure, and close collaboration with the surgeon is necessary. Indications in which permanent success can be exspected are rare, but with these reservations, appropriate embolization is a valuable and safe interventional neuroradiological technique.

References

1. Stoeter P (1980) Computertomographic, scintigraphic, and histological control studies after embolization of cranio-facial tumors. In: Veiga-Pires JA, Martins da Silva M, Oliva L (eds) Intervention radiology. Excerpta Medica, Amsterdam, pp
2. Stoeter P, Reinshagen G, Voigt K (1979) Interventionale Neuroradiologie cranialer Tumoren bei inoperablen Alterspatienten. Janssen, Düsseldorf (Gerontopsychiatrie 7)
3. Voigt K (1978) Neuroradiologische Diagnostik und Therapie von duralen Carotis-Cavernosus-Fisteln. Arch Psychiatr Nervenkr 225:359–377
4. Voigt K, Stoeter P (1980) Indikation und Befunde neurologischer Embolisationen. Neurol Psychiatr 6:64–78
5. Voigt K, Schwenzer N, Stoeter P (1978) Angiographic, operative, and histological findings after embolisation of cranio-facial angiomas. Neuroradiology 16:424–427
6. Voigt K, Thron A, Mironov A (1981) Interventionale Neuroradiologie. I. Kranio-faziale Embolisationen. Radiologe 21:215–226

Embolization of Spinal Angiomas

H. Vogelsang

Abteilung für Neuroradiologie, Zentrum Radiologie, Medizinische Hochschule, Konstanty-Gutschow-Strasse 8, 3000 Hannover 61, FRG

Among vertebrospinal vascular malformations, arteriovenous angiomas and vertebral angiomas are especially accessible to therapeutic embolization under certain conditions. This can be indicated as a preoperative measure or as a single measure. Thus, for example, small retromedullary angiomas with only one or two feeding arteries can mostly be readily embolized. In larger angiomas, especially in younger patients, the surgical procedure should be preferred, possibly with embolization as a preoperative measure. On the other hand, in older patients with large angiomas, embolizations are indicated. Patients displaying a vertebral hemangioma with or even without neurologic deficits constitute a further indication for therapy by means of embolization.

Preconditions are as follows:

1. There must be good localization of the catheter tip in the lumen of the feeding artery. The caliber of the artery to be embolized must be large enough to receive the embolization particles.
2. The angioma may not be fed via the anterior spinal artery.
3. The procedure should not be attempted in angiomas with a shunt which is so large that the embolization mass can pass into the draining veins, possibly resulting in their occlusion, congestion, and edema of the spinal cord.
4. In the cervical region, only external carotid arteries and subclavian arteries feeding the lesion may be embolized, not vessels from the vertebral arteries or from the internal carotids.
5. Each potential case must be discussed with the neurosurgeon.

As a rule, spinal arteriography is only performed after prior myelography with a nonionic contrast medium and tomography. Preconditions for embolization are an exact visualization of the vascular malformation with its feeding and draining blood vessels, precise localization, and analysis of the pictures obtained by means of the subtraction technique. Spinal arteriographies have been carried out for more than 1 year using the stereomagnification technique in our department in cases of angioma. In contrast to other study groups, we perform superselective spinal arteriography and embolization without anesthesia so that complications can be detected in good time.

Up to the middle of 1980 either Gelfoam or lyophilized dura was used as the embolization material. Since then, Tachotop-Flokuli (Hormonchemie, Munich) have been used; at our request, they were manufactured with diameters of 1.8–4 mm. Tachotop-Flokuli are fibrils of collagenous fiber bundles 0.1–0.5 µm thick, isolated from equine connective tissue, processed, and comminuted to a foam.

Our experience is based on a total of 40 demonstrated spinal angiomas, ten of which were embolized. In some cases, the embolization was performed as the sole measure and in some cases as a preoperative measure. Four patients were embolized twice within 3–6 months because of a recurrence. A rigid schedule for the embolization cannot be observed; it must be adapted individually to each patient. The results of embolization are as varied as the angiomas visualized and partly depend on the neurologic status and duration of the disease. On the other hand, excellent results can be attained even in patients with a high degree of paraplegia. In some cases, a relapse and demonstration of fresh collaterals occurred after a few weeks or months. In some cases, no reaction to the embolization could be discerned.

This can be illustrated by a few brief examples:
In a 17-year-old male patient, there was a spinal angioma the size of a walnut at the level of the thoracolumbar transition with several feeding arteries (see Fig. 1). Increasing paraparesis of the legs with sensory disorders had begun 3 months prior to arteriography.

Radiology Today 2. Ed. by F. H. W. Heuck and M. W. Donner

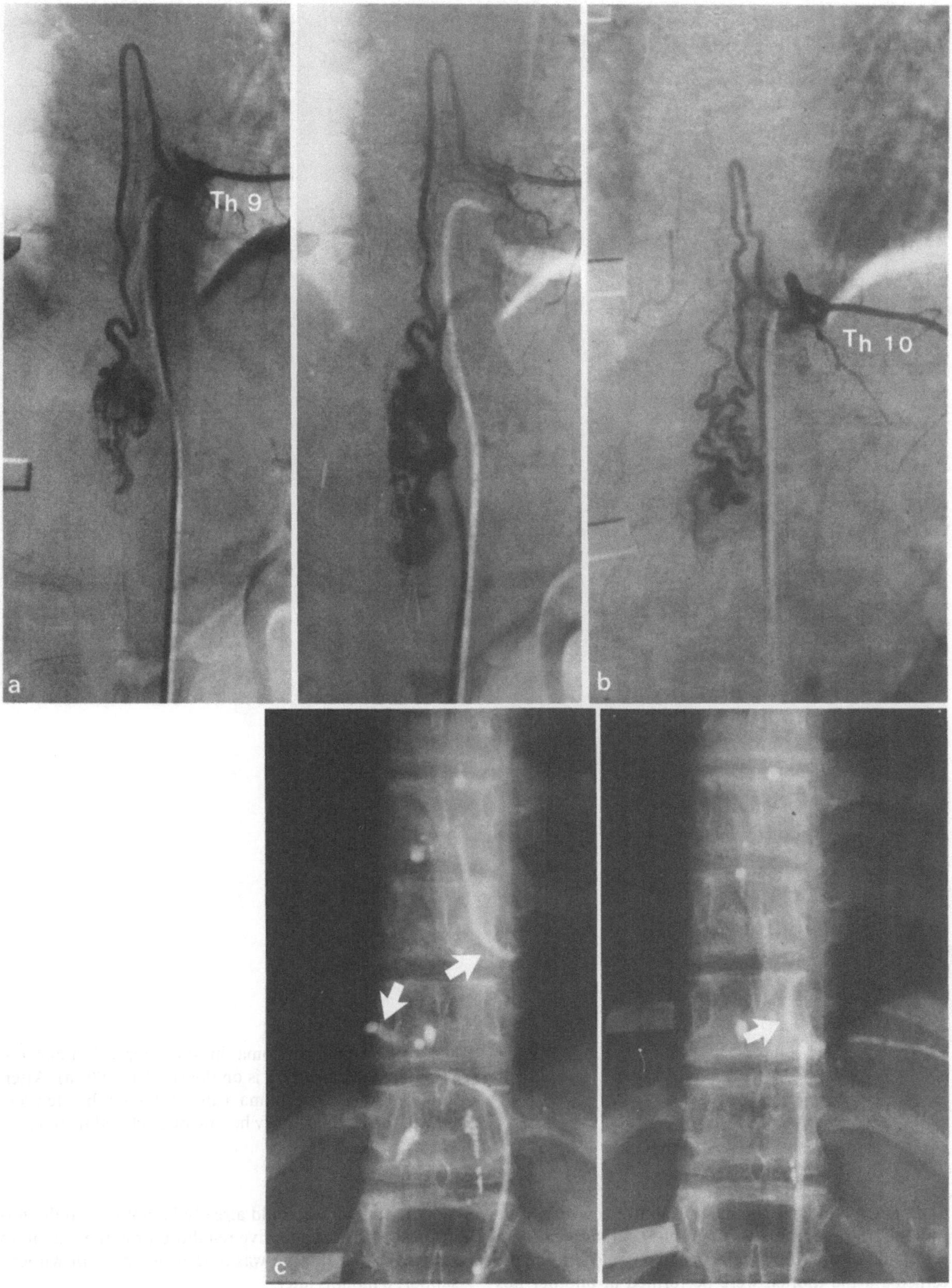

Fig. 1 a–c. Spinal angioma in the thoracic region. The feeding arteries are on the left Th9 (**a**) and Th10 (**b**) and on the right Th10 (not demonstrated). After embolization (**c**) the feeding arteries are closed (*arrows*)

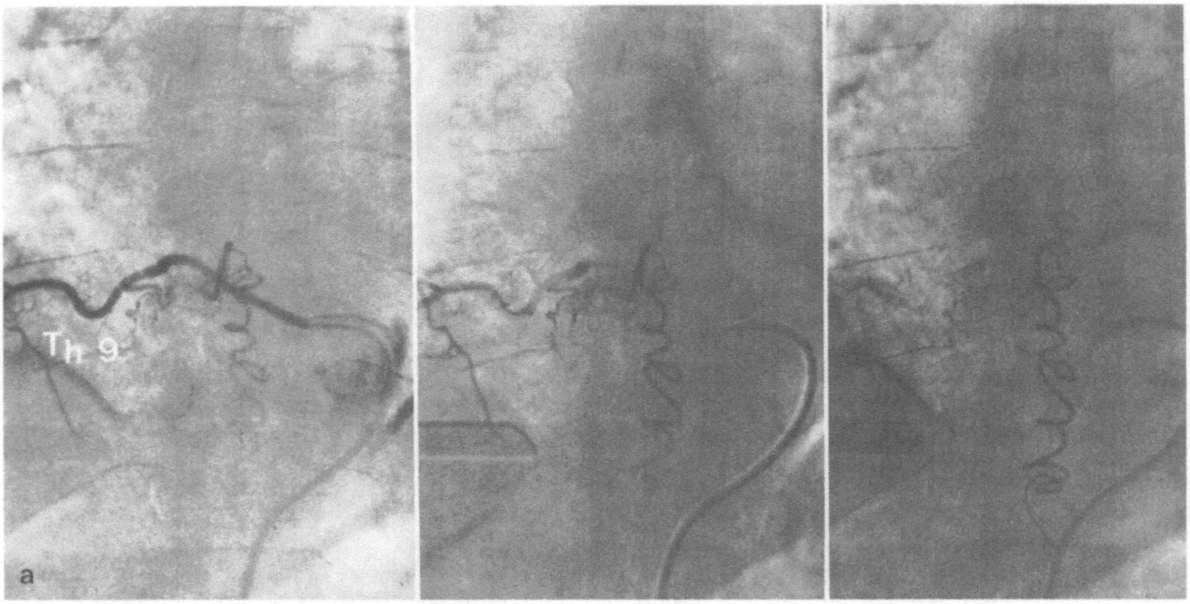

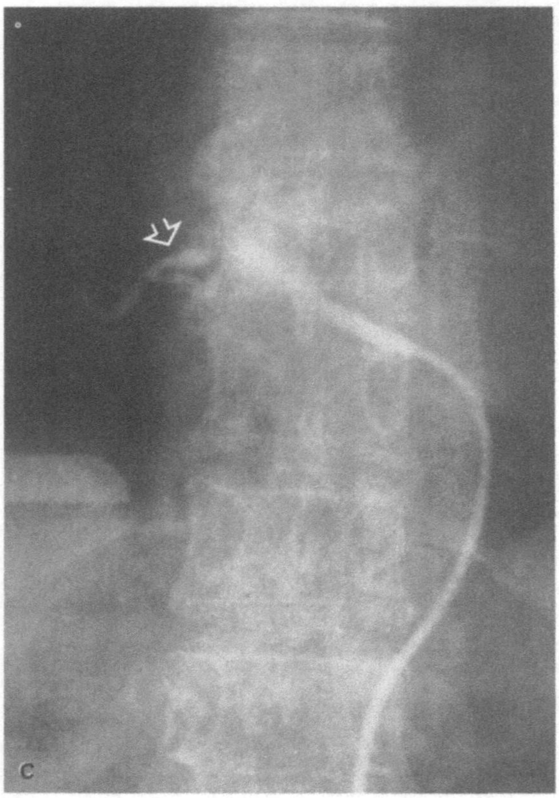

Fig. 2 a, b. Spinal angioma in the thoracolumbar region. The feeding artery is on the right at Th9 (**a**). After embolization the angioma can no longer be demonstrated, the feeding artery having been closed (*arrow*)

The patient had been unable to walk for 3 weeks at the time of arteriography. Myelography and surgical demonstration of the filling defect, which could also be discerned via the thorax, were performed at another hospital; high thoracic surgery was carried out. The correct localization of the angioma was only shown by subsequent spinal arteriography in our department. Embolization was performed in two sessions. Increasing mobility in the legs could already be noticed on the following day. After intensive rehabilitation, the patient to such an extent that he was able to walk again without support 6 months later.

A 45-year-old male patient, in whom embolization was performed because of clinically incomplete paraplegia with complete vesicorectal paresis in the lower thoracic region, showed similar results. There was a slight im-

provement in the mobility in the region of the upper leg after only a few hours. Now, 2 years after the operation, the patient is once again able to run his agricultural enterprise even though he has certain neurologic deficits.
A 66-year-old female patient showed the clinical and myelographic signs of a spinal angioma dorsally in the middle thoracic region. In the first angiography, only one feeding vessel (right intercostal artery Th7) could be demonstrated. Embolization was carried out. Both subjectively and objectively, there was a marked improvement in paraspasticity and sensory disturbance (especially in vesicorectal disorders). However, 2 months later there was fresh increase in the deficits and numerous collaterals to the angioma were detected in a control angiography; occlusion of the embolized vessels had largely persisted. Surgery with removal of the angioma was then performed, in view of the good general state of the patient and her own desire for the operation. After rehabilitation, the intensity of the deficits declined. The patient is once more able to walk.
In a 57-year-old patient with an intradural thoracolumbar spinal angioma fed by three vessels of small caliber and draining in the basal direction, embolization was performed in an almost complete transverse lesion syndrome. There was then a marked improvement in the mobility of the legs even within 24 h. In the course of the following weeks and months, he was again able to climb stairs alone, to go for walks, even though there were transient manifestations of fatigue. Seven months later, there was a relatively sudden recurrence of paraplegia, which subsequently developed into complete transverse syndrome. Control angiography showed recanalization of the right ninth intercostal artery; this was embolized once more. According to a report from an outside hospital 6–7 months later, there has been no further improvement.

References

1. Djindjian R (1978) Treatment of spinal angiomas by embolization. In: Pia HW, Djindjian R (eds) Spinal angiomas. Springer, Berlin Heidelberg New York, pp 189–200
2. Djindjian R, Merland JJ, Djindjian M, Houdart R (1978) Place de l'embolisation dans le traitement des malformations arterio-veineuses medullaires. A propos 38 cas. Neuroradiology 16:428–429
3. Doppman JL (1978) Embolization of spinal arteriovenous malformations. In: Pia HW, Djindjian R (eds) Spinal angiomas. Springer, Berlin Heidelberg New York, pp 201–208
4. Hilal SK, Sane P, Michelson WJ, Kosseim A (1978) The embolization of vascular malformations of the spinal cord with low-viscosity silicon rubber. Neuroradiology 16:430–433
5. Merland JJ, Riche MC, Chiras J, Bories J (1981) Therapeutic angiography in neuroradiology: Classical data, recent advances and perspectives. Neuroradiology 21:111–121
6. Vogelsang H (1981) Angiographische Untersuchungen von Wirbelsäule, Spinalkanal und Rückenmark. In: Diethelm L, Wende S (eds) Röntgendiagnostik des Zentralnervensystems. – Roentgendiagnosis of the central nervous system. Springer, Berlin Heidelberg New York (Handbuch der medizinischen Radiologie, vol 14/1B, pp 177–267)
7. Voigt K, Stoeter P (1980) Indikation und Befunde neuroradiologischer Embolisationen. Neurol Psychiatr 6:64–78

Workshop
Bone Tumors: Radiologic-Pathologic Correlations

H. D. Dorfman, M. T. Freedman, and W. Bessler

Department of Pathology, Sinai Hospital of Baltimore, Baltimore, MD 21215, USA

Case 1 (Sinai Hospital 79-1855)

A girl was first examined in 1976 at the age of 2 because of anterior bowing of the right leg. X-rays showed an intracortical radiolucent lesion in the midshaft of the tibia and a small lytic lesion in the distal fibula. Further X-rays taken in 1977 and in December 1978 showed slow progression of the tibial lesion with thickening of the anterior cortex. Excision of the tibial lesion and biopsy of the fibula were performed in February 1979.

Radiographic Findings and Comments

In this child there is anterior bowing of the tibia. Several well-demarcated lytic lesions are present within and widen the cortical bone of the anterior tibia. Each lesion has a well-defined sclerotic margin. There is no evidence of calcification within the matrix (Fig. 1 a).

There are two diagnoses that should be considered in this case: osteofibrous dysplasia and adamantinoma. Osteofibrous dysplasia occurs in young children and is usually a predominantly cortical lesion, with foci of decreased ossification lying within a thickened and sclerotic tibial cortex. The radiographs in this case are typical of the lesion. Adamantinoma of the long bones us usually intramedullary, but less commonly can appear cortically oriented. Although adamantinoma has been reported in patients as young as 8 years

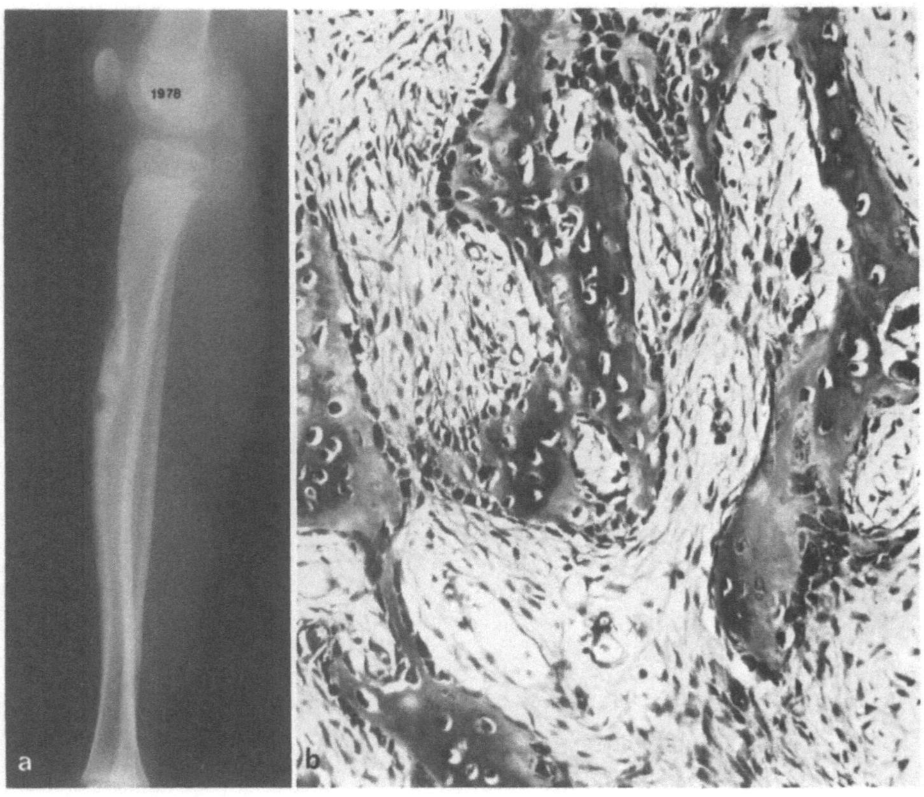

Fig. 1 a, b. Osteofibrous dysplasia of tibia and fibula. **a** Radiography; **b** pathology

Radiology Today 2. Ed. by F. H. W. Heuck and M. W. Donner

of age, the more common presentation is in the fourth decade. With this radiographic appearance at this patient's age, the most likely diagnosis is osteofibrous dysplasia.

Pathology

This is a fibro-osseous lesion in both the tibial and fibular sites (Fig. 1b). There is osteoblastic rimming of bone trabeculae with osteoclastic resorption in a moderately cellular fibrous tissue. The lesion is intracortical and is associated with cortical thickening, formation of new bone in the periosteum, and sclerosis of adjacent cancellous bone trabeculae. There is no extension to the adjacent soft tissue. This rare lesion should be distinguished from fibrous dysplasia on the basis of its predilection for the anterior tibial cortex in the midshaft and occasional simultaneous involvement of the lower fibula. It also appears in the literature under other names (ossifying fibroma of long bone, intracortical fibrous dysplasia). It can present as early as the 6th month of life and is usually seen in children below the age of 15. It may produce progressive deformity and lead to pathologic fractures, but most cases do not show any continued development after puberty. Treatment should be conservative.

In this case the patient suffered a pathologic fracture of the tibia 3 years after operation (1982) at the age of 8. At internal fixation of the fracture, biopsy material showed tissue identical to that removed in 1979 (age 5).

Diagnosis: Osteofibrous dysplasia of the tibia and fibula.

Further Reading

1. Campanacci M (1976) Osteofibrous dysplasia of long bones. A new clinical entity. Ital J Orthop Traumatol 2:221–237
2. Campbell CJ, Hawk T (1982) A variant of fibrous dysplasia (osteofibrous dysplasia) J Bone Joint Surg [Am] 64:231–236
3. Kempson RL (1966) Ossifying fibroma of the long bones. A light and electron microscopic study. Arch Pathol 82:213–233
4. Schoenecker PL, Swanson K, Sheridan JJ (1981) Ossifying fibroma of the tibia. Report of a case and review of the literature. J Bone Joint Surg 63-A: 483–488

Case 2 (Sinai Hospital 82-5573)

A 4-year-old boy with a limp of 3 months' duration complained of pain in the left thigh which was worse at night. There was no history of significant trauma. Acetaminophen gave incomplete relief of symptoms. Radiographs were obtained.

Radiographic Findings and Comments

There is a well-defined lytic lesion approximately 1 cm in diameter in the distal lateral femoral cortex. The lesion is rimmed by sclerosis which fades into the surrounding bone. Several lamellae of moderately thick new periosteal bone surround the lesion. There is no evidence of a surrounding soft tissue mass (Fig. 2a).

The radiographic pattern seen in this case is not specific. Osteoid osteoma and focal bone abscess could both have this appearance.

Osteoid Osteoma. When calcification is present in the nidus of an osteoid osteoma, the diagnosis is almost certain, but in the many cases in which the nidus is lytic, the appearance overlaps that of osteoblastoma and focal bone abscess. Periosteal reaction is common in osteoid osteomas; however, it is usually thick and often merges with the cortex, giving an appearance of cortical thickening. While thinner lamellae of new periosteal bone can be seen, this would be an unusual pattern for osteoid osteoma. Osteoblastoma, which is a larger lesion than osteoid osteoma, is usually a lytic process, more often medullary than cortical when it occurs in the long bones. It is usually not surrounded by as much bone sclerosis as osteoid osteoma, but their patterns can overlap.

Focal Bone Abscess. A focal cortical abscess has a radiolucent center, is surrounded by increased reactive bone, and can cause formation of lamellar periosteal bone; usually the lamellae are quite thin.

In this case a decision cannot be made between a cortical abscess and an osteoid osteoma. Cortical abscess is considered more likely from the radiographic appearance, but the history is more suggestive of osteoid osteoma.

Pathology

En bloc excision was carried out in the area of radiolucency and the lesion was found to contain nidus tissue (Fig. 2b), as well as reactive new bone of periosteal origin and cortical bone. The nidus is recognized microscopically by the cellu-

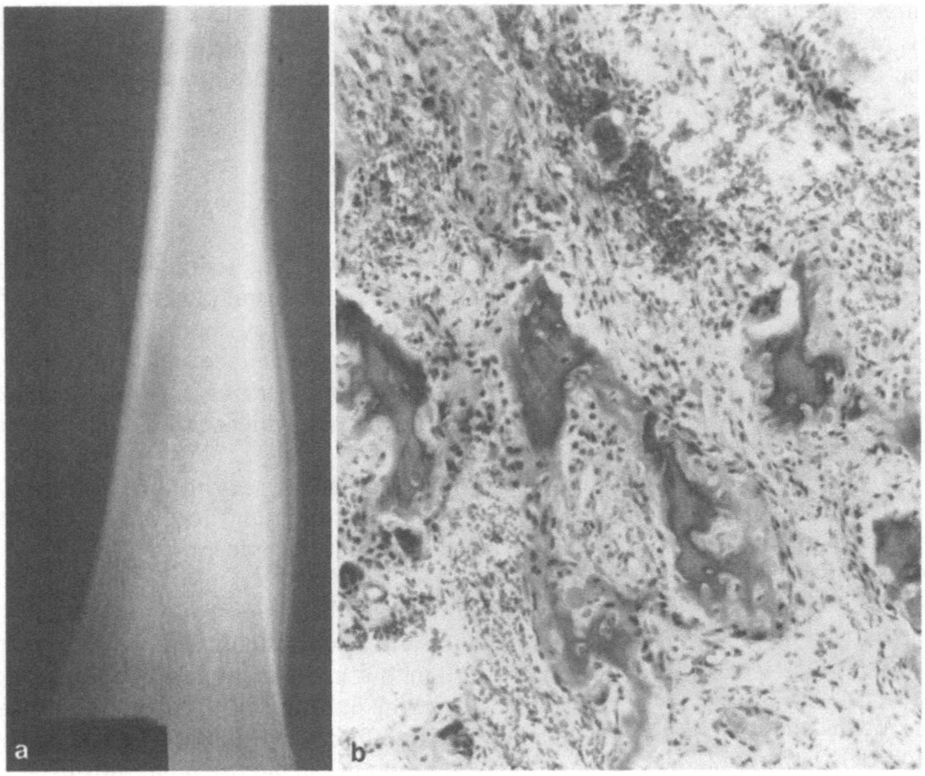

Fig. 2a, b. Osteoid osteoma of femur with extensive lamellar periosteal reaction. **a** Radiography; **b** pathology

lar osteoblastic tissue, which is richly vascularized and contains small irregular trabeculae of osteoid and woven bone. The pathogenetic mechanism for the extensive reactive bone formation in areas adjacent to an osteoid osteoma is not well understood.

Diagnosis: Osteoid osteoma of femur with extensive lamellar periosteal reaction.

Further Reading

1. Norman A, Dorfman HD (1975) Osteoid osteoma inducing pronounced overgrowth and deformity of bone. Clin Orthop 110:233–238
2. Schajowicz F, Lemos C (1970) Osteoid osteoma and osteoblastoma. Closely related entities of osteoblastic derivation. Acta Orthop Scand 41:272–291
3. Sim FH, Dahlin DC, Beabout JW (1975) Osteoid osteoma, diagnostic problems. J Bone Joint Surg [Am] 57:154–159
4. Winter PF, Johnson PM, Sadek KH, Feldman F (1977) Scintigraphic detection of osteoid osteoma. Radiology 122:177–178

Case 3 (Sinai Hospital 78-7364)

A 13-year-old girl complained of dull aching pain in the region of the left hip for 2 months. Radiographs were obtained.

Radiographic Findings and Comments

There is an approximately 3 × 5 cm lytic lesion of the body of the left ilium with a thick zone of surrounding sclerosis. The lytic area may contain foci of calcified matrix material. Irregular and somewhat spiculated bone is present along the lateral margin of the ilium. This is predominantly new periosteal bone, but a portion inferiorly is more likely tumorous bone (Fig. 3a).

The presence of the calcified matrix and the existence of tumorous bone lateral to the ilium indicate that this tumor is of the osteoid-forming series. The differential diagnosis is between osteosarcoma and osteoblastoma. On the radiograph, there is little information to aid in differentiation. The computed tomogram is helpful, however, in that it does not demonstrate a soft tissue mass extending beyond the limits of the visu-

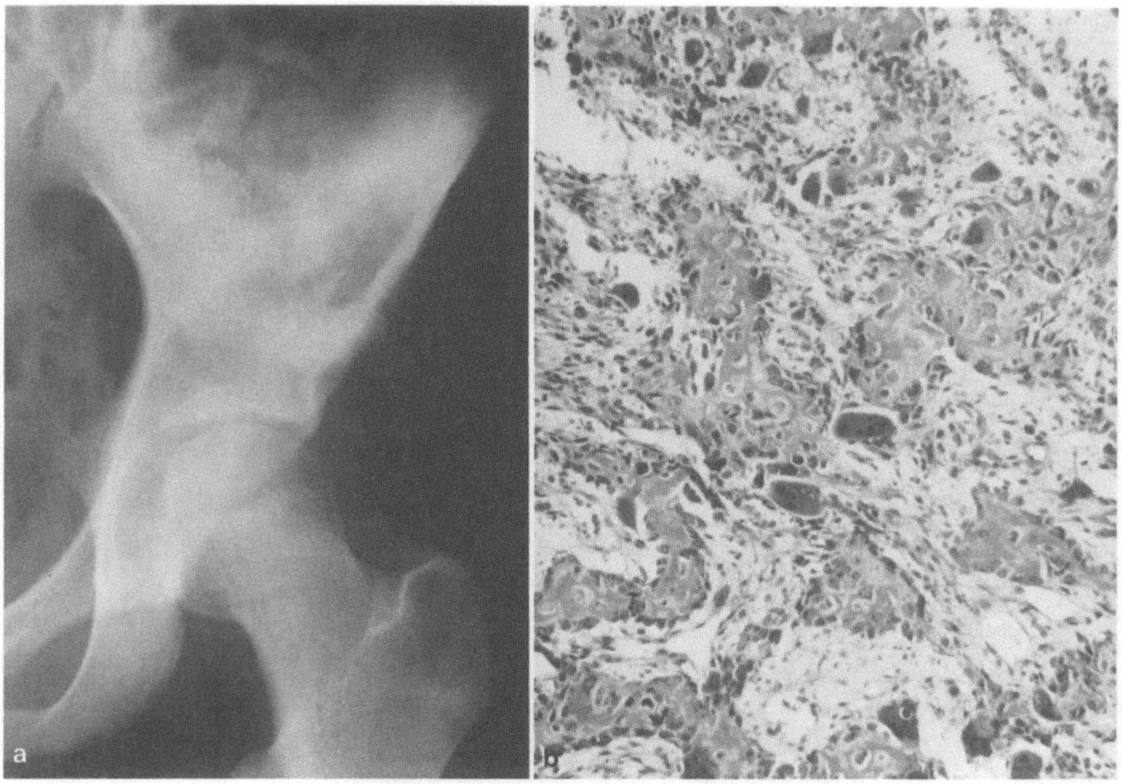

Fig. 3a, b. Benign osteoblastoma of ilium. **a** Radiography; **b** pathology

alized periosteal bone. In a lesion this big, the lack of such a soft tissue mass increases the probability that this is a benign lesion: osteoblastoma.

Pathology

A biopsy of the lesion (Fig. 3b) showed a benign bone-forming neoplasm characterized by trabeculae of osteoid and woven bone rimmed by osteoblasts and osteoclasts with a cellular intervening stroma even more rich in small blood vessels than the osteoid osteoma, which is otherwise histologically identical. There is no nuclear atypism and only occasional normal mitoses are present. There is no cartilage formation in the tumor. A rim of reactive bone could be found surrounding the lesion.
Diagnosis: Benign osteoblastoma of left ilium (supra-acetabular).
This tumor recurred locally 14 months after removal and a second wide excision was performed. There has been no further recurrence as of 1982, 3½ years later. Unlike osteoid osteoma, the larger osteoblastoma shows a progressive pattern of growth, though this is contained within a shell of reactive bone. Some osteoblastomas, especially those showing epithelioid osteoblasts, may recur aggressively, but they do not metastasize.
Diagnosis: Benign osteoblastoma of ilium.

Further Reading

1. Dorfman HD (1980) Case records of the Massachusetts General Hospital, CPC #40-1980. N Engl J Med 303:866–873
2. Marsh BW, Bonfiglio M, Brady LP, Enneking WF (1975) Benign osteoblastoma. Range of manifestations. J Bone Joint Surg [Am] 57:1–9
3. McLeod RA, Dahlin DC, Beabout JW (1976) The spectrum of osteoblastoma. AJR 126:321–335

Case 4 (Sinai Hospital 82-6260)

A 12-year-old male had a 2-month history of pain and a sense of fullness in the distal thigh. Radiographs were obtained.

Radiographic Findings and Comments

The anteroposterior view (Fig. 4a) reveals an expansile lytic lesion of the cortex with a thin rim of

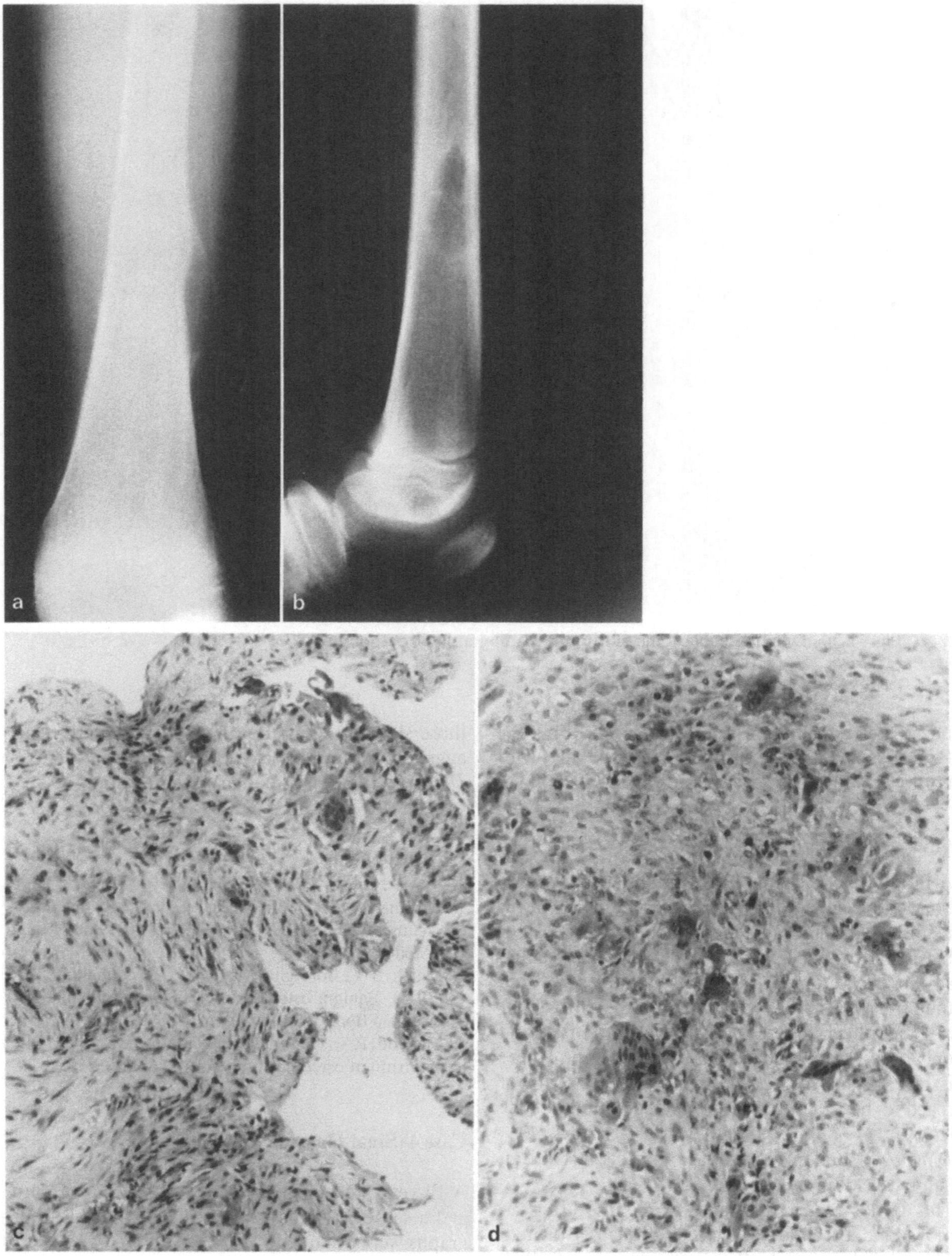

Fig. 4a–d. Aneurysmal bone cyst on nonossifying fibroma. **a** Anteroposterior view; **b** lateral view; **c, d** pathology

new periosteal bone. At the corners of the lesion there are several lamellae of new periosteal bone in a Codman's triangle shape.

The lateral view (Fig. 4b) demonstrates the shape of the lesion in the cortex. The lesion is elongated along the long axis of bone and has minimal sclerosis along the posterior margin.

This expansile lesion with a thin rim of new periosteal bone is almost certainly an aneurysmal bone cyst. The Codman's triangles and the thinness of the periosteal bone indicate the rapid expansion, but also show that the lesion is not expanding freely within the soft tissues.

Aneurysmal bone cysts may arise from other lesions. In this patient, the lateral view demonstrates an elongated lesion of the cortex with minimal sclerosis along a portion of its edge. This appearance is closest to that of a nonossifying fibroma – fibrous cortical defect – and it is likely that this is the nature of the preexisting lesion.

Pathology

The biopsy material removed from this expanded lesion had a hemorrhagic spongy appearance grossly, and microscopically showed two distinct patterns. The bulk of the tissue was composed of cellular connective tissue septa forming the walls of large blood-filled channels. Numerous multinucleated giant cells were present in the septa and some formed the linings of the blood spaces (Fig. 4c). These are the characteristic features of an aneurysmal bone cyst with no cell atypism in the walls. The second pattern consisted of proliferating fibroblasts with interlacing bundles of collagen fibers and scattered multinucleated giant cells, which is diagnostic for either metaphyseal fibrous cortical defect or nonossifying fibroma (Fig. 4d). Aneurysmal bone cysts are secondary vascular alterations, superimposed on a recognizable precursor lesion in ⅓–½ of cases. They may progress very rapidly, often contain trabeculae of osteoid and woven bone in the septa, and may radiologically mimic a malignant process. They are sometimes difficult to distinguish microscopically from giant cell tumors or teleangiectatic osteosarcomas.

Diagnosis: Aneurysmal bone cyst engrafted onto a benign fibrous lesion (nonossifying fibroma).

Further Reading

1. Biesecker JL, Marcove RC, Huvos AG, Mike V (1970) Aneurysmal bone cyst. A clinicopathologic study of 66 cases. Cancer 26:615–625
2. Jaffe HL, Lichtenstein L (1942) Solitary unicameral bone cyst with emphasis on the roentgen picture, the pathologic appearances and pathogenesis. Arch Surg 44:1004–1025
3. Levy W, Miller AS, Bonakdarpour A, Aegerter E (1975) Aneurysmal bone cyst secondary to other osseous lesions. Report of 57 cases. Am Jour Clin Pathol 63:1–8
4. Steiner GC, Kantor EB (1977) Ultrastructure of aneurysmal bone cyst. Cancer 40:2967–2978

Case 5 (Sinai Hospital 81-15157)

A 19-year-old male had an entirely unsymptomatic lesion of the right humerus discovered incidentally on films taken following a motor vehicle accident. He had been a weight lifter in the past but had noted no palpable mass or pain. A Craig needle biopsy was done.

Radiographic Findings and Comments

There is a 1.5-cm well-defined area of lysis of the posterior margin of the proximal humeral diaphysis. The lesion has destroyed the bone from its periosteal surface and abundant sclerotic bone surrounds the lesion on all but the periosteal margin. No bone is present along the periosteal margin. No calcification is seen within the matrix of the lesion (Fig. 5a).

This lesion has almost certainly arisen from the periosteum. The thick band of adjacent sclerosis indicates that the lesion has been present for a long time, indicating its nonaggressive nature. A lesion with this appearance can be a periosteal chondroma or a periosteal fibroma: a periosteal chondrosarcoma can occasionally look similar. No calcification is seen within the matrix of the lesion, preventing precise identification. However, since periosteal chondromas show this pattern of cortical erosion more often than periosteal fibromas do, periosteal chondroma is radiologically the most likely diagnosis.

Pathology

The biopsy established that a cartilaginous lesion was present, and en bloc excision revealed a well-circumscribed lobulated mass of hyaline cartilage which was moderately cellular (Fig. 5b). The cortical bone was thickened, as was the adjacent cancellous bone. A rim of intact periosteum surrounded the lesion, a benign cartilage tumor

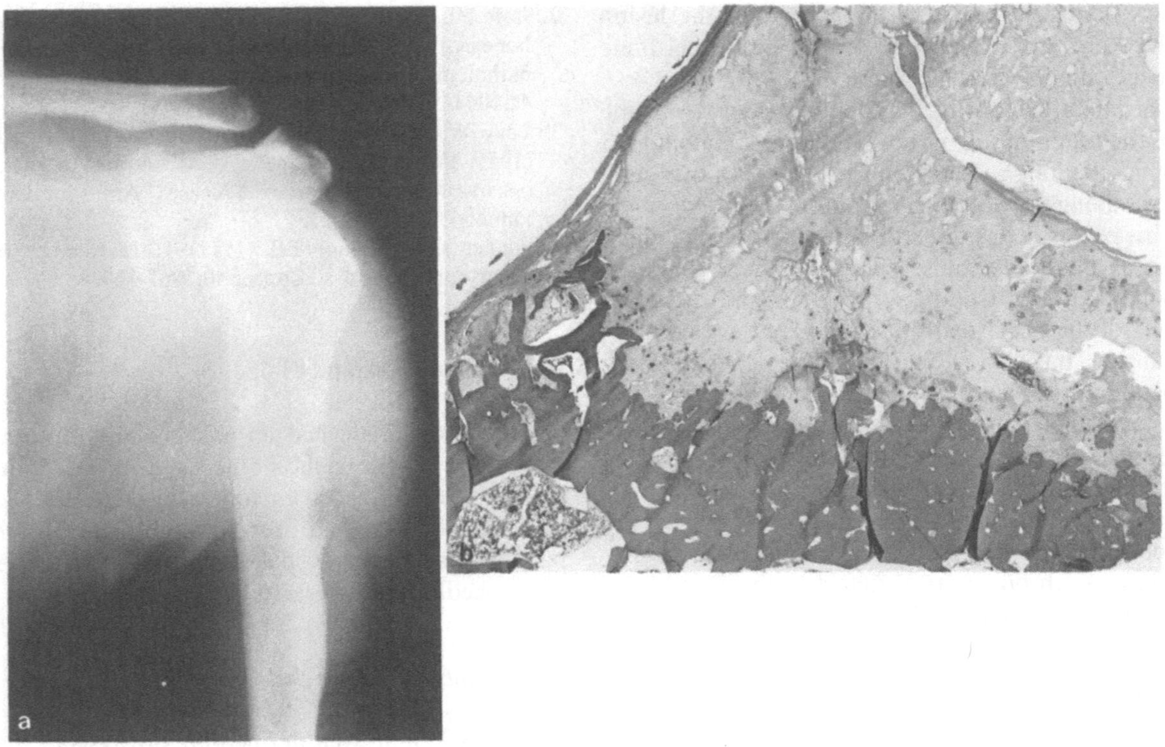

Fig. 5a, b. Periosteal chondroma of humerus. **a** Radiography; **b** pathology

growing just beneath the periosteum and derived from it. This neoplasm is sometimes microscopically mistaken for a chondrosarcoma because of increased cellularity. It does not usually recur after resection.

Periosteal chondromas are among the rarest cartilage tumors. They occur on the surface of tubular bones in their metaphyseal areas, the most common site being the proximal humerus. Saucerization of the cortex with buttress-like periosteal bone formation is the common radiographic appearance.

Diagnosis: Periosteal chondroma of humerus.

Further Reading

1. De Santos LA, Spjut HJ (1981) Periosteal chondroma: a radiographic spectrum. Skeletal Radiol 6:15–20
2. Lichtenstein L (1955) Tumors of periosteal origin. Cancer 8:1060–1069
3. Marmor L (1964) Periosteal chondroma (juxtacortical chondroma). Clin Orthop 37:150–153

Workshop
Skeletal Dysplasias: An Analytic Diagnostic Approach

H. J. Kaufmann

Abteilung für Pädiatrische Radiologie, Universitäts-Kinderklinik KAVH, Heubnerweg 6, 1000 Berlin 19, FRG

The field of skeletal dysplasias and dysostoses is still considered by many as enigmatic and puzzling. Admittedly this was the situation a generation ago, but then the efforts of a number of particularly interested specialists led to the first Paris nomenclature in 1969 and its updating in 1977 (see Appendix). Order has been imposed on this large group of skeletal disorders, only a handful of which can be diagnosed reliably by clinical examination, the remaining vast majority requiring careful radiological analysis.

Role of the Radiologist

The radiologist can be confronted by different actual patient-related situations:

1. Confirmation is requested of a clinically suspected diagnosis. For example, the clinician thinks that a patient is suffering from achondroplasia and a definite answer must be given. If the radiologist cannot confirm the clinicians's impression, it is of considerable importance that he offers either the correct diagnosis or a firmly negative statement leaving the actual diagnosis open.
2. A skeletal dysplasia is vaguely suspected and it is up to the radiologist to correctly identify the pathological condition. Only thus will it be possible to offer individual and genetic counselling.
3. Clinically a skeletal dysplasia is incorrectly suspected. Here the radiologist will orient the further diagnostic approach toward a metabolic disorder, the Battered child syndrome, or other conditions.
4. A skeletal dysplasia is not suspected but a chest film, a film requested for analysis of bone age, or another skeletal X-ray reveals to the radiologist that a given patient suffers from a skeletal dysplasia or a dysostosis. Such a situation is most rewarding for the astute radiologist!

In order to be able to offer a reliable diagnostic opinion a radiologist must be familiar with this large and continuously expanding special field. In our attempts to fill this role we must observe several ground rules:

1. All X-ray findings, together with the clinical changes, must fully fit the diagnostic criteria for any one of the well over 100 listed conditions (updated Paris nomenclature 1977 and subsequent publications).
2. Without adequate X-ray documentation no diagnosis can be made.
3. Quite often even experienced radiologists find themselves unable to diagnose a skeletal dysplasia correctly. We must know our individual limits and those of the field under discussion.

Adequate Radiological Documentation

Without adequate radiological documentation the task of the radiologist becomes very difficult if not impossible to fulfill. As soon as the clinician suspects skeletal dysplasia, X-ray documentation should be obtained, Ideally a complete skeletal survey, but if this is not possible the following minimal documentation must be obtained: skull AP and lateral, spine AP and lateral, chest PA, pelvis AP, one upper and one lower extremity AP, and one hand PA. For reliable interpretation of the X-ray manifestations of a suspected skeletal dysplasia, all pertinent clinical information must be available to the radiologist.

Variable Diagnostic Approach

In his approach to the diagnosis of a given patient the radiologist can proceed in different ways. De-

Radiology Today 2. Ed. by F. H. W. Heuck and M. W. Donner

pending on his individual experience he will start with one of the following:

1. Recognition of reliable, fully diagnostic findings
2. Systematic analytic search
3. Horizontal analysis (Rubin)
4. Correlation with clinical findings – Gamut approach

Reliable Diagnostic Findings

This is the so-called first-sight or on-the-spot diagnosis. Reliable diagnostic findings are present in only about 25% of all skeletal dysplasias, the pelvic and spinal changes of achondroplasia being the prime example. A further important point is that some diagnosis, for instance achondroplasia, are excluded by the absence of some of these reliable findings. An important aspect to keep in mind is the variability in time of some radiological findings in skeletal dysplasias. It is occasionally necessary to offer only a differential diagnosis, with a comment that further investigations will have to be undertaken in order to arrive at the correct diagnosis.
Even in the presence of reliable radiological findings we must still carefully analyze all available documents. On-the-spot diagnoses based on one or two specific findings can be dangerous and must be avoided.

Systematic Analytic Search

Conducting a systematic analytic search is the best way to avoid overlooking important information. Every film and all previous documents must be systematically analyzed.
The following schematic approach is recommended (in variable sequence):

- Location of lesion(s)
- Timing of lesion(s)
- Timing of manifestation(s)
- Contours (shape of individual bones such as pelvis and skull, bowing of long bones, etc.)
- Proportions (spine/extremities, segments of extremities)
- Density (individual bones, generalized, partial, or systematized)
- Function (restricted joint mobility, localized or generalized)
- Pattern of pathology recognized
- Correlation with clinical manifestations

A regional systematic sequence should also be followed:

1. Skull
2. Spine
3. Thorax
4. Pelvis
5. Limbs
6. Hands and feet
7. Joints
8. Areas of special interest, e.g., atlanto-occipital joint, base of skull

If a patient is obviously too small (in the range of well below − 2 SD to − 5 SD) the first question to be answered is whether we are dealing with a proportionate or disproportionate disorder. The ratio between the length of the spine and the length of the lower extremities must be established. The individual parts of the upper and lower extremities must be carefully evaluated (rhizomelic, mesomelic, or acromelic shortening).
Every long bone has to be approached carefully to determine if there is individual or general pathology in the development of the epiphyses, metaphyses, and diaphyses. Here the initial list of questions should be carefully answered.
The next step should clarify whether we are dealing with a disorder with combined spinal and extremity pathology (spondyloepiphyseal, spondylometaphyseal or spondyloepi/-metaphyseal). In similar fashion, if there is pathology of the skull, we should ascertain whether there is associated pathology of the metaphyses or diaphyses.
A careful analysis of the hands is always mandatory since much information can be derived from shortening of individual elements. Poznanski's pattern profile analysis [8] has proved extremely informative and can be reliable in a number of rare disorders. Of equal interest and value is the recognition of cone-shaped epiphyses of the short bones of the hand. According to Giedeon's schematic analysis [2] it can also be possible to pinpoint a disorder. Again, all recognized abnormal findings must be fully compatible with a suspected diagnosis.
On the basis of the positive or negative findings it should be possible to narrow down the diagnostic possibilities considerably. In the presence of only localized bony abnormalities, however, the orientation is much easier, although it should always be ascertained that indeed no other skeletal lesions exist.

Horizontal Analysis (Rubin)

By this approach an individual patient can be correctly diagnosed on the basis of the main radiographical features. Rubin has put logic and order into this field by compiling extensive listings. It must be noted, however, that these and even newer books may be incomplete in their listing of differential diagnoses.

An example is mesomelic dysplasia. This is a rapidly expanding field and new conditions with mesomelic shortening have recently been described. It is therefore important not only to consult the established literature [2], but also to read recent articles in the respective speciality journals [20, 33] (*Radiology, Pediatrics, Orthopedics, Genetics*). Historically, one of the major steps forward was Rubin's *Dynamic Classification of Bone Dysplasias.* It is still beneficial to read this classic book today, but unfortunately Rubin has never published an updated second edition.

Correlation with Clinical Findings – Gamut Approach

Occasionally it can be helpful to review the possibilities established by the clinical findings, for instance when a patient has lead symptoms involving the eye, hearing loss, malformations of ear, face, hands, or feet, fragility of bones, dermatological alterations, etc.

In reviewing the gamuts and the appropriate literature one may arrive at the correct diagnosis, perhaps from abnormal skeletal findings mentioned but not emphasized in the original report.

Recognition of Our Diagnostic Limitations

Over the years every radiologist sees cases that he finds difficult if not impossible to diagnose. This may be due partly to his own limitations, but it is also the result of the fact that the variability of skeletal dysplasias is such that hardly a month passes without the published or unpublished report of a previously unrecognized combination of skeletal findings or of manifestations of a disease affecting the skeleton not covered by any of the present listing of 125 individual disorders.

A number of radiologists have established themselves as experts in this field and now function as individual reference centers. Most radiologists, pediatricians, and geneticists have recognized this and consult an expert of their choice when faced with difficult diagnostic problems.

There is one major new development that may turn out to be an important step in a new direction. At the *Hôpital des Enfants Malades* in Paris, on the initiative of Jacques Sauvegrain and Pierre Maroteaux, a data bank for the storage of information on constitutional disorders of the skeletal system has been successfully put to work [26]. The stored information is presently available in French and English, and other languages will be added. It is hoped that in the future access to the pioneer work of the French group will be open to radiologists throughout Europe and beyond. The recognition of new disease entities will be greatly facilitated by the storage of information, since the computer will easily ascertain whether or not clinical and radiological findings correspond to information already coded. The need for such a service to the profession is clear if one considers that in every reference center, on average only one in three diagnostic problems submitted meets with a satisfactory response.

References

Reference Books for Diagnostic Approach

1. Beighton P (1978) Inherited disorders of the skeleton. Churchill/Livingstone, Edinburgh
2. Giedion A et al. (1981) Osteochondrodysplasien und andere konstitutionelle Skeletterkrankungen. In: Schinz HR et al. (eds) Lehrbuch der Röntgendiagnostik, vol. II/2, 6th edn. Thieme, Stuttgart, pp 1–186
3. Kaufmann HJ (ed) (1971) Intrinsic diseases of bones. Karger, Basel
4. Konigsmark BW, Gorlin RJ (1976) Genetic and metabolic deafness. Saunders, Philadelphia, pp 135–228
5. Maresh MM (1955) Linear growth of long bones of extremities from infancy through adolescence. Am J Dis Child 89:725–742
6. Maroteaux P (1979) Bone diseases of children. Lippincott, Philadelphia
7. McKusick VA (1978) Mendelian inheritance in man, 5th edn. Johns Hopkins Press, Baltimore
8. Poznanski A (1974) The hand in radiologic diagnosis. Saunders, Philadelphia
9. Rimoin DL (1979) International nomenclature of constitutional diseases of bone with bibliography. Birth Defects 15 (10)
10. Rubin P (1964) Dynamic classification of bone dysplasias. Year Book Medical Publishers, Chicago
11. Spranger J, Langer LO, Wiedemann HR (1974) Bone dysplasias. Fischer, Stuttgart

Publications on New Syndromes with Skeletal Manifestations

12. André M, Vigneron J, Didier F (1981) Abnormal facies, cleft palate, and generalized dysostosis: a lethal x-linked syndrome. J Pediatr 98:747–752
13. Beighton P, Cremin BJ, Kozlowski K (1980) Osteoglophonic Dwarfism. Pediatr Radiol 10:46–50
14. Dinno ND, Shearer LT, Weisskopf B (1980) An unusual case of short limbed dwarfism and thoracic dystrophy with normal spine, hands and feet. Pediatr Radiol 9:105–108
15. Fuhrmann W, Fuhrmann-Rieger A, De Sousa F (1980) Poly-, syn- and oligodactyly, aplasia or hypoplasia of fibula, hypoplasia of pelvis and bowing of femora in three sibs – a new autosomal recessive syndrome. Eur J Pediatr 133:123–129
16. Gruhn JG, Gorlin RJ, Langer LO (1978) Dyssegmental dwarfism. A lethal anisospondylic camptomicromelic dwarfism. Am J Dis Child 132:382–386
17. Hall BD, Spranger J (1980) Congenital bowing of the long bones. A review and phenotype analyses of 13 undiagnosed cases. Eur J Pediatr 133:131–138
18. Khajavi A, Lachman R, Rimoin D, Schimke N, Dorst J, Handmakers S, Ebbin A, Perreault G (1976) Heterogeneity in the campomelic syndromes. Long and short bone varieties. Radiology 120:641–647
19. Kozlowski K, Bützler HO, Galatius-Jensen F, Tulloch A (1978) Syndromes of congenital bowing of the long bones. Pediat Radiol 7:40–48
20. Löhr H, Wiedemann HR (1981) Mesomelic dysplasia – associated with other abnormalities. Eur J Pediatr 137:313–316
21. Majewski F, Ranke M, Kemperdick H, Schmidt E (1981) The Weaver syndrome: a rare type of primordial overgrowth. Eur J Pediatr 137:277–282
22. Maroteaux P (1980) L'osteomesopycnose – une nouvelle affection condensante de transmission dominante autosomique. Arch Fr Pediatr 37:153–157
23. Robinow M, Chumlea WC (1982) Standard for limb bone length ratios in children. Radiology 143:433–436
24. Saint-Martin J, Peborde J, Dupont H, Beguere A, Labes A (1979) Malformations osseuses complexes d'évolution letale. Un nouveau syndrome a caractère familial. Arch Fr Pediat 36:188–193
25. Sauvegrain J, Maroteaux P, Ribier J, Garel L, Tato L, Rochiccioli P, De Magalhaes J, Duhamel B (1980) Chondromes multiples avec atteinte rachidienne (spondyloenchondroplasie et autres formes). J Radiol 61:495–501
26. Sauvegrain J, Garel L, Maroteaux P, Garel P, Faure Cl, De Heaulme M (1982) Une banque de données: radiologie des maladies osseuses constitutionnelles. Arch Fr Pediatr 39:1–2. English translation (1981) Radiologic data bank for congenital bone diseases. Pediatr Radiol 11:121–123
27. Scott JE, Taor WS (1979) The "small patella" syndrome. J Bone Joint Surg (Br) 61:172–175
28. Stanescu R, Stanescu V, Bordat C, Maroteaux P (1980) La dysplasie spondylo-epiphysaire congenitale et son heterogeneite. Arch Fr Pediatr 37:527–530
29. Stöss H, Pesch HJ, Pontz B, Otten A, Spranger J (1982) Wolcott-Rallison syndrome: diabetes mellitus and spondyloepiphyseal dysplasia. Eur J Pediatr 138:120–129
30. Theander G, Ekberg O (1981) Congenital malformations associated with maternal osteodysplasty. A new malformation complex. Acta Radiol. [Diagn] (Stockh) (3B) 22:369–377
31. Vanek J (1981) Ischiopatellare dysplasie (Syndrom der „kleinen Patella" von Scott und Taor). Fortschr Geb Röntgenstr Nuklearmed (Ergänzungsband) 135 (3):354–356
32. Weisswichert PH, Knapp G, Willich E (1981) Accelerated bone maturation syndrome of the Weaver type. Eur J Pediatr 137:329–333
33. Wendler H, Schwarz R (1980) Carraro-syndrom. Fortschr Geb Röntgenstr Nuklearmed (Ergänzungsband) 133 (1):43–46

Appendix

International Nomenclature of Constitutional Diseases of Bone*
(Revision, May, 1977)

I. Osteochondrodysplasias

Abnormalities of cartilage and/or bone growth and development

A) Defects of Growth of Tubular Bones and/or Spine

a) Identifiable at Birth

1. Achondrogenesis type I (Parenti-Fraccaro)
2. Achondrogenesis type II (Langer-Saldino)
3. Thanatophoric dysplasia
4. Thanatophoric dysplasia with clover-leaf skull
5. Short rib-polydactyly syndrome type I (Saldino-Noonan) (perhaps several forms)
6. Short-rib polydactyly syndrome type II (Majewski)
7. Chondrodysplasia punctata
   a) Rhizomelic form
   b) Dominant form
   c) Other forms
   Exclude: symptomatic stippling in other disorders (e.g. Zellweger syndrome, Warfarin embryopathy)
8. Campomelic dysplasia
9. Other dysplasias with congenital bowing of long bones (several forms)
10. Achondroplasia
11. Diastrophic dysplasia
12. Metatropic dysplasia (several forms)
13. Chondro-ecto-dermal dysplasia (Ellis Van Creveld)
14. Asphyxiating thoracic dysplasia (Jeune)
15. Spondylo-epiphyseal dysplasia congenita
   a) Type Spranger-Wiedemann
   b) Other forms (see b. 11–12)
16. Kniest dysplasia
17. Mesomelic dysplasia
   a) Type Nievergelt
   b) Type Langer (probably homozygous dyschondrosteosis)
   c) Type Robinow
   d) Type Reinhardt
   e) Others
18. Acromesomelic dysplasia
19. Cleido-cranial dysplasia
20. Larsen syndrome
21. Oto-palato-digital syndrome

b) Identifiable in Later Life

1. Hypochondroplasia
2. Dyschondrosteosis
3. Metaphyseal chondrodysplasia type Jansen
4. Metaphyseal chondrodysplasia type Schmid
5. Metaphyseal chondrodysplasia type McKusick
6. Metaphyseal chondrodysplasia with exocrine pancreatic insufficiency and cyclic neutropenia
7. Spondylo-metaphyseal dysplasia
   a) Type Kozlowski
   b) Other forms
8. Multiple epiphyseal dysplasia
   a) Type Fairbanks
   b) Other forms
9. Arthro-ophthalmopathy (Stickler)
10. Pseudo-achondroplasia
   a) Dominant
   b) Recessive
11. Spondylo-epiphyseal dysplasia tarda
12. Spondylo-epiphyseal dysplasia, other forms (see a. 15–16)
13. Dyggve-Melchior-Clausen dysplasia
14. Spondylo-epi-metaphyseal dysplasia (several forms)
15. Myotonic chondrodysplasia (Catel-Schwartz-Jampel)
16. Parastremmatic dysplasia
17. Tricho-rhino-phalangeal dysplasia
18. Acrodysplasia with retinitis pigmentosa and nephropathy (Saldino-Mainzer)

B) Disorganized Development of Cartilage and Fibrous Components of Skeleton

1. Dysplasia epiphysealis hemimelica
2. Multiple cartilaginous exostoses
3. Acrodysplasia with exostoses (Giedion-Langer)

* *List of participants:* Drs. J. Dorst, C. Fauré, A. Giedion, J. Hall, H. J. Kaufmann, K. Kozlowski, L. Langer, L. Lenzi, P. Maroteaux, A. Murphy, A. K. Poznanski, D. Rimoin, J. Sauvegrain, F. Silverman, J. Spranger, R. Stanescu, V. Stanescu.

4. Enchodromatosis (Ollier)
5. Enchodromatosis with hemangioma (Maffucci)
6. Metachondromatosis
7. Fibrous dysplasia (Jaffé-Lichtenstein)
8. Fibrous dysplasia with skin pigmentation and precocious puberty (McCune-Albright)
9. Cherubism (familial fibrous dysplasia of the jaws)
10. Neurofibromatosis

C) Abnormalities of Density of Cortical Diaphyseal Structure and/or Metaphyseal Modeling

1. Osteogenesis imperfecta congenita (several forms)
2. Osteogenesis imperfecta tarda (several forms)
3. Juvenile idiopathic osteoporosis
4. Osteoporosis with pseudo-glioma
5. Osteopetrosis with precocious manifestations
6. Osteopetrosis with delayed manifestations (several forms)
7. Pycnodysostosis
8. Osteopoikilosis
9. Osteopathia striata
10. Melorheostosis
11. Diaphyseal dysplasia (Camurati-Engelmann)
12. Cranio-diaphyseal dysplasia
13. Endosteal hyperostosis
    a) Autosomal dominant (Worth)
    b) Autosomal recessive (Van Buchem)
14. Tubular stenosis (Kenny-Caffey)
15. Pachydermoperiostosis
16. Osteodysplasty (Melnick-Needles)
17. Fronto-metaphyseal dysplasia
18. Cranio-metaphyseal dysplasia (several forms)
19. Metaphyseal dysplasia (Pyle)
20. Sclerosteosis
21. Dysosteosclerosis
22. Osteo-ectasia with hyperphosphatasia

II. Dysostoses

Malformation of individual bones, singly or in combination

A) Dysostoses with Cranial and Facial Involvement

1. Craniosynostosis (several forms)
2. Cranio-facial dysostosis (Crouzon)
3. Acrocephalo-syndactyly (Apert) and others
4. Acrocephalo-polysyndactyly (Carpenter) and others
5. Mandibulo-facial dysostosis
    a) Type Treacher-Collins, Franceschetti
    b) Other forms
6. Oculo-mandibulo-facial syndrome (Hallermann-Streiff-François)
7. Nevoid basal cell carcinoma syndrome

B) Dysostoses with Predominant Axial Involvement

1. Vertebral segmentation defects (including Klippel-Feil)
2. Cervico-oculo-acoustic syndrome (Wildervanck)
3. Sprengel anomaly
4. Spondylo-costal dysostosis
    a) Dominant form
    b) Recessive forms
5. Oculo-vertebral syndrome (Weyers)
6. Osteo-onychodysostosis
7. Cerebro-costo-mandibular syndrome

C) Dysostoses with Predominant Involvement of Extremities

1. Acheria
2. Apodia
3. Ectrodactyly syndrome
4. Aglossia-adactyly syndrome
5. Congenital bowing of long bones (several forms) (see also osteochondrodysplasias)
6. Familial radio-ulnar synostosis
7. Brachydactyly (several forms)
8. Symphalangism
9. Polydactyly (several forms)
10. Syndactyly (several forms)
11. Poly-syndactyly (several forms)
12. Camptodactyly
13. Poland syndrome
14. Rubinstein-Taybi syndrome
15. Pancytopenia-dysmelia syndrome (Fanconi)
16. Thrombocytopenia-radial-aplasia-syndrome
17. Oro-digito-facial syndrome
    a) Type Papillon-Léage
    b) Type Mohr
18. Cardiomelic syndrome (Holt-Oram and others)
19. Femoral facial syndrome
20. Multiple synostoses (includes some forms of symphalangism)
21. Scapulo-iliac dysostosis (Kosenow-Sinios)
22. Hand foot genital syndrome
23. Focal dermal hypoplasia (Goltz)

III. Idiopathic osteolyses

1. Phalangeal (several forms)
2. Tarso-carpal
   a) Including François form and others
   b) With nephropathy
3. Multicentric
   a) Hajdu-Cheney form
   b) Winchester form
   c) Other forms

IV. Chromosomal aberrations

V. Primary metabolic abnormalities

A) Calcium and/or Phosphorus

1. Hypophosphatemic rickets
2. Pseudo-deficiency rickets (Prader, Royer)
3. Late rickets (McCance)
4. Idiopathic hypercalciuria
5. Hypophosphatasia (several forms)
6. Pseudo-hypoparathyroidism (normal and hypocalcemic forms, include acrodysostosis)

B) Complex Carbohydrates

1. Mucopolysaccharidosis, type I (alpha-L-iduronidase deficiency)
   a) Hurler form
   b) Scheie form
   c) Other forms
2. Mucopolysaccharidosis, type II – Hunter (sulfoiduronate sulfatase deficiency)
3. Mucopolysaccharidosis, type III – San Filippo
   Type A (Heparin sulfamidase deficiency)
   Type B (N-acetyl alpha-glucosaminidase deficiency)
4. Mucopolysaccharidosis, type IV – Morquio (N-acetylgalactosamine-6-sulfate-sulfatase deficiency)
5. Mucopolysaccharidosis, type VI – Maroteaux-Lamy (aryl sulfatase B deficiency)
6. Mucopolysaccharidosis, type VII (beta-glucuronidase deficiency)
7. Aspartylglucosaminuria (aspartylglucosaminidase deficiency)
8. Mannosidosis (alpha-mannosidase deficiency)
9. Fucosidosis (alpha-fucosidase deficiency)
10. GM1-Gangliosidosis (beta-galactosidase deficiency)
11. Multiple sulfatases deficiency (Austin, Thieffry)
12. Neuraminidase deficiency (formerly Mucolipidosis I)
13. Mucolipidosis II
14. Mucolipidosis III

C) Lipids

1. Niemann-Pick disease
2. Gaucher disease

D) Nucleic Acids

1. Adenosine-deaminase deficiency and others

E) Amino Acids

Homocystinuria and others

F) Metals

Menkes kinky hair syndrome and others

Selected Chapters on New Imaging Techniques

Technical Aspects of Digital Fluoro Imaging (Subtraction Angiography)

M. Pfeiler and P. Marhoff

Siemens AG, Unternehmensbereich Medizinische Technik, Henkestrasse 127, 8520 Erlangen, FRG

Introduction

In recent years, digital radiography – especially in the form of subtraction angiography – has not only attracted attention at all radiological congresses, but has also been the particular subject of a series of symposia. Many interesting images have been shown at these meetings, documenting in chronological sequence the considerable increase in clinical and technical experience. Figure 1a shows a recent (spring 1982) intravenous subtraction angiogram of the aorta and bifurcation. Comparison with Fig. 1b a similar image taken in September 1981, shows the improvement of image quality achieved within less than a year here with a 512 × 512 pixel matrix.

At the meetings mentioned, the principle and technique of digital radiography were presented and discussed in detail. At one of them we made a contribution [8], referring to several key papers [1, 2, 4–7, 9, 11, 12], and therefore, after referring to some terms necessary for definition, this paper will restrict discussion of principle and technique to a summary. The technical consequences of fluoroscopic and fluorographic subtraction will be discussed with respect to both raw data storage application and exposure technique. The central theme will be an examination of the so-called signal-to-noise ratio, since this has clinical as well as technical consequences.

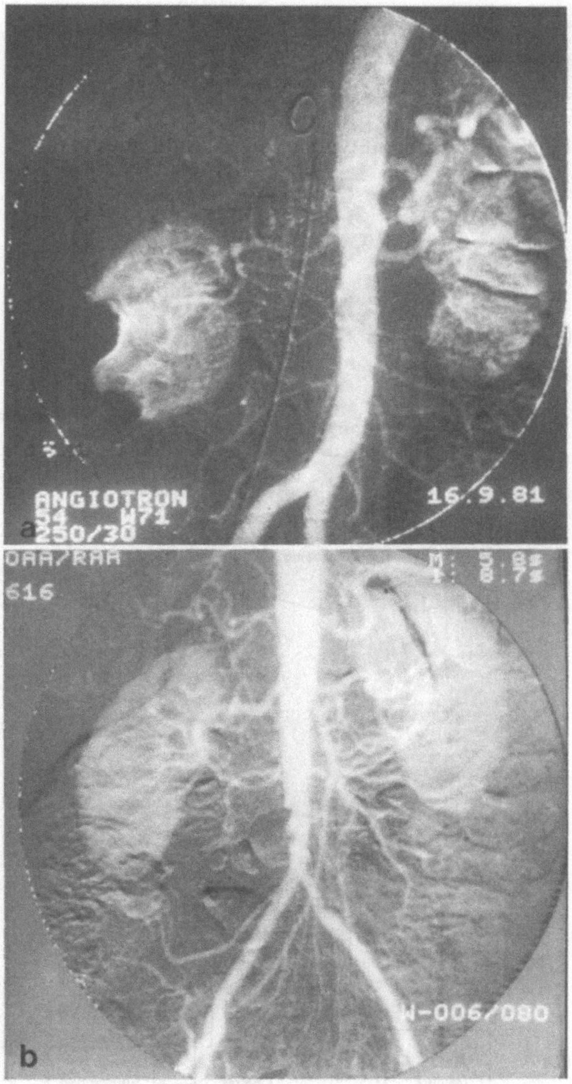

Fig. 1a, b. Development of subtraction angiography: imaging of the aorta and bifurcation. **a** State of the art, spring 1982. **b** Comparable case about 9 months earlier. In both cases 40 cc contrast medium was injected intravenously. (Images courtesy of Dr. Walter Seyferth, Diagnostic Department, Radiology Center, Klinikum Nürnberg)

Digital Radiography and Digital Subtraction Angiography

Under the term "digital radiography" (Fig. 2), three fundamentally different procedures are to be understood. Only computer tomography (CT) and computer radiography or scanned projection radiography, usually performed with a CT installation, are fully digitized procedures, in that the image is constructed from digitally recorded data.

Radiology Today 2. Ed. by F. H. W. Heuck and M. W. Donner

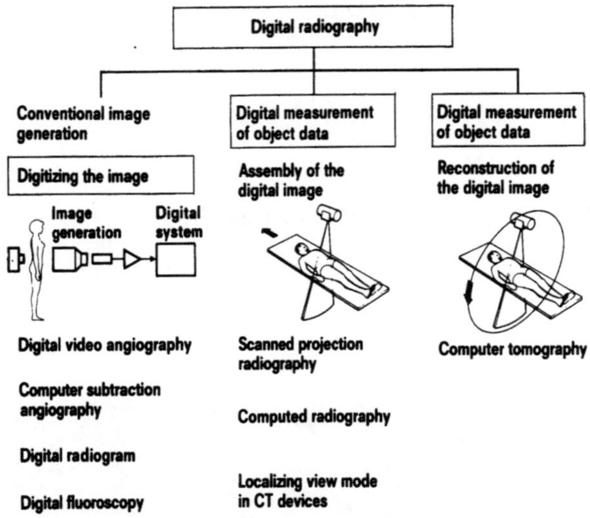

Fig. 2. The different types of digital radiography

In fluoro imaging, in our particular case in digital subtraction angiography, the image is produced in the conventional manner and then transmitted to the digital system in the form of an analog video signal (Fig. 3) which is then digitized. These digitized signals are subsequently available for postprocessing.

Naturally, at this point the question arises: What advantage does digital processing offer over the old (late 1960s and early 1970s), well-known radiological procedure of image subtraction which includes (analog) electronic subtraction of X-ray or fluoroscopic images (pathfinder technique)?

The answer gained from experience to date is twofold, and both points are very important. The digital technique provides survey image subtraction with an "instant subtraction image" and also

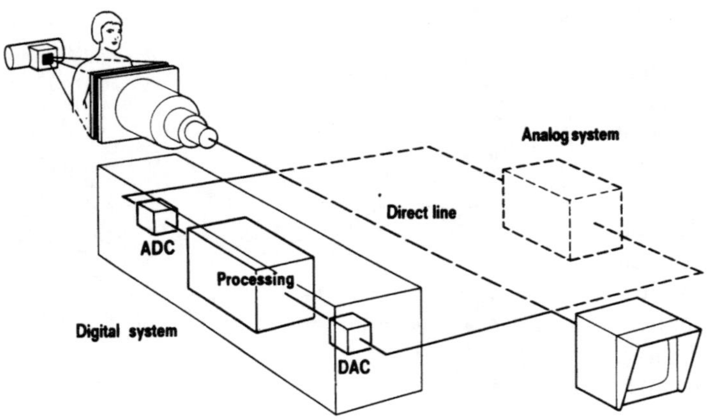

Fig. 3. Principle of digital radiography. Digitization or analog-to-digital conversion (ADC), processing, digital-to-analog conversion (DAC)

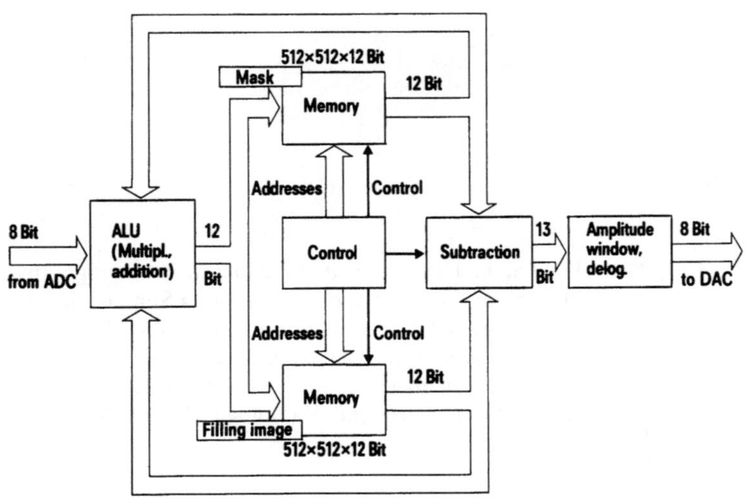

Fig. 4. Digital subtraction angiography: block circuit and data flow

permits total reproducibility and fully determinable signal storage and processing. As opposed to analog methods, reproducibility and precision are not a question of physics or technology, but only of cost.

Principle and Technique

The subtraction angiography system itself (Fig. 4) includes basically at least two digital working memories, or stores: one for the mask image and the other for the filling image. From these stores the desired image is produced by the calculation process of subtraction. It should be noted that Fig. 4 represents digital fluoroscopy. The analog-to-digital conversion (ADC) of the individual TV frames coming from the X-ray TV installation is performed with 8 bits, that is, by assigning one out of 256 signal values to each pixel, although the store can accommodate 12 bits (one out of 4096 values per pixel) which then is the actual gray scale of the unit. This expanded gray scale or contrast resolution is appropriate and efficient) because in the fluoroscopic mode, the mask or filling image does not consist of one individual TV image but is obtained from the average value of an image sequence of, for example, 16 images. The determination of the average value (Fig. 5) takes place in the store itself by means of a feedback or recursive method, resulting in a weighted

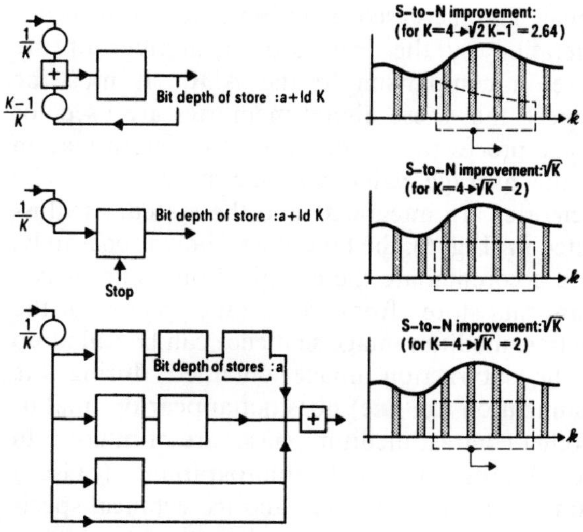

Fig. 5. Digital averaging and summation. The sketches at the right show for an evaluation factor K of 4 how the input images contribute to one output image

or sliding average, or by summating the individual images of a predetermined image sequence. (A "sliding" summation, as shown in the lower part of Fig. 5, cannot be performed by a single store.)

This "assembling", or integration of mask or filling images from a number of individual images, means an increased effective dose for the latter and thus an improvement in the signal-to-noise ratio, i.e., the noise reduces in comparison to the

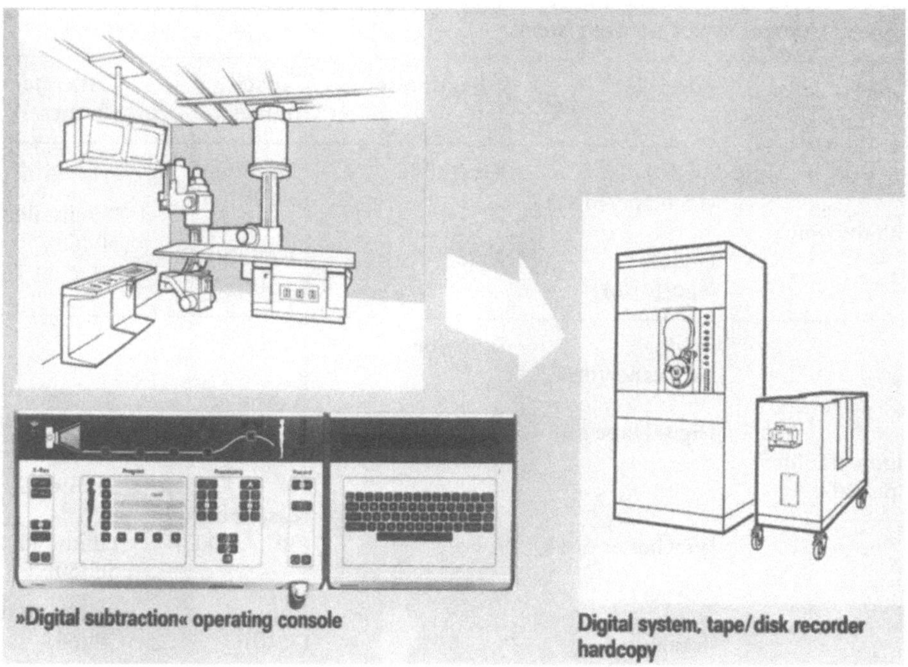

Fig. 6. Angiographic installation with digital subtraction system

signal. The increased precision is taken into consideration by the increased bit-number of the store in comparison to the ADC. It must be stressed that these digital memories are used for image processing; in this case, for determination of the average value and for subtraction. The memories are integrated into the system as illustrated in (Fig. 6); the tape store, shown separately, is to accommodate the examination scene. It is a "raw data store" from which other phases of the contrast medium image sequence can be called up if the subtraction image obtained during the examination (on line) does not appear optimal or if other contrast medium phases are of interest. In the fluoroscopic and fluorographic (pulsed) modes, this raw data store and its technical specifications play an important role in the comparison of digital systems.

The Difference between the Fluoroscopic and Fluorographic Modes

Figure 7 illustrates the essential technical difference between a fluoroscopic system, with, e.g., a standard frame rate of 50 or 60 Hz, and a fluorographic or pulsed system. This difference is expressed by the connection between the X-ray generator and the central system control which triggers the generator-set X-ray pulse sequences at the required time, with correct temporal lengths and, of course, rates. The pulse mode also has the consequences indicated for the primary image storage device from which the digital system can retrieve the most appropriate images to be used in subtraction. There may be a straightforward explanation for the use of different types of storage devices. For example, we can say that a 50-Hz fluoroscopic system generates many more images in total and per unit time than a two-pulse-per-second machine. The pulse mode system would easily meet our principal requirement of obtaining distortionless image storage, but would involve costly digital storage. Fluoroscopic systems, due to the numerous single images produced, preferably use a videotape or videodisk with the attendant low-cost image storage (Table 1). An analog videotape or videodisk adds some noise to the image from its internal noise sources, but as long as this additional noise is small compared with the quantum noise of the original single images, it has only a small influence on the resulting filling or mask images.

Only when storing integrated images produced by an effective dose of significantly above 300 µR does the noise from the storage medium contribute noticeably to the overall noise level. Since in our studies an integrated image results from approximately 30 individual images or TV frames, we can conclude that in such a single (stored) frame with an individual dose up to 10 µR the additional noise from a high-quality analog operating storage medium does not exceed the quantum noise.

Table 1. Comparison of storage systems

Type	Principle	Storage noise	Capacity (frames)	Data rate (frames/s)	Costs (k $)
Fluoroscopic	Analog videotape/(disk)	Perceptible	Unlimited (> 10^5)	"Unlimited" 50 (60)	Low (> 10)
	Digital tape/(disk)	None	"Unlimited" (> 10^4)		Very high (> 100)
Fluorographic ("pulsed")	Analog videotape/(disk)	Annoying	As above	As above	As above
	Digital tape disk				
	Winchester disk	None	reasonable (30 . . . 1000)	Limited 2 to unlimited 50 (60)	Reasonable (> 10) to high (> 50)
	Solid-state storage		Limited (< 10)	"Unlimited" 50 (60)	High (> 50)

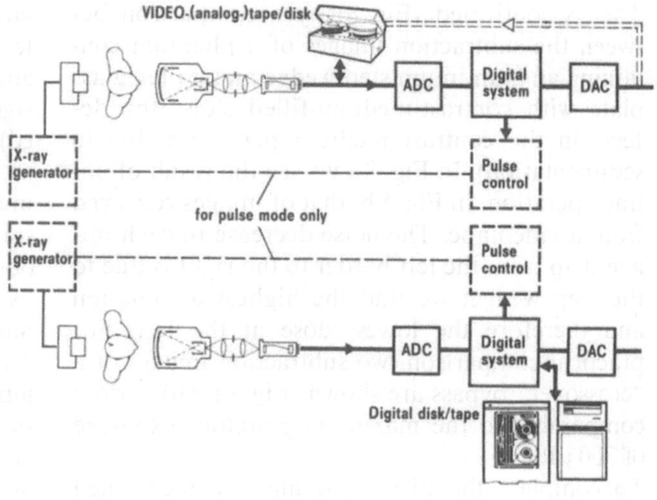

Fig. 7. Digital radiography. Diagrams of fluoroscopic and fluorographic systems

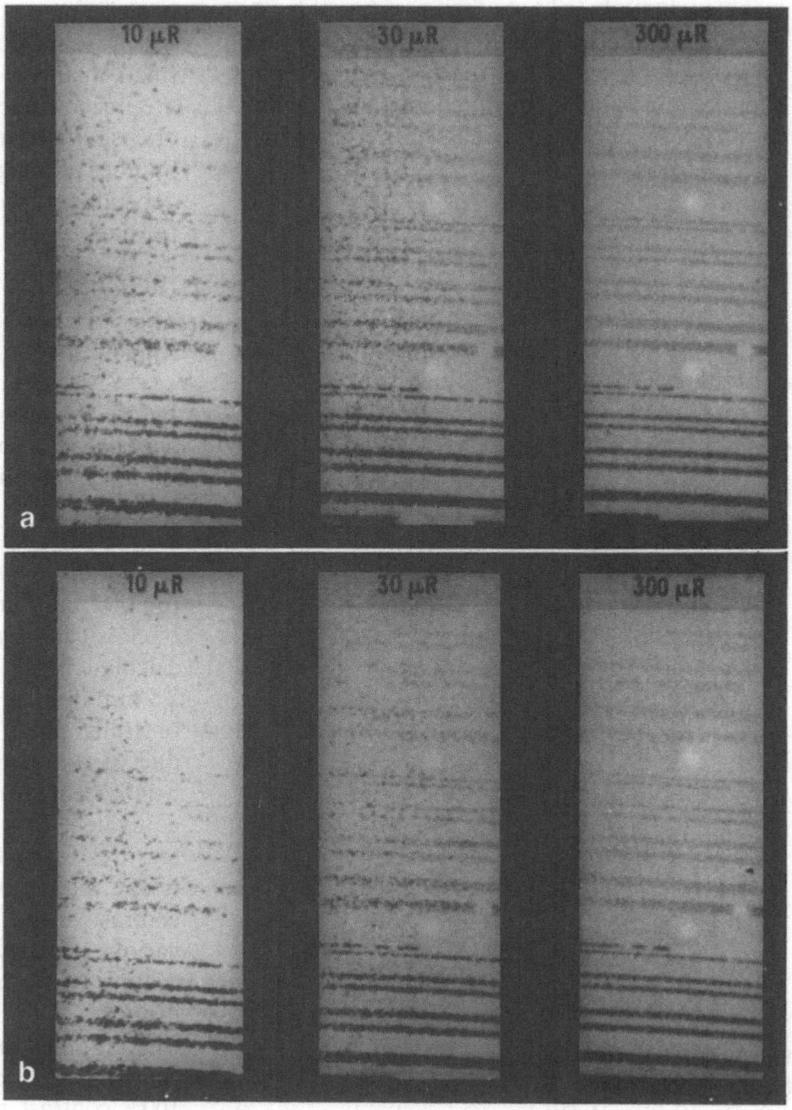

Fig. 8 a, b. Digital subtraction angiography. Subtraction images of an object phantom (aluminium step wedge with contrast medium structure superimposed; ratio of intensity behind the last and the first steps of the step wedge is 15:1) with varying image dose. **a** On-line images: a_0, filling image; a_1, a_2, a_3 subtraction images of varying effective dose (evaluation factor $K = 16$, i.e., about 30 single frames contribute to the filling and mask images). **b** Subtraction images as in *a* but with videotape intermediate raw data storage (off line)

This is confirmed (Fig. 8) by a comparison between the subtraction images of a phantom containing an aluminium step wedge and a plexiglass plate with contrast-medium-filled slots (the defects in the contrast medium paths are due to sedimentation). In Fig. 8a we see the result of online operation, in Fig. 8b, that of images retrieved from a videotape. The noise decrease in each image strip from the left border to the right is due to the step wedge; we find the highest attenuation and therefore the lowest dose at the left. For practical comparison two subtraction images of a "crossover" bypass are shown (Fig. 9) with a dose comparable to the maximum phantom exposure of 300 μR.

To complete the picture, it may be mentioned that the influence of the analog storage device noise can be reduced by a factor of 2 to 4 by storing only subtracted images (double dashed line in Fig. 7). This results from the fact that after subtraction, the signal (ideal conditions assumed) consists of less gray steps and can therefore be enlarged or amplified to fill all the available gray levels of the system. Thus the noise added by analog recording is smaller in comparison to the signal than to the recorded original (nonsubtracted) data. Also, the original information is not lost, as it can be retrieved by adding the subtracted images to a separately stored mask. However, this solution can obviously only work with nonmoving objects, otherwise some information may be lost by saturation effect in the subtracted image.

Summarizing the situation, we can say that for a digital system of the fluoroscopic type, the videotape or videodisk is an appropriate raw data store: many images can be stored without limitation on the frame rate but, depending upon the dose situation, certain additional noise has to and can be tolerated. In the case of the fluorographic or pulse mode however, the use of a digital working raw data store is practically a must, due to the small quantum noise in the single images which are not averaged before subtraction. For reasons of cost, we have here to compromise between the number of images to be stored and the image rate, depending upon the intended application, e.g., cardiac studies.

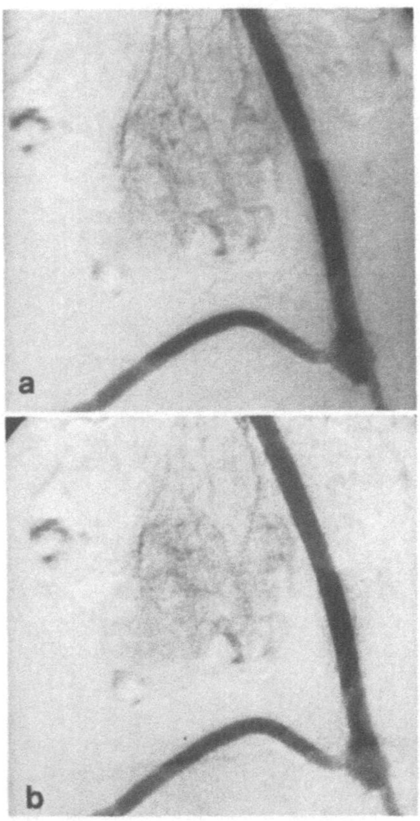

Fig. 9a, b. Digital subtraction angiography. Subtraction images of a crossover bypass. Effective dose 300 μR. **a** On line; **b** Off line (Original videotape courtesy of Dr. Walter Seyferth, Diagnostic Department, Radiology Center, Klinikum Nürnberg)

The Signal-to-Noise Ratio in Subtraction Angiography

Before a more specific discussion as to when and why the fluoroscopic and fluorographic modes should be applied, the signal-to-noise ratio must be discussed.

Figure 10 serves for orientation. It demonstrates first of all the usual meaning of the normal signal-to-noise ratio, using for visualization the example of classical arteriography. These signal curves are calculated for a object containing an artery 2.5 mm in diameter opacified by either an arterial or transvenous injection of Urografin (selected due to the availability of absorption data from Schoknecht [10]). The pixel size of 0.5 × 0.5 mm is equivalent to a 24-cm input diameter image intensifier with a fully utilized (high-resolution TV) image matrix of 512 × 512. Figure 10 shows the contrast of the vessel and the quantum noise for various dose levels and contrast medium concentrations; the ribbon indicates the RMS value of the noise.

The graphics for classical arteriography (Fig. 10) confirm what our experience tells us; close to 100% contrast medium concentration in the observed vessel means practically a "total contrast" or extinguishing of the original native signal. For

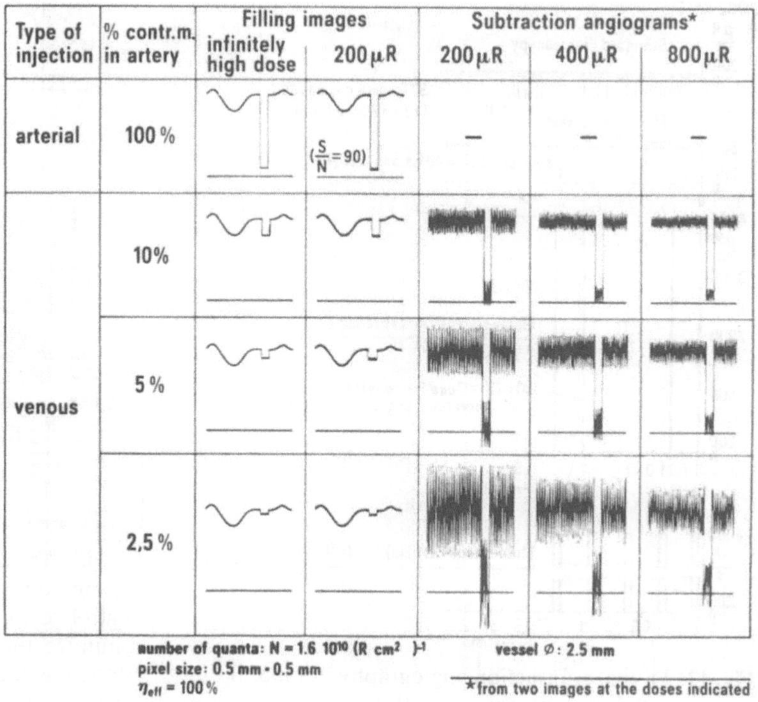

Fig. 10. Signal-to-noise ratio for conventional radiographs and subtraction angiograms. Visualisation for different doses and contrast medium concentrations

a normal angiographic system and a dose of 200 µR (measured at the input of the image receptor) we see a modest quantum mottle, calculated in accordance with the well-known signal-to-noise formula of radiology.

Assuming now a dilution of the contrast medium in the same artery of down to between 10% and 1% with intravenous injection the contrast of the vessel decreases dramatically. This is the chance for digital subtraction, during which the non-opacified mask is subtracted from the arteriogram and the difference signal expanded to the full gray scale of the TV system.

What works reasonably with a 200-µR dose in the case of 10% concentration looks nonusable in the case of 2.5% dilution. The desire to increase the dose can be understood by looking at the 800-µR column in Fig. 10.

It is essential to realize that in contrast to a normal radiogram, where the signal and noise are only correlated by dose, in the subtraction image the signal-to-noise ratio is determined additionally by the contrast medium concentration (Fig. 11) here expressed by a formula. The simple consequence is that an improvement of the signal-to-noise ratio can be brought about either by increasing the contrast medium concentration or by increasing the dose. Thus, for example, an increase in the concentration by a factor of 2, say from 2.5% to 5%, is equivalent to a dose increase by a factor of 4 in respect of the signal-to-noise ratio due to the square-root dependence of noise on dose.

We cannot report experiences on the difficulties associated with increasing the contrast medium concentration by improved contrast media or injection techniques. However, we wish to touch on the problems of generating a 1000-µR dose at the input of a system, if it is desired that this dose should not be accumulated from subsequent frames of a fluoroscopic or continuous mode but generated within a pulse time as short as possible.

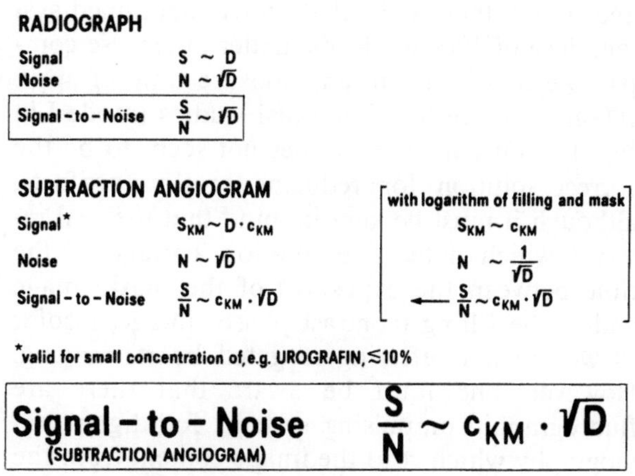

Fig. 11. Signal-to-noise ratio for subtraction angiograms, corresponding to the graphics in Fig. 10. *D*, dose, C_{KM}, contrast medium concentration (derivation of the formula in brackets in accordance to Fig. 13)

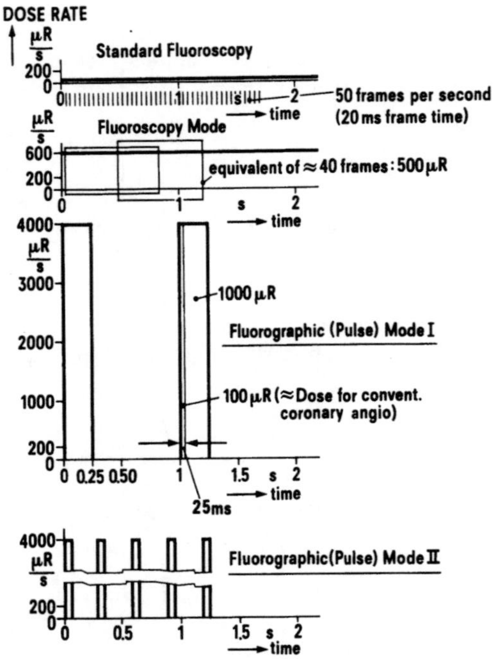

Fig. 12. Digital subtraction angiography: temporal diagram for the fluoroscopic and fluorographic (pulse) modes

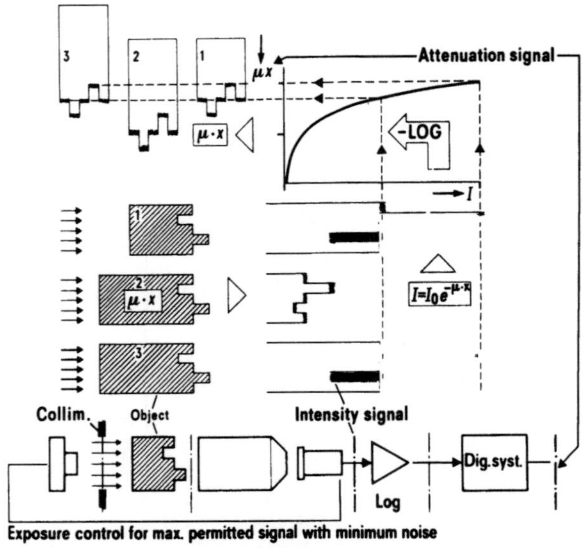

Fig. 13. Transformation of the intensity signal into the attenuation signal by logarithms (before). Exposure control compensates increased patient thickness to minimize the noise (transfer from case 2 to case 3). With reference to Fig. 11, the logarithmic curve transforms small signal variations caused by contrast medium, noise), multiplying by a factor proportional to the inverse of the actual dose (differential quotient of the logarithmic function)

Why is it then questionable to call such an exposure a real pulse? Let us recall Melvin Judkins' efforts, at Loma Linda Hospital, California, around 1970, to achieve exposure times as short as possible for coronary studies on the imaging basis of film changers. He ended up, – remarkably considering the technology available at that time – with exposure times of about 10 ms, although he selected a very sensitive film-screen combination requiring a system dose of only about 100 μR and technique factors like 80 kV and over 1000 mA. So that above-mentioned system dose of 1000 μR leads, under otherwise comparable conditions, to an exposure time of appr. 100 ms or more for abdominal studies (mode I in Fig. 12). Of course, this does not seem to be the correct solution for reducing motion artifacts, although it must be kept in mind that the real interval which determines motion artifacts is the time between the exposures of the mask image and of the filling (contrast phase) image, insofar as we are not referring to gated heart imaging. However, one must be aware that there are fluorographic or pulsing systems for digital angiography which read the image content from the TV pick-up tube during this so-called pulse time, using the standard TV mode, or integrate digitally stored frames from a series of shorter pulses (mode II in Fig. 12, necessary and useful for ECG-gated heart imaging). This raises the question of whether the continuous or fluoroscopic mode is the more natural one to be applied to any high-dose, non-cardiac study. Some digital subtraction angiography systems offer both modes; the fluoroscopic and the fluorographic or pulse.

Returning to dose, and to the fact that fluoroscopic systems are able to collect a high dose per image by integration, not only the technical viewpoint, but also the dose to patient and personnel has to be considered.

The principle of exchanging contrast medium concentration and radiation dose with respect to signal-to-noise ratio in a subtraction angiogram is a common problem for radiologists and physicists as well as for the contrast media chemist.

Noise Minimization: Exposure Technique and Postprocessing

To obtain the maximum signal-to-noise ratio for a preset exposure mode, it is of advantage to use the system in such a way that the maximum signal permitted, or the maximum operational system dose, is obtained. Figure 13 shows the logarithm of the input signals as preparation for subtraction

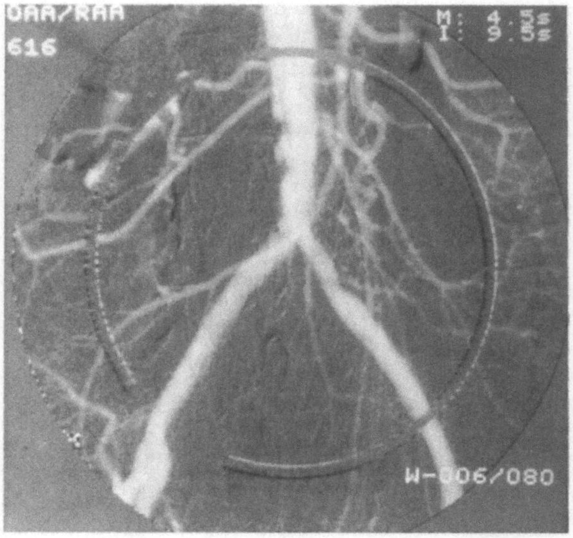

Fig. 14. Digital subtraction angiography with rubber balloon as compressorium. The ring in the image indicates the area of the balloon in contact with the patient. (Courtesy of Dr. Walter Seyferth, Diagnostic Department, Radiology Center, Klinikum Nürnberg)

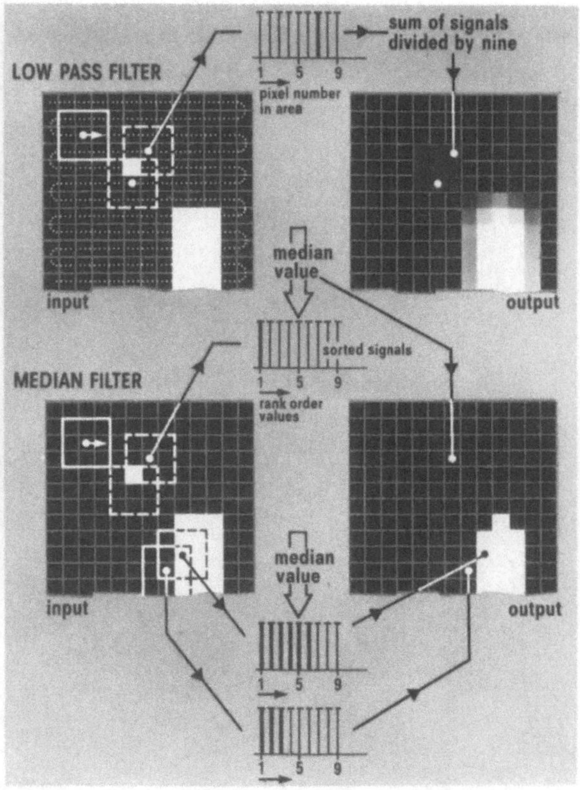

Fig. 15. The principle of noise diminution by low-pass and median filtration. Low-pass filtration is a blurring or smoothing procedure affecting both noise grain and fine signal detail, e.g., edges. A median filter selects the median value from the signal values in the actual filter area: edges are essentially preserved (or even "reconstructed," which could mean false information)

and illustrates two situations. First, it shows the decrease of the dose and increase of noise as a consequence of increased patient thickness. This situation can be handled satisfactorily with an automatic exposure control, which of course needs proper collimation to the field of interest. Second, it is advantageous for image quality to have object transmission or object thickness with little or no variation in the irradiated object field. To obtain maximum flatness, including gas bubble suppression, a large rubber balloon may serve as compressorium (Fig. 14); the ring visible in the image indicates the area of the balloon in contact with the patient. Therefore careful collimation ("semitransparent," or, better expressed, space-variant collimation could be of advantage: direct radiation should be absolutely avoided) and compression are very helpful in keeping the noise as low as possible.

Nevertheless, depending upon the type of examination and imaging system, enough noise could be left to consider noise suppression by postprocessing, especially by filtering. Based on the progress in communication theory, filters are being discussed which are more sophisticated than the well-known and well-proved "smoothing" or spatial low pass filter, a so-called linearly operating filter which reduces noise by a smooth blurring but also blurs edges and small details, because it replaces every pixel in an image by the average of the pixel itself and the other pixels in its neighborhood. Looking at the smoothed edges in the resulting image which should be sharp ones, the observer can easily, what type of other fine detail in the image could be suppressed. This is a sort of inbuilt warning; not only noise but also diagnostically useful and interesting information could be diminished by smoothing.

One of the more sophisticated methods is median filtration (Fig. 15), a so-called nonlinear type. It is known that nonlinear filtration's effect on the image is generally not spatially invariant, as in common smoothing filtration (which blurs the image in the same way at every point), but depends strongly upon the image content. Frieden [3] has been selected from the literature as a representative reference.

A median filter can really suppress the noise grains while preserving edges and lines in the image. In an area around each pixel, the filter checks the signal values of it and the other pixels

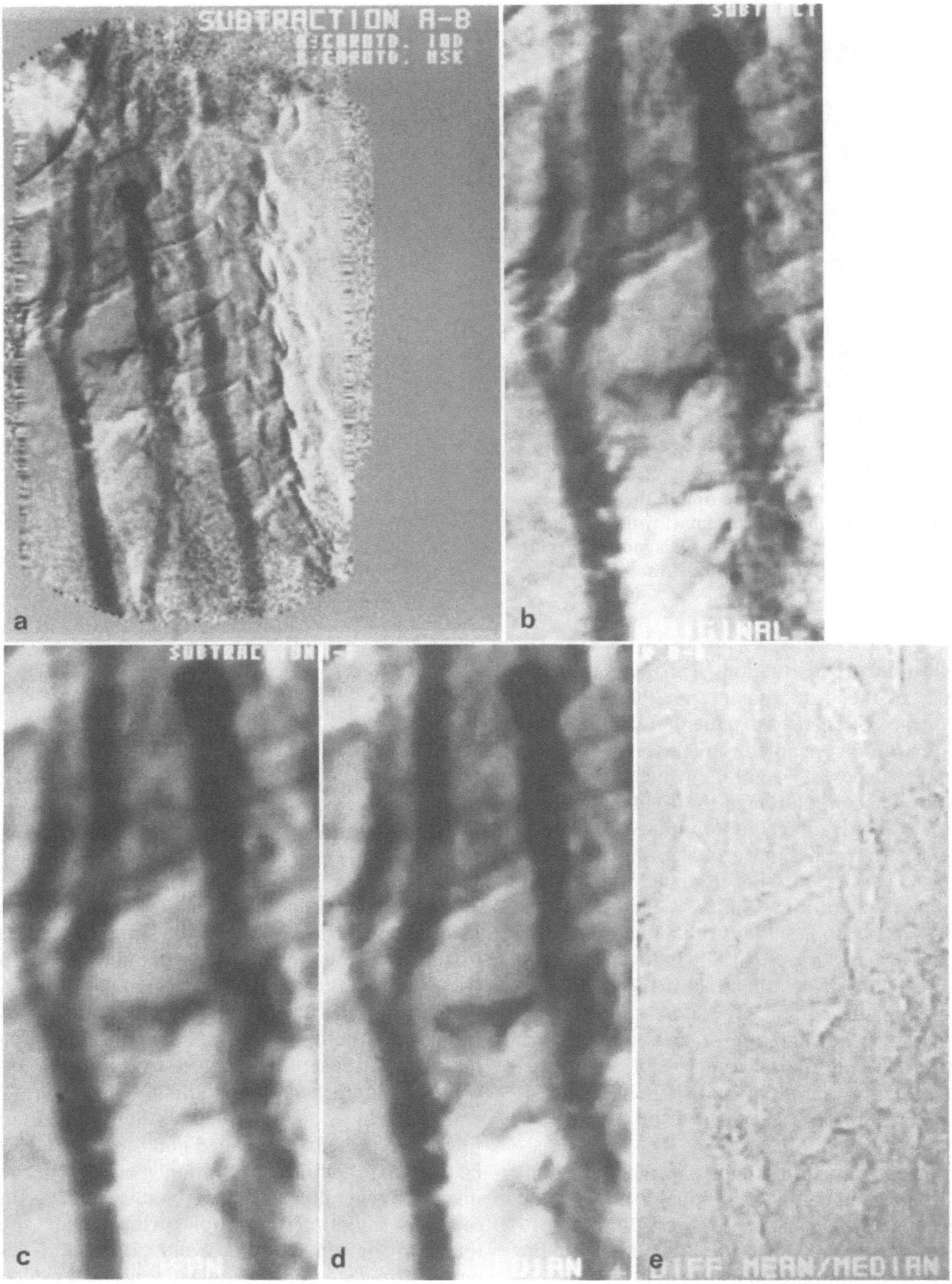

Fig. 16 a–e. Example of noise diminution by low-pass and median filtration: carotid subtraction angiogram (256 × 256 pixel image) **a** Original angiogram; **b** section of original; **c** low-pass filtration; **d** median filtration; **e** subtraction of low-pass and median filtered samples. The (digitally taped) mask and filling images from which the original was produced were kindly provided by Dr. Ronald G. Evens, Director of the Mallinckrodt Institute of Radiology, St. Louis, Missouri. The procedure of median filtration was performed with a computer program from Dr. Michael W. Vannier, Mallinckrodt Institute and sorts the values into rank order, starting with the largest. From the row of values the procedure selects the middle or median value to replace the value of the central pixel. The problem with this type of filtrations is that a filtered image itself gives us only little information to help us to assess what other information could have been suppressed with the noise. In the filtered image in this example (Fig. 15), there appears something which could be interpreted as a sharply contoured microaneurysm, whereas in the nonfiltered image only a straight vessel wall is seen. Conversely, the filtered image may show a straight vessel wall where in the original image a small stenosis is seen. Nevertheless, median filtration seems to be a very promising postprocessing procedure, especially for angiographic imaging.

The effect of low-pass filtration can be demonstrated by means of a clinical example (Fig. 16) taken by pulse mode as a 256 × 256 pixel image. One can observe the lowered noise and also the blurred edges. Median filtration follows, and the edge-preserving effect of the median filter is proved by the subtraction of the median and low-pass filtered images.

It is not the intention here and now to stress the subject of filtration, even though postprocessing is of increasing interest. The rule holds and will continue to hold with digital imaging: What has been done well during the imaging itself generally does not need correction by postprocessing.

References

1. Brennecke R, Brown TK, Bürsch J, Heintzen PH (1976) Digital processing of videoangiocardiographic image series. In: IEEE Catalog No 76 CH 11 60-1 C, Computers in Cardiology, pp 255–260
2. Feist JH, Sternglass EJ (1970) Application of TV subtraction techniques to clinical fluorographic procedures. Phys Med Biol 15:182
3. Frieden BR (1976) A new restoring algorithm for the preferential enhancement of edge gradients. SPIE/OSA vol 74, Image Processing, pp 44–48
4. Frost MM, Fisher HD, Nudelman S, Roehrig H A digital video acquisition system for extraction of subvisual information in diagnostic medical imaging. SPIE vol 127, Optical Instrumentation in Medicine VI
5. Groh F (1967) Ein elektronisches Subtraktionsgerät. Röntgenpraxis 20:43–51
6. Mistretta CA, Kruger RA, Houk TL, Riederer SM, Shaw CG, Ergun D, Kubal W, Crummy AB, Zwiebel W, Rowe G, Zornstorff W, Flemming D (1978) Computerized fluoroscopy techniques for non-invasive cardiovascular imaging. SPIE vol 152, Recent and Future Developments in Medical Imaging, pp 65–71
7. Mistretta CA, Crummy AB, Strother CM (1981) Digital angiography: a perspective. Radiology 139:273–276
8. Marhoff P, Pfeiler M (1982) Digital fluorography. Frontiers in European Radiology vol 2. Springer, Berlin Heidelberg New York, pp 41–61
9. Paulson B (1979) Television is moving fast from A to D. Broadcast communications, Sept, 26–49
10. Schoknecht G (1966) Strahlenabsorption durch Kontrastmittellösungen. Röntgenpraxis 19:123–130
11. Schüßler HW (1973) Digitale Systeme zur Signalverarbeitung. Springer, Berlin Heidelberg New York
12. Ziedses des Plantes BG (1935) Subtraktion. Eine röntgenographische Methode zur separaten Abbildung bestimmter Teile des Objekts. Fortschr. Röntgenstr 52:69–79

Possibilities of New Image Storage Modalities

D. Meyer-Ebrecht

Philips GmbH, Forschungslaboratorium, Vogt-Koelln-Strasse 30, 2000 Hamburg 54, FRG

Introduction

Information storage is, alongside transmission and processing, one of the basic functions of systems assisting medical diagnostics. State-of-the-art distributed computer systems are now supplying these functions, but only in the domain of alphanumeric information. Complementary to alphanumeric information, pictorial information is the basis for several medical disciplines. Unfortunately, the digital representation of a picture requires several orders of magnitude more basic units of information (bits) than an alphanumeric document. This is due to the fact that a picture has to be resolved into a matrix of picture elements (pixels), each of which described by the binary representation of its grayness or color shade. The matrix has to be large enough to allow the reconstruction of the finest picture details, and thus depends on the 'MTF' of the imaging process [5]. Table 1 gives some examples.

Digital processing of pictures – at least of those of moderate resolution – has become an established technique. Fast digital transmission systems have also become available (e.g., based on optical fiber cables). The greatest hurdle, however, was digital storage, because the number of bits per picture multiplied by the annual production of pictures (no less than several hundred thousand X-rays in a single medium-size hospital!) and the legally laid down number of years for retention results in a total required storage capacity of $10^{13}-10^{14}$ bits. Digital optical disk storage technology will now lead to mass data stores which will outdo conventional computer storage systems by several orders in density and in cost per bit. The introduction of this technology will not just provide an electronic alternative to the current hospital X-ray archive, but will probably have a tremendous impact on the integration of imaging and image processing modalities [3], thus leading to more efficient and extended use of pictorial information in medical diagnostics.

Table 1. Data volumes of digitized pictures

Type	Volume
Large-format X-ray film	2000^2 pixels @ 8 bits = 32 Mbits
High-resolution X-ray TV frame	1000^2 pixels @ 8 bits = 8 Mbits
CT scan	512^2 pixels @ 12 bits = 3 Mbits
Ultrasound scan	512^2 pixels @ 4 bits = 1 Mbits
Radionuclide scan	256^2 pixels @ 6 bits = 0.4 Mbits
for comparison:	
Typewritten A4 page	2500 characters @ 8 bits = 20 kbits

Digital Optical Disk Recording

The Philips digital optical recorder (DOR) uses a 30-cm glass disk to store 1.6×10^{10} bits. The bits are written into a metal layer and read out by means of lasers [1, 2, 4, 9]. The DOR disk is formed from two glass substrates placed back to back in a sealed airtight "sandwich" construction (Fig. 1 top). The sensitive metal layers are fitted to the inner surfaces of both substrates on top of a spiral groove. The DOR disk is thus in principle an empty disk similar to a magnetic disk except for the groove, which is necessary to track the laser spot. The groove is equivalent to 32000 tracks, and is partitioned off into 64 sectors per revolution. Each sector is headed by a prewritten sector address code (Fig. 2 left).

The laser can write about 4000 bits into each sector (Fig. 2 right). The total 1.6×10^{10} user bits on both sides of the disk are saved for more than 10 years. The disk is not erasable. High-power solid-state lasers are used to write the user bits and, at a lower power level, to read sector headers and user

Radiology Today 2. Ed. by F.H.W. Heuck and M.W. Donner

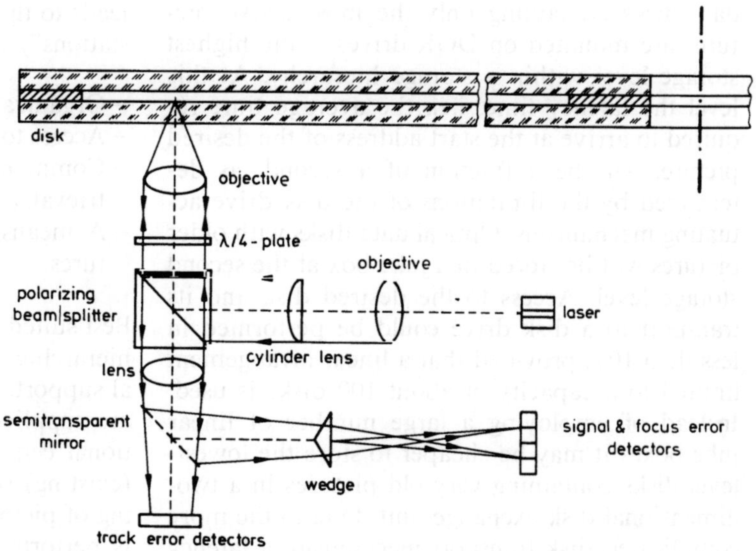

Fig. 1. The DOR mechanism: disk sandwich (*top*) and laser and detector optics for write and read (*bottom*)

bits (Fig. 1 bottom). They are positioned and focused by means of an electromechanical deflection system with a mean access time of 135 ms and a continuous data rate of 2 Mbits/s. Handling of the disks is convenient due to their compact size and rugged design. There is no problem in installing mechanical disk exchange units ("juke boxes") to arrive at an overall archive of some thousands of disks. A disk access time of around 10 s has already been achieved with an experimental 64-disk unit.

The "Picture Base"

A DOR alone does not form an electronic picture archive, although it will obviously be the key component. When considering archives of several million pictures (e.g., a hospital's production over a period of 10 years), appropriate structuring into a hierarchy of storage levels becomes necessary.

The basic storage medium will be the digital optical disk with a storage capacity of 1.6×10^{10} bits, corresponding to between 10^3 and 10^4 pictures per disk. A complete electronic picture archive will therefore contain several thousand disks. How can access to one picture in that number of disks be made sufficiently fast? Fortunately, in general there is a marked decrease in the average retrieval frequency as a function of the age of the pictures. Pictures are retrieved most frequently during a patient's stay, less frequently during the first 2–3 years, when regular follow-up investigations may occur, and far less frequently thereafter. Although this situation may change to some degree as a result of faster and more convenient access to electronic picture archives, it will still be an acceptable archive strategy to have access time increase as duration of storage increases.
This feature results in a picture-base structure (see Chap. 4.3 in [1]) where one or more optical

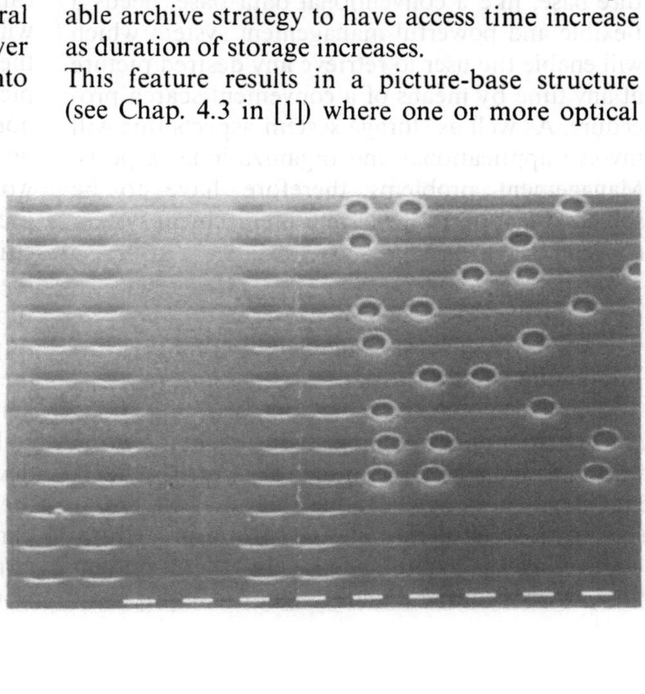

Fig. 2. Electron-microscope photograph of DOR disk surface: holes of less than 1 μm in diameter burned by the laser (*top right*), prewritten sector address codes (*left*), three empty grooves, and scale of micron units (*bottom*)

data disks containing only the most active pictures are mounted on DOR drives – the highest storage level within a storage hierarchy. At this level the latency time, i.e., the average time required to arrive at the start address of the desired picture, will be a fraction of a second, as determined by the limitations of the disk drive actuating mechanisms. Optical data disks with older pictures will be stored in a juke box at the second storage level. Access to the desired disk and its transport to a disk drive could be performed in less than 10 s, provided that a linear arrangement limited to a capacity of about 100 disks is used. Instead of employing a large number of linear juke boxes it may be cheaper to store the lowest-level disks containing very old pictures in a two-dimensional disk exchange unit. Due to the more complicated disk transport mechanism, a latency time beyond 10 s will probably have to be tolerated at this level.

If nonerasable optical data disks are used throughout the picture base it would not be convenient to reorganize the archive. As a result, in some applications related pictures which are filed at different times will be located on different disks at different storage levels. The retrieval of sets of related pictures (e.g., when scanning the case history of a patient over a period of several years) may be speeded up by means of a management and control system which transfers pictures anticipated to be needed next into a magnetic disk foreground memory at the highest storage level immediately after the first picture of a sequence has been accessed.

Supplementary to the mass storage system, a picture base, like a conventional data base, needs a flexible and powerful management system which will enable the user to retrieve any desired picture at any time by means of a convenient search procedure. As well as storage system aspects this will involve applicational and organizational aspects. Management problems therefore have to be solved at a superior level in a hierarchical system concept.

Toward the Integrated Diagnostic Picture Information System

A system to support radiologists during their routine work must be adaptable to the user's requirements in a given environment rather than making him a slave of a set structure and operating procedure. Unraveling the complicated network of patient flow, work routines, and diagnostic equipment leads to the definition of functional nodes ("work stations"). At these nodes the user should have:

- Organizational support information
- Access to patient data
- Command of picture transactions (filing, retrieval, and possibly communication)
- A means of manipulating and evaluating pictures

Best suited to fit these different user functions is a hierarchical system concept [6]. The organizational support, patient data, and picture management are supplied on the top system level by conventional centralized data processing hardware and (existing) software [8]. Transactions and processing of pictorial information, as well as its control, is performed on lower system levels. Dedicated hardware on these levels is distributed and located at dedicated work stations or central facilities (picture storage system). Provided that interface conditions have been standardized, any given or future digital imaging device or image processing device could be adapted to the system on its lower levels (Fig. 3).

Appropriate peripherals, such as X-ray film scanners, and hard copy devices which produce transparent film copies of X-ray quality, would serve as a link to present radiologic practice [7].

Impact on the Use of Pictures

It is quite obvious that convenient and fast access to a comprehensive picture archive will significantly increase the use of old X-rays. Radiologists will not longer be forced into the situation where they have to choose between dispensing with old pictures or interrupting their diagnostic work for hours or days. Because pictures can be retrieved on demand with a negligible waiting time, many work routines can be made more efficient. Less preparation will be necessary, and work on a specific subject can be carried out in a continuous logical sequence instead of having to be interrupted for time-consuming picture retrievals.

A pictorial information system which integrates the diverse diagnostic imaging modalities will help to overcome the present isolation of the specialities which has been caused by the individual development of different imaging processes for the various diagnostic methods. Simple and transparent access to *all* pictures from each retrieval terminal will certainly stimulate interdisciplinary work.

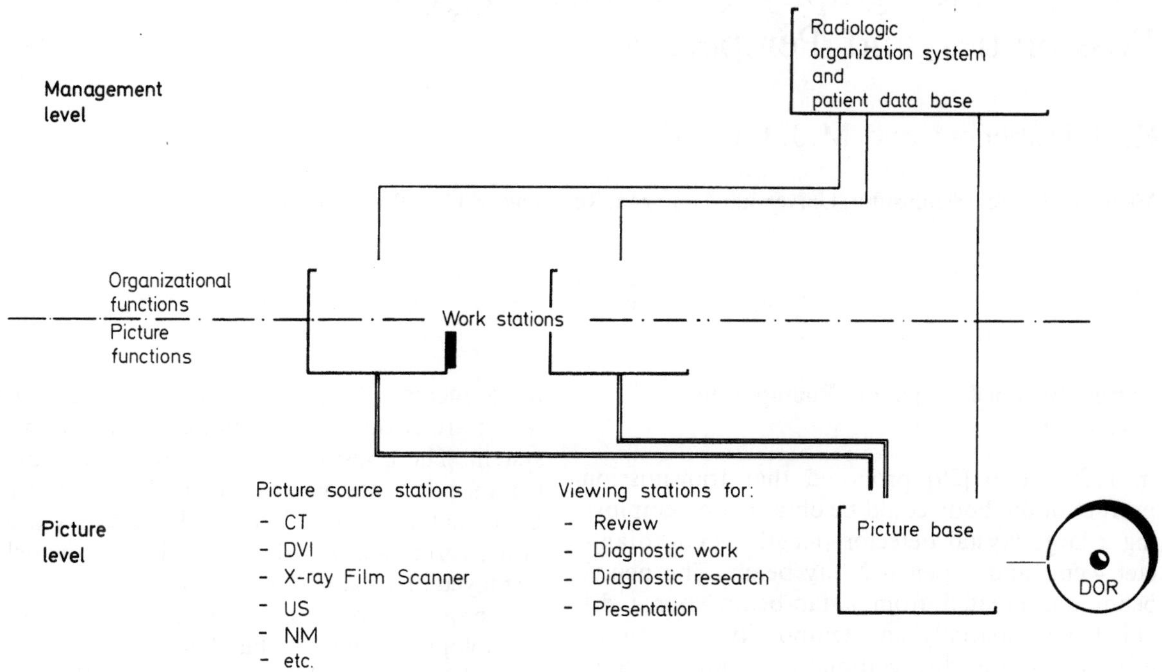

Fig. 3. Hierarchical concept for a distributed pictorial information system

The lack of convenient distribution and storage of pictorial information has resulted in procedures where pictures (or the relevant parts of them) are converted into clumsy verbal descriptions, even in those cases where the picture itself, alone or in combination with a simple hand-drawn overlay, would be more definitive and much easier to understand. This will certainly change if pictorial information can be handled as conveniently and as fast as alphanumeric information.

Finally, the availability of sophisticated picture processing will introduce the use of picture enhancement and analysis methods into many routine procedures. This will certainly yield a better subjective and objective evaluation of pictures, and thus further stimulate their use.

References

1. Bell AE (ed) (1982) High density optical recording. Van Nostrand Reinhold, New York
2. Bulthuis K, et al. (1979) Ten billion bits on a disk. IEEE Spectrum 16/8:26–33
3. Duerinckx AJ (ed) (1982) Proceedings of the 1st international conference and workshop on picture archiving and communication systems (PACS) for medical applications. SPIE Proc 318
4. Kenney GC, et al. (1979) An optical disk replaces 26 mag tapes. IEEE Spectrum 16/2:33–38
5. Killat U (1982) Modern optical methods for the storage of radiographs. In: Orton CG (ed) Progress in medical radiation physics. Plenum, New York, pp 323–376
6. Meyer-Ebrecht D (1980) The management and processing of medical pictures: an architecture for systems and processing devices. In: Proc. IEEE Workshop on Picture Data Description and Management, Asilomar. pp 202–206
7. Meyer-Ebrecht D, et al. (1981) Medical picture base systems. In: Höhne K-H (ed) Digital image processing in medicine. Springer, Berlin Heidelberg New York (Lecture notes in medical informatics, vol 15, pp 133–148)
8. Meyer-Ebrecht D, et al. (1982) A laboratory prototype system for the archiving of CT pictures on optical disks. SPIE Proc 318:308–310
9. Digital optical recording: introduction to DOR. Philips Data Systems Nederland B. V., Den Haag

Digital Radiography (Scanning Projection): Possibilities and Perspectives

K. H. Hübener* and M. J. Lipton**

Medizinisches Strahleninstitut, Universität Tübingen, Röntgenweg 11, 7400 Tübingen, FRG

Current Scanned Projection Radiography Technique

In 1975, Stein [29] proposed that transmission profiles of the body could be obtained by employing a large-crystal detector (length 54 cm, diameter 4 cm) and a pencil X-ray beam. The pencil beam was created from a fan-beam source divided both spatially and temporally into pulses using a rotating disc collimator containing slits. This system, although of simple design, elegantly demonstrated the remarkable advantages of this technique, namely extremely low radiation dose coupled with greatly improved contrast resolution, the latter due to an almost total lack of scattered radiation. This concept was further developed and improved by AS & E. Today scanned projection radiography (SPR) is mostly performed using a computed tomographic (CT) scanner. The attenuated X-ray beam is recorded by the detector array which is held stationary throughout the exposures. The pulsed X-ray tube is placed in a frontal, lateral, or oblique position and generates a fan-shaped beam of radiation; each pulse is 2–5 ms in duration. The attenuated X-ray beam is collimated and aligned with an array of detectors. This ensures that only a beam 1 mm in width can be transmitted through the patient. The narrow transverse transmission profile which is produced is measured and stored. Longitudinal attenuation measurements can also be recorded to obtain complete digital radiograph. The patient is transported through the imaging plane at a speed of 20–75 mm/s, which corresponds to an exposure time of between 5 and 20 s and provides a complete SPR image. During the patient's movement the X-ray tube emits radiation in defined increments, generally of 1, 1.5 or 2 mm, which are critical for the spatial resolution of the system. The transmission files obtained form the basis for data storage and are available for further mathematical manipulation. This process results in the formation of a digital radiograph which is displayed on a cathode-ray oscilloscope.

Numerous improvements appear feasible as the technology advances. The detection system, for example, can be tailored to the SPR system, which is not the case with present CT data acquisition systems. This would greatly reduce the complexity and cost of such instruments compared with CT scanners. In order to obtain a suitable measuring signal in the detector array, and especially for the complete utilization of the measured values (more than 20000), a minimum number of quanta are required at the detectors to achieve an adequate signal-to-noise ratio. Furthermore, a large spectrum of more than 20000 attenuation values must be differentiated. In the radiographic installation described by Stein [29], where one large sodium iodide crystal was used, almost 100% of the radiation could be expected and thus the radiation dose attained a minimum of 2.5–3.5 μGy. Our type of installation (Topogramm, Somatom SF, Siemens AG) 520 cesiumiodide crystals with a volume of 1.2 × 13.5 × 10.0 mm are used.

Their radiation utilization efficiency is approximately 77%; this corresponds to a radiation dose of 59 μGy [14], maximum skin dose of 125 kVp, and field size of 256 × 270 mm. Using xenon detectors where the utilization efficiency is on the order of 56% – as in the General Electric CT/T 8800 unit termed "scout view" – the maximum skin dose reported is approximately 300 μGy [12].

The spatial and density resolution of any imaging system is characterized by the quality and efficiency of its images. All imaging systems which rely on transmission should reproduce object contrast as faithfully as possible. The transmission of

* Dr. Hübener's work was kindly supported by the Deutsche Forschungsgemeinschaft

** Dr. Lipton is the recipient of a Public Health Service Research Career Development Award, Grant No. 5K04 HL00360, NHLBI

Radiology Today 2. Ed. by F. H. W. Heuck and M. W. Donner

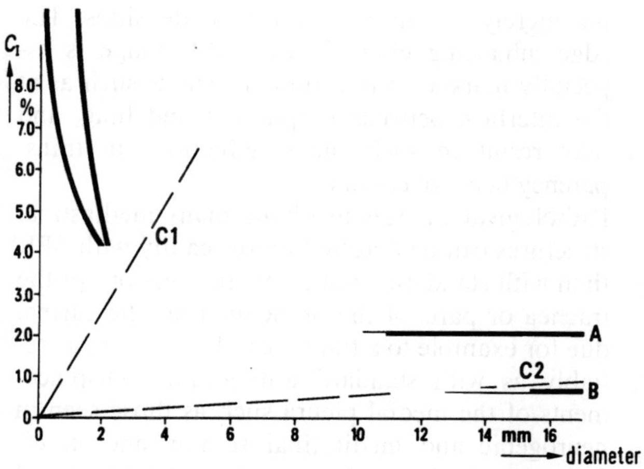

Fig. 1. Contrast-detail diagram using an Alderson phantom, abdominal slices. **A**, Standard film-screen system, surface dose 6.8 mGy (680 mrad). **B**, Digital radiography, surface dose 59 μGy (5.9 mrad). **C**, Contrast of a "tissue" cube ($\varrho = 1.0\ \mathrm{g\ cm^{-3}}$) with respect to "lung" ($\varrho = 0.3\ \mathrm{g\ cm^{-3}}$; *C1*) and "denser tissue" ($\varrho = 1.05\ \mathrm{g\ cm^{-3}}$; *C2*)

contrast resolution frequently depends also upon the size of the object under study. Therefore the assessment of an imaging system should include variation in these two parameters, object size and contrast. This information is best recorded in the form of a contrast-detail diagram and will enable the efficiency of any given system to be compared with that of other systems. In order to determine spatial resolution, particularly with low contrast, a phantom was designed to provide a contrast-detail diagram for the SPR as well as for standard film radiographs (Fig. 1). The conventional film radiograph is clearly superior to the SPR for small objects (1.5 mm) when there is adequate contrast. For objects larger than 2 mm, however, the better density resolution renders SPR superior to standard radiography (Fig. 1). The spatial resolution of SPR depends primarily on the detector size and table incrementation, and further improvements can be achieved by reducing the detector size. Improvements of the SPR technique are also possible by means of dual-energy subtraction, in which different radiation absorption factors of bone, soft tissue, and iodinated tissue are imaged at different X-ray energies [5–8]. Switching the X-ray energy frequent (e.g., 50–60 times per second) between 125 kVp and 85 kVp and subtracting the corresponding recorded transmission profiles allows "bone" or "soft tissue" radiographs to be recorded. This technique exploits the energy-dependent radiation absorption of different dense tissues to separate superimposed structures. Clinical experience with this technique is discussed below in the next section.

Digital SPR images can be readily manipulated and offer considerable opportunity for later processing of data. The diagnostic value of SPR could be optimized by developing different algorithms than those currently used by CT scanners, which are merely concerned with the production of a localizing projection radiograph. Two classes of filter functions and arbitrary combinations of the filtered and unfiltered images have been evaluated [20]. Results of early clinical experience using this technique are presented below.

Clinical Experience with SPR

The assessment of any emerging diagnostic modality must be based on practical criteria. Climbing the slow learning curve of such an innovative form of imaging is initially required. This was accomplished by performing SPR in patients with known and proven pathology, so that the SPR findings could be validated. Experience is necessary before one can fully exploit the many advantages of this technique. The physician learns to use the gray scale on the display monitor to appreciate the remarkable diagnostic capabilities of electronic image manipulation. Relatively few papers have been published which compare SPR with standard radiography [2, 11, 12, 14, 15, 16, 23, 25, 26]. The disadvantages and advantages of CT should be scientifically evaluated both in the laboratory and also by carefully designed clinical trials. The advantages of SPR compared with standard film technique may be stated as follows:

1. Low radiation exposure
2. Small scattered radiation component
3. High density and contrast resolution
4. Incorrect exposures impossible
5. Recording and reproduction of a large absorption value spectrum
6. Rapid radiography of large areas of the body
7. Electronic storage of the radiographs
8. Electronic manipulation of the image
9. Distortion-free imaging in the longitudinal axis of the body
10. Additional software available for image manipulation
11. Transmission of radiographs possible via cable or radio
12. Further possibilities for the development of the system

At the present, the disadvantages of SPR are:

1. Low spatial resolution
2. Long exposure times, therefore dynamic studies are impossible
3. Variability of the imaging format restricted
4. Radiographic capability only for the recumbent patient

Chest

The extensive range of spectral absorption values always permits the representation of both skeletal structures and soft tissues. The normal chest digital radiograph, unlike standard chest X-rays, images mediastinal contours simultaneously with the trachea, main bronchi, pleural reflections, and aorta.

One major advantage of the technique's superior contrast resolution is that the pulmonary vessels can be seen and followed almost to the lateral wall of the chest. The recognition of circumscribed pulmonary lesions in the conventional X-ray image depends upon their size, contrast, and localization. Dense lesions (e.g., calcified tuberculomas) are not difficult to diagnose, but weakly contrasted lesions in close proximity to the pleura can easily escape detection. The large differences in density between circumscribed lesions and the pulmonary parenchyma give maximum contrast, so that a spatial resolution of about 1 mm can be achieved. This means that a spatial resolution of 1 mm or less as present in routine films may not improve diagnostic accuracy, and is therefore not necessarily a limiting factor. This is in agreement with the observations of Foley et al. [13], who digitized chest films using different pixel sizes. They reported that an increase of pixel size from 0.2 to 1.0 mm^2 had no significant influence on diagnostic accuracy; hence the visualization of structures less than 1 mm^2 will only be of critical and diagnostic value on rare occasions.

Many diffuse pulmonary diseases can be diagnosed on the basis of a characteristic increase in density. Both interstitial and alveolar exudates can be distinguished in the SPR image. Regions which are extremely difficult to interpret in the plain chest X-ray include the medial and basal pleural reflections. The SPR system readily reveals displacements of these structures, which are usually easier to interpret using the digital technique. Medial and lateral pleural effusions can be detected and differentiated from pneumothorax. However, in the recumbent patient, small infrapulmonary effusions may not be obvious, presenting merely as minimal abnormal densities. The edge-enhancing effect in the SPR image is especially marked in transitional regions such as at the interface between diaphragm and lung, and may result in such small reductions in transparency being overlooked.

Pathological changes involving many mediastinal structures can be detected more readily with SPR than with standard chest films. Impressions of the trachea or parts of the bronchus near the carina, due for example to a tumor, can be detected as reliably as with standard tomography. Displacements of the medial pleura such as those seen in neurogenic and mediastinal tumors and in effusions or mediastinal prolapse can be diagnosed as well by SPR as by conventional radiography.

An adequate digital radiographic representation of the esophagus is not possible at present because the spatial resolution is inadequate for a detailed assessment of mucous membranes. Only large lesions, tumors, fistulas and diverticula can be demonstrated with the aid of the patient swallowing undiluted Gastrografin.

The value of the digital technique was determined in a comparative study of 250 patients who underwent both SPR and standard plain film of the chest within 1–5 days [16]. The study was performed after experience with more than 1800 SPR examinations since 1979. SPR was performed before routine radiography in one half of the 250 patients studied; after it in the other half.

The findings were normal in 100 patients. In 94% of cases (235/250) the diagnosis could be established by SPR, in 90% (225/250) the diagnosis was evident from the standard film. The slight superiority of SPR was especially evident in demonstrating lung metastases and mediastinal masses. When discrete linear changes were present in the lungs, such as in bronchiectasis and enlargement of the pulmonary vessels, the standard chest film proved marginally more efficient. This emphasizes the point mentioned earlier that further improvements can be expected not from improved spatial resolution, but rather from special reconstruction procedures specifically designed from SPR and perhaps by means of dual-energy subtraction techniques.

Kalender et al. [20] noted that several factors, namely convolution filter kernels, functional design, and other mathematical parameters, provide a simple means of accentuating structural detail. This processing is usually linear in the mathematical sense, and necessarily produces artificial "overshoots" when applying a high-pass filter to a large sharp contrast difference, for example at the

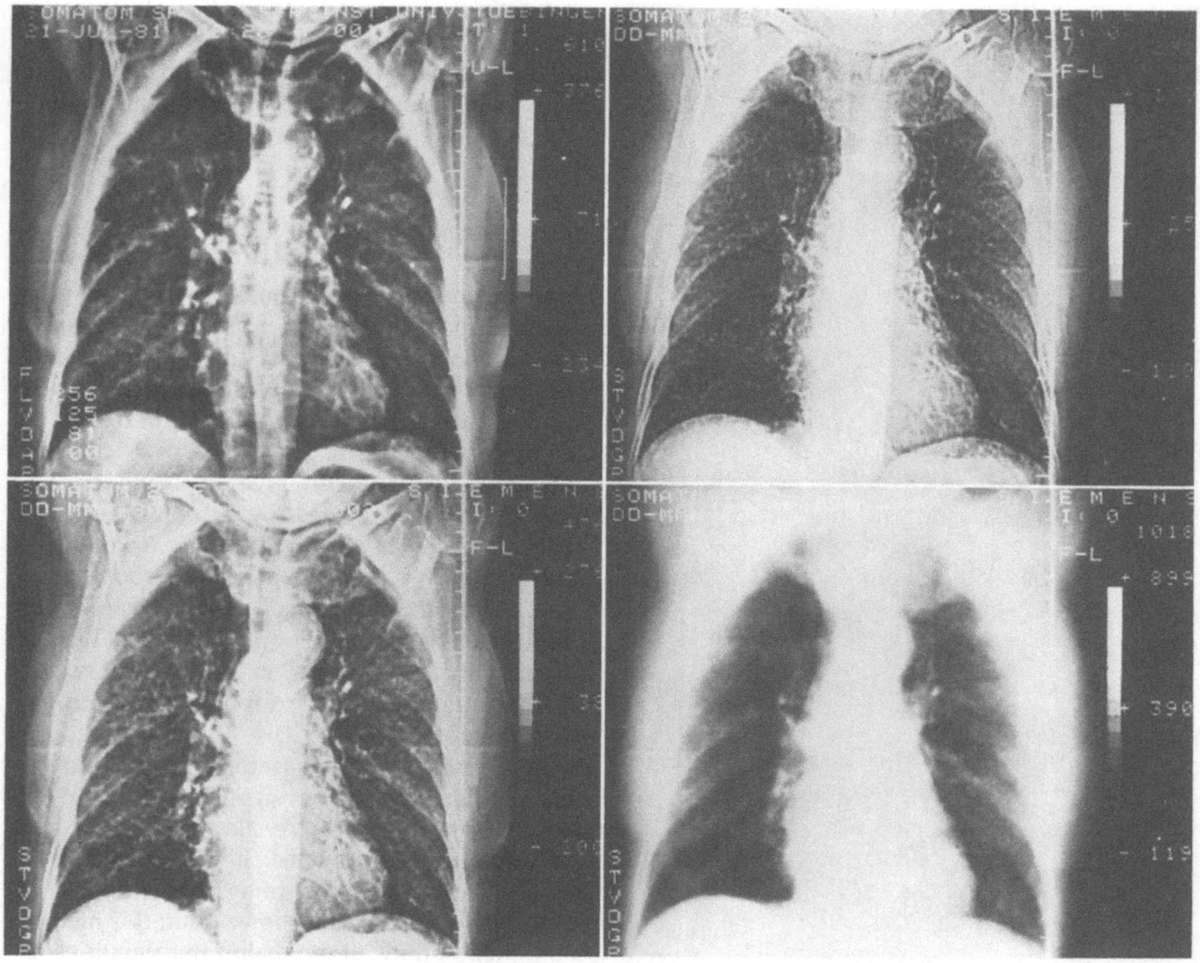

Fig. 2. Digital chest radiographs, using one exposure and four different reconstruction algorithms in order to optimize visualization of lung, vessels, and mediastinal structures

border between mediastinum and lung. As such regions may be of primary interest, the filter and parameters have to be chosen carefully and appropriately for a given diagnostic problem. In order to demonstrate and establish these facts in the clinical setting, a series of 70 investigations using four to ten different reconstruction types for SPR was performed. Clinical experience showed that results can be optimized for specific applications, e.g., for chest diagnosis (Fig. 2) or for abdominal imaging (Fig. 3). For chest diagnosis a further slight improvement of diagnostic accuracy could be obtained using three different reconstruction algorithms [16].

Both the heart and the thoracic aorta can be visualized with SPR just as readily as with conventional film radiography. The important difference is that owing to the long exposure time of about 5–20 s and to the pulsed X-ray beam, the cardiac contour is represented in a kymographic form. The movement of the patient's body, however, limits the kymographic study in a temporal manner, allowing analyses of only a few heartbeats, and consequently little or no information is available concerning myocardial motility. An interesting concept for such studies is the Chronogram techniques [18, 19, 24].

Abdomen and Pelvis

Digital radiography has the potential of playing an important role in supplementing and replacing plain films. Its wide dynamic range ensures a diagnostic exposure unlike that of the equivalent supine plain radiograph of the abdomen, which is particularly prone to inadequate exposure due to great variations in tissue depth and the widely

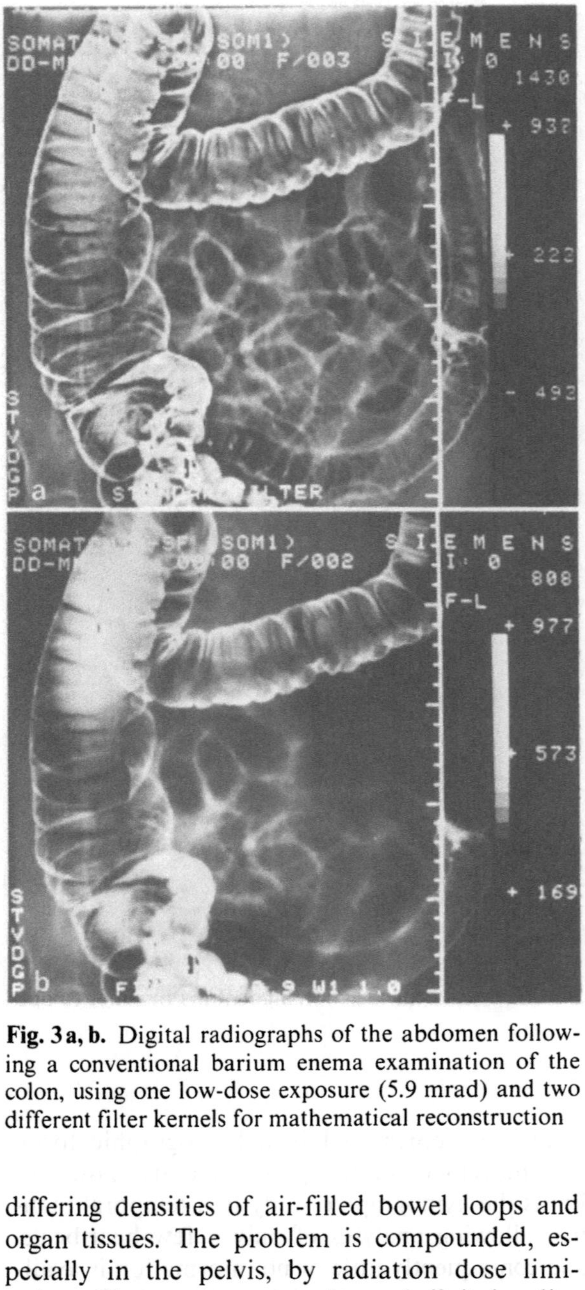

Fig. 3 a, b. Digital radiographs of the abdomen following a conventional barium enema examination of the colon, using one low-dose exposure (5.9 mrad) and two different filter kernels for mathematical reconstruction

differing densities of air-filled bowel loops and organ tissues. The problem is compounded, especially in the pelvis, by radiation dose limitations. The non-contrast-enhanced digital radiograph of the abdomen provides good delineation of most organs, including the urinary bladder as well as the bony structures. The kidneys may be obscured by a gas-filled colon [21], but when this occurs it is worth adjusting the window setting, as this often provides improved edge enhancement of the renal outlines.

The digital radiograph is helpful in evaluating patients presenting with an acute abdomen. Lateral decubitus exposures will allow "free air" localization and can frequently distinguish large from small bowel loops, which may be useful in separating atonia from mechanical small bowel obstruction. The digital approach is also superior to routine films in defining free air in the abdominal wall and is particularly helpful if the free air is small in quantity and/or the patient is obese [14].

Skeletal Applications

Bone diagnosis requires analysis of both gross structure and fine detail. The spatial resolution of conventional film/screen systems provides five line pairs per millimeter, while present line-scanned radiographs have a resolution on the order of between one and two line pairs per millimeter [9]. Despite this great discrepancy, line scanning systems can readily demonstrate major bone lesions such as fractures. The technique is therefore well suited to emergency room problems, as the trauma patient can receive a rapid skeletal survey and radiology staff will not need to concern themselves with exposure factors. All anatomical areas can be examined and appropriately "windowed".

Delay in managing the severely traumatized patient is not uncommon in the radiology department, as reported by Ayella [1]. It was indeed this study which stimulated Stein [29] to develop his digital radiographic imaging technique. A study by Curtis et al. [10] showed that this method could demonstrate all the major abnormalities requiring treatment. The relatively short exposure, small radiation dose, and large possible field size, are distinct advantages – besides having the confidence of knowing that the exposure was satisfactory. Finally, there is less scattered radiation with SPR studies, hence reduced exposure of both the patient and all personnel involved in patient care.

Utilization of Contrast Medium

Angiographic Applications

Line-scanned digital radiography has been successfully applied to imaging the carotid arteries. Brody et al. [6–8] used large boluses of 0.6–0.75 ml/kg diatrozoate meglumine 66%, sodium 10% (Renografin 76) injected at 7.5–12 ml/s using a pressure injector. The contrast medium was delivered through a 16-gauge intravenous cannula placed in the right antecubital vein. Pre- and postcontrast images were obtained. Initially only two postcontrast images were possible, but the system was subsequently modified to permit four exposures in rapid succession following administration of the contrast agent. The carotid region was typically imaged in a 20°–30° oblique projection. Hard film copies were then made from the cathode-ray oscilloscope display using a multiformat camera. One problem encountered with this approach is the limitation imposed by temporal resolution due to difficulties in timing exposures to coincide with the arrival of contrast agent in the field of interest [17]. This is related to circulation time variations due to obstruction in central venous pathways – thrombosis was present in 20% of Brody's patients. Another major problem is artifacts due to the subtraction process; variations in X-ray source intensity cause horizontal streaks. This fluctuation does not affect CT images because image reconstruction is quite different for that technique. The precise nature of these band-shadow artifacts in projection radiography is uncertain, but noise in the detectors may contribute to artifact appearance and magnitude. Motion artifacts, a fundamental problem with all types of temporal subtraction, may be another cause of image degradation. The exposure time of line scanning instruments is relatively long and depends on the area being scanned. Obviously adequate time must be allowed for sufficient X-ray quanta to reach the detectors for imaging each scan line. There is, therefore, a trade-off between scatter reduction, image quality, and scan time. Sources of registration artifacts are mechanical; patient translation, motion of high-contrast structures like calcium or metallic prosthetic materials, and of course movement of the patient in the imaging field.

The technique has also been used in aortography and venography. Phlebographic examination of both extremities can diagnose major thrombi even with moderately small volumes of contrast agent (20 ml of a 30% agent). Conventional radiography with intravenous angiography [30] and xeroradiography of extremities, described by Kramann [22], are alternative imaging techniques which preceded digital imaging. The major limitation of line-scanned digital radiography is long exposure time, a problem not shared by fluoroscopic subtraction systems [17]. The superiority of contrast resolution of digital radiography over digital fluoroscopy is, however, considerable and accounts in large part for the diagnostic value of this imaging method.

Contrast Enhancement Outside the Vascular System

Contrast agents used for identifying the esophagus and bowel have very limited value, as only gross lesions are likely to be seen. Standard fluoroscopic techniques with spot film are the practical answer at present. Likewise, cholegraphic agents have little value in digital radiography because the interpretation of fine detail is inadequate. This also applies to detailed anatomical display of renal structures. However, the low radiation dose given during computed radiography may be useful in special situations such as pregnancy and perhaps in children in whom delayed function (i.e., ureteric obstruction) is present and contrast agent has time to accumulate in regions of interest. This technique will have to compete with and complement ultrasound in the clinical setting if it is to be of practical use.

It should be noted that the systems with which the studies just described were performed were not optimized for these purposes. Where a line-scanned system to be built specifically for intravenous arteriography, then spatial resolution and quantum efficiency of the detector system could be vastly improved. Finally, despite the technical difficulties discussed here, there are definite pos-

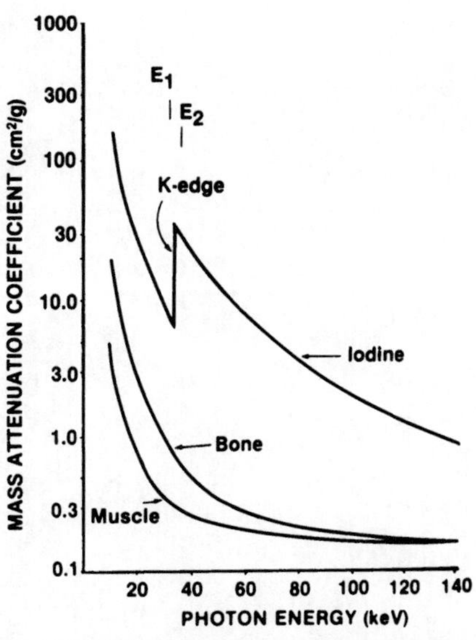

Fig. 4. Relation between X-ray energy and mass attenuation coefficient for different dense tissues. For dual-energy subtraction, X-ray energy is usually switched from 55 to 80 keV (85–120 kVp), 50–60 times per second. In future it seems possible to use dual-energy subtraction for visualization of vessels and iodinated tissue at the K-edge of iodine, switching X-ray energy between E_1 and E_2

sibilities for significant improvements in diagnosis with computed radiography.

Dual-Energy Digital Computed Radiography

The bility of digital systems to perform image subtraction allows superimposed tissues to be removed. Temporal subtraction has become familiar to radiologists in angiographic studies and continues to capture the imaginations of the medical profession and of manufacturers. The initial surge of enthusiasm has given way to more critical concern for diagnostic images of vascular structures using peripheral intravenous injections of contrast agent. Unfortunately, the areas of perhaps the greatest interest and highest risk during angiography, namely the cardiac chambers and coronary arteries, are the most difficult to image due to their continuous motion. Furthermore, even the carotid arteries – the object of 70% of all digital studies at the moment – have a failure rate. This is due either to reflex swallowing related in contrast medium effects or to movement of the patient in the field during the interval (4–12 s) between data collection for the mask and the postcontrast frames. This fundamental problem is inherent to time-dependent subtraction. A solution is the application of energy subtraction.

Energy subtraction techniques depend upon tissues having different X-ray attenuation. The graph in Fig. 4 shows the variation in the X-ray attenuation of iodine, compact bone, and water as a function of the radiographic beam energy. Photoelectric absorption is seen to occur for iodine across the whole diagnostic X-ray spectrum,

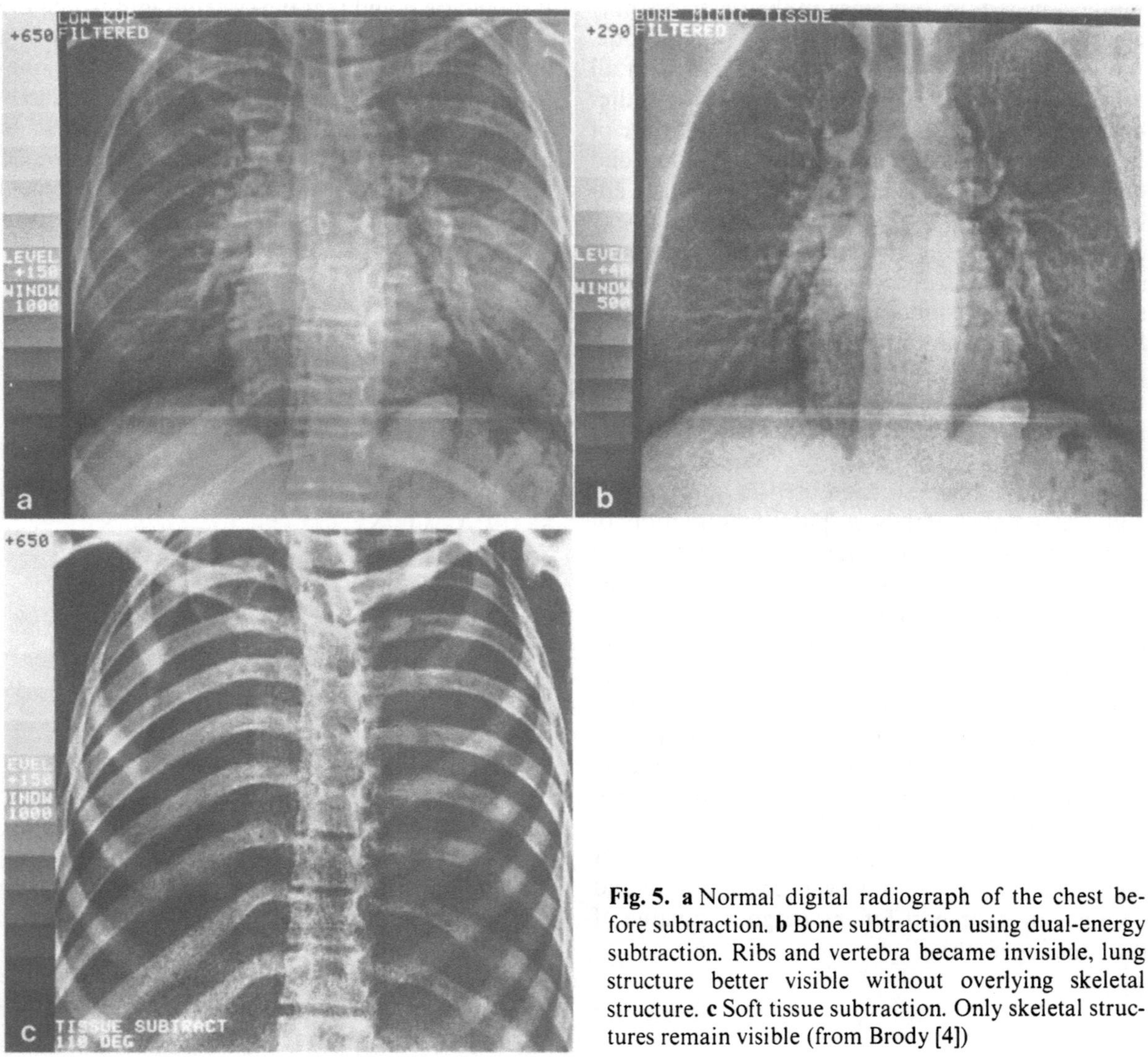

Fig. 5. a Normal digital radiograph of the chest before subtraction. **b** Bone subtraction using dual-energy subtraction. Ribs and vertebra became invisible, lung structure better visible without overlying skeletal structure. **c** Soft tissue subtraction. Only skeletal structures remain visible (from Brody [4])

Compton scattering predominates for fatty tissue, and for bone and water there is a combination of both. Dual-energy subtraction involves selective removal of different tissues by subtracting images obtained of the same subject field at two kVp energy levels. This separates Compton from photoelectric effects. Brody [3–8, 27] recently utilized line-scanned computed radiography in conjunction with dual-energy subtraction to obtain images of the thoracic aorta and the visceral and iliofemoral arteries. Two images were obtained at 85 kVp and 135 kVp initially in dogs after intravenous contrast injection. Subtraction results in the cancellation of either soft tissue or bone. The major advantage of this technique is that the two images are obtained almost simultaneously, the delay between them being in the order of milliseconds. The delay between images obtained by temporal subtraction is usually several seconds, as the mask image must be obtained before contrast agent arrives in the field under investigation. Dual-energy subtraction is therefore particularly exciting and promises to be the technique of choice for regions where motion is always present. Dual-energy subtraction methods can also be used without contrast agents, for example in the abdomen, where bowel gas shadows can be cancelled, or in the chest, where ribs can be subtracted from the soft tissue (Fig. 5), allowing greater diagnostic potential. It seems clear that considerably more research is needed both in the development of newer systems and in the methods used by radiologists to optimize the exploitation of this remarkable technique.

The future is certainly bright for this field. There is now a greater need than ever for close collaboration between physicists, engineers, and radiologists involved in the development and application of digital diagnostic subtraction imaging. Only time will tell what place this new diagnostic technique will take among the many competing invasive and noninvasive modalities now available to the clinician.

References

1. Ayella RJ (1978) Radiologic management of the massively traumatized patient. Williams & Wilkins, Baltimore, pp 1–4
2. Baker HJ Jr (1981) Screening for brain lesions with digital radiography of the head using a CT scanner. J Comput Assist Tomogr 5/1:54–59
3. Brody WR (1981) Hybrid subtraction for improved intravenous arteriography. Radiology 141:828–831
4. Brody WR (1982) Energy-selective radiography (Walter W. Herbert Memorial Lecture). In: Margulis AR, Gooding CA (eds) Diagnostic radiology. University of California, San Francisco, pp 207–216
5. Brody WR, Macovski A, Lehmann L, et al. (1980) Intravenous angiography using scanned projection radiography: preliminary investigation of a new method. Invest Radiol 15/3:220–223
6. Brody WR, Cassel D, Sommer FG, et al. (1981) Dual-energy projection radiography: initial clinical experience. AJR 137:201–205
7. Brody WR, Butt G, Hall A, et al. (1981) A method for selective soft tissue and bone visualization using scanned projection radiography. Med Phys 8:659–667
8. Brody WR, Enzmann DR, Deutsch LS, et al. (1981) Intravenous carotid arteriography using line scanned digital radiography. Radiology 139:297–300
9. Cohen G, Wagner LK, Amley SR, et al. (1979) Contrast-detaildose evaluation of computed radiography: comparison with computed tomography and conventional radiography. Proceedings: Application of Optical Instrumentation in Medicine VII:41–47
10. Curtis DJ, Ayella RJ, Whitley J, et al. (1979) Digital radiology in trauma using small dose exposure. Radiology 132:587–591
11. Federle MP, Cohen HA, Rosenwein MF, et al. (1982) Pelvimetry by digital radiography: a low-dose examination. Radiology 143:733–735
12. Foley WD, Lawson TL, Scanton GT, et al. (1979) Digital radiography of the chest using a computed tomographic instrument. Radiology 133:231–234
13. Foley WD, Wilson CR, Keyes GS, et al. (1981) The effect of varying spatial resolution on the detectability of diffuse pulmonary nodules. Radiology 141:25–31
14. Hübener KH (1980) Digitale Radiographie: Möglichkeiten und Perspektiven einer neuen radiologischen Technik. *Habilitationsschrift,* University of Tübingen
15. Hübener KH (1982) Digital radiography using a computed tomography instrument. Front Eur Radiol 1:126–170
16. Hübener KH (1983) Scanning projection radiography of the chest versus standard X-ray film: a comparison of 250 cases. Radiology, in press
17. Hübener KH, Klott KJ (1980) Statisches und dynamisches Kontrastmittelenhancement der Körperstamm-Computertomographie. RoFo 133/4: 347–354
18. Hübener KH, Metzger HOF, Kalender W (1982) Erste klinische Erfahrungen mit der schnellen digitalen Aufnahme von Röntgentransmissionsprofilen beim Menschen (Chronogramm). CT Sonographie 2:83–91
19. Hübener KH, Kalender W, Metzger HOF (1982) Fast digital recording of X-ray attenuation profiles: a preliminary evaluation. Radiology 145,2:545–547

20. Kalender W, Hübener KH, Jass W (1983) Optimization of image characteristics in digital scanned projection radiography. Radiology, in press
21. Katragadda CS, Fogel SR, Cohen G, et al. (1979) Digital radiography using a computed tomographic instrument. Radiology 133:83–87
22. Kramann B (1979) Transvenous xeroarteriography for demonstrating peripheral arteries. AJR 133:245–250
23. Kruger RA, Armstrong JD, Sorenson JA, et al. (1981) Dual-energy film subtraction technique for detecting calcification in solitary pulmonary nodules. Radiology 140:213–219
24. Kruger RA, Anderson RE, Koehler PR, et al. (1981) A method for the noninvasive evaluation of cardiovascular dynamics using a digital radiographic device. Radiology 139:301–305
25. Lawson TL, Foley WD, Imray TJ, et al. (1980) Abdominal computed radiography: evaluation of low-contrast lesions. Invest Radiol 15/3:215–219
26. Metzger HOF, Hübener KH (1980) Bestrahlungsplanung mit computerisierter digitaler Radiographie. Strahlentherapie 156:684–688
27. Sommer FG, Brody WR, Gross D, et al. (1981) Excretory urography using dual-energy scanned projection radiography. Radiology 141:529–532
28. Sommer FG, Brody WR, Gross D, et al. (1982) Renal imaging with dual energy projection radiography. AJR 138:317–322
29. Stein JA (1975) X-ray imaging with a scanning beam. Radiology 117:713–716
30. Steinberg I, Finby N, Evans JA (1959) A safe and practical intravenous method for abdominal aortography, peripheral arteriography and cerebral arteriography. AJR 82:758–771

Functional Possibilities with the DVI System

J. W. Ludwig, P. H. C. Engels, and T. T. C. Overtoom

St. Antonius Ziekenhuis, Jan van Scorelstraat 2, 3500 Utrecht, The Netherlands

With digital angiography, functional as well as morphological examinations are possible. The functional methods are based on one hand on the lessening or enhancement of contrast after administering the contrast medium, and on the other hand on the availability of information in digital form. Furthermore the functional examination is based on the transport, the flow of the contrast medium.

Possible functional examinations, not yet all available in our institution, include the following:

1. Evaluation of density of certain organs after administration of contrast medium
2. Assessment of relative flow
3. Measurement of absolute flow
4. Examination of ejection fraction and wall motion with the aid of the time interval difference (TID) mode

Evaluation of Density

An exact determination is not yet possible in our institution, but we can obtain a rough visual approximation. One examination of the aortic arch revealed a hypervascular hyperfunction of the thyroid gland (Fig. 1). Another example is the demonstration by the absence of contrast in a certain part of the lung of a lung embolus in the capillary phase (Fig. 2). The absence of contrast enhancement is clearer on DVI than on conventional angiography.

Relative Flow Assessment

Comparison of speed and degree of enhancement in left and right vessels can reveal a stenosis or occlusion on one side, for an example the complete occlusion of an iliac artery (Fig. 3) or a left and/ or right carotid artery (Fig. 4). The washout of

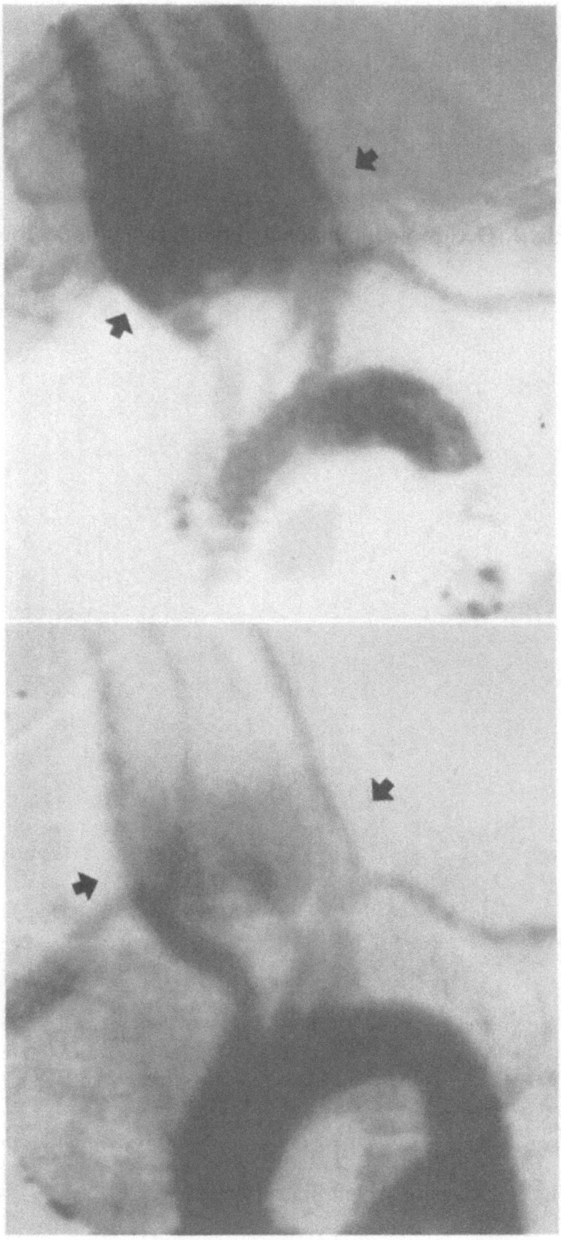

Fig. 1. Hypervascularity (→) of thyroid gland as expression of hyperfunction

Radiology Today 2. Ed. by F. H. W. Heuck and M. W. Donner

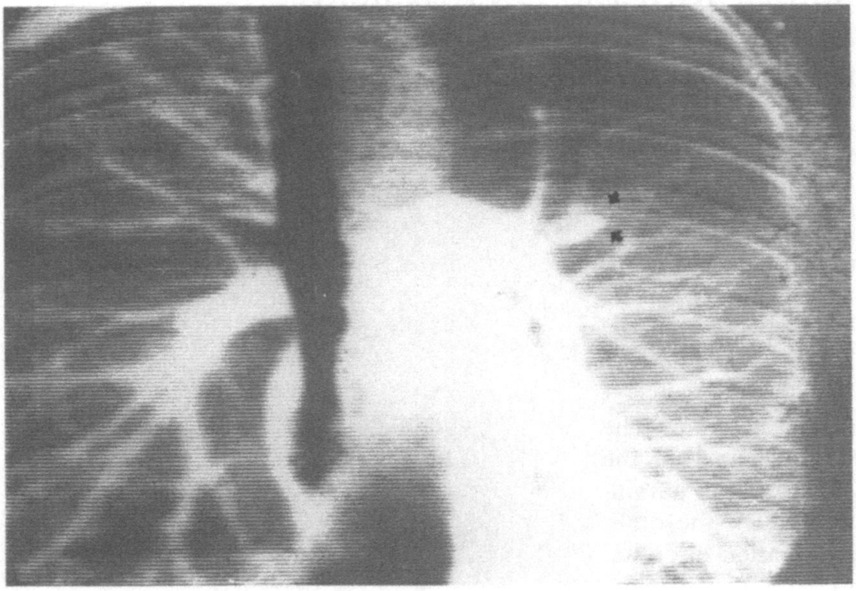

Fig. 2. Occlusion of pulmonary branch to left upper lobe (→)

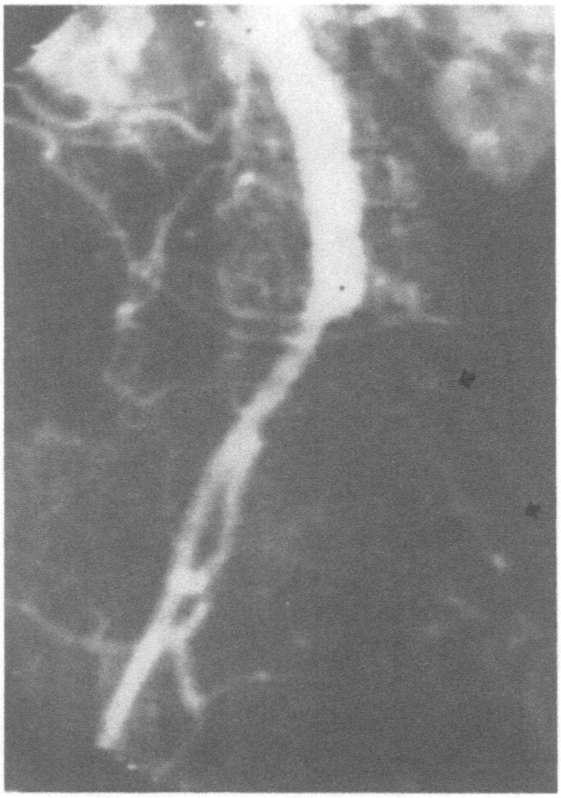

Fig. 3. Occlusion of left iliac artery

contrast medium also gives an impression of the functional condition of an organ.

Measurement of Absolute Flow

As the information is in digital form, video densitometry can be applied, enabling flow measurement in a determined blood vessel, probably be a very important addition to assessment of the quality of the blood vessel and the significance of any existing stenosis. This method is not yet available in our institution but we intend to employ it soon.

Examination of Ejection Fraction and Wall Motion with TID

To assess TID we performed a comparative study. We measured ejection fraction and wall motion on one hand by injection of contrast medium into the left ventricle via a catheter, and on the other by the TID technique after injection of contrast medium into a peripheral vein. Each patient was examined on two consecutive days. The left ventricular angio images were recorded on an analog disc and afterwards on 16-mm film at 50 frames per second. The projection angle was the same for both techniques, and the dose was very similar. The films of both studies were evaluated with the aid of a Menno Greatbatch Analyzer. Endsystole

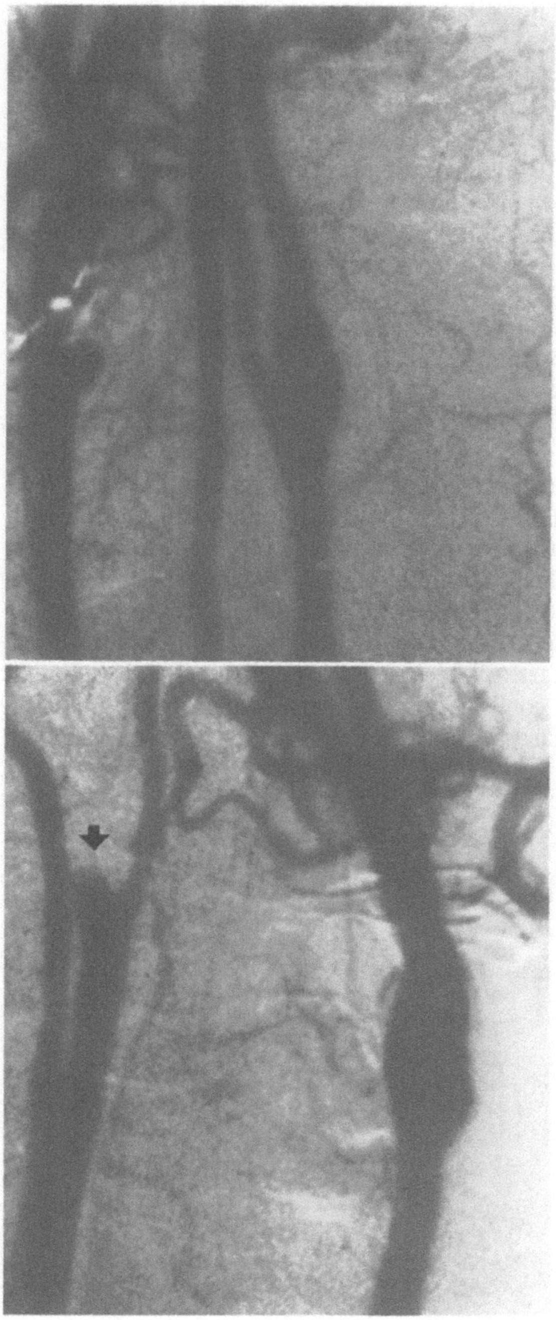

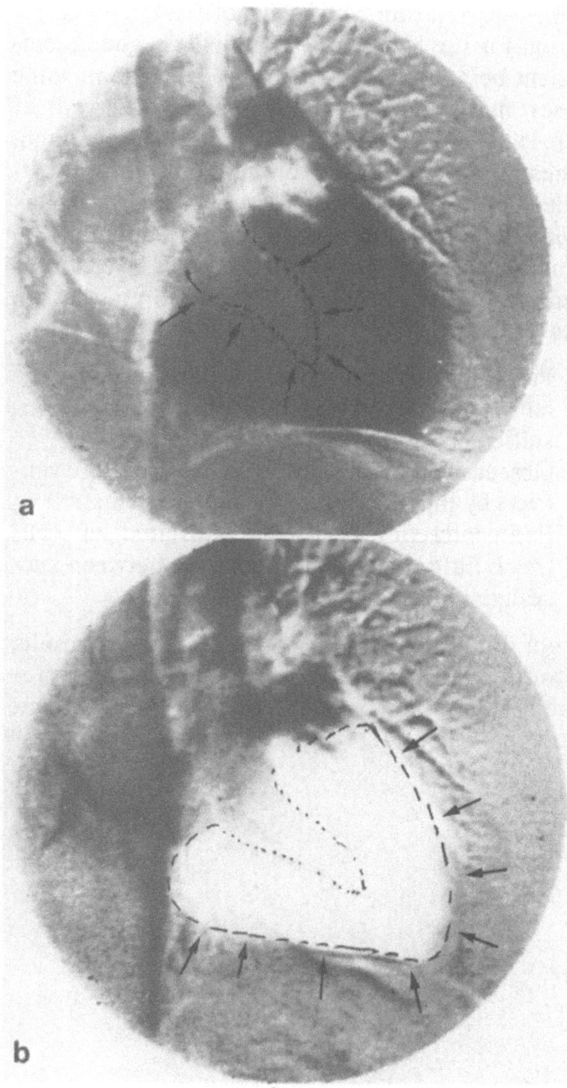

Fig. 5a, b. TID technique for imaging of left ventricle (*arrows*). **a** Maximum systole; **b** maximum diastole

Fig. 4. Occlusion of right internal carotid artery (→)

and enddiastole contours were drawn, and with a minicomputer ejection fraction and wall motion were calculated by the Leighton method. Altogether, 40 patients were examined, 20 retrospectively in regard to the judgement of the amount of contrast medium, the projection angle, and the interpretation of images and 20 prospectively, with one examiner evaluating the left ventricular angiograms and an other the TID images.

Ejection Fraction. The correlation of the ejection fraction determination of the two methods is good. The correlation coefficient is 0.81.

Wall Motion. The measurements of the front wall, lower wall, and apex and the average percentages of wall shortening are calculated for each patient using both methods. The correlation between the left ventricular angiograms and the TID method are excellent for the front wall and the lower wall, with a correlation coefficient of 0.89. The correlation for the lower wall alone is less good, coefficient being 0.62. This is partly because in some cases, mainly on TID images, the lower wall of the left ventricle is not visualized well enough. The diaphragm is overprojected and the contrast-filled left atrium also partly obscures the back wall of the left ventricle, so that the boundary of that part of the left ventricle is less clear. In summary, difficulties of TID interpretation are caused by:

1. Partial transposition of the left atrium over the left ventricle, mainly in mitral valve insufficiency.
2. Obscuration of the lower wall of the left ventricle by the diaphragm in some patients.
3. Bad contraction of a severely dilated left ventricle; little difference in contrast between successive images.

From this study one can conclude that the results from the TID technique are better and more reliable than the conventional left ventricle angiography. The TID method has clear advantages:

1. It is relatively noninvasive.
2. No catheterization is needed for assessment of the left ventricle, so it is very suitable, for examination of high-risk patients and in follow-up studies.
3. Injection of contrast medium into a peripheral vein is more physiological than injection into the left ventricle; left ventricular function is less disturbed.

Figure 5 gives an impression of the diagnostic possibilities in the heart after intravenous injection of contrast medium.

The functional results obtainable with the aid of the DVI system are in part still insufficient, and further development is required. Functional studies of ejection fraction and wall motion with intravenous injection of contrast medium already afford valuable and reliable results. As soon as the extension to functional analytical programs in the DVI system is available, examination of the heart will become less complicated, and we intend to continue with further evaluation of functional examinations.

First Experience with a New 57-cm (22-in.) Image Intensifier for Chest Examinations

G. Friedmann, K. F. R. Neufang, P. E. Peters, F. H. W. Heuck, and F. W. Hofmann

Radiologisches Institut und Poliklinik, Universität Köln, Ebene 6, Joseph-Stelzmann-Strasse 9, 5000 Köln 41, FRG

Chest X-ray is the most frequently carried out roentgen examination; accounting for 40%–50% of all such examinations performed in hospitals in Western countries [4, 8]. Any reduction in the radiation dose required for chest examinations should, therefore, contribute to the reduction in the radiation exposure to the entire population. For this reason, intensified photofluorography, which is known to require very low radiation doses per exposure [1, 5], must be considered a very interesting alternative in chest radiology compared with nonintensified photofluorography and conventional film-screen techniques.

Intensified (or "indirect") photofluorographic exposures of the entire thorax are made possible by a recently developed X-ray image intensifier with a 57-cm image-field diameter. A square field of 40 cm by 40 cm can be inscribed into this circular field. The output screen diameter is 10 cm. Hence the electron-optical magnification at full-field size is 5.7:1 and correspondingly less at smaller (i.e., "zoomed") input fields. The imaged field can be reduced by varying the potentials of the three focusing electrodes to 33 cm. The vacuum envelope of the image-intensifier tube consists of a steel mantle, a convex entrance window of 1.8-mm aluminum, and a glass output window. The loss of contrast due to scattering by the entrance window is minimized by this choice of window material. The output image is focused by a pair of tandem objectives onto the film plane of a 100-mm sheet film camera. Figure 1 shows the 57-cm image-intensifier camera assembly, suspended from the ceiling by a telescopic mounting. The X-ray source assembly is similarly suspended and is electrically centered on the image intensifier.

Spatial resolution of the 57-cm image intensifier was measured to be 4.5–5.2 line pairs (LP)/mm at the output phosphor (Table 1). The spatial resolution of the 100-mm photofluorographic images was measured to be 2.6–3.8 LP/mm in the center and 2.1–3.2 LP/mm at the periphery. Thus the spatial resolution of the new large-field image intensifier is better than in nonintensified photofluorography, but of course is lower than in conventional chest films [2]. The spatial resolution at the periphery is 15%–20% poorer than in the center, which is typical for image intensifiers [5]. The mean exposure time was 11.4 ms for sagittal views at 125 kVp. The mean skin dose measured by thermoluminescent dosimetry was 6.3 mrad in PA projections, which is lower than the values registered at the automated chest unit by a factor of 5 and lower than with nonintensified photofluorography by a factor of 20–50 [3, 6] (Table 2).

Table 1. Spatial resolution

Nonintensified photofluorography	2.0 LP/mm
Large-fied image intensifier	
Center	2.6 – 3.8 LP/mm
Periphery	2.1 – 3.2 LP/mm
Film-screen combinations	5 – 9 LP/mm

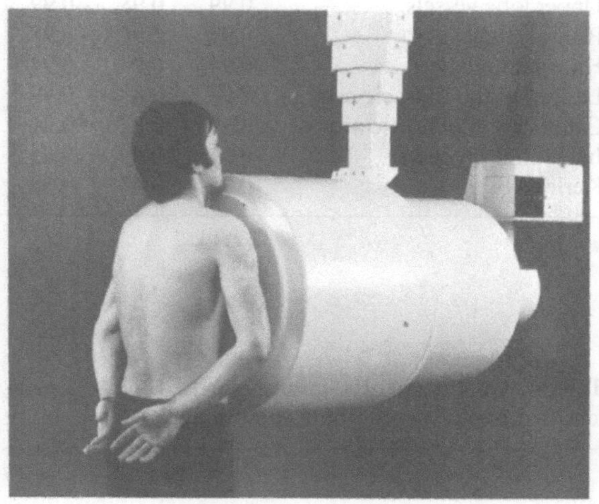

Fig. 1. The 57-cm image intensifier with 100-mm camera in exposure position. Telescopic ceiling suspension

Radiology Today 2. Ed. by F. H. W. Heuck and M. W. Donner

Table 2. Skin doses (sagittal view)

Non-intensified photofluorog-raphy		Conventional chest film		Large-field image intensifier exposure
200 – 500 mrad		31 mrad		6.3 mrad
50	:	5	:	1
(100%)		(10%)		(2%)

Table 3. Visualization of investigated parameters by 100 mm intensified photoflourographic chest images (Neufang et al. [7])

Parameters	Accu-racy	Sensi-tivity	Spe-cifity
Right paratracheal stripe	1.00	1.00	1.00
Coin lesions	0.95	1.00	0.93
Upper lobe vessels	0.99	0.98	0.99
Pleural changes	0.97	0.96	0.98
Hilar pathology	0.94	0.94	0.94
Lesions of the thoracic cage	0.97	0.83	0.99
Calcification of aortic arch	0.89	0.82	0.91
Interstitial processes	0.91	0.79	0.95
Kerley's B lines	0.95	0.48	0.98

$n = 350$

Table 4. Quality of 100 mm intensified and non-intensified photofluorographic chest images

		+	(+)	–
A	Intensified	0.83	0.16	0.01
	Nonintensified	0.28	0.69	0.03
B	Intensified	0.74	0.24	0.02
	Nonintensified	0.30	0.67	0.03
C	Intensified	0.82	0.17	0.01
	Nonintensified	0.36	0.62	0.02
D	Intensified	0.97	0.03	0.00
	Nonintensified	0.20	0.80	0.00
E	Intensified	0.54	0.38	0.08
	Nonintensified	0.38	0.54	0.08

A, Demonstration of the cortical lung structures; *B*, visibility of the lung borders; *C*, clear delineation of the lung vessels; *D*, sharp outlines of the heart and the diaphragm; *E*, good penetration of the heart shadow and visibility of the left lower lobe vessels and the lower thoracic spine
+ good and very good; (+) moderate; – poor
$n = 237$

Using the large-field image intensifier, up to now a total of 3300 patients have been studied. For comparison, conventional biplane chest films were obtained for 350 unselected patients by means of an automated chest unit [7]. Nonintensified photofluorographic images were obtained, also for comparison, for another 500 patients referred for mass-screening chest examination. In 350 unselected patients, a comparative blind analysis of the conventional biplane chest films and the biplane 100-mm intensified photofluorographic chest images revealed a high degree of accuracy for all parameters investigated (Table 3). The highest sensitivity (more than 95%) was obtained for the detection of the normal and pathologic right paratracheal stripe, the evaluation of coin lesions, pulmonary vasculature, and pleural changes. All lung nodules of more than 4 mm in diameter were detected with the intensified photofluorography. Fairly good agreement was obtained in hilar pathology, lesions of the ribs, and calcifications of the aortic arch. Subtle interstitial changes, including Kerley's B lines, were often missed in full-field images but became visible on zoomed films centered upon the lower lung fields. According to Stender [9] and Stender and Saure [10] five parameters characteristic of chest film quality can be evaluated: (a) demonstration of the cortical lung structures; (b) visibility of the lung boundaries; (c) clear delineation of the lung vessels; (d) sharp outlines of the heart and the diaphragm; and (e) good penetration of the heart shadow and visibility of the left lower lobe vessels and the lower thoracic spine. In nearly all cases, these criteria were fulfilled on the intensified 100-mm photofluorographic chest images (Table 4). The images obtained with the large-field image intensifier were, in most cases, equal or superior to the nonintensified photofluorographic images (Table 4). There was a marked haziness of the hilar vessels and the heart borders in nonintensified images, whereas the intensified images showed a clear delineation even of the smaller pulmonary vessels (Fig. 3).

In conclusion, the advantages of the large-field image intensifier over nonintensified photofluorography for imaging of the chest are significant reduction in radiation dose to less than 5% and improved image quality (Figs. 2–7). Compared with conventional film-screen techniques, intensified images provide a significant reduction in radiation dose to less than 20% and a reduction in film and storage costs. Indications for intensified photofluorography of the chest are admission chest films, mass-screening examinations,

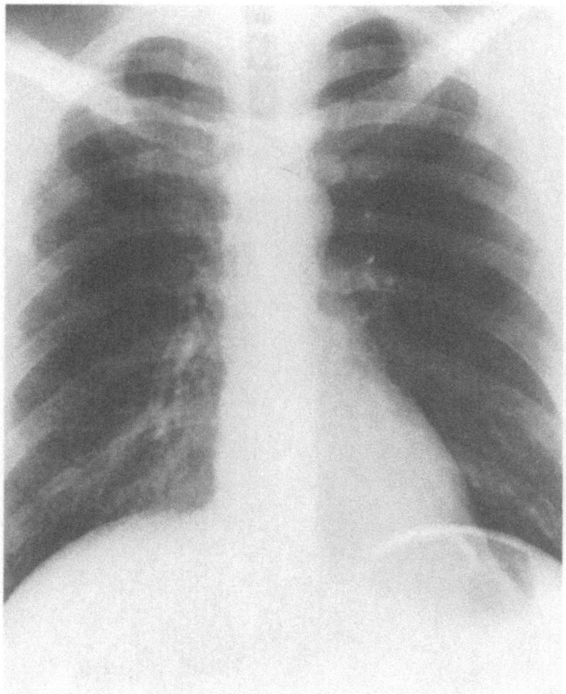

Fig. 2. Normal intensified photofluorographic chest image, taken at 125 kVp

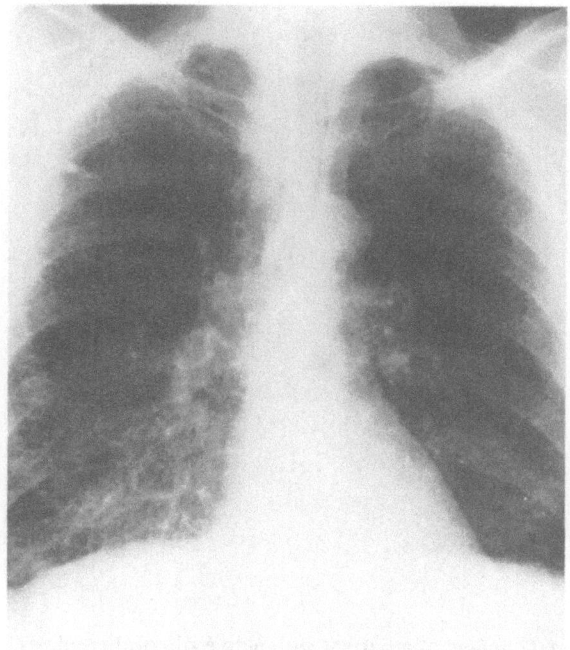

Fig. 4. Image of a patient with gastric cancer and lymphangiosis carcinomatosa in the lower lung fields. Kerley's B lines

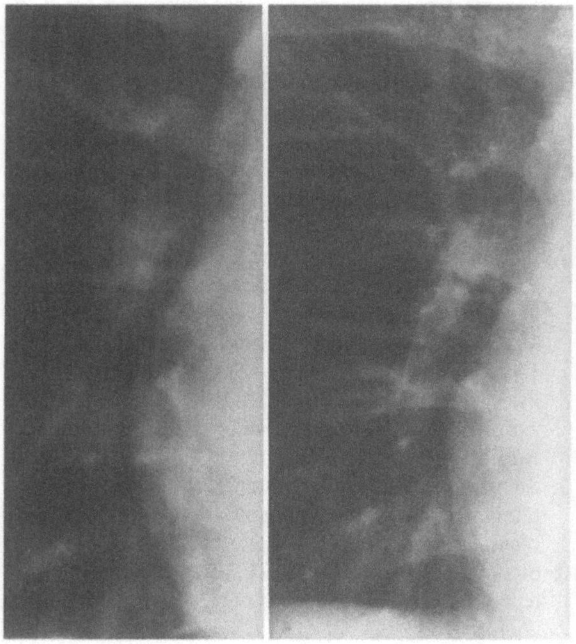

Fig. 3. Differences in image quality between nonintensified (*left*) and intensified (*right*) photofluorographic chest images. There is a marked haziness of the hilar vessels and the heart border in nonintensified images, while the intensified images show a clear delineation even of the smaller pulmonary vessels

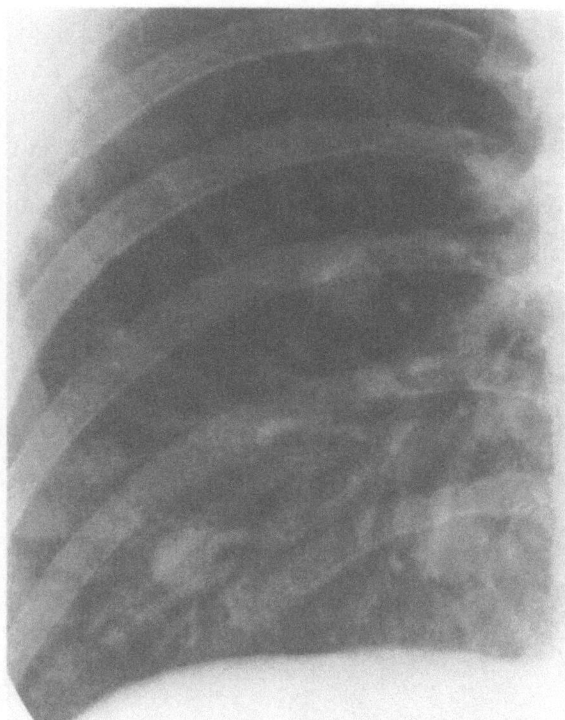

Fig. 5. Multiple coin lesions due to meastases. Image taken with electronic magnification. Even very small nodules of only 2 mm diameter are clearly visible

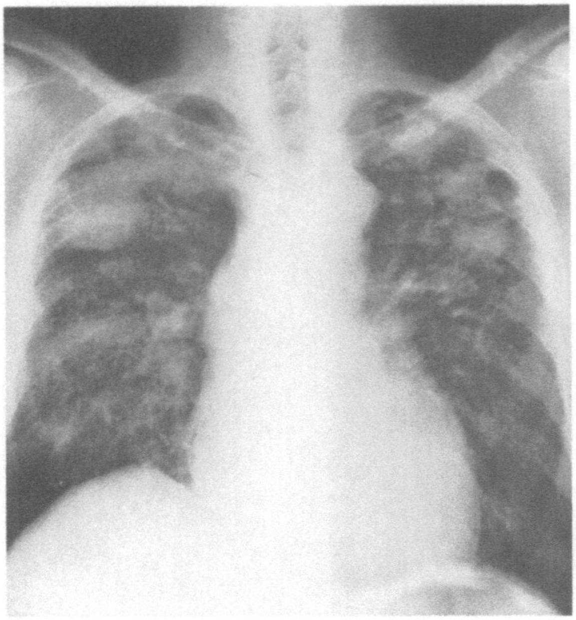

Fig. 6. Image of a patient with active silicotuberculosis

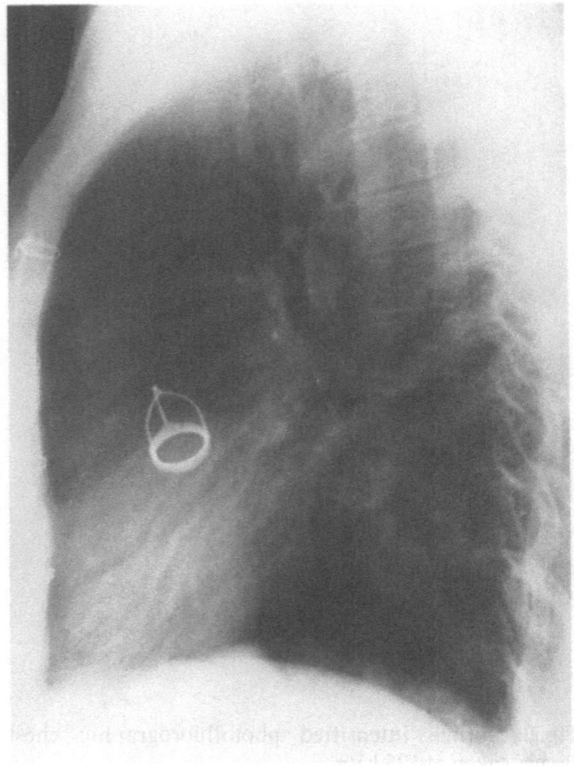

Fig. 7. Lateral view of a patient with aortic valve replacement. Sharp outlines of the prosthesis due to very short exposure time

and follow-up studies. There will be limitations only in subtle interstitial changes and in the lateral view in obese patients.

References

1. Bischoff K, Gellinek W (1965) Geräte für die Anwendung ionisierender Strahlen. In: Vieten H (ed) Physikalische Grundlagen und Technik. – Physical principles and techniques. Springer, Berlin Heidelberg New York (Handbuch der medizinischen Radiologie, vol 1/2, pp 226–230)
2. Ewen K, Schmitt G (1975) Grundlagen des praktischen Strahlenschutzes. Enke, Stuttgart
3. Ewen K, Schmitt G, Kaufmann H (1972) Gonadenexpositionen bei drei röntgendiagnostischen Standarduntersuchungen. RoFo 116: 808–817
4. Ewen K, Steiner H, Jungblut R, Günther D, Schoppe WD (1980) Die Bestimmung von Organdosen bei Röntgenaufnahmen und computertomographischen Untersuchungen sowie die Berechnung der somatisch signifikanten Dosisindizes. RoFo 133:425–429
5. Gebauer A, Lissner J, Schott O (1974) Das Röntgenfernsehen. Thieme, Stuttgart
6. Muth H (1957) Zusätzliche Strahlenbelastung durch zivilisatorische Einflüsse. In: Wissenschaftliche Grundlagen des Strahlenschutzes. Braun, Karlsruhe, pp 197–216
7. Neufang KFR, Friedmann G, Peters PE, Fischer PG, Kronholz HL (1982) Erste klinische Erfahrungen mit einem neuen Großbildverstärker (Siemens Optilux 57) in der Thoraxdiagnostik. RoFo 137:535–539
8. Plewes DB, Wandtke JC (1982) A scanning equalization system for improved chest radiography. Radiology 142:765–768
9. Stender HS (1980) Zur praktischen Qualitätssicherung in der Röntgendiagnostik. Roentgenblaetter 33:618–625
10. Stender HS, Saure D (1982) Röntgenologische Untersuchungstechnik der Lunge. Roentgenblaetter 35:158–164

The Slot Technique

P. Grotemeyer, N. Schad, and G. Seyler

Radiologische Abteilung, Städtisches Krankenhaus, Bischof-Pilgrim-Strasse 1, 8390 Passau, FRG

Although scattered radiation is usually reduced by the use of a conventional grid; another method is the so-called slot technique. The principle is almost as old as radiology itself. In 1903 Pasche [4] described "A New Shutter for the Roentgen Technique." In 1959 Vuorinen [5] summarized the different methods of exposure with the use of slits. He concluded that "the roentgenographic slit methods are not to be expected to became part of everyday roentgenology." The reasons for this assertion probably lay in the limited capacity of the X-ray tubes available at that time and in the generators that did not produce a constant output and lacked sensitive automatic exposure controls. At the end of the 1970s Moore and Amplatz [3] took up the problem, developing a slot technique with a moving X-ray source. The considerations drawn from their experience induced Siemens to develop equipment for the slot technique, which we have been testing in our institution since April 1981. The main goal was to simultaneously improve image quality and reduce radiation to the patient [1].

Material and Methods

The principle of the technique is represented in Fig. 1. The scatter is reduced not by a conventional grid but by two small shutters with slots. The slots, one close to the X-ray tube and the other close to the film, are moved in synchronized fashion over the examined organ. They are connected to the X-ray tube, which rotates around the focal spot as its center. The size of the slot close to the film is 10 mm. The radiation, emanating from a focal spot of 0,6 × 0,6 mm, is collimated by the slot in one direction. The reduction of scattered radiation is demonstrated in Fig. 2. The ratio of primary to scatter image-producing radiation is twice as high with the slot technique as with the usual grid technique when a 10 mm slot is used. Comparing the radiation passed when using a slot to that passed through a moving 12/40 grid, one obtains a value of 1.00 for the slot against 0.57 for the grid. Table 1 shows measurements on a 20-cm water phantom. The skin dose with the grid is used as the reference value. With a comparable slot image the reduction in dose is 23–38%.

Considering the fact that with the slot technique one obtains improved transparency and better contrast, it can be stated that clinically the skin dose amounts to 50% of that with a 12/40 grid.

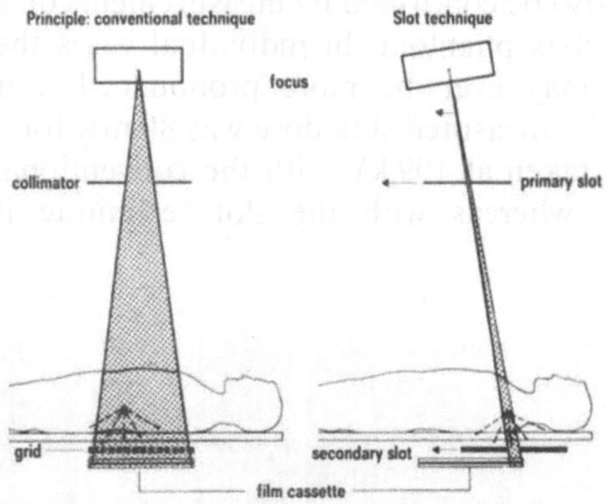

Fig. 1. Conventional roentgen technique compared with the slot technique (from Grotemeyer et al. [1])

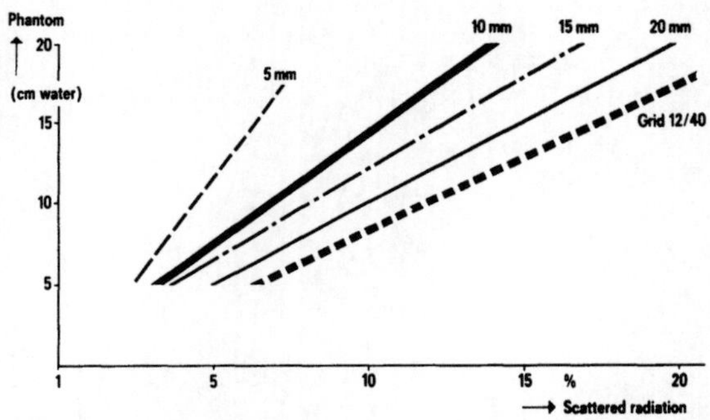

Fig. 2. Reduction of scatter with various slots compared with a 12/40 grid (from Grotemeyer et al. [1])

Radiology Today 2. Ed. by F. H. W. Heuck and M. W. Donner

Table 1. Skin radiation dose comparison between 12/40 grid and 10-mm slot

kV	Dose (%)	
	12/40 grid	10-mm slot
70	100	62
100	100	75
120	100	77

That can also be confirmed by measurements on a skull or pelvis phantom. In individual cases the reduction may even be more pronounced. For example, the measured skin dose was 80 mR for a chest film taken at 109 kV with the conventional technique, whereas with the slot technique it amounted to only 32 mR. These measurements approximately agree with the results of Korbuly et al. [2].

Results

We have exposed over 700 films using the slot technique, concentrating on bone, heart, and lung examinations. We have also examined the stomach and bowels and the kidneys and biliary tract, which are combined under "Other" in Table 2. The results obtained with the technique can be illustrated by films of a normal ankle (Fig. 3). It is immediately obvious that better delineation of bone structures is obtained with the slot technique than with a conventional grid. The reduction of scattered radiation also leads to an improved

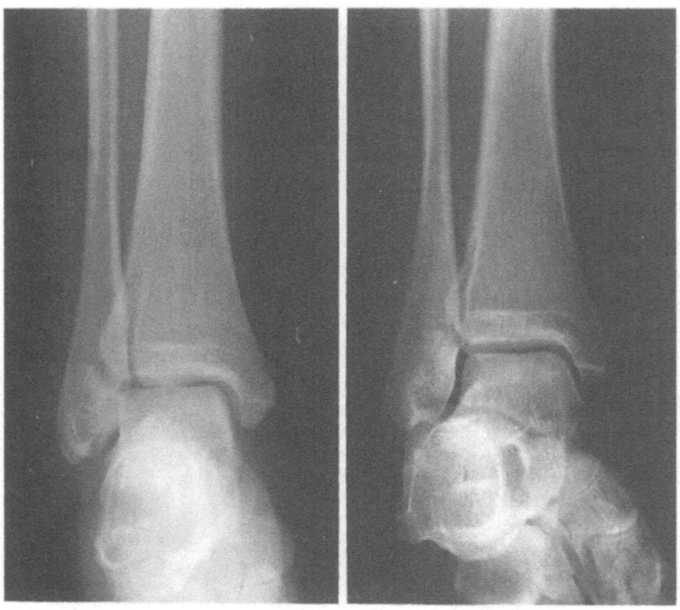

Fig. 3. Film of an ankle. *Left:* Conventional technique; *right:* slot technique

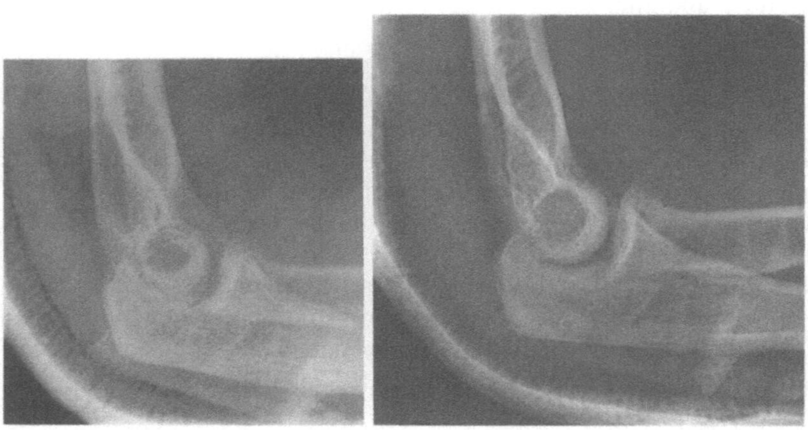

Fig. 4. Fracture of a head of radius in a cast. *Left:* Conventional technique; *right:* slot technique

Table 2. Plain films using the slot technique

Organ	*n*
Skull	43
Vertebral column	60
Pelvis	51
Extremities	439
Chest	117
Other	30
Total	740

evaluation of fractures and of the position of fragments within the cast (Fig. 4), and to a better transparency of the cranial base, almost giving a three-dimensional impression.
The advantages of the slot technique in bone films are as follows:

- Better delineation of structures
- Small lesions more easily detectable
- Improved separation of the basis of the skull
- Transparency of casts

In the field of chest films the advantages are also obvious:

- Better delineation of vascular and interstitial structures
- Improved differentiation of hilar components (lateral view)
- Less penetration of highly aerated zones
- No kymographic effect

Summary

The advantages of the slot technique are twofold: image quality is considerably improved and radiation dose to the patient is at the same time significantly reduced. In contrast, until now improved visualization of detail has been always achieved by an increase of the dose. The great benefits of the technique have already been described by Moore and Amplatz [3], who emphasize the reduction of scattered radiation by the use of slot shutters.

References

1. Grotemeyer P, Schad N, Seyler G (1982) Slot-Technik: Verbesserte Bildqualität bei reduzierter Strahlenbelastung. Roentgenpraxis 35:186
2. Korbuly D, Moore R, Formanek A, Castaneda-zuniga W, Justich E, Amplatz K (1980) Scanography with rotation of the radiographic tube: A new method. Radiology 135:495
3. Moore R, Amplatz K (1981) Schlitzaufnahmetechnik mit mitgeführtem Strahler. Electromedica Siemens 1:34
4. Pasche O (1902/1903) Über eine neue Blendenvorrichtung in der Röntgentechnik. Fortschr. Roentgenstr 6:210
5. Vuorinen P (1959) The roentgenographic slit methods. A survey and analysis of procedures based on the use of a narrow bundle of roentgen rays (scanography). Acta Radiol (Stockh) 177:1–88

Chronogram: A Method for Dynamic Measurements by CT

U. J. Reiser and F. H. W. Heuck*

Zentrum für Radiologie, Katharinenhospital, Radiologisches Institut, Kriegsbergstrasse 60, 7000 Stuttgart, FRG

In the field of digital X-ray imaging the Chronogram presents a novel development. A description of the underlying principles, technical and physical parameters, model experiments, and first clinical results will be given in this report.

Prototypes of the Siemens Chronogram mode are under investigation in the departments of Professor Felix in Berlin [3] and Professor Frommhold in Tübingen [5] and in our department [11]. Kruger et al. [10] designed a comparable experimental set-up in Salt Lake City.

Since the introduction of computed tomography (CT) to diagnostic radiology, there has been the requirement for higher spatial and temporal resolution. Besides the implementation of powerful computers and highly sophisticated reconstruction software, various measuring techniques have been developed, for example the method of dynamic CT with segmental or "image-split" reconstruction. In this mode, images with different temporal centers of gravity are reconstructed by using overlapping segments from a 360° scan. But there is still dead time between the successive scans and therefore information is lost (Fig. 1). To avoid this disadvantage, a mode similar to that of digital radiography, known as topogram, scanogram, scout view or pilot scan was implemented. To get computed radiographs using a CT device, the tube is kept stationary and the patient is moved through the X-ray beam. The Chronogram is a variant of this imaging mode in which both the X-ray tube and the patient remain stationary (Fig. 2a). Consequently the attenuation profile of one slice is measured for each of the consecutive X-ray pulses and stored digitally. To generate a two-dimensional image of the measured values, each attenuation profile is displayed as one column of the image matrix. Thus the x-direction corresponds to the time axis and each point in a column represents one detector element (Fig. 2b). As a reference beam passing outside the object is measured at the same time as the attenuation profiles, the quality obtained in each pixel is the absolute attenuation value of the total path through the object. The Chronogram (Fig. 3a) presents measured attenuation values versus time and does not give a common anatomical image. For interpretation, the corresponding CT image of the examined slice (Fig. 3b) and further processing are needed. The first step is to subtract all time-invariant background structures, so that for example changes of attenuation after injection of contrast medium can be visualized (Fig. 3c). The invariant background can be obtained by averaging the attenuation values of some precontrast profiles. The remaining values after subtraction then represent the change in attenuation with time. For each pixel of the CT image of the examined slice, the corresponding line number of the Chronogram can be determined.

Enhancement curves can thus be plotted for all structures seen in the CT image, not only for

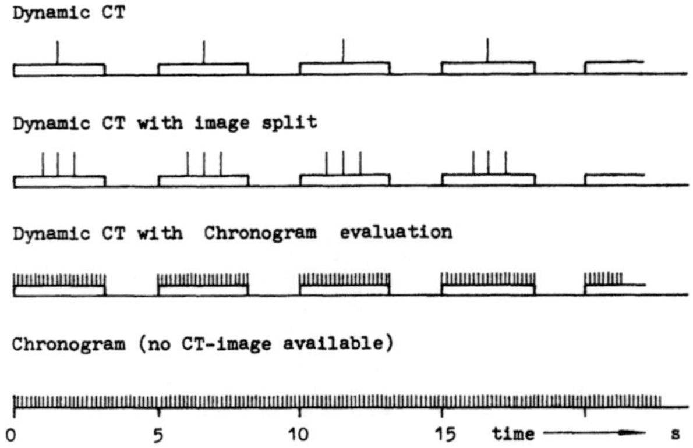

Fig. 1. Comparison of sampling rates for the Siemens Somatom DR CT scanner

* The authors would like to thank Dr. W. A. Kalender, Siemens AG Medical Division, Erlangen, for the help given in the performance of this study and for providing Figs. 1 and 2a

Radiology Today 2. Ed. by F. H. W. Heuck and M. W. Donner

blood vessels but also for soft tissue. As an example, the enhancement curve of the pulmonary artery after intravenous injection of contrast medium is shown in Fig. 4a. The heartbeat moves the artery and thus modulates the enhancement curve. In Fig. 4b smoothed enhancement curves for the pulmonary artery and the ascending aorta are plotted together. The bolus arrival times after injection and the bolus passage time can easily be read off.

Before presenting the results of our first clinical examinations, a few words about the technical and physical parameters of the Chronogram mode.

In the Chronogram prototype being tested in our institution, temporal resolution can be varied from 20-ms pulse intervals, which results in a 5.1-s examination time for 256 pulses, up to a 51.2-s examination with a sampling rate of 200 ms. Detector width and geometry limit the spatial resolution to a sampling distance of about 1.1 mm at the object center and to a slice thickness of 8 mm. Contrast sensitivity is determined by the X-ray dose, object thickness, and CT system used. In model experiments a minimum concentration of 2.3 mg iodine/ml could be detected. Patient dose in a Chronogram is comparable to that of a 5-s 230-mAs CT scan.

Figure 5 briefly summarizes the theory of absolute contrast medium measurements. As the primary energy I_0 and the energy I of the X-ray after passing the object are measured at the same time,

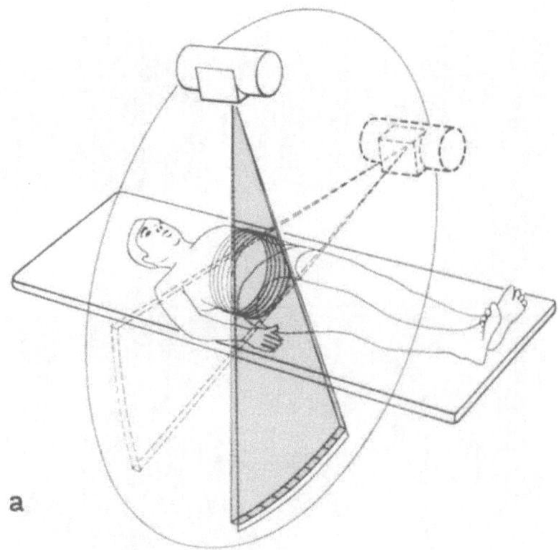

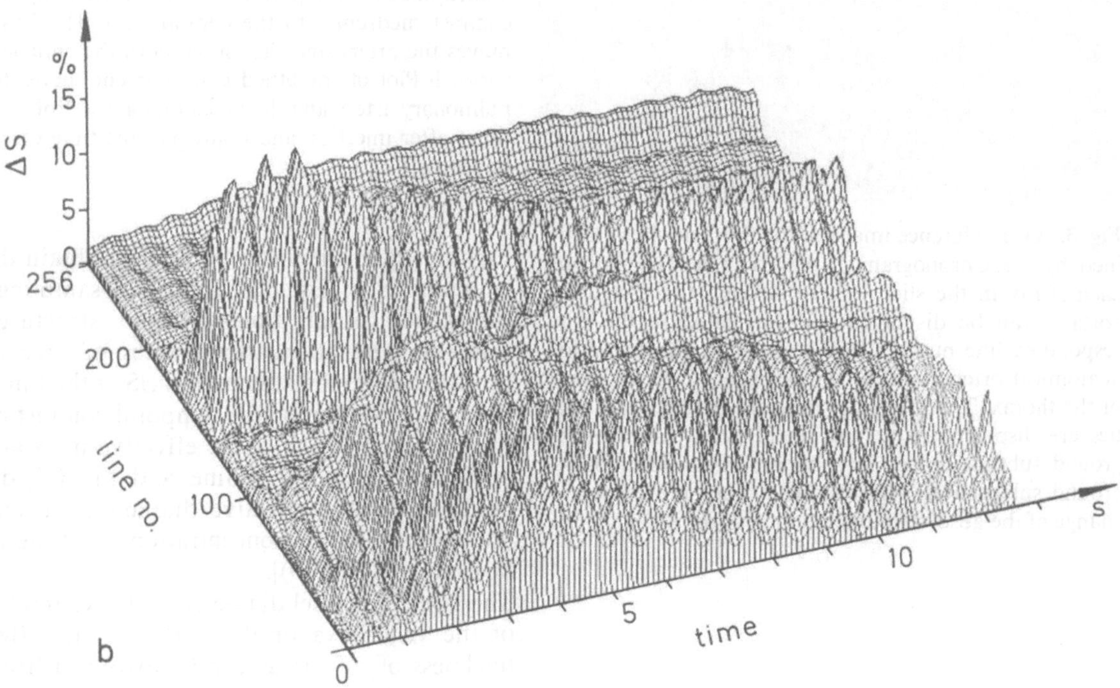

Fig. 2. a Scanning mode for the Chronogram projection radiography method. **b** Pseudo 3D map of the Chronogram data. Each of the measured 256 attenuation profiles is displayed as one column of the 256 × 256 image matrix (columns correspond to the time axis)

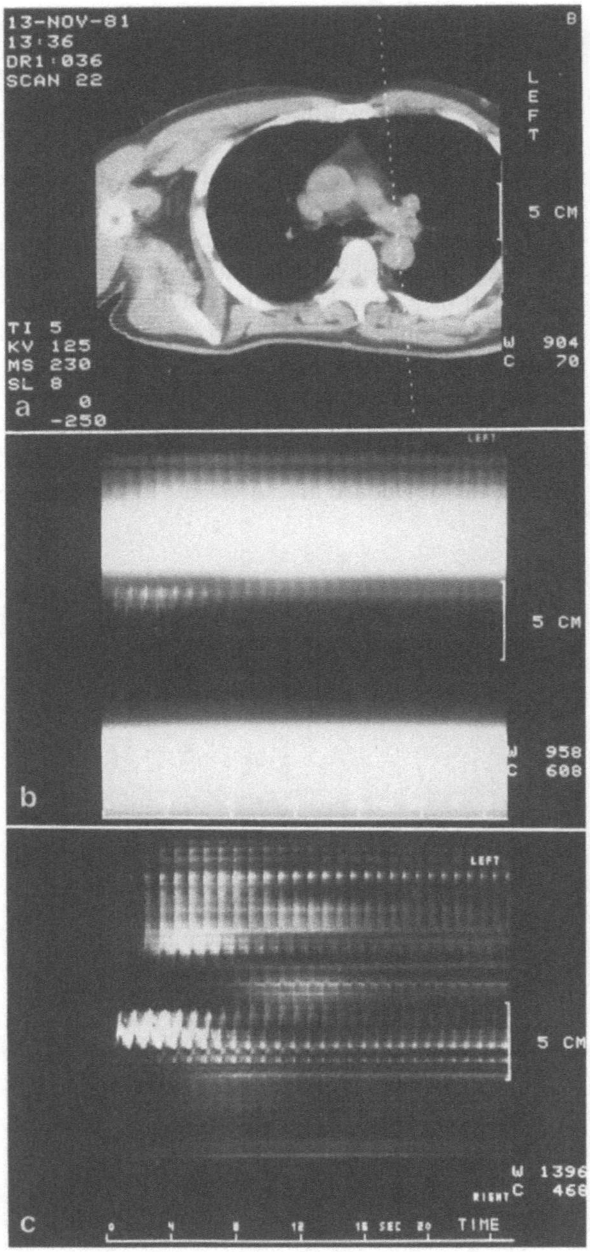

Fig. 3. a CT reference image of the thoracic slice examined by the Chronogram displayed in **b**. The path of each X-ray in the slice – here through the ascending aorta – can be displayed and correlated to the corresponding line number in the Chronogram image for anatomical orientation. **b** Chronogram of an AP study of the thorax. The originally measured attenuation values are displayed as a function of time before background subtraction. **c** Chronogram image after background subtraction. The residual values represent the change of the absolute attenuation with time

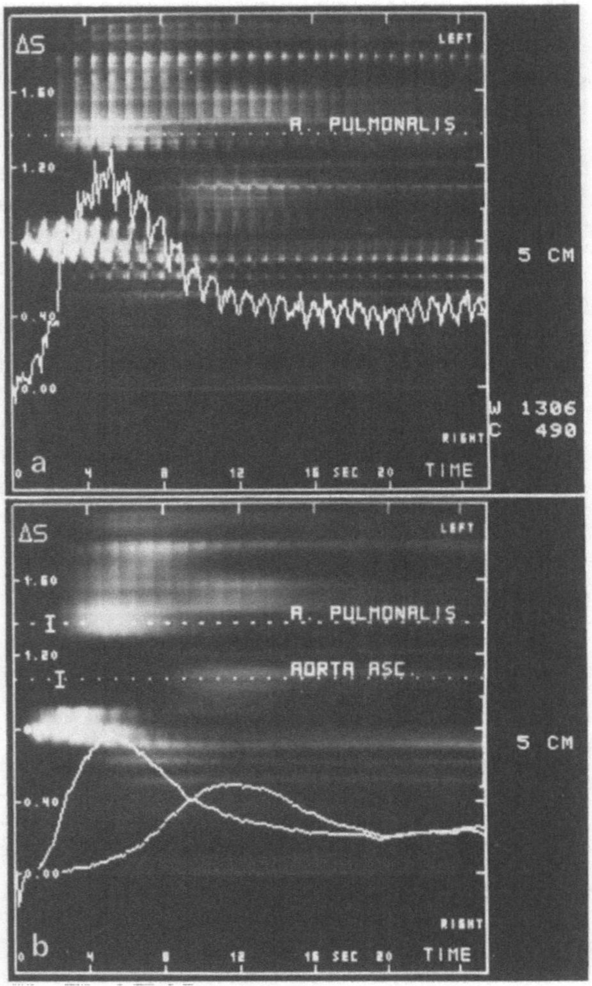

Fig. 4. a Plot of the enhancement curve (data from the *dashed line*) for the pulmonary artery after injection of contrast medium into the cubital vein. The heartbeat moves the artery and thus modulates the enhancement curve. **b** Plot of smoothed enhancement curves for the pulmonary artery and the ascending aorta. Bolus arrival times after injection and bolus passage time can easily be read off

Lambert-Beer's law can be used to obtain the attenuation S in Eq. (2). Temporal sampling and subtraction of all time-invariant structures by averaging the attenuation values of precontrast profiles lead to the attenuation ΔS at the time t_i in Eq. (4), dependent on the temporal contrast medium concentration. If α, the effective mass attenuation coefficient for iodine and the CT device used, and d, the effective diameter, are known, the absolute iodine concentration c at time t_i can be evaluated [Eq. (5)].

The effective vessel diameter, as for example that of the vena cava or the aorta, or the effective thickness of soft tissue can be extracted from the corresponding CT image. Another way of obtaining vessel diameter is to integrate the attenuation across the vessel in one attenuation profile of the Chronogram. As we proved in model experiments, both methods work well for vessel diameters of more than 4 mm.

The coefficient α has to be evaluated separately for each CT device by means of model experiments, in which the attenuation ΔS has to be measured for known iodine concentration and known vessel diameter. For our CT device, α has been evaluated to 3.26 cm^2/g.

As the Chronogram is intended for dynamic studies with quantitative evaluation, this potential has been exploited for model experiments and clinical studies.

In application of all types of digital radiography device, as well as in dynamic CT, precise timing of exposure is necessary in order to hit the maximum contrast concentration at the required part of the body after intravenous injection of contrast medium. In a first study, the arrival times of the maximum contrast medium concentration have been measured after intravenous injection of 30 ml contrast medium at 8 ml/s into the cubital vein. Mean peak arrival times (Fig. 6a) only vary within a small range, but the range becomes larger as the bolus passes the pulmonary circulation. Figure 6b demonstrates the relation between injection flow, contrast medium concentration, and enhancement. In model experiments a doubling of the injection flow caused a linear increase of the enhancement. In contrast, in vivo studies showed that augmentation of the injection flow to more than 8 ml/s does not increase the enhancement to the same degree. It is assumed that in this case the lungs work as a buffer. Thus it is not worthwhile to introduce contrast media into the cubital vein at a rate greater than 8 ml/s; this only inflicts unneccessary suffering on the patient.

To demonstrate the relation between contrast medium concentration and dispersion as a bolus passes the pulmonary circulation, bolus transit times were measured (Fig. 7). After standard injection – 30 ml contrast medium with 300 mg iodine/ml and an injection flow of 8 ml/s – into the cubital vein, concentration decreases to a value of 20 mg/ml as measured in the descending aorta (7% of the injected concentration), while bolus mean transit time doubles from 4 to 8 s. These results correlate with quantitative considerations. It could be observed that a lower injection flow increases the mean bolus transit time and decreases the iodine concentration passing the aorta. If a sharp bolus of contrast medium is required, an in-

Theoretical aspects of absolute contrast medium measurements

Lambert-Beer's law

$$\boxed{I = I_0 \cdot \exp\left(-\frac{\mu}{\varrho}\varrho d\right)} \quad \mu\left[\frac{1}{cm}\right] \text{ absorption coefficient} \tag{1}$$

Attenuation $S = \ln\frac{I_0}{I}$ $\quad \varrho\,[g/cm^3]$ density

$$\boxed{S = \frac{\mu}{\varrho}\varrho d} \quad d\,[cm] \text{ effective diameter} \tag{2}$$

$$\alpha = \frac{\mu}{\varrho} \quad \alpha\left[\frac{cm^2}{g}\right] \text{ effective mass att. coefficient}$$

Changes in attenuation with time and contrast medium

$$\boxed{S(t) = \alpha\, c(t)\, d} \quad c\,[g/ml] \text{ concentration of contrast medium} \tag{3}$$

Subtraction of time-invariant background structures

$$S(t_i) - S(t_0) = \alpha\, c(t_i)\, d - \alpha\, c(t_0)\, d$$

Attenuation caused by contrast medium ($c(t_0) = 0$)

$$\boxed{\Delta S(t_i) = \alpha\, c(t_i)\, d} \tag{4}$$

$\Rightarrow$ If α (effective mass attenuation coefficient for iodine and the used CT-device) and d (effective vessel diameter) are known, the absolute iodine concentration $c(t_i)$ at time t_i can be evaluated.

Absolute iodine concentration

$$\boxed{c(t_i) = \frac{1}{d}\frac{1}{\alpha}\Delta S(t_i)} \tag{5}$$

Effective vessel diameter

Can be taken from 'normal' CT-image or by integration across vessel in the Chronogram

$$d = \frac{4}{\pi}\int\frac{S(x)\,dx}{S_{max}}$$

Effective mass attenuation coefficient for iodine and the used CT-device

Evaluation by model experiments with known iodine concentration and known vessel diameter

$$\boxed{\alpha = \frac{1}{d}\frac{1}{c}\Delta S} \quad \alpha\left[\frac{cm^2}{g}\right] \tag{6}$$

e.g. Siemens Somatom at the Stuttgart Katharinenhospital

$$\alpha = 3.26\,\frac{cm^2}{g}$$

Fig. 5. Summary of the equations for evaluating contrast medium concentration after intravenous injection using the CT Chronogram mode jection flow of 8 ml/s gives the best iodine concentration with the lowest dispersion or shortest mean transit time obtained in the descending aorta.

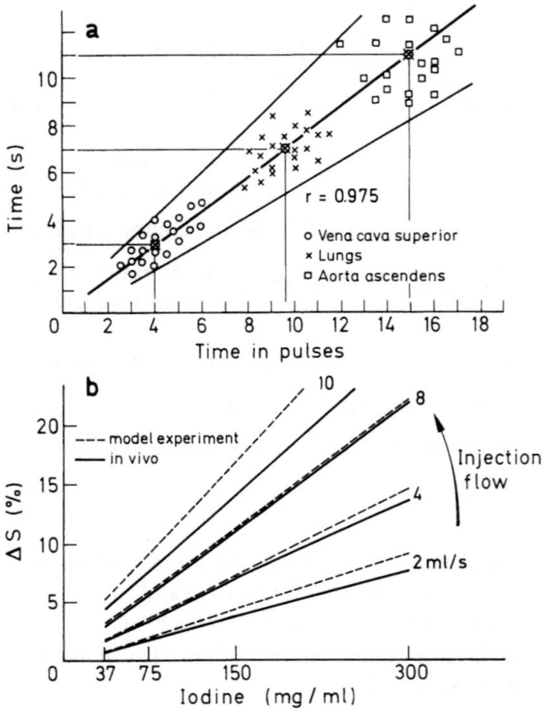

Fig. 6. a Arrival times of the maximum contrast medium concentration after bolus injection into the cubital vein. Time plotted over pulses. **b** Attenuation ΔS in relation to contrast medium concentration and injection flow. Comparison of in vivo measurements in the ascending aorta after bolus injection into the cubital vein and model experiments

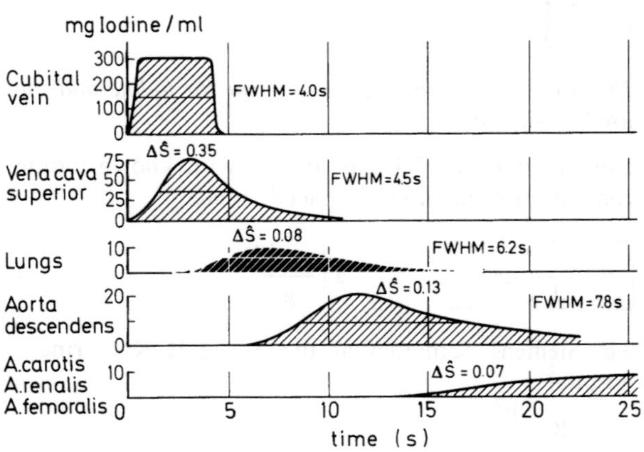

Fig. 7. Comparison of contrast medium transit time and iodine concentration after bolus injection into the cubital vein (FWHM = full width at half maximum, $\Delta\hat{S}$ maximum attenuation)

Conclusions

A major advantages of the Chronogram is that it enables the measurement of the absolute attenuation as it changes with time for all structures with the high precision required for CT. It has the potential to quantify physiological parameters such as enhancement, passage times, relative blood flow through pairs of arteries, and absolute iodine concentration in all body regions.

The major disadvantage is that patient motion can prevent quantitative evaluation. This is true for all imaging procedures which depend on background subtraction, but the effect is more dramatic for the Chronogram because we do not

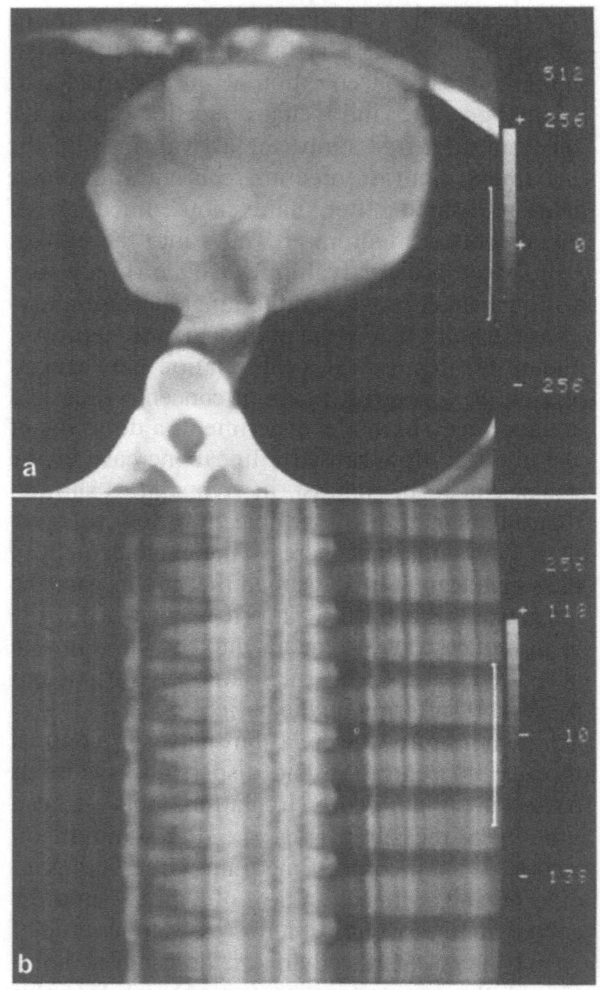

Fig. 8. a CT reference image of the heart for the Chronogram displayed in **b** Chronogram (examination time 5.15 s) of an AP study of the heart. The originally measured attenuation (no contrast medium used) is displayed without background subtraction. Time progresses from top to bottom. Cardiac activity can easily be read off

obtain individual images with each X-ray pulse and can only evaluate a complete study. However, this apparent drawback can be turned to advantage in that all kinds of motion can be measured, for example movement and thickening of the heart wall (Fig. 8).

Other disadvantages are that no spatial information, for example on stenoses, can be obtained; blood flow velocities cannot be measured directly; and only a slice of 8 mm in thickness can be investigated at any one time.

Other studies more extensive than those outlined here could be performed utilizing the Chronogram, but all such work has to be considered in the light of the fact that applications of digital radiography are still in their initial stages.

References

1. Amtey SR, Morgan C, Cohen G, et al. (1979) Applications of digital processing in computer radiography. In: Recent and future developments in medical imaging. Proceedings of the Society of Photo-optical Instrumentation engineers 206:190–192
2. Brody WR, Macovski A, Lehmann L, Dibianca FA, Volz D, Edelheit LS (1980) Intravenous angiography using scanned projection radiography: preliminary investigation of a new method. Invest Radiol 15/3:220–223
3. Claussen C, Linke G, Felix R, Lochner B, Weinmann H-J (1982) Bolusgeometrie und -dynamik nach intravenöser Kontrastmittelinjektion. RöFc 137/2:212–216
4. Hübener KH (1982) Digital radiography using a CT instrument. Front Eur Radiol 1:120–177
5. Hübener KH, Metzger HOF, Kalender W (1982) Erste klinische Erfahrungen mit der schnellen digitalen Aufnahme von Röntgentransmissionsprofilen bei Menschen („Chronogram"). Computertomographie 2:83–91
6. Kalender WA, Linke G, Pfeiler M (1979) German patent application P 2928 825.3, July 17
7. Katragadda CS, Morgan C, Cohen G, et al. (1979) Computed radiography – a new imaging system. IEEE, New York, pp 74–80
8. Katragadda CS, Fogel SR, Cohen G, et al. (1979) Digital radiography using a computed tomographic instrument. Radiology 133:83–87
9. Kruger RA (1981) Estimation of the diameter of and iodine concentration within blood vessels using digital radiography devices. Med Phys 8/5:652–658
10. Kruger RA, Anderson RE, Koehler PR, Nelson JA, Sorenson JA, Morgan T (1981) A method of the noninvasive evaluation of cardiovascular dynamics using a digital radiographic device. Radiology 139:301–305
11. Reiser UJ Study of bolus geometry after intravenous contrast medium injection – dynamic and quantitative measurements using an X-ray CT device ("Chronogram"). Accepted for publication by J. of Computer assisted Tomography

Basics of Contrast Enhancement in Computed Tomography

M. Kormano*

Department of Diagnostic Radiology, University Central Hospital, 20520 Turku 52, Finland

Introduction

Since the successful use of contrast media (CMs) to enhance the visibility of certain brain lesions in the first clinical computed tomography (CT) scans, contrast enhancement (CE) has become a standard procedure in most CT examinations. For many years CE was practiced with no systematic approach to optimize the result. When fast, dynamic CT equipment became available, more attention was paid to the dynamics of CE. Few approaches toward the logical use of CMs in CT have been presented [3, 5, 12], largeley because of insufficient knowledge and lack of control of the pharmacokinetics of CMs after intravenous injection.

Purposes and Methods of CE with Intravascular CM

The iodine atoms introduced into the blood and extracellular fluid increase the linear attenuation coefficient of all tissues which have a blood supply and/or a rapidly exchangeable extracellular fluid compartment [7]. CE is performed in the hope that different tissues will accumulate different amounts of CM, and in fact various components of the normal anatomy are seen more clearly and differentiated more distinctly from lesions barely or not at all visible on plain scans. Avascular (cystic) lesions are also well characterized by their total lack of CE. If several CT scans of the same body section are taken in a rapid sequence, CE allows evaluation of blood flow and tissue perfusion [6, 12]. The more CM given, the higher CE will be. Toxicity and volume of injection in the case of dynamic studies set certain limits to the amount administered. Furthermore, the absolute CE values, given in Hounsfield units, only have meaning when related to the CE values of the neighboring tissues.

Contrast media have been administered by more or less rapid bolus injection or by infusion into the vein. Intra-arterial injections will not be considered in this chapter. The highest temporal blood iodine concentrations are achieved by a rapid intravenous bolus injection, which is considered helpful for diagnosis in many abdominal lesions [1]. After the bolus phase, a nonequilibrium phase of about 1 min may also be useful for diagnosis [2]. A rapid bolus injection is a prerequisite for successful dynamic CT examination. If the time sequence of CM accumulation and clearance from a given organ and a lesion is correctly predicted, a tailored CE using a rapid intravenous bolus can be performed even without a dynamic CT facility.

Comparison of Different CMs for CE

The pharmacokinetic properties of conventional angiographic/urographic CMs are virtually identical. Newer CMs differ from them and from each other in molecular structure, osmotic effect, and liposolubility [10]. Our experimental studies with rats have shown that these differences may influence the blood concentration and accumulation of CM in some organs as follows [4]: The nonionic CM iopamidol resulted in higher blood concentrations than conventional CMs. The uptake of nonionic CM in the liver had a positive correlation to liposolubility. In the kidney the parenchymal iodine concentration was directly related to the number of iodine atoms per molecule or ion. Thus a ratio-6 CM (ZK 38005, a nonionic dimer, Schering) produced a calculated twice as high CE of the renal parenchyma than the ratio-3 CMs, the nonionic monomers and the monoionic

* The studies reported here were supported financially by the Sigrid Jusélius Foundation, Helsinki, Finland

Radiology Today 2. Ed. by F. H. W. Heuck and M. W. Donner

dimer ioxaglate. Nonionic dimers, primarily developed for myelography, would therefore be superior for renal CE. Unfortunately, they may all present significant nephrotoxicity in large intravascular doses (Sovak, personal communication, 1982). In all other organs except for bowel wall and skeletal muscle the concentration of iodine produced by equal doses of various CMs closely followed blood concentrations, and there seems to be little hope that any one of them would be superior to the others from the CE point of view.

In clinical patients iopamidol produced the highest average peak and 2-min aortic CE, significantly higher than diatrizoate, ioxaglate, or ioxithalamate [9]. Thus the nonionic CMs appear to have the best dose efficiency in the vascular phase of dynamic CT (and in digital subtraction angiography).

Differences in the CE of parenchymal organs with different CMs are so small that they are unlikely to have clinical significance.

Timing of CT Scans After Intravenous CM Administration

Infusion of dilute (ca. 30%) CM is a suitable method of CE whenever prolonged delineation of vascular structures, namely veins from the site of infusion into the heart, pulmonary blood vessels, and systemic arteries, is desired. In systemic veins CE is substantially lower due to the uptake of CM into the large extracellular space of the tissues. Since the nonequilibrium phase disappears rapidly after infusion is stopped [2], infusion should be continued as long as vascular opacification is desired. Infusion is also useful in CE of highly vascularized muscular tissues like the uterus [2, 8]. Both uptake and washout of CM in muscular tissue are delayed compared to those in most other tissues [4].

Peak aortic CE is attained 10–30 s after the beginning of a rapid intravenous bolus injection of CM (25–50 ml within 10 s or less). Peak CE of the spleen and other abdominal organs, excluding the liver, usually occurs in scans finished not more than 10 s later. Peak liver CE occurs 20–40 s after peak aortic CE [9]. This delay is caused by the portal venous supply, which substantially adds to the liver CE. In dynamic CE scans such events are easily detected, and any abnormality of the time-density curve may provide diagnostic information. Single or multiple nondynamic scans should be timed to hit the highest CE of the normal tissue, when, with the rare exception of some hypervascular lesions, the abnormal portion of the tissue is best outlined. Even gross differences between CE of normal and abnormal tissue may disappear within 2 min.

Differential Diagnostic Potential of CE

Homogeneous tissues, whether normal or pathological, have a typical cellular structure. It can be assumed that their extracellular space and fluid dynamics in this space are also characteristic. If the resolution of the CT scanner were high enough, the uptake and washout of CM in tissues could give diagnostic information comparable to microscopy. Unfortunately most pathological tissues are inhomogeneous, thir vascularization is bizarre, and the resolution of CT scans is notoriously poor. Some relatively homogeneous processes, such as liver cirrhosis or diffuse lymphomatous infiltration of the spleen, give clearly abnormal dynamic enhancement curves. Without clinical information, such deviations from the normal are not characteristic enough to provide definite diagnosis.

Tumors and their metastases are a special problem. In experimental Rous sarcomas in the rat, we correlated the uptake and topographical distribution of CM to tumor size and histology [11]. All tumors, independent of their diameter, showed the same pattern of CM pharmacokinetics. Uptake of CM was faster in the periphery than in the center of the tumor. The iodine concentration at the center was constant from 5 to 120 min after the intravenous injection, but did not exceed that of the periphery within this period. Solid and cystic parts of the tumor contained roughly equal CM concentrations. Thus topographical variation of tumor histology and vascularity was poorly reflected by the pharmacokinetics of CM at the level of spatial resolution achieved by CT scanning. The best time for detecting the tumor appeared to depend also on the vascularity and CE of the surroundings, not only on the CE of the tumor itself.

Clinically, most metastases and some primary tumors to be detected on CT are located in the liver. They are seen as less enhancing areas in the very early phase after CM injection, independent of the histology of the lesion. Carcinoid tumor, its metastases, and hemangiomas are exceptions; they show characteristic high CE at the early phase and can in most cases be diagnosed on the basis of their CE patterns.

Limitations of Quantitative Measurement of CE

CT scans are useful for visual inspection of the anatomy and estimation of relative densities. Quantitative measurements are often made pointless by various obvious or subtle artifacts which are frequently present, in addition to the inaccuracies inherent to the CT device itself. In the case of abdominal CT, such artifacts are often caused by the gas content of the anterior abdomen or by voluntary or involuntary motion by the patient. In dynamic CT scans this is easily detected, as it causes a bizarre course of the time-density curve not compatible with any pharmacokinetic phenomenon [9]. One should not rely on abnormal quantitative readings of CE of the anterior part of the liver and the spleen unless the scans are totally devoid of gas-induced artifacts and the readings consistent from scan to scan. Diaphragmatic motion may have a similar influence on the posterior aspect of the upper abdomen if aerated lung is included in the scan.

As many pixels as possible should be included in the region of interest to be measured, since a small region of interest adds to statistical variation. In small organs such as the adrenal, the combination of the partial volume effect and motion usually makes quantitative measurements highly unreliable. In the vena cava, CM may be inhomogeneously distributed or even layered and the diameter of the vessel may vary from scan to scan. It is therefore advisable to use the aorta, rather than the inferior vena cava, as the reference for blood CE levels.

Conclusions

With fast CT equipment the total amount of CM required for CE will decrease. Bolus injections tailored for the organ to be studied should be used to improve the detectability of localized lesions. Occasionally, dynamic studies will reveal the nature of localized lesions or detect subtle diffuse abnormality, but in most cases CE will not be able to provide histological diagnosis, even if it improves the detectability of lesions. A nontimed injection or infusion of CM is indicated only in certain areas such as the blood vessels and the uterus.

Nonionic CMs may give improved dose efficiency in the vascular phase but are of no significant help in parenchymal CE, which is impaired by the inaccuracy of quantitative measurements, interindividual variations, and assorted artifacts.

References

1. Baert AL, Usewils R, Marchal G, Wilms G, Ponette E (1981) Contrast enhancement of the liver. Excerpta Med Int Congr Ser 56:259–261
2. Burgener FA (1981) Contrast agents for body computed tomography. In: Fuchs WA (ed) Contrast enhancement in body computerized tomography. Thieme, Stuttgart New York, pp 5–19
3. Dean PB, Kivisaari L, Kormano M (1978) The diagnostic potential of contrast enhancement pharmacokinetics. Invest Radiol 13:533–540
4. Dean PB, Kivisaari L, Kormano M (1983) Contrast enhancement pharmacokinetics of six ionic and non-ionic contrast media. Invest Radiol, in press
5. Felix R, Kazner E, Wegener OH (eds) (1981) Contrast media in computed tomography. Excerpta Med Int Congr Ser 56
6. Galanski M, Cramer BM, Drewes G (1980) Möglichkeiten der Kontrastmittelanwendung bei der Computertomographie. RoFo 132:139–144
7. Kormano M, Dean PB (1976) Extravascular contrast material: the major component of contrast enhancement. Radiology 121:379–382
8. Kormano M, Goske MJ, Hamlin DJ (1981) Attenuation and contrast enhancement of gynecologic organs and tumors in CT. Eur J Radiol 1:307–311
9. Kormano M, Partanen K, Soimakallio S, Kivimäki T (1983) Dynamic contrast enhancement of the upper abdomen: effect of contrast medium and body weight. Invest Radiol, in press
10. Mützel W (1981) Properties of conventional contrast media. Excerpta Med Int Congr Ser 56:19–26
11. Sattler BW, Kormano M (1981) Pharmacokinetics of iopamidol in experimental Rous sarcoma of the rat. 67th Annual Meeting of the Radiological Society of North America, Chicago, Nov. 15–20, data available from the authors
12. Young SW, Turner RJ, Castellino RA (1980) A strategy for the contrast enhancement of malignant tumors using dynamic computed tomography and intravascular pharmacokinetics. Radiology 137: 137–144

Iopromide: A New Contrast Substance for Angiography

K.-J. Wolf

Abteilung für Radiologie, Chirurgische Universitätsklinik, Calver Strasse 7, 7500 Tübingen, FRG

One of the basic steps forward for modern angiography was the further development of the di-iodinated organic contrast media [2], leading to the tri-iodinated organic ionic contrast substances with considerably better tissue tolerance and excretion almost exclusively by glomerular filtration. In spite of this improved tolerance, a number of side effects may occur which are attributable to toxic reaction to the physicochemical properties of the contrast medium molecule and its solution. The problems of anaphylactoid reactions are not discussed here.

The tissue injury caused by the physicochemical properties of the contrast medium is essentially due to two factors, hyperosmolality and chemotoxicity. The kidney, heart, central nervous system, and blood vessels are the best-examined organs.

Known forms of kidney injury are tubular nephrotoxicity [14], proteinuria and enzymuria [7], and increase in the mitosis rate of the tubule cells after selective nephroangiography in the rabbit [19], which is considered mainly to be due to chemotoxicity. The effects on the heart can roughly be divided into injury of the muscle cells and those of the conducting system [10]. In the mechanical functional impairment of the muscle cells it is hyperosmolality which is one of the main factors, while the effects on the stimulus-conducting system are more probably a question of chemotoxicity [4, 21]. According to Higgins and Schmidt [11] and Pfister and Hutter [16], ECG changes at intravenous urography are due to both factors.

Hyperosmolality is held mainly responsible for the severe pain occurring in some cases during peripheral angiography [20]. Chemotoxicity should also be mentioned with regard to the occurrence of endothelial injury [17]. Disturbances of the central nervous system can occur as a result of injury to the blood-brain barrier, the carotid endothelium, or the nerve tissue itself, with hyperosmolality probably the main factor, although chemotoxicity is also a contributor [3, 8, 9, 18]. Chemotoxicity can be lowered by means of excellent water solubility, which can be achieved by extension of the substituent. This method has been chosen in the development of preparations from Angiografin or Conray to Telebrix and Rayvist.

A double-blind study (Table 1) on 90 patients undergoing leg arteriography shows the success of improved hydrophilicity. Premedication is necessary. There is an obvious reduction of severe pain and severe heat. Telebrix and Rayvist are still the most frequently used contrast substances.

The decisive advance, however, was the introduction of the nonionic contrast medium in the form of metrizamide (Amipaque) [1, 6, 13]. There is no longer a cation, so the number of dissolved particles and the osmotic pressure have been reduced by half.

In comparing the ionic Angiografin with the nonionic Amipaque, no premedication was given. Amipaque caused no severe pain or severe heat (Table 2). As is known, the extremely high price and the lack of stability in solution prevented the further spread of this well-compatible contrast medium [12], but the gap has been filled by ioxaglate (Hexabrix). In linking two iodinated benzene rings, only half the number of molecules were necessary to have the same iodine content. Ioxaglate is an ionic contrast medium [12].

This point in the development of contrast media used in angiography was reached about 3 years ago. This stage was characterized by the continuous improvement of hydrophilicity, i.e., the increase in the number of hydroxyl groups, and by the consequent reduction of osmotic pressure.

The next step had to be the nonionic, ready-for-injection contrast medium. In 1977 Felder [5] introduced iopamidol, available as Solutrast since October 1981. We have had the opportunity of testing another new nonionic preparation with on-

Radiology Today 2. Ed. by F. H. W. Heuck and M. W. Donner

Table 1. Side effects of Angiografin, Telebrix, and Rayvist in 90 patients undergoing leg arteriography in the Department of Radiology, University of Tübingen

Side effect		Diatrizoate Angiografin $n = 30$		Ioxitalamate Telebrix 300 $n = 30$		Ioglicinate Rayvist 300 $n = 30$	
		%	(patients)	%	(patients)	%	(patients)
Pain	moderate	33	(10)	37	(11)	27	(8)
	severe	17	(5)	3	(1)	7	(2)
Heat	moderate	37	(11)	43	(13)	47	(14)
	severe	50	(15)	27	(8)	20	(6)
Other		10	(3)	7	(2)	0	(0)

Premedication: Fortral (86 patients); Valium (68 patients); Rohypnol (10 patients)
Dose: 80 ml
Flow rate: 18 ml/s

Table 2. Side effects of Angiografin and Amipaque in 20 patients undergoing leg arteriography in the Department of Radiology University of Tübingen

Side effect		Diatrizoate Angiografin $n = 10$ %	Metrizamide Amipaque $n = 10$ %
Pain	moderate	40	0
	severe	60	0
Heat	moderate	30	100
	Severe	70	0
Other		30	10

Premedication: none
Dose: 65 ml
Flow rate: 16–18 ml/s

Table 3. Side effects of Hexabrix and iopromide in 262 patients undergoing leg arteriography in the departments of radiology of the Universities of Berlin (Charlottenburg), Nürnberg, and Tübingen

Side effect		Ioxaglate Hexabrix $n = 133$		Iopromide $n = 129$	
		%	(patients)	%	(patients)
Pain	moderate	44	(58)	48	(62)
	severe	5	(6)	10	(13)
Heat	moderate	83	(110)	74	(96)
	severe	17	(22)	23	(30)
Other		11	(14)	2	(2)

Premedication: none
Dose: 80 ml
Flow rate: 18 ml/s

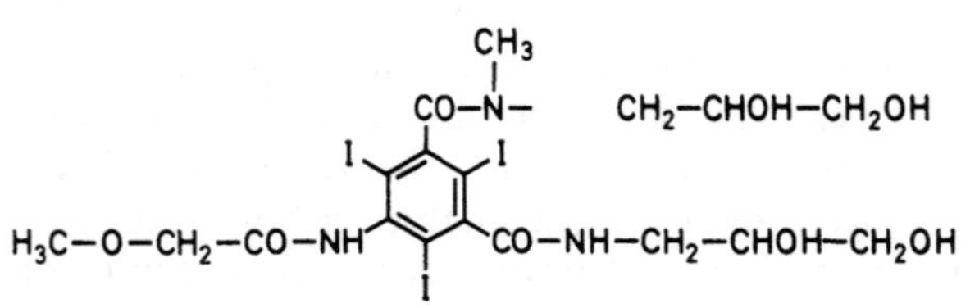

Fig. 1. Structure of iopromide

ly a slight difference in the substituents, iopromide (Fig. 1). The question was whether the non-ionic iopromide has any advantages over the ionic dimer Hexabrix.

In a multicenter study (Table 3) there were no great differences in the occurrence of slight pain. As regards severe pain, there were seven patients

Table 4. Side effects of Hexobrix, Solutrast, and iopromide in 50 patients undergoing leg arteriography in the Department of Radiology, University of Tübingen (study not complete)

Side effect		Ioxaglate Hexabrix $n = 20$		Iopamidol Solutrast $n = 14$		Iopromide $n = 16$	
		%	(patients)	%	(patients)	%	(patients)
Pain	moderate	5	(1)	21	(3)	0	(0)
	severe	0	(0)	0	(0)	0	(0)
Heat	moderate	100	(20)	93	(13)	100	(16)
	severe	0	(0)	7	(1)	0	(0)
Other		5	(1)	7	(0)	0	(0)

Premedication: none
Dose: 80 ml
Flow rate: 18 ml/s

Table 5. Side effects of different types of contrast medium

Side effect		Ionic monomer $n = 90$ %	Ionic dimer $n = 153$ %	Nonionic monomer $n = 169$ %
Pain	moderate	32	39	39
	severe	9	4	8
Heat	moderate	42	71	63
	severe	32	14	18
Other		9	9	2
		with premedication	without premedication	without premedication

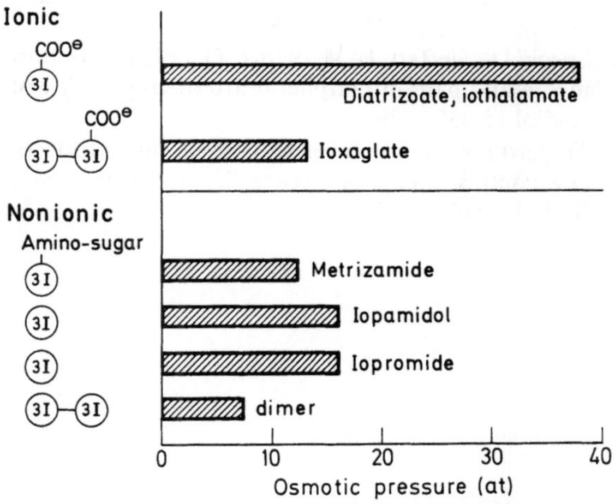

Fig. 2. The osmotic pressures of various contrast media at a solution of 300 mg iodine/ml

more with iopromide, and the sensation of heat shows similar figures. However, in contrast to the study with ionic contrast substances (Table 1), no premedication was necessary. The number of patients with the normal side effects is less with iopromide than with Hexabrix.

Regarding sensations of pain and heat, then, there is no obvious difference between these two new preparations. We have therefore begun an extended double-blind study, comparing Hexabrix, Solutrast, and iopromide (Table 4). Up to now, no convincing difference between the three substances has been seen. We have not been able to test the other new nonionic contrast medium, Iohexol (Nyegaard), but similar results may be expected.

Taking all our studies together, according to the group or generation of the contrast substances, i.e., dividing them into ionic monomers, ionic dimers, and nonionic monomers (Table 5), the current situation may be defined as follows: With the introduction of the low-osmolality contrast media, premedication is only sometimes necessary. Concerning pain and heat, there is no convincing difference between ionic dimers and nonionic monomers.

There is however, an obvious tendency toward reduction of other side effects with nonionic preparations.

The next step will probably be the development of the nonionic dimer (Fig. 2). This solution will be isotonic to blood, so a good tolerance may be expected.

References

1. Almen T (1980) Experience from 10 years of development of water-soluble nonionic contrast media. Invest Radiol 15:283–288
2. Binz A (1930) The chemistry of Uroselectan. Br J Urol 2:348–351

3. Broman T, Olsson O (1948) The tolerance of cerebral blood vessels to a contrast medium of the diodrast group. Acta Radiol [Diagn] (Stockh) 30:326–342
4. Brooks WW, Paulin S, Bing OHL, Laraia PJ (1980) Effect of angiographic contrast agents on the mechanical performance of the isolated rat papillary muscle preparations. Invest. Radiol. 15:203–207
5. Felder E (1977) Preclinical studies with a new nonionic contrast agent. Second congress of the European Society of Cardiovascular Radiology, Uppsala, May 25–27
6. Golman K, Almen T (1973) Metrizamide in experimental urography. 1. Iodine concentration and flow of urine following intravenous injections of an ionic and a non-ionic contrast medium in rabbits. Acta Radiol [Suppl] (Stockh) 335:312–322
7. Golman K, Holtas S (1980) Proteinuria produced by urographic contrast media. Invest Radiol 15:61–65
8. Gonsette RE, Anore-Balisaux G (1967) La perméabilité des vaisseaux cérébraux. Etude de la tolérance pour les produits de contraste. Acta Radiol [Suppl] (Stockh) 270:228–243
9. Gonsette RE, Liesenborgh L (1980) New contrast media in cerebral angiography: animal experiments and preliminary clinical studies. Invest Radiol 15:270–274
10. Higgins CB (1980) Overview and methods used for the study of the cardiovascular actions of contrast materials. Invest Radiol 15:188–193
11. Higgins CB, Schmidt W (1978) Alterations in calcium levels of coronary sinus blood during coronary arteriography in the dog. Circulation 58:512–519
12. Holm M, Praestholm J (1979) Ioxaglate, a new low osmolar contrast medium used in femoral angiography. Br J Radiol 52:169–172
13. Holtermann H (1973) Metrizamide. Introduction. Acta Radiol [Suppl] (Stockh) 335:1–4
14. Moreau J-F, Droz D, Noel L-H, Leibowitch J, Jungers P, Michel J-R (1980) Tubular nephrotoxicity of water-soluble iodinated contrast media. Invest Radiol 15:54–60
15. Nyman U (to be published) Pain and hemodynamic effects in aorto-femoral arteriography. Clinical comparison of Iohexol, Ioxaglate and Metrizamide. Acta Radiol
16. Pfister RC, Hutter AM (1980) Cardiac alterations during intravenous urography. Invest Radiol 15:239–242
17. Raininko R (1979) Role of hypertonicity in the endothelial injury caused by angiographic contrast media. Acta Radiol [Diagn] (Stockh) 20:410–416
18. Rosenberg FJ, Romano JJ, Shaw DD (1980) Metrizamide, Iothalamate, and Metrizoate: Effects of internal carotid arterial injections on the blood-brain barrier of the rabbit. Invest Radiol 15: 275–279
19. Skalpe JO, Evensen A (1973) Toxicity of metrizamide, meglumine iocarmate and sodium metrizoate in selective nephroangiography. Acta Radiol [Suppl] (Stockh) 335:175–185
20. Speck U, Sieffert H-M, Klink G (1980) Contrast media and pain in peripheral arteriography. Invest Radiol 15:335–339
21. Trägardh B (1980) Investigation of the effects of new contrast media on myocardial function. Invest Radiol 15:194–195

Contrast Quality of Ionic and Nonionic Contrast Media in Computed Tomography to Test Suitability for Digital Subtraction Angiography

H. Tschakert

Knappschafts-Krankenhaus, Röntgen- und Radiumabteilung, Westerholter Weg 82, 4350 Recklinghausen, FRG

The new nonionic X-ray contrast media, such as iohexol and iopamidol, have among other features, a lower osmolality than the older ionic media. The fact that dilution due to the osmotic pressure gradient between the intravascular and extravascular spaces is less marked makes it likely that there will be measurably greater enhancement within the vessels than with the ionic media [2]. The purpose of this study was to establish, with special reference to digital subtraction angiography, to what extent nonionic X-ray contrast media provide improved enhancement of blood vessels after intravenous cubital injection where the medium also passes through heart and lungs.

Two double-blind studies were performed, involving computed tomography (CT) examination of ten patients in one case, and nine in the other. To improve the statistical value of the studies and to exclude differences due to the individuals concerned (details below), we used the crossover technique, reexamining each patient after an interval of at least 10 days with an ionic standard preparation instead of the nonionic preparation employed the first time. The dosage was 1.5 ml/kg body weight, administered at a rate of 5 ml/s (Fig. 1 a, b).

In the first group the patients received iohexol (Omnipaque, Schering) with meglumine ioglicinate (Rayvist, Schering) as the ionic standard; in the second group the nonionic preparation was iopamidol (Solutrast, Byk Gulden Lomberg) and the ionic standard was meglumine ioxithalamate

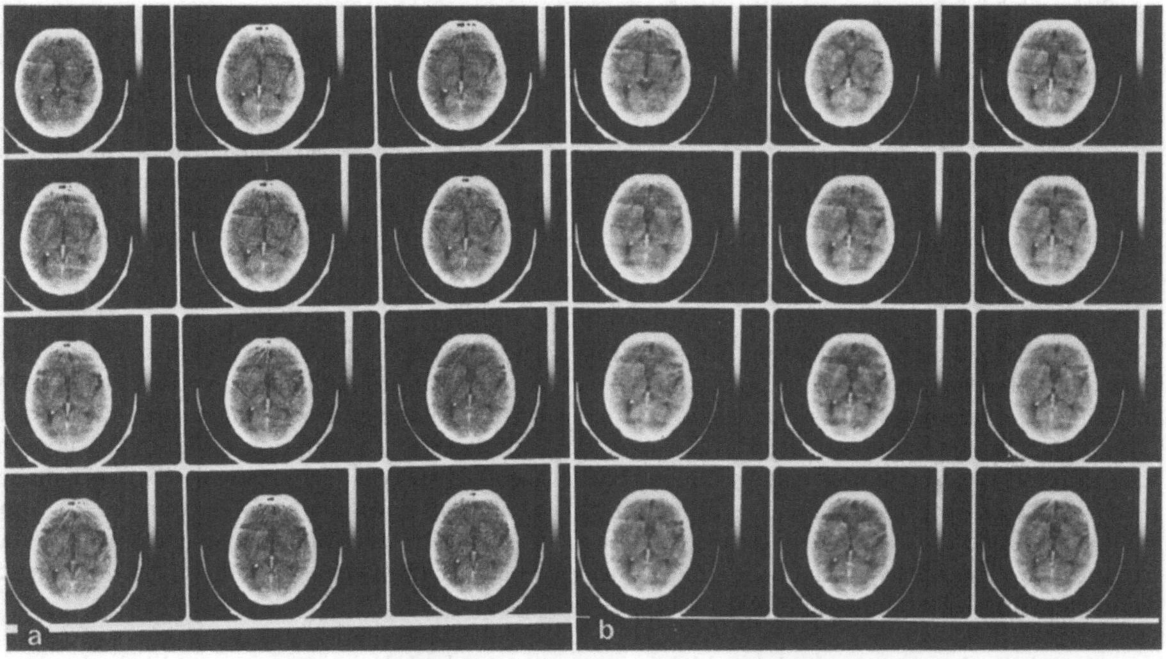

Fig. 1 a, b. The density of a central point of the sinus rectus was measured before and 0.45, 1.45, 2.45, 3.45, 4.45, 5.45, 6.45, 10.00, 15.00, 20.00, and 30.00 min after bolus injection of contrast medium. **a** Ionic contrast medium; **b** nonionic contrast medium (12 days later)

Radiology Today 2. Ed. by F. H. W. Heuck and M. W. Donner

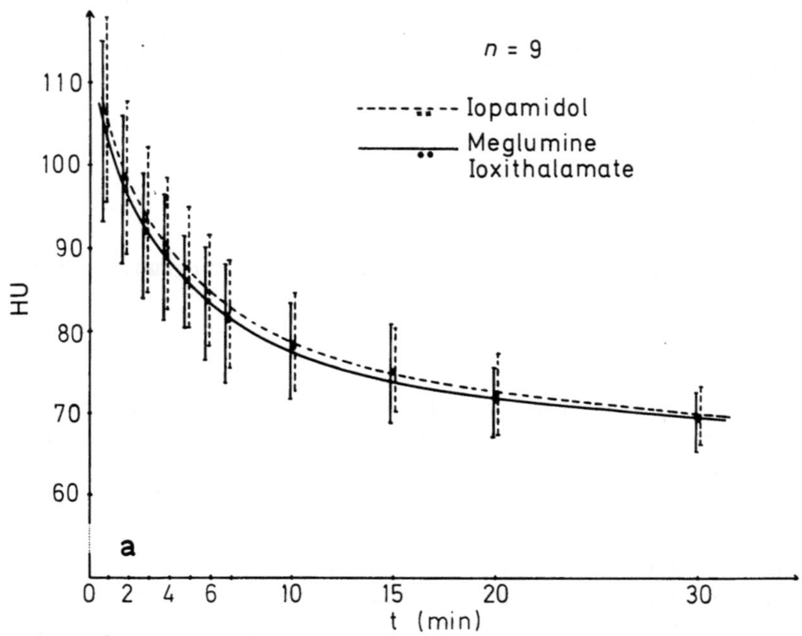

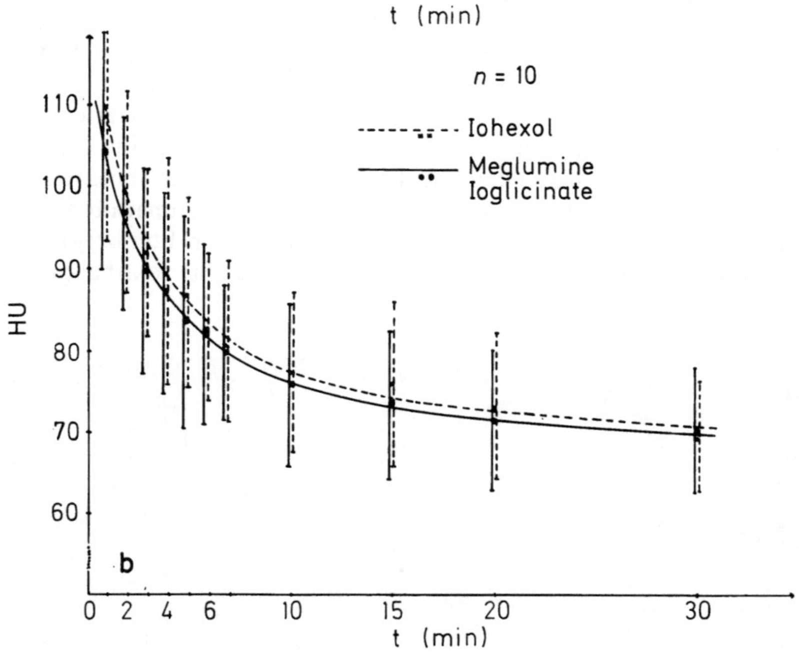

Fig. 2 a, b. Contrast enhancement (HU) of the sinus rectus with standard deviation in relation to the time after bolus injection of ionic and nonionic contrast media. **a** Iopamidol vs. meglumine ioxithalamate; **b** iohexol vs. meglumine ioglicinate. For detail see text

(Telebrix, Byk Gulden Lomberg). All preparations were at a concentration of 300 mg iodine/ml. The CT examination was performed on the ON 50 FS [Ohio-Nuclear Inc, Ohio, N.A.) with a scan time of 18 s and 8-mm wide sections. The plane, marked by means of three dots of indelible ink spaced round the skull circumference, was selected to show the whole length of the sinus rectus. Throughout the CT examination (at least 30 min), the patient's head was kept perfectly still to ensure that the volumes measured would be constant. At various times after injection of the contrast medium the absorption in the same vein was ascertained.

The absorption data were collated and the standard deviations computed. As Fig. 2a, b shows, both the ionic and nonionic media had in principle the same absorption pattern. The nonionic agents displayed a marginally better enhancement, but since this only accounted for about 2%–3% difference on average, and since the standard deviations were wide, there was no statistical significance.

The wide interindividual variance – expressed as the standard deviation – is most likely due mainly to the partial volume effect of the tomogram and to the dosage, which was based exclusively on individual body weight and not on blood volume

[1]. In addition, other individual characteristics such as heart rate, state of hydration, age, and condition of the arteries make for varying contrast enhancement [2].

Provisional results show that there is no significantly greater enhancement in the venous intravascular space after two passages through the circulation; the only finding in this context is a slight average improvement in intravascular enhancement, amounting to about 2%–3%, with both nonionic contrast media. This difference can scarcely be of practical importance, as the examining physician will not be able to detect it. In respect of the tomogram timing it may be said that the 45-s wait between the start of injection and the first tomogram section (about two passages of the circulation) means that the arterial contrast pattern should not be expected to vary – at least during this period after injection – on account of the fact that intravascular mixing is almost complete. This assumption was confirmed with the aid of a small control group in which we determined arterial absorption levels in the aorta at the same time. As a result of the very long scan times, the subsequent lateness of measuring, and the wide intervals between measurements, it is not possible to make any definite statement about contrast agent behavior during the first passage through the circulation. Further investigations must be carried out to ascertain what differentiation can be made between ionic and nonionic contrast media in respect of contrast achieved during their first passage through the circulation, to establish which of the two types is more suitable for digital subtraction angiography.

References

1. Dean PB, Kivisaari L, Kormano M (1978) Contrast enhancement: diagnostic significance from a statistical point of view. J Comput Assist Tomogr 2:314–318
2. Gardeur D, Lautron J, Millard JC, Berger M, Metzger J (1980) Pharmacokinetics of contrast media: experimental results in dog and man with CT implications. J Comput Assist Tomogr 4:178–185

Nuclear Magnetic Resonance with a 3.5 KG Superconducting Imager

A. R. Margulis

Department of Radiology, University of California, San Francisco, CA 94143, USA

Nuclear magnetic resonance (NMR) is the newest imaging modality and has created tremendous excitement throughout the medical community, combining as it does the advantages of X-ray computed tomography (CT), superb resolution and tomography, with those of ultrasound, the use of nonionizing radiation and the possibility of imaging in any desired plane, sagittal, coronal, or oblique. Like nuclear medicine, it provides data on metabolic processes and the physiologic status of tissues. The absence of biologic risks in the energy range in which NMR imaging is performed further enhances its attraction. In addition, information on blood flow is obtainable.

The imager at UCSF is a superconducting machine with a field strength of 3.5 kG. At present, head images are obtained with a matrix of 128×128 pixels and body images with 256×128 pixels. The pixel size is usually 1.7×1.7 mm, but in the body some are 1.9×1.9 mm or 2.5×2.5 mm. The section thickness varies from 3 mm to 7 mm. In a period of 13 min, five sections of the subject are imaged. Each section is obtained with four permutations, TE = 28 ms or 56 ms and TR = 0.5 s or 1.0 s (TE the interval between excitation and observation; TR, the interval between excitations). Thus a total of 20 images are obtained. Using inversion recovery, five sections are imaged in 8.5 min. Each section is imaged with TE 28 ms and TE 56 ms. In this mode TR is 1.0 s and the recovery time is 0.4 s. Fifteen sections can also be obtained with the same imager, with TE 28 ms and TR 1.5 s in 6.5 min in the head and 6.5 min or 13 min in the body. By obtaining the four permutations in the pulse echo mode, T-1 and T-2 values can be calculated by the computer and imaged, as can the H values. Subtracting T1 information and only using that from T2 and H, a so-called asymptote image can be produced by the computer.

The field of imaging can be sagittal, coronal, or oblique, as well as the usual transverse. Multiple images can be obtained with spin echo or inversion recovery techniques.

Human Experience with NMR

NMR appears to offer all the capabilities of X-ray CT, with a number of advantages in the head and neck. Imaging is possible along coronal and sagittal planes in a direct manner, avoiding the need for reformatting from multiple sections. Bones do not produce artifacts, so NMR is better for imaging in the posterior fossa of the skull. Aside from the improved versatility of NMR imaging, when compared with X-ray CT it clearly, offers improved diagnostic efficacy in degenerative brain disorders. It seems to offer more information regarding infarcts, areas of edema, and particularly demyelinating diseases. It is still necessary to develop the best imaging techniques for presentation and study of the findings in many of these diseases. In demyelinating diseases such as multiple sclerosis, in our experience intensity pulse echo images show the abnormalities better then inversion recovery images. In the chest, mediastinal structures and blood vessels are seen to excellent advantage. The accuracy of the method promisses to be greater than that of CT, as tumors appear to be distinguishable from normal tissues even without contrast media, particularly when calculated T-1 and T-2 images are also obtained and studied.

Ungated images of the heart have shown dyskinetic regions (the regions of the myocardium that move rapidly are blurred, and only slow or nonmoving regions are imaged). Other groups, notably the one of Case Western Reserve University Medical School at Cleveland, Ohio, have presented excellent gated NMR images of the heart. Carcinoma of the lung is well visualized and there have been excellent demonstrations of pulmonary infarcts and of pneumonia. In the abdomen, the

Radiology Today 2. Ed. by F. H. W. Heuck and M. W. Donner

area where NMR offers most advantages appears to be the kidneys, where tumors, cysts, hydronephrosis, etc. have been studied and the usefulness of the method has been well demonstrated. There is also a great deal of promise in diseases of the adrenal glands, as well as of the prostate, where it appears that carcinoma can be distinguished from benign prostatic hypertrophy. Whether NMR is more accurate and offers advantages over CT in the liver has yet to be demonstrated. There is little question that NMR imaging is more sensitive than X-ray CT in the detection of soft tissue lesions, but the ability to characterize these lesions with a high level of confidence (malignant vs. benign, abscess vs. hematoma, etc.) remains to be demonstrated. NMR promises to be accurate in demonstrating lesions in the spine and intervertebral discs. Detail in cancellous bone where there is an abundance of bone marrow can be studied closely.

There are areas where NMR imaging seems to offer less diagnostic accuracy than X-ray CT. For instance, calcifications are seen only if they are large and extensive. Solid bone and air produce no signal, and in certain areas of the head like the petrous pyramid it is difficult or impossible to separate these two.

Future Developments

It is expected that NMR will become very important, probably complementing or even replacing many of the currently used imaging modalities, and it is particularly in diseases of the brain and soft tissues, in the heart, and in study of tumors throughout the body (except perhaps the liver) that NMR will threaten CT. However, CT still has the advantages of greater speed and resolution, and the promised development of a millisecond X-ray CT scanner may change some present impressions of the relative values of NMR and X-ray CT. With contributions regarding chemical environment of tissues in various disease processes, a new breed of radiologists will have to be developed who are cognizant of physiology and biochemistry and think in terms of quantitative analysis. Cooperative research projects with internists, neurologists, physiologists, biochemists, physicists, etc. will speed up the rate of progress and will allow earlier determination of the best NMR imaging technique for the display and study of information.

Missed Diagnosis Conference

The Missed Diagnosis as a Powerful Teaching Device

P. S. Wheeler, O. Pohlenz, H. Hacker, and M. T. Freedman

Department of Radiology, The Johns Hopkins Hospital, 601 N. Broadway, Baltimore, MD 21205, USA

The Recognized Error is the Best Teacher

Diagnostic errors can harm patients and the legal consequences can harm physicians and hospitals. Some medicolegal compensation settlements run as high as a million dollars, and in these terms one simple mistake could prevent a hospital from being able to buy a new nuclear magnetic resonance unit or computed tomography scanner, and in some instances might even threaten bankruptcy.

Over the last 3 years we have developed a conference in our radiology department which deals primarily with mistakes or cases which could have been missed without a very keen eye, some critical clinical information, or just plain luck. Cases with false-positive and false-negative diagnoses are analyzed and reasons for the mistakes are identified. The best examples are presented at the conference and discussed openly, with emphasis on ways to prevent such mistakes in the future.

It takes a firm departmental commitment to gather missed diagnoses, because they naturally evoke shame and anxiety in the radiologist responsible. For that reason, we maintain absolute anonymity at our conference so that members of the department will feel free to contribute as the cases are discovered.

A number of interesting developments have come from the conference. We have identified "difficult diagnosis zones" on various types of X-ray examinations. On the chest X-ray, for example, the mediastinum from top to bottom poses the most difficult diagnosis zone of all, with the pleural reflections a close second. Also of interest are the problems caused by high-kV technique: calcifications in pleural plaques, granulomas calcified heart valves, and in some instances even metal foreign bodies are totally obscured.

Another revelation is the amount of misleading clinical data. This is particularly a problem because we are always asking for more information.

Finally, in America, the Joint Accreditation Commission for hospitals has demanded a "Quality Assurance Program" from all hospitals. We found during the commissioners' visit that our missed diagnosis conference is exactly what they desired.

Radiology Today 2. Ed. by F. H. W. Heuck and M. W. Donner

General Considerations

O. Pohlenz and D. Bartelt

Allgemeines Krankenhaus St. Georg, Albers-Schönberg-Institut, Abteilung für Strahlendiagnostik, Lohmühlenstrasse 5, 2000 Hamburg 1, FRG

Most of us have spent many years improving our diagnostic accuracy, yet we still make mistakes. There are no reliable objective data on the number of false diagnoses made, broken down by the individual physician or department. Careful analysis would probably reveal rather frightening information.

Basically, each abnormality not recognized on X-ray must be called a missed diagnosis. Incorrect reports can be broken down into three general categories:

1. Nonpathologic variations (Normal variants), e.g., congenital bone deformities, certain "humps" and "bumps" of the kidney, and accessory pleural fissures. They are usually of no clinical significance, but are included since strictly speaking they do represent deviations from the normal and therefore should not be missed or misinterpreted.
2. Pathologic findings which are of little or no relevance to the patient's current problem(s) but will possibly be important in the future, e.g., degenerative joint disease, vascular calcifications, and diverticula of the GI tract.
3. Pathologic findings of direct or indirect greater importance to the patient's *current* problem(s): (a) being the key to his diagnosis, (b) leading to an explanation of this present situation, or (c) being of major importance for the future.

Only missed diagnoses belonging to the third category will be dealt with here.

Differential and final diagnosis are the result of a well-organized series of actions (technical procedures) and thought (interpretation). The reliability of this system is rather high and predictable, as long as the stages are gone through systematically and logically. Missed diagnoses (mistakes), however, are usually unpredictable and often due to breaks in this chain. Although in theory it is fairly easy to learn and teach a system for arriving at a diagnosis, it is in fact difficult to establish a foolproof way of avoiding mistakes.

Misinterpretation or overlooking of findings is usually an *individual* occurrence with an *individual* history; cases are difficult to classify, which, for a presentation like this, would mean a collection of *individual* case reports. Nevertheless, certain mistakes can be classified as repetitions, so-called typical pitfalls, since they occur again and again (e.g., luxation/subluxation of the lunatum, lesions of the epiphysis in the growing skeleton, infiltrations or masses in certain areas of the chest). However, even knowledge of these typical pitfalls will not prevent mistakes in general.

Let us look at a system as foolproof as possible. We will first establish five major *preconditions*, then correlate them with five *essential steps* in the process of film interpretation. The five major preconditions are:

I. Good image *quality*.
II. Examination with the *appropriate* method in the *appropriate* area at the *appropriate* time.
III. Clinical *information* and interdisciplinary *cooperation* (patient's history). Clinical information should be looked at with caution, since it may be highly unreliable or misleading for many different reasons.
IV. *Care*, *System*, and *Logic* in image analysis and in retrieval from previous or other images.
V. *Knowledge* and experience.

The essential steps for logical interpretation are the so-called five D's:

Detection
Description
Differentiation
Discussion
Diagnosis

Correlation and combination of the five preconditions and the five essential steps in interpretation leads to the final result: the *diagnosis* (Fig. 1).

Radiology Today 2. Ed. by F.H.W. Heuck and M.W. Donner

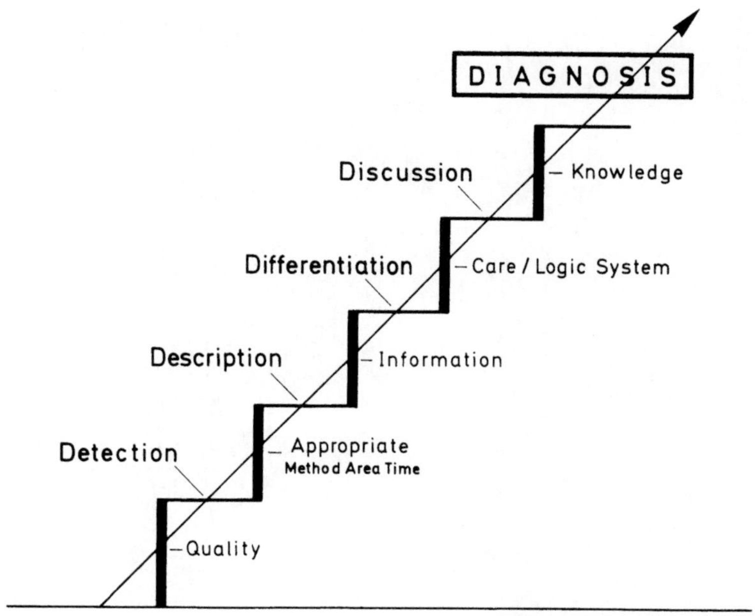

Fig. 1. Diagnostic staircase: exemplar

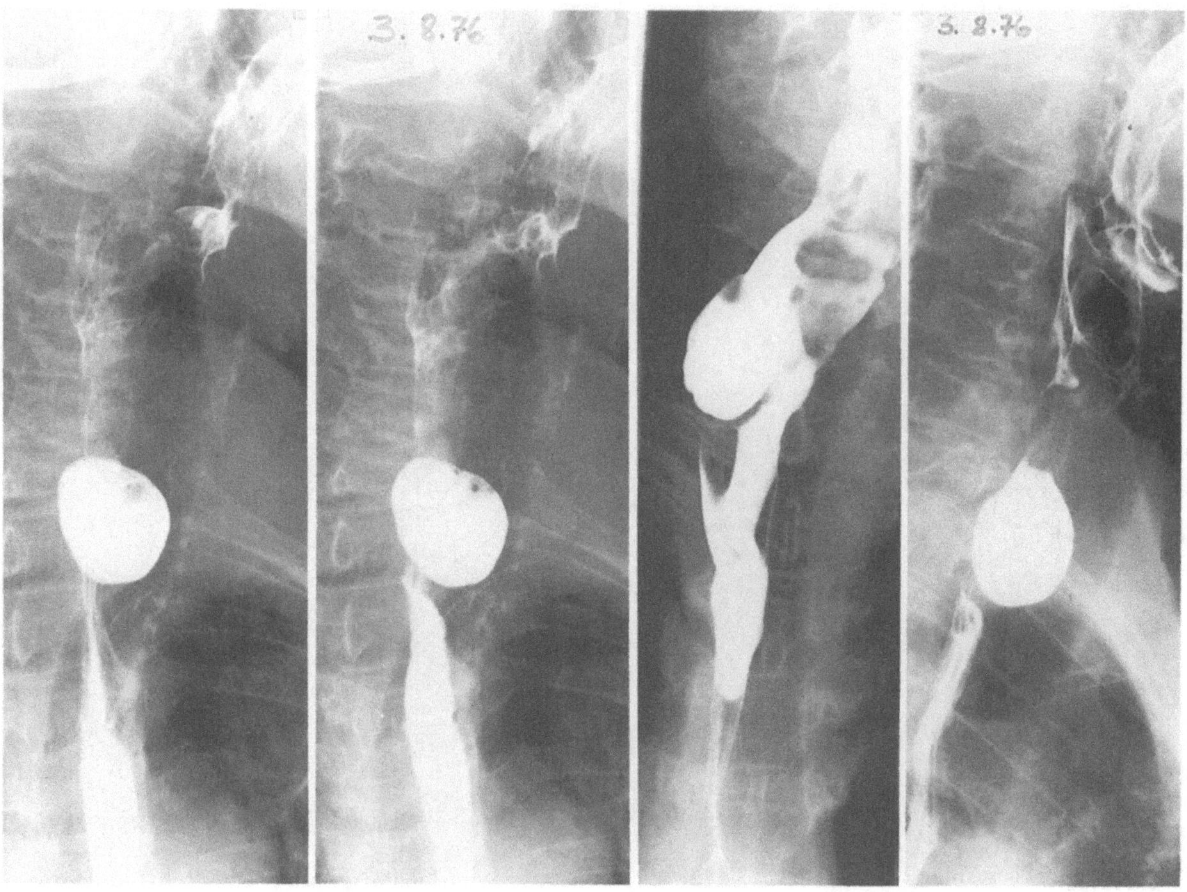

Fig. 2. Large Zenker diverticulum

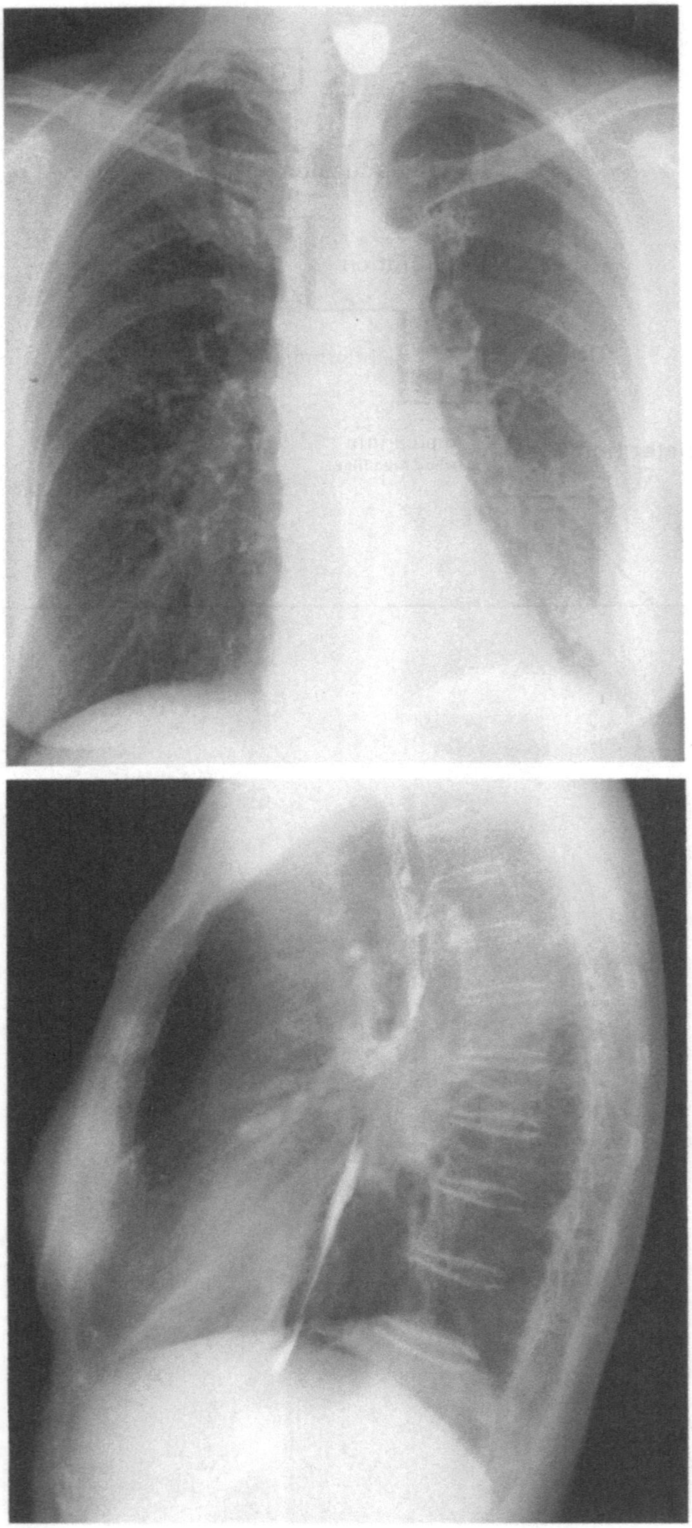

Fig. 3. Pre-op chest film

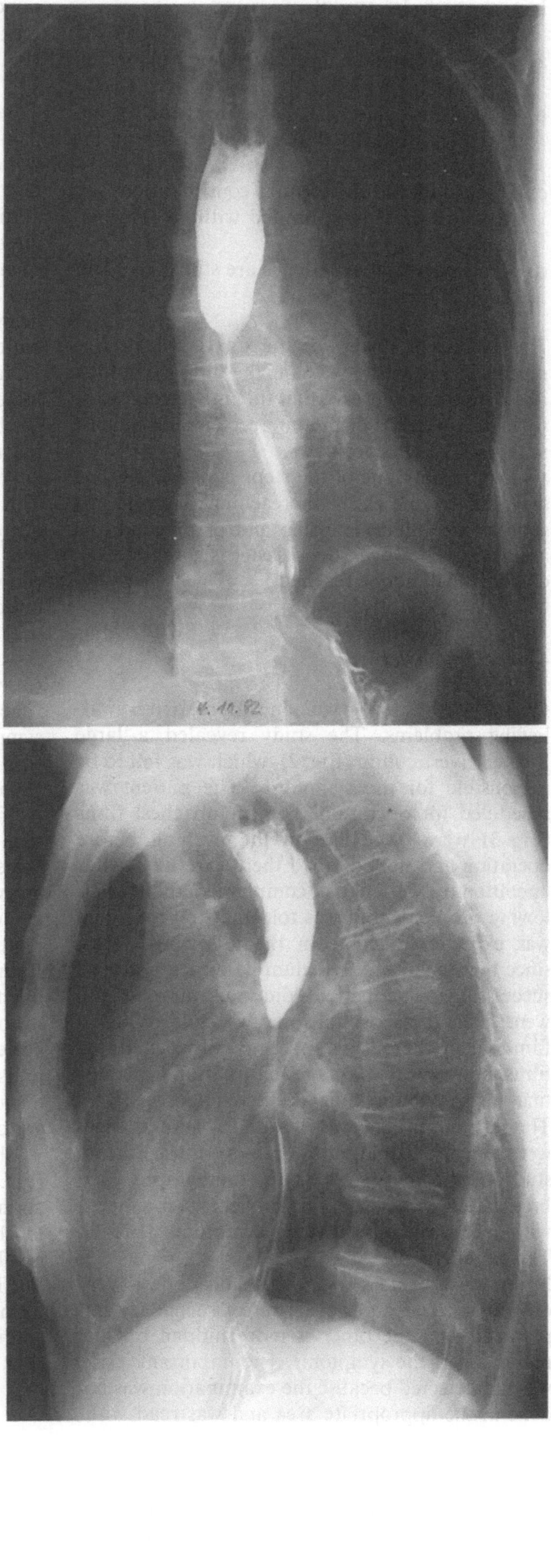

Fig. 4. Chest film 8 weeks later

It is easy to understand that:

a) With bad film quality, detection can be impossible.
b) Good film quality has no value if the examination is done in the wrong area or at the wrong time.
c) Discussion and differential considerations are worthless or at least limited without information.
d) Knowledge and experience are still the key for the final result.

The five essential steps on the x-axis and the five preconditions on the y-axis make the system look like a staircase. Observe that the intellectual quality and experience of the interpreter rank highest in the system of coordinates.

As long as only one of the steps is neglected, one *may* still be successful in reaching the goal. As soon as more than one step and/or precondition are missing, however, the disaster is complete: the diagnosis will not be reached.

Clinical Examples

Case 1. A 50-year-old woman suffered from swallowing problems. The study revealed a large Zenker diverticulum (Fig. 2), which was felt to be responsible for the symptoms. The patient was scheduled for operation. The pre-op chest films (Fig. 3) were done late in the evening before operation and nobody read them carefully. After operation the patient still complained about swallowing problems, but was told that improvement was expected to come in the following weeks, since the Zenker diverticulum had been removed successfully. The patient did *not* improve and went to another hospital some weeks later. Chest films taken there (Fig. 4), especially penetrated films, now revealed a large left hilar and mediastinal mass, compressing the esophagus (Fig. 5). The left diaphragm was elevated. These changes were already visible on the pre-op films. Barium study of the *lower* esophagus, tomography, and bronchoscopy revealed a bronchial carcinoma with metastases causing the symptoms (Fig. 6). The patient died!

In this case we deal with *two* lesions: one is very obvious and easy to detect but of secondary importance, and the other is more hidden but the real cause of the symptoms. The important lesion was not detected because the examination was not done in the appropriate area and was read without care. The patient's history was not taken properly; she coughed and had lost weight for months (Fig. 7).

Case 2. A 65-year-old man noticed severe chest pain immediately after lifting a heavy weight. He was admitted with the diagnosis of myocardial infarction. From the beginning, clinicians felt an aortic aneurysm to be possible. Myocardial infarction was excluded clinically. There were no roentgen signs indicating aortic aneurysm, no mediastinal widening (Fig. 8). The clinicians heard a mild murmur between the shoulders, the patient still complained of belt-like chest pain. Ultrasound revealed "suspicion" of a double lumen in the ascending aorta. The radiologist did *not* believe this because his X-rays were normal, but could be persuaded to do an aortogram. A large dissection was shown (Fig. 9).

This could have been a radiologically missed diagnosis because there was nothing to detect on film and because without other information and cooperation the appropriate method (aortogram or computed tomography) would not have been used (Fig. 10).

Case 3. A 40-year-old woman came for routine "check-up" chest X-ray (Fig. 11). No clinical symptoms, no complaints. The chest films were read as normal in the presence of the patient. "What about all my fractures?" the patient asked. No fractures were seen on the X-ray. Then the patient told about a car accident she had had some years previously with multiple fractures of both arms, lower ribs, both legs, and pelvis (high energy-deceleration polytrauma). She had altogether more than 20 orthopedic operations with at least 15 different pre-op chest films, all looking exactly like this one, all reported to be normal. With this history, one quick glance at the aortic arch revealed a double contour, minimal tracheal compression from behind, and downward displacement of the left main stem bronchus. The aortogram – the patient had to be persuaded! – showed a typical post-traumatic aneurysm (Fig. 12). The patient was operated on, and the aorta ruptured immediately when the surgeon touched the area. The patient could be saved and is still in good health.

The lesion was not detected because of lack of information (no history) and lack of care in film reading (no adequate request – "routine chest") (Fig. 13).

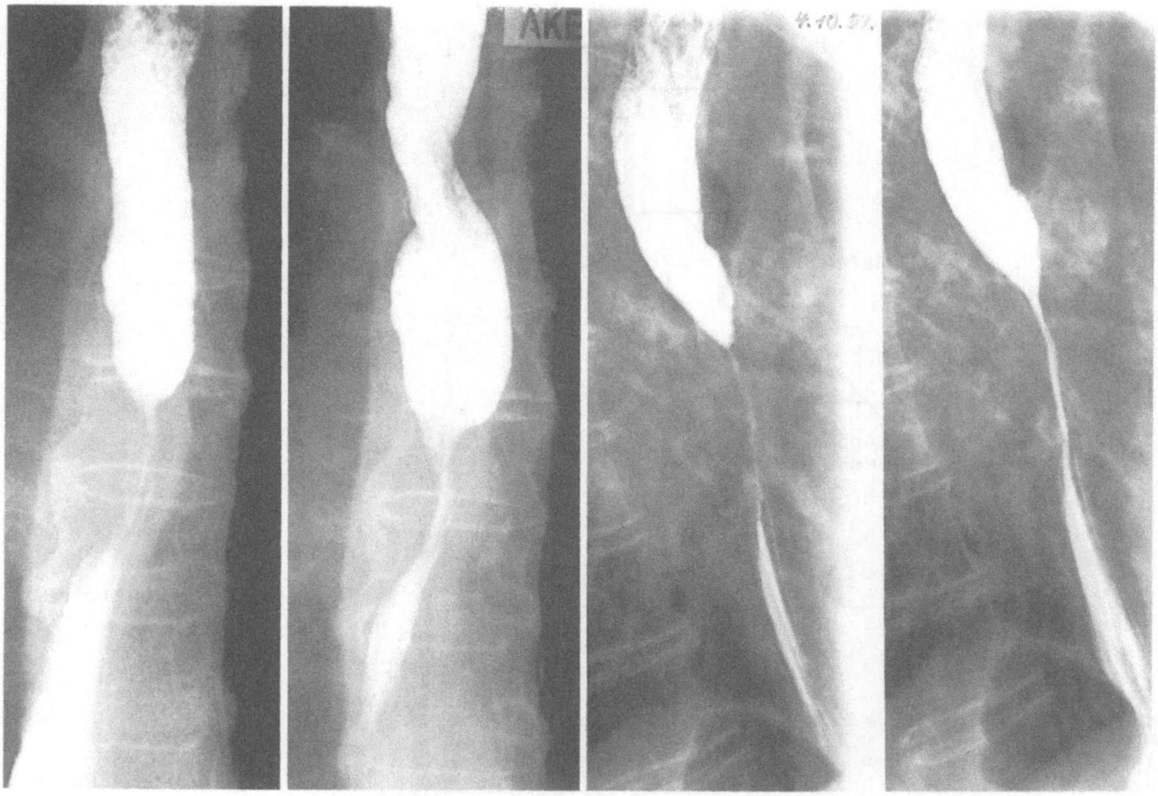

Fig. 5. Middle esophagus with narrowing caused by mediastinal mass

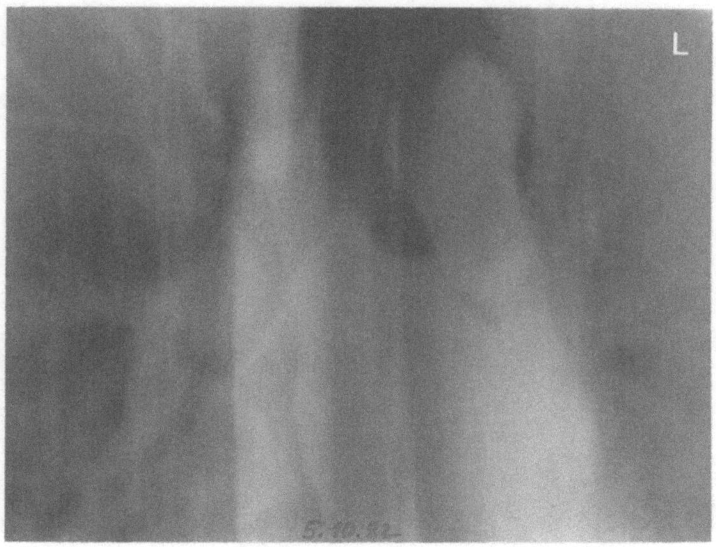

Fig. 6. Hilar tomography with high-grade left main stem bronchus stenosis

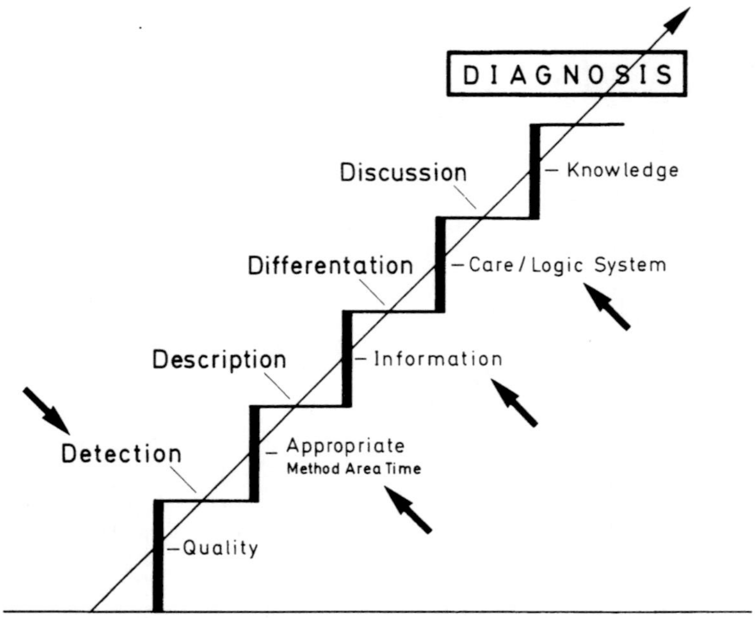

Fig. 7. Diagnostic staircase: case 1

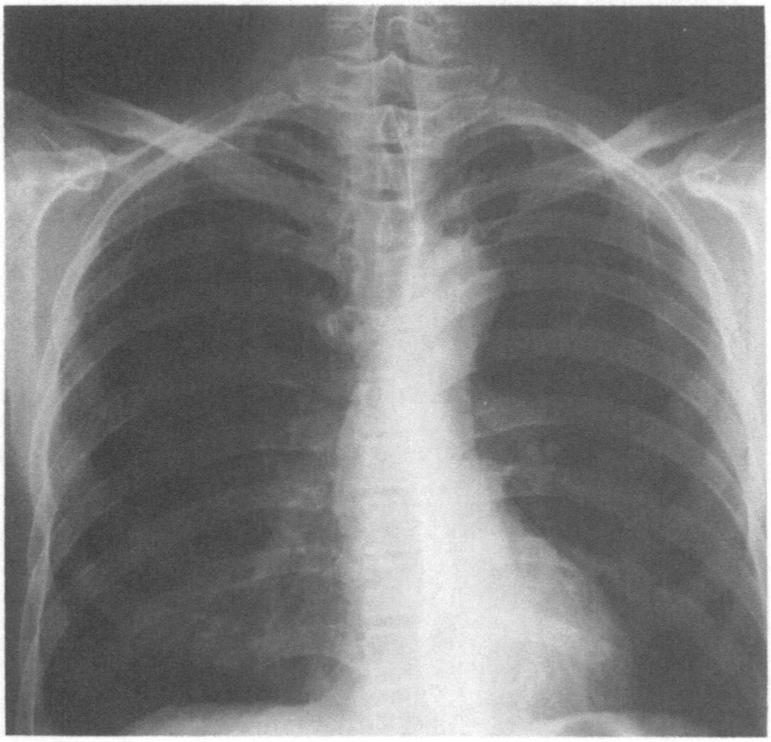

Fig. 8. Chest film 2 weeks after admission with severe chest pain. No evidence of aortic widening or mediastinal hematoma, no changes in comparison to previous films

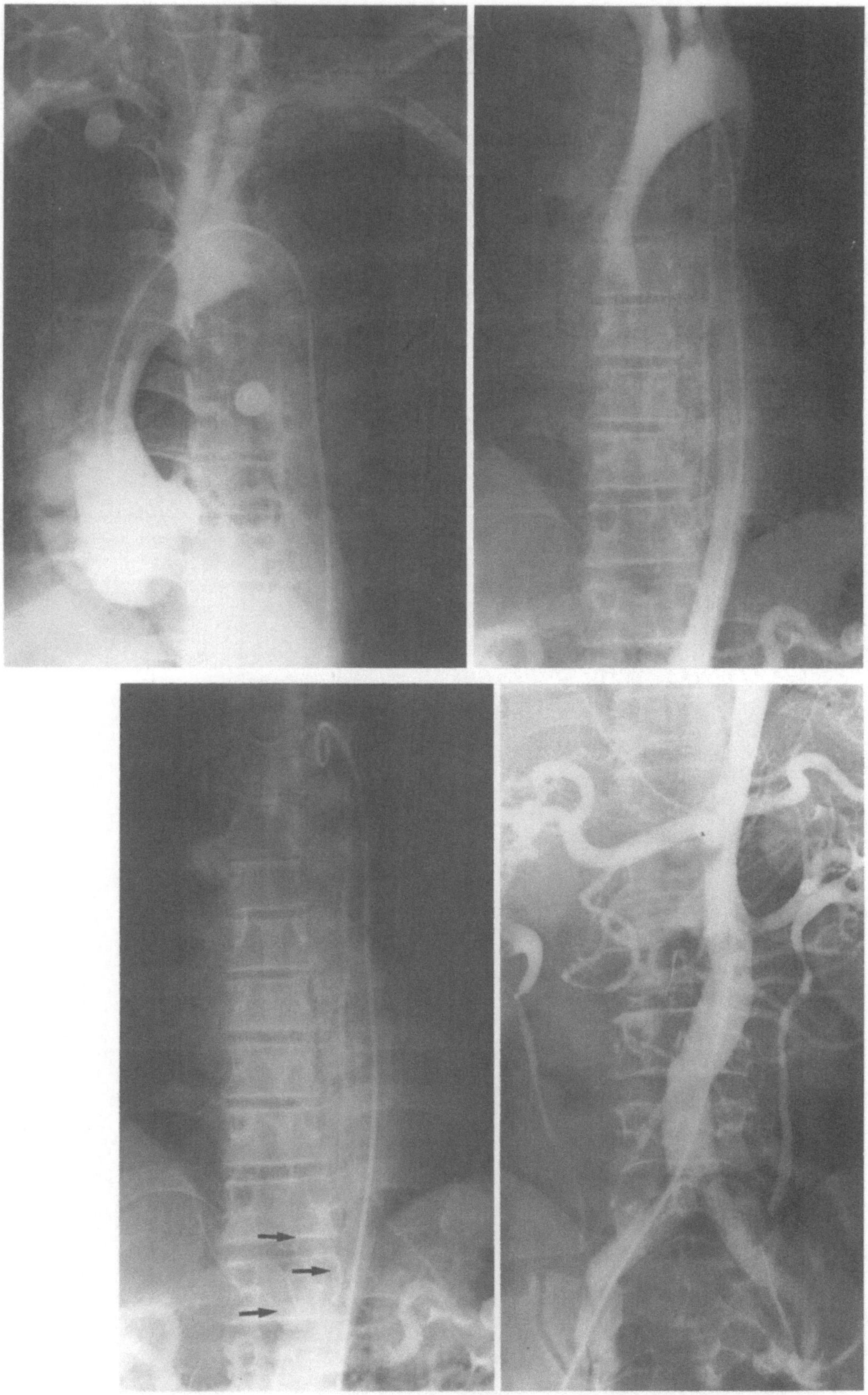

Fig. 9. Aortic dissection from root to abdomen, involving the right renal artery. True and false lumen marked by *arrows*

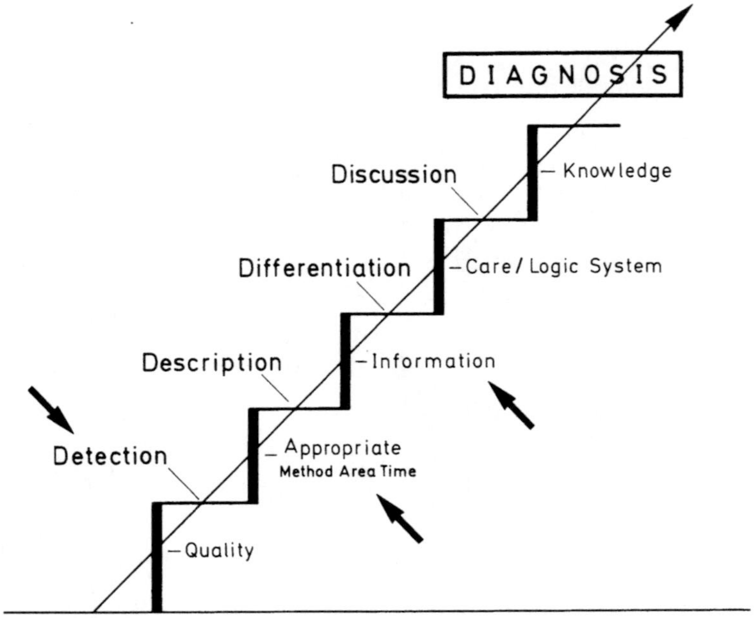

Fig. 10. Diagnostic staircase: case 2

Fig. 11. see p. 349

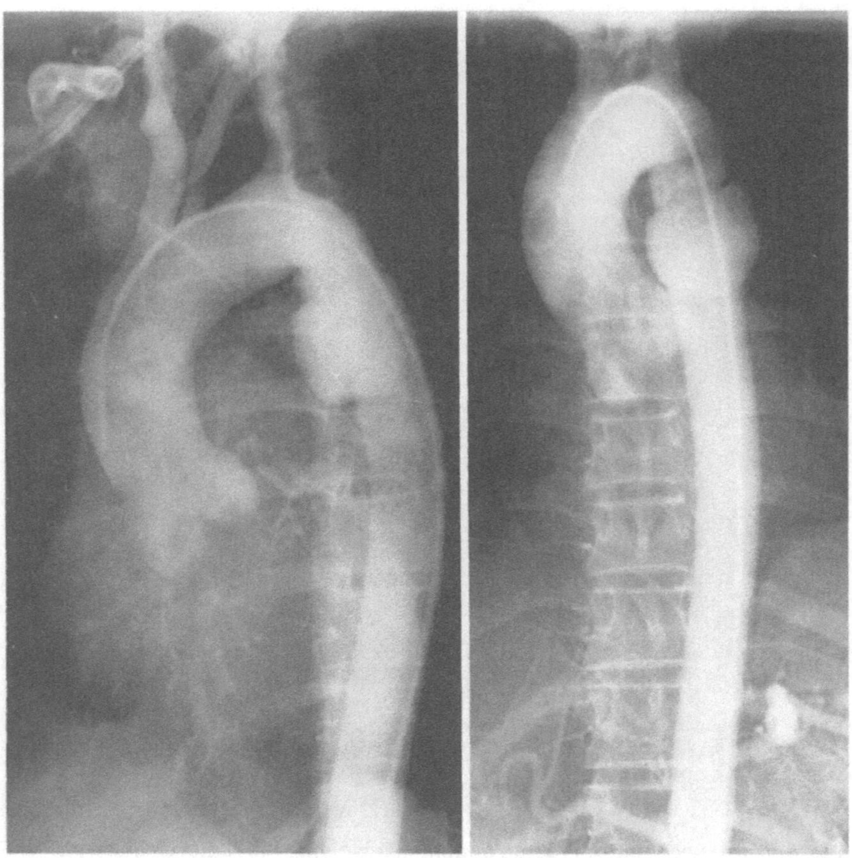

Fig. 12. Aortogram. Typical (post-traumatic) aneurysm of the arch area

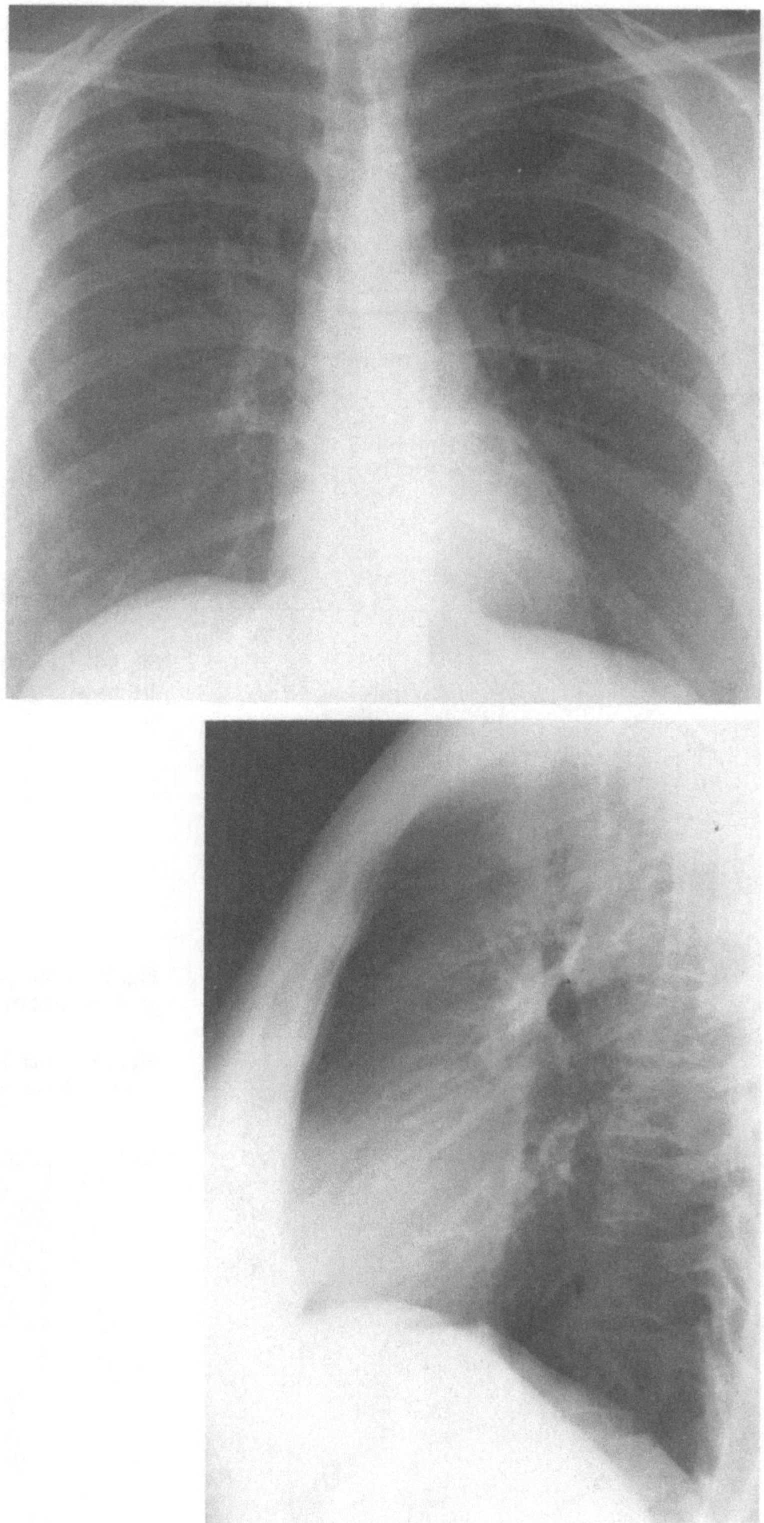

Fig. 11. Routine chest film for "check-up," no symptoms. Double contour of aortic arch, moderate depression of left main stem bronchus, mild compression of lower trachea from behind

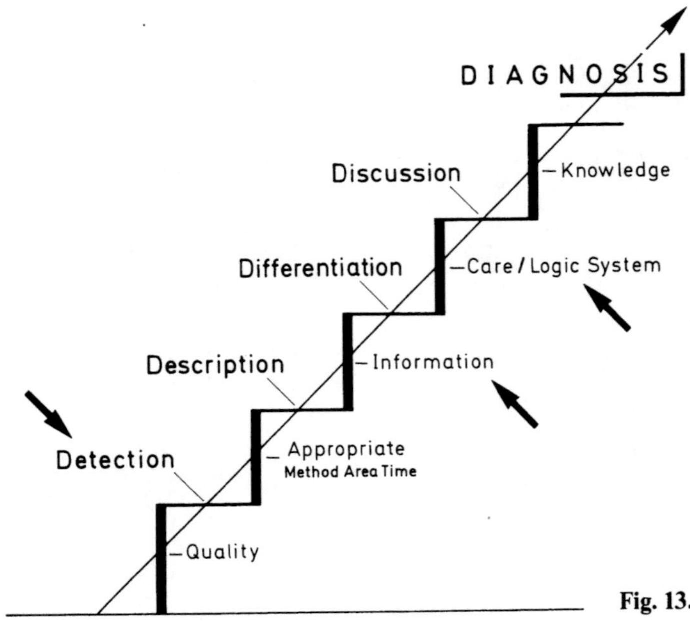

Fig. 13. Diagnostic staircase: case 3

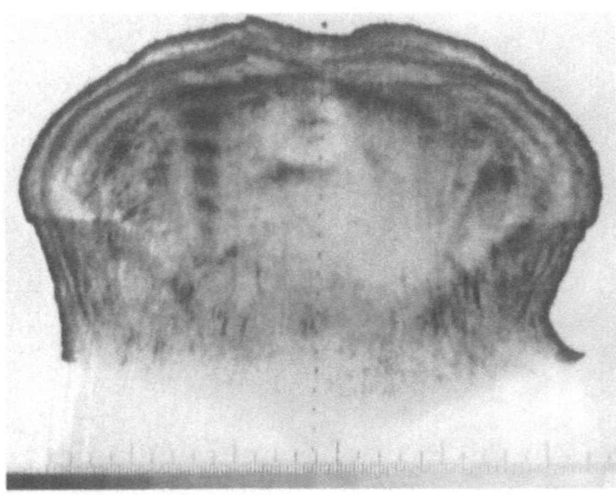

Fig. 14. Ultrasound transverse section demonstrating the mass ◄

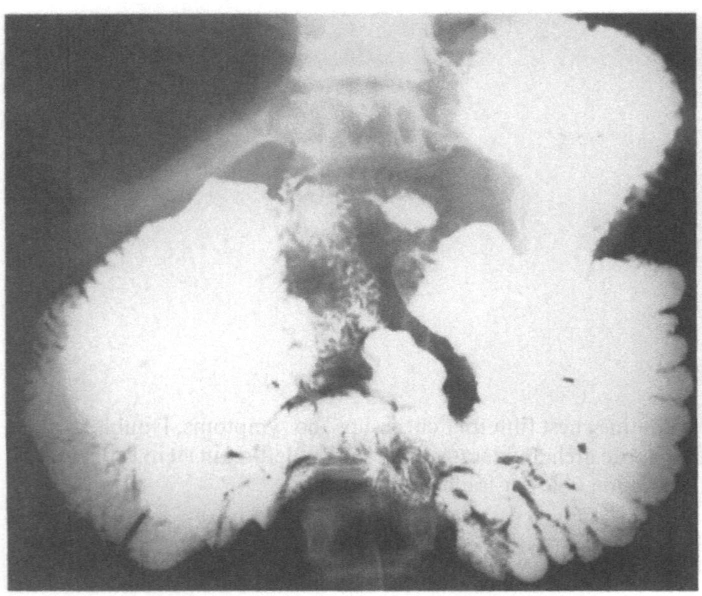

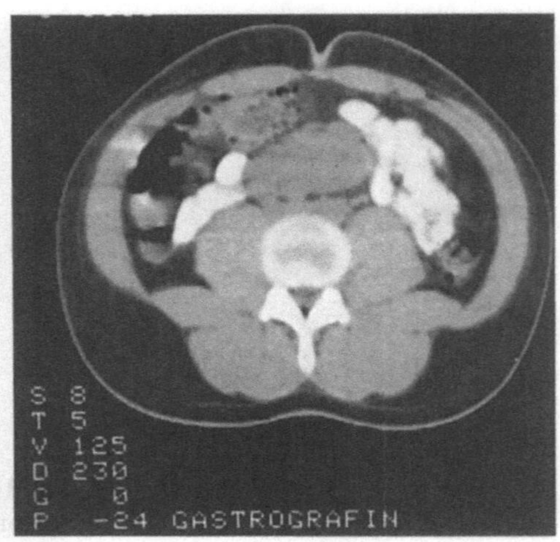

Fig. 15 (*lower left*). Barium meal, small bowel. Low-grade malrotation, no bowel in lower abdomen

Fig. 16 (*lower right*). Computed tomography. Mass in front of the spine; no enhancement

Case 4. A young man of 25 one day discovered a lump in his abdomen. He had no further symptoms. His doctor, owner of a recently purchased ultrasound machine, could "see" the mass (Fig. 14). The patient was sent to a radiologist for a barium meal that was reported to be normal (Fig. 15). Infact it is *not* normal since there is evidence of minor malrotation. The next stage: radiologist no. 2 for computed tomography (Fig. 16). Again the lump was identified but without differential considerations. No further recommendations, no contrast enhancement. Then on to radiologist no. 3 for barium enema. The report mentioned bad preparation (feces), otherwise normal. The last stage was surgery! A young surgeon thought this lump to look very much like a kidney. He was right. A later IVP revealed malposition of the left kidney (Fig. 17).

What were the reasons for this error? There was no correct differential discussion in the beginning when the mass was detected; the appropriate method (IVP/contrast enhancement in computed tomography) was not used; and the patient saw several doctors who obviously never communicated properly.

No information – no cooperation – no diagnosis!

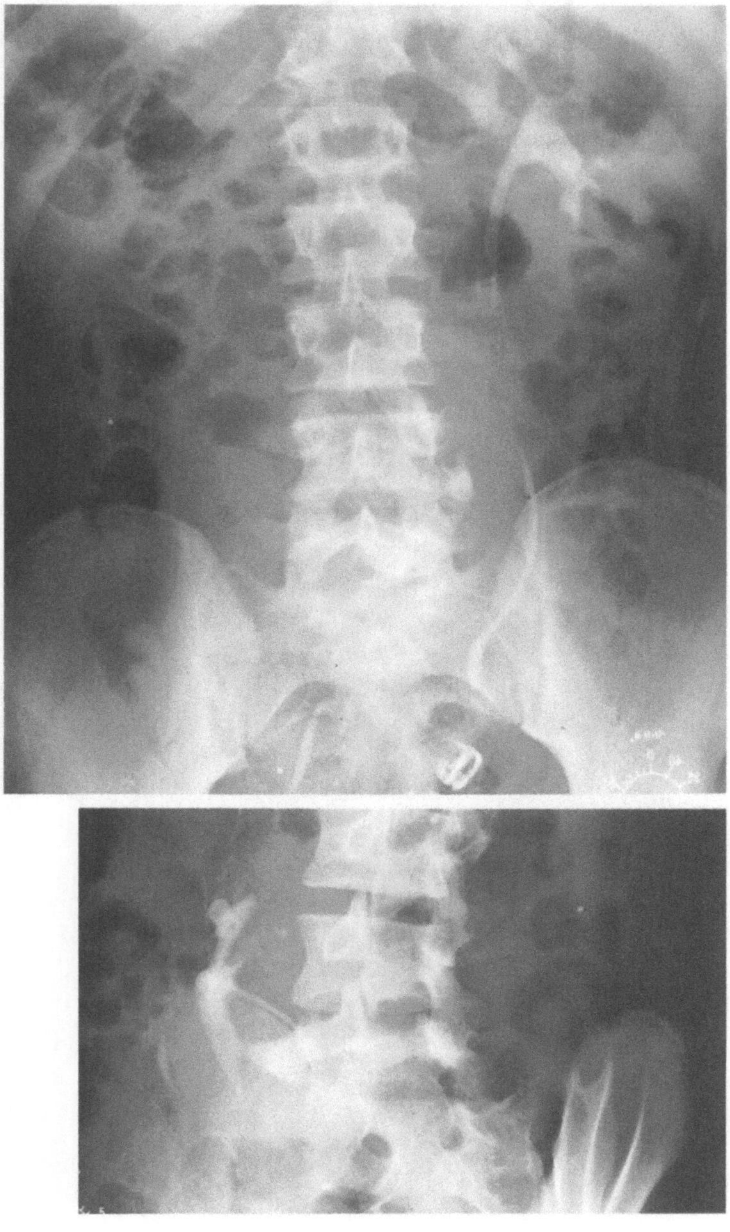

Fig. 17. IVP Malposition of left kidney, representing the palpable mass

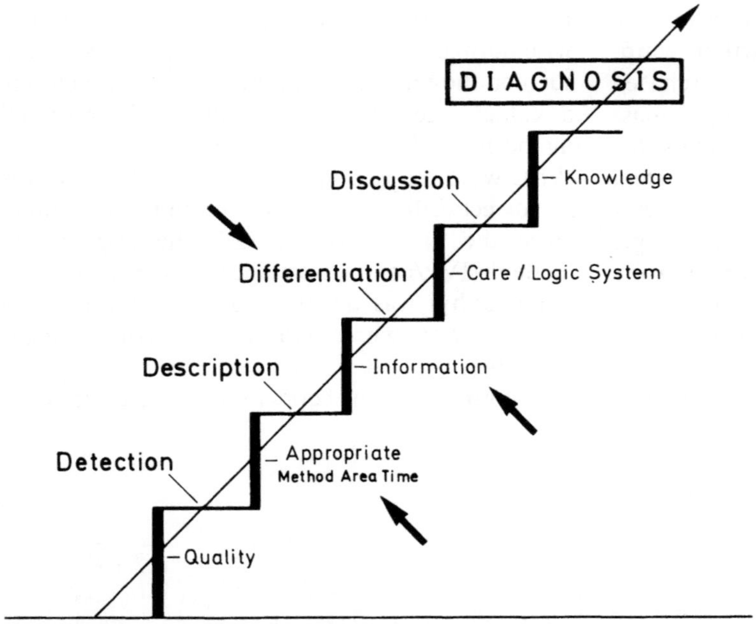

Fig. 18. Diagnostic staircase: case 4

Summary of Dr. Hacker's Presentation

H. Hacker

Abteilung Neuroradiologie, Zentrum Radiologie, Klinikum der Johann-Wolfgang-von-Goethe-Universität, Schleusenweg 2–16, 6000 Frankfurt, FRG

Dr. Hacker stressed the point that general radiologists frequently allow themselves to be tempted into making more exact diagnoses from CT scans and other specialized imaging procedures then would be attempted even by neuroradiologists. He emphasized that precision of diagnosis is best attained by serious specialization; generalists usually lack the knowledge to make highly specific statements on anatomy and pathology. In essence, Dr. Hacker strongly supports Alexander Pope's famous words "A little knowledge is a dangerous thing."

Missed Diagnosis in Bone Radiology

The four sources of problems that I see which often result in missed diagnoses are (a) improper film technique, (b) improper selection of area to be viewed, (c) failure to detect minimal changes of disease, and (d) casts.

Improper Film Technique

The detection of minimal disease requires that the film show both the bone and soft tissue. Salter I transepiphyseal injuries, if undisplaced, may show only edema adjacent to the growth plate. A wide-latitude film is most helpful in searching for subtle injuries. Underexposure, particularly on lateral views of the wrist and AP views of the patella, has resulted in missed diagnoses in our institution.

Improper Selection of Area

Improper selection of the area to be viewed is an important cause of missed diagnoses. The most common mistake is to request a hand when the injury is to a finger, or a foot when the injury is to a toe. Our technician are instructed to take the patient's history and to modify the requested study when they believe this would better serve the patient, and in cases of doubt, to have one of the radiologists examine the patient and decide which study to obtain.

Failure to Detect Minimal Changes

The detection of minimal changes of disease is always a problem. An undisplaced chip fracture, the early changes of inflammatory arthritis or hyperparathyroidism, the impacted femoral neck fracture; each causes its own type of problem. Often the film-screen combination used does not yield sufficient detail for elucidation.

Casts

Radiologists and orthopedists often fail to inspect the image of the cast adequately. Fracture of a cast can permit the displacement of fragments and pinching of skin, which can result in tissue necrosis. Coins and wires can also result in foci of tissue necrosis. While cast problems are not often present, when present they are usually missed.

Radiology Today 2. Ed. by F. H. W. Heuck and M. W. Donner

Continuing Medical Education in Europe

J. H. Middlemiss (†)

Department of Radiodiagnosis, University of Bristol, Bristol Royal Infirmary, Marlborough Street, Bristol BS2 8HW, Great Britain

The concept of continuing medical education (CME) has not yet had any significant impact in European countries, whereas in the United States, in its organized form, it has had during the past 10 years a very great effect, though not always, some believe, the desired effect or a beneficial effect. In order to discuss CME in Europe, I must first review the experience in the United States, for it is in the context of what has happened there that we must consider the present situation.

United States of America

In America, a medically qualified doctor is unable to practise independently or obtain a senior hospital post in radiology, or indeed in any specialized branch of medicine, until he has passed an *examination* held by the appropriate board, in our case the American Board of Radiology, and has been certified as a specialist. He is then eligible to be licensed to practise in any individual state. The idea that he will remain competent for the remainder of his professional life without further "input" has been questioned, and so the idea of periodic recertification has been put forward. Tied to the idea of recertification is the practice of CME. In order to qualify for recertification, a specialist must accumulate over a period of say 3 years a certain number of credits. If he gains the necessary credits he can be recertified, and if he is recertified he can be relicensed to practise.

Beginning about 10 years ago, CME, which would enable the specialist to gain his credits, became a big item in medical life. The American Medical Association began with the Physician's Recognition Award, a voluntary effort on the part of the doctor. Various types of learning experience were grouped in categories of credit. Category I referred to that type of educational activity resulting in the acquisition of new knowledge, the upgrading of current knowledge or the reinforcement of past knowledge. CME activities became progressively more widespread and complicated. Institutions such as medical schools, national societies, state societies etc. were accredited for conducting or sponsoring category I courses or programs. In some states, but not all, the earning of CME credits became part of medical relicensing. In some medical societies, CME credits became a necessity for the continuation of membership. Conducting CME courses became big business. This has also had its impact on educational boards like the Board of Radiology, which conducts the examination for certification as a specialist. The boards have been urged to implement procedures for granting certification for a limited period (e.g. 7–10 years) with a requirement for the specialist to seek recertification at the end of the period. This has not yet happened in radiology.

There are many other activities which gain CME credits, such as teaching; the writing of articles and books; unsupervised educational activities; self-instruction with, for example, audiovisual programs, the reading of journals or the use of scientific exhibits; consultation; participation in programs for evaluation of patient care; and self-assessment examinations. It is not relevant to the present discussion to do anything but mention these facets of CME, which continue in the US in great profusion and confusion.

The general atmosphere now appears to be less urgent than was apparent 3–4 years ago. It seems possible that the original impetus came from politicians and from their allegations that there were many physicians or doctors of only borderline competence. The doctors then became the favourite "whipping boys". Now, however, political attention seems to have been diverted to the realm of medical care costs and the push is for cost containment of medical care. CME is not irrelevant in considering medical care costs, for in the end all

Radiology Today 2. Ed. by F. H. W. Heuck and M. W. Donner

costs, all money spent, has to be recovered from some source, either by taxation or by passing on the cost to the patient or the insurance company. When considering the cost of CME one has to consider everything: journals and books, time away from practice, travel, accommodation, courses, rented educational programs etc.

There are a number of problems related to CME which remain unresolved. There are no valid studies as to its effectiveness, it is not known whether attendance at courses changes practice methods or habits, and it is not clear whether courses are designed round the needs of the students or the wishes of the teachers. Finally, is it worth all the money being spent?

Europe

Nowhere in Europe is there any system even remotely resembling what takes place in the US. Indeed, there is no uniformity as to training or assessment of the successful completion of training, no general pattern of certification and no generally agreed criteria on the quality of training or of training departments. Countries where diagnostic radiology embraces all organ imaging and other countries where, for instance, nuclear medicine imaging and ultrasound lie in the hands of other clinicians – non-radiologists. Assessment of the completion of training by *examination* occurs only in France, Britain, Ireland, Italy and Switzerland. The completion of training is marked in some countries by the presentation and defence of a thesis or dissertation, and in some there is no formal conclusion to training. It is not surprising, therefore, that there has been no call for recertification in the American style or for the organized CME that goes with it. In Europe the medical "mystique", the aura of authority that may go with medicine, is still with us. And the hierarchical system still rules; in Europe the professor is still supreme. That is not to say that there is no CME. What is this gathering if not CME? The kind of refurbishing that we all engage in by attending professional society meetings, postgraduate courses, symposia, seminars, workshops, lectures and so forth are all CME. This method, however, does not require the individual to demonstrate the fact that he has learned the material to which he has been exposed. But Europe is awash with meetings of national societies and occasionally there are regional meetings, such as a joint meeting of the Scandinavian societies. There are meetings of specialist groups like the European Society of Neuro-radiologists, the European Society of Paediatric Radiologists or the European Society of Angiology. Regularly there are courses like the gastro-enterology one held annually in Leeds or this forward-looking one in Salzburg. Spontaneous seminars like those on foetal echocardiology (this year in Strasbourg), abdominal ultrasound (this year in Besancon), digital radiology (in Kiel) or planning (in Copenhagen) are organized frequently. Specialist societies like the Skeletal Society and the Fleischner Society organize courses in Europe in alternate years. There are many more that I have no time to mention. All are well attended and go from strength to strength. And so CME is available to all those who are motivated to benefit from it. Motivation is probably the prime factor in encouraging the organization of such activities. And of course the journals and books are as available in Europe as they are anywhere else.

Language is our greatest problem. English is slowly becoming the language of scientific communication, but the multiplicity of tongues in Europe produces difficulties.

European Diploma

I must now tell you of one other European activity which may in time have some effect. Eleven or twelve years ago the Commission on Education of the European Association of Radiology, under its president, Professor van der Schueren of Belgium, decided to institute diploma examinations in radiodiagnosis and radiotherapy. The preparation – drawing up the regulations, the examination structure and the syllabus in a committee with, at that time, members from 19 different countries – took several years, but finally in December 1977 all was agreed at a plenary session held in Hamburg. Professor van der Schueren was ill at the time and I took his place as president, and when he died shortly afterwards I was asked to implement the decisions of the Commission. We have held the examination twice, in 1979 and 1981, and will be holding it again in September 1982. To be a candidate a radiologist must be a certified specialist in a European country with a minimum of 4 years' training. The examination consists of a multiple choice paper and an essay-type paper which are written at the same time on the same day in the candidate's own language in all countries in Europe where there are candidates. To date, the greatest number of countries at one time has been 11, when the paper had to be translated into eight languages for the candidates. The multiple choice papers are returned to me at Bristol University for marking. The essay-type papers are marked by a panel of "internal" examiners appointed by the national society in the candidate's own country and the marks are returned to me. Then two "external" examiners, from other countries than the candidate's own, travel to his country and hold an oral (viva voce) examination together with the internal examiners. Marks are allocated at the oral examination. Finally all the external examiners meet in some central city such as Paris under my chairmanship and consider the marks and examiners' reports on each candidate individually. Thus some degree of uniformity is achieved throughout Europe. This is a postgraduate diploma, and radiology is the first branch of medicine in which such a "European standard" has been achieved, although at present this is to be regarded largely as experimental. It is not clear what the standing of the diploma will be eventually, but in some countries very senior radiologists have entered for the examination. Already we have had heads of departments in such countries as Germany, Portugal and Greece, and this year the past president of one National Society of Radiology is a candidate. In such company, it will be good to see many of you younger radiologists enter as candidates. I hope you will come forward. In the end it is you who will decide the value and the future of this embryo form of CME.

That, then, is a review of CME in Europe against the background of what has been organized and instituted in the United States.

Subject Index

Radiology Today

Volume 1

Editors: **M.W. Donner, F.H.W. Heuck**

1981. 290 figures, 61 tables. XIX,431 pages
ISBN 3-540-10099-7

Contents: Cardiovascular Radiology. – Pulmonary Radiology. – Gastrointestinal Radiology. – Urinary Tract Radiology. – Skeletal Radiology. – Mammography. – Lymphography. – Ultrasound. – ENT Radiology. – Neuroradiology. – Subject Index.

Radiology Today presents the most recent advances in all areas of diagnostic radiology, with internationally renowned specialists reviewing the progress made in their fields during the last 2 years. Oriented primarily to the needs of practicing radiologists, it contains descriptions of new procedures from a broad range of radiologic disciplines including diagnostic radiology, nuclear medicine and ultrasound.

Volume One encompasses the results of a highly successful post-graduate course attended by more than 200 radiologists from 17 countries. Each of the subjects covered was presented in broad overview by an acknowledged expert in his field, and was followed by more detailed papers on further aspects of the topic. The concept of the course as a whole – ranging from the selection of subjects to the high caliber of the speakers and the active interest in workshop discussions – was enthusiastically received. The attendance at the course was large enough to be viable and small enough to be friendly. As a result, the participants were drawn together into a cohesive group that could engage fully in the educational pursuit of open communication among colleagues.

Springer-Verlag
Berlin
Heidelberg
New York
Tokyo

Frontiers in European Radiology

Editors-in-Chief:
A. L. Baert, E. Boijsen,
W. A. Fuchs, F. H. W. Heuck

Frontiers in European Radiology aims
- to provide a platform for European radiological research
- to strengthen the position of radiology in clinical medicine by integrating the various approaches to clinical and experimental radiology

Frontiers in European Radiology (FER) addresses radiologists all over the world with the goal of improving the international exchange of information on all aspects of radiological research. This exchange has unfortunately been limited in the past, especially by the language barriers involved. As a result, Europe's contribution to scientific progress in this interdisciplinary specialty has influenced only regional developments. A first step toward rectifying the situation was taken in Hamburg in September 1979, when the formation of the association of European University Radiologists was discussed and decided upon.

FER is the logical continuation of that initiative; it will provide a forum for scientists in European clinical experimental radiology where important reports on progress in the field can be presented in a depth not possible in a journal. It will be a concise source of detailed information for those wanting to keep abreast of the scientific progress in this field.

Volume 1

1982. 113 figures in 187 separate illustrations. V, 170 pages
ISBN 3-540-10753-3

Contents: *I. Fernström, B. Johansson:* Percutaneous Extraction of Renal Calculi. – *R. Günther, P. Alken:* Percutaneous Nephropyelostomy and Endo-Urological Manipulations. – *R. Pasariello, G. P. Feltrin, D. Miotto, S. Pedrazzoli, P. Rossi, G. Simonetti:* Transhepatic Portal Catheterization with Pancreatic Venous Sampling Versus Angiography in the Localization of Pancreatic Functioning Tumors. – *G. M. Kauffmann, G. Richter, J. Rassweiler, R. Rohrbach:* New Topics in Embolization. Effects of Central, Peripheral or Capillary Occlusion Type in Animal Models Simulating Tumor Embolization. – *F. Brunelle:* Electric Transcatheter Vascular Obliteration: Electrothrombosis. Electrolysis or Electrocoagulation. – *V. Hegedüs, O. Winding, J. Grønvall, P. Faarup:* Manufacturing-Derived Impurities in Angiography. – *K.-H. Hübener:* Digital Radiography Using a Computed Tomography Instrument.

Volume 2

1982. 70 figures in 84 separate illustrations. V, 103 pages
ISBN 3-540-11349-5

Contents: *W. Loeffler:* NMR as an Imaging Method. – *R. E. Steiner, G. M. Bydder:* Initial Clinical Experience with NMR Imaging. – *F. W. Smith:* NMR Imaging of the Liver and Kidney. – *P. Marhoff, M. Pfeiler:* Digital Fluorography. – *M. P. Capp, S. Nudelman, D. Fisher, T. W. Ovitt, G. D. Pond, M. M. Frost, H. Roehrig, J. Seeger, D. Oimette:* Digital Radiography. – *A. B. Crummy, C. A. Mistretta:* Digital Subtraction Arteriography (DSA). – *T. F. Meaney, M. A. Weinstein, E. Buonocore, J. H. Gallagher:* Digital Subtraction Angiography: Cleveland Clinic Experience.

Springer-Verlag
Berlin
Heidelberg
New York
Tokyo

MIX
Papier aus verantwortungsvollen Quellen
Paper from responsible sources
FSC® C105338

If you have any concerns about our products,
you can contact us on
ProductSafety@springernature.com

In case Publisher is established outside the EU,
the EU authorized representative is:
Springer Nature Customer Service Center GmbH
Europaplatz 3, 69115 Heidelberg, Germany

Printed by Libri Plureos GmbH
in Hamburg, Germany